GUILLAIN-BARRÉ SYNDROME

CONTEMPORARY NEUROLOGY SERIES AVAILABLE:

Fred Plum, M.D., *Editor-in-Chief*
***Series Editors:* Sid Gilman, M.D.**
Joseph B. Martin, M.D., Ph.D.
Robert B. Daroff, M.D.
Stephen G. Waxman, M.D., Ph.D.
M-Marsel Mesulam, M.D.

19 The Diagnosis of Stupor and Coma, Edition 3
Fred Plum, M.D., and
Jerome B. Posner, M.D.

21 Disorders of the Cerebellum
Sid Gilman, M.D.,
James R. Bloedel, M.D., Ph.D. and
Richard Lechtenberg, M.D.

24 Disorders of Peripheral Nerves
Herbert H. Schaumburg, M.D.,
Peter S. Spencer, Ph.D., MRC Path., and
P. K. Thomas, M.D., D.Sc., F.R.C.P.

25 Neuromuscular Manifestations of Systemic Disease
Robert B. Layzer, M.D.

26 Principles of Behavioral Neurology
M-Marsel Mesulam, M.D., *Editor*

27 The Acute Stroke
Vladimir Hachinski, M.D., F.R.C.P.(C), and
John W. Norris, M.D., F.R.C.P.

28 Clinical Neuroendocrinology, Edition 2
Joseph B. Martin, M.D., Ph.D., F.R.C.P.(C), and
Seymour Reichlin, M.D., Ph.D.

29 Advances in Contemporary Neurology
Fred Plum, M.D., *Editor*

30 The Wernicke-Korsakoff Syndrome and Related Neurologic Disorders
Due to Alcoholism and Malnutrition, Edition 2
Maurice Victor, M.D.,
Raymond D. Adams, M.D. and
George H. Collins, M.D.

31 Seizures and Epilepsy
Jerome Engel, Jr., M.D., Ph.D.

32 Clinical Neurophysiology of the Vestibular System
Robert W. Baloh, M.D., and
Vicente Honrubia, M.D.

33 Spinal Cord Compression
Thomas N. Byrne, M.D. and
Stephen G. Waxman, M.D., Ph.D.

35 The Neurology of Eye Movements, Edition 2
R. John Leigh, M.D., and
David S. Zee, M.D.

GUILLAIN-BARRÉ SYNDROME

ALLAN H. ROPPER, M.D.
Professor of Neurology
Tufts University School of Medicine
Chief, Division of Neurology
St. Elizabeth's Hospital
Boston, Massachusetts
Formerly:
Director, Neurological/
Neurosurgical Intensive Care Unit
Massachusetts General Hospital
Harvard Medical School
Boston, Massachusetts

EELCO F.M. WIJDICKS, M.D.
Visiting Neurologist
Neurology-Neurosurgery Intensive Care Unit
Massachusetts General Hospital
Boston, Massachusetts
and
Consultant Neurologist
Department of Neurology
University Hospital
Utrecht, The Netherlands

BRADLEY T. TRUAX, M.D.
Clinical Associate Professor of Neurology
School of Medicine and Biomedical Sciences
State University of New York at Buffalo
and
Director of Neurology
Erie County Medical Center
Buffalo, New York

F.A. DAVIS COMPANY • Philadelphia

Printed in the United States of America

Last digit indicates print number: 10 9 8 7 6 5 4 3 2 1

NOTE: As new scientific information becomes available through basic and clinical research, recommended treatments and drug therapies undergo changes. The author(s) and publisher have done everything possible to make this book accurate, up-to-date, and in accord with accepted standards at the time of publication. The authors, editors and publisher are not responsible for errors or omissions or for consequences from application of the book, and make no warranty, expressed or implied, in regard to the contents of the book. Any practice described in this book should be applied by the reader in accordance with professional standards of care used in regard to the unique circumstances that may apply in each situation. The reader is advised always to check product information (package inserts) for changes and new information regarding dose and contraindications before administering any drug. Caution is especially urged when using new or infrequently ordered drugs.

Library of Congress Cataloging-in-Publication Data

Ropper, Allan H.
Guillain-Barré syndrome / Allan H. Ropper, Eelco F.M. Wijdicks, Bradley T. Truax.
p. cm. -- (Contemporary neurology series ; 34)
Includes bibliographical references and index.
ISBN 0-8036-7572-0 (Hardbound : alk. paper)
1. Polyradiculoneuritis. I. Wijdicks, Eelco F. M., 1954- . II. Truax, Bradley T., 1948- . III. Title. IV. Series.
[DNLM: 1. Polyradiculoneuritis. W1 CO769N v. 34 / WL 400 R785g]
RC416.R67 1991
616.8'7--dc20
DNLM/DLC
for Library of Congress 90-15721
CIP

DEDICATION

We devote this book to our wives, Sandy, Barbara, and Beth, and to our children, who patiently waited for our return on those many nights we worked late to complete the project.

FOREWORD

The appearance of this monograph will be welcomed by a large readership, once its content is known. Its importance lies in the great clinical material, all personally observed, which is retrospectively and prospectively viewed, and in the description and critical evaluation of current modes of therapy.

Many practicing neurologists still remember how grim was the outlook for victims of this disease 20 or 30 years ago. At the Massachusetts General Hospital as many as 25% died, even after the introduction of the old Drinker tank respirator. The fault lay in the inadequacy of care of the quadriplegic patient needing respiratory assistance. Dr. Allan Ropper came upon the scene in our hospital at the time when this sorry state of affairs was being appreciated and he has played a major part in establishing a critical care facility for neurological patients. The mortality rate in the several hundred patients who were admitted to the unit with Guillain-Barré disease has been reduced to 3% to 4%. This has been one of the most significant advances in patient management in our hospital and others like it in North America and Europe. The authors' description of how the patient needing respiratory support should be managed and how certain problems related thereto can be averted is commendable.

Other more specific therapies about which there is considerable uncertainty—plasmapheresis, high-dose steroids, intravenous gammaglobulin—are also appraised, again based on both personal experience and collaboration in multi-institutional studies. The reader will find their observations sound and authoritative.

And finally, access to such a large group of patients has enabled the authors to perceive many subtle and overlooked features of this disease, including a number of variant syndromes. This has provided a wider perspective on the entire category of closely related infective and autoimmune inflammatory diseases of the peripheral nervous system.

RAYMOND D. ADAMS, M.D.

ACKNOWLEDGMENTS

The authors are grateful to several individuals and medical units for their help and support in investigating these patients with Guillain-Barré syndrome and composing this book. Dr. Raymond Adams, Chairman Emeritus of the Department of Neurology at the Massachusetts General Hospital, was most helpful in reviewing the entire text and offering many suggestions for the chapter on pathology. Dr. M. Vermeuelen and Dr. A. Brand kindly reviewed the sections on immunology and chronic inflammatory demyelinating polyneuropathy (CIDP). Dr. Léger of the Praticien Des Hôpitaux and Ms. Véronique Leroux-Hugon, Librarian at the Hôpital de la Salpétrière, spent long hours in the libraries of their medical school to obtain for us the beautiful photographs of Guillain, Barré, and Strohl that appear in Chapter 1. The New England Rehabilitation Hospital in Woburn, Massachusetts, has had a close relationship with our unit, has taken care of many of our GBS patients, and has supplied many of the pictures of orthotic devices and physical therapy in Chapter 18.

Ms. Bernice Wissler and Dr. Sylvia Fields were unfailingly helpful and kind in their editorial handling of the text. We are also most grateful to Dr. Sid Gilman, Chairman of Neurology at the University of Michigan, for reviewing drafts of the book and spending many hours annotating margins with his excellent comments.

The greatest credit, and our profound thanks, goes to Miss Dolores Altavilla, who, besides composing the book on a word processor, was also an invaluable research assistant. Her administrative skills played a major part in the completion of the text.

We thank Mr. and Mrs. Joseph Quick for their support and encouragement in this and other academic projects in our Neurological Intensive Care Unit.

CONTENTS

INTRODUCTION

The acute inflammatory polyneuropathy Guillain-Barré syndrome (GBS) has been recognized under different names for more than 100 years. The widely accepted syndromic eponym has persisted because the illness is easy to identify from clinical features delineated in a seminal report in 1916. Other more descriptive names such as idiopathic polyneuritis, acute inflammatory polyneuropathy (polyneuritis), postinfectious (infectious, infective) polyneuropathy (polyneuritis), Landry's (ascending) paralysis, Landry-Guillain-Barré syndrome (with or without Strohl's name attached), Osler's febrile polyneuritis, and a bewildering variety of other designations[39,1023] all denote the same disease, whether in English, its native French, or other languages. For the sake of brevity and simplicity we have chosen to use the term *GBS*. The "S" can be taken to designate "Strohl" or "syndrome," with concern that the historic slight of Strohl's omission may be propagated (see Chapter 1). The same disease occurring after infectious mononucleosis, hepatitis, human immunodeficiency virus (HIV), other identifiable infections, surgery, or associated illness such as systemic lupus erythematosus or lymphoma, is generally agreed to be GBS rather than a specific consequence of the precipitating or preceding event.

The typical illness consists of (1) relatively symmetric weakness evolving over one to several weeks in the hips and legs, later the arms, frequently involving the face and respiratory muscles, and less often eye movements; (2) paresthesias in the toes and fingertips that advance proximally; (3) eventual loss of deep tendon reflexes; (4) spontaneous gradual recovery over several weeks to months; and (5) elevated spinal fluid protein concentration with few cells in most cases. To these classic descriptors, electrophysiologic abnormalities—particularly conduction block and abnormal late responses—can be added. An association with a preceding viral or other infection is common. The illness occurs at any age, including neonates and octogenarians.

As a result of the eradication of poliomyelitis and the rarity of other acute polyneuropathies such as diphtheria, the typical disease can be correctly identified by most physicians. Atypical presentations of GBS that simulate other diseases are more common than typical presentations of these rarer illnesses. Diagnostic criteria have been offered by many authors through the years, as discussed in Chapter 2; the most recent, by Asbury, have been adopted by the NINCDS.[51] While criteria have been useful for research and epidemiologic work, the diagnosis can be (and usually is) deduced fairly easily on clinical grounds. An appreciation of the breadth of clinical presentation of GBS and diseases that stimulate it is therefore more helpful in practice than are rigid criteria. Munsat and Barnes[829] astutely noted, ". . . the Guillain-Barré syndrome is easy to diagnose but impossible to define." As long as the disease must be recognized by a variable constellation of signs of an acute peripheral neuropathy, this clinical dependence and the ambiguity it embodies will remain.

There is enough experience recounted in the literature and from our own patients to give a fairly complete clinical accounting of GBS. The main goal of this book is to provide a comprehensive clinical source on GBS and to collect all the relevant information necessary for the physician and others to understand the disease and to care effectively for these patients. The many small clinical and electrophysiologic details that punctuate the book, especially in Chapters 7 through 9 and 14, are meant to enrich the experience of caring for and contemplating individual cases. The most interesting parts of the illness have to do with the patients themselves, their clinical presentations, the travails of the course, and the struggles of physical improvement. A wide variety of symptoms and signs, the psychologic aspects of immobilization, the likelihood of spontaneous recovery, and the inextricable ties to general medical and respiratory care, all require special physician and nursing skills not usually called for with other neurologic diseases.

The details in this book are based on years of observation and care delivered personally (AHR) to over more than 250 patients with Guillain-Barré syndrome from 1979 to 1988. One hundred twenty of these patients admitted consecutively to the inpatient services of the Massachusetts General Hospital (MGH) between 1980 and 1988 had clinical and electrophysiologic data recorded prospectively. They constitute the prospective series referred to throughout the book and are the basis for most of the original numerical data. Insights gained from the other patients seen in the office, at other hospitals, or after the closure of systematic data collection in late 1988 are interjected where appropriate. Information in the prospective series was obtained in a uniform manner, by personal examination, and only by our laboratories, mainly the Clinical Electrophysiology Service of Dr. Bhagwan Shahani, who assisted in preparing Chapter 13 on electrophysiology in GBS. (One hundred fourteen of the 120 prospectively studied patients had electrophysiologic testing performed at the MGH.) A retrospective series of 169 patients admitted to the MGH in the pre–plasma exchange era from 1962 to 1978, gathered from chart review largely by Dr. Truax, is the basis for much of the additional data, especially in the tables. This material has guided the organization of data for the prospective series. The precise denominator for some statements and tables is at times slightly less than 120 (prospective) or 169 patients (retrospective) because of absent or uncertain data. The prospective series may be biased toward sicker, more severely affected patients because many were referred directly to our Neurological Intensive Care Unit (ICU) facility.

A plethora of variants and elaborations of the typical disease have been reported and may create diagnostic difficulty. Several chapters deal with cases that have a bias toward early regional distributions of the weakness (arms, cranial nerves, eye movements); inconstant features such as respiratory failure, autonomic dysfunction, ataxia, or a peculiar triad of limb ataxia, ophthalmoplegia, and areflexia called Fisher's syndrome; normal spinal fluid protein concentration, or spinal fluid pleocytosis; and a chronically persistent or relapsing type of illness. Chronic inflammatory polyneuropathy, closely related to acute GBS, has many illuminating clinical differences that require separate consideration. During the period of the prospective series we cared for 30 patients with the chronic form of the disease, drawing the data in Chapter 10 from this group.

A watershed event for GBS has been the demonstration of the benefit of plasma exchange, now a relatively routine treatment for the illness. The unanimity of its acceptance is based on several well-designed therapeutic trials that provided much ancillary data, summarized in Chapter 15 and other appropriate sections. In contrast, the ambiguous role of corticosteroids in inflammatory neurologic disease is still spawning clinical trials.

The pathology of acute GBS has been relatively well settled as a widely distributed perivenular inflammatory lesion in peripheral nerves, with adjacent demyelination (Chapter 4). The inflammation and demyelination are almost certainly due to a cellular immunologic response that is incited by a variety of agents. Some demyelination, however, appears at a distance from, or before the appearance of, inflammatory cells and may be the result of damage by antibodies. The immunologic mechanisms underlying the inflammatory lesions, and several other clinical and elctrophysiologic phenomena, are not yet fully understood, but the general nature of the immune problem is being approached by several groups. An experimental model, experimental autoimmune neuritis (EAN), closely resembles GBS, and a complete discussion of GBS requires an analysis of what has been learned through this laboratory work. For reasons of limited space and our desire to maintain a clinical emphasis, we have not provided a definitive review of the rapidly changing field of immunology, but we have collected the data that pertain to the clinical understanding of GBS in Chapter 5. One of the aims of the book is to synthesize what is known of the pathology and immunology with clinical features.

The psychologic facets of GBS and the stresses of caring for these patients are discussed in Chapter 16. One of the most useful pieces written on the care of patients with GBS is the personal account of Denise Bowes,[130] a Canadian physician who had Fisher's syndrome that progressed to cause generalized weakness. The combination of knowledgeable medical and lay insights makes this excellent piece salient reading that accurately reflects our own sense of our patients' experiences. The importance of attention to the mundane details of daily care, such as the technique of suctioning, mouth care, routine blood testing, professional behavior, courtesy, and communication are transmitted without the drama and superficiality of some other accounts of GBS. Bowes' story is worth reading by all physicians and nurses who care for these patients.

Several other physicians have had GBS and have given valuable accounts in professional terms of the sensory distortions, pain, and helplessness engendered by the illness. Rice[983] has emphasized the myriad types of common and sometimes devastating pain, and curious alterations of body image that a few of our patients have reported. The importance of liberal analgesic doses, especially at night, was reported poignantly:

> What a difference that made to comfort and relief when compared with the rigid regimens in some hospitals. . . . Hours are just as long between 3 AM and 7 AM as at any other time and the pains of peripheral neuritis are most severe in the night and early morning.

He recounted the slow and deliberate course of recovery, dwelling appropriately on the importance of small things such as a handle over the head of the bed to allow him to turn, or to grip if the pain became unbearable, and the "help, understanding, and encouragement" from staff. He also offered an insight into the exigencies of caring for a physician with GBS by alluding to maintaining his own professional interest by some shop talk and the occasional solicitation of his own opinion. Another physician and his wife have recorded a personal account of his illness through first-person narratives.[1093] Fear and helplessness were dominant emotions for both—a reminder that medical familiarity does not protect one from the psychologic disorganization of a painful and immobilizing illness. These articles have at times been valuable to the families of our own patients because they demonstrate that their concerns are appropriate and appreciated.

We cared for an internist with a particularly long and painful course of GBS that left enough residual deficit to impede his practice. Despite his own anxiety, he offered helpful insights into his illness and was calmed by having a hand in the management of some small details, usually involving nursing, that otherwise would have received cursory attention. Other patients who have consulted us after the acute illness had passed have related similar sentiments. Confidence in the attending physician and involvement in matters of pain control, hygiene, turning, physical therapy, and a daily routine were critically important. The uncertainty of recovery, and its timing, seem particularly difficult for physicians (perhaps as much as nonmedical patients) to accept.

There are several allusions to GBS in the nonmedical literature (including GBS as the focus of novels), the most prominent a recent autobiographic account by Heller and Vogel,[508] in which Heller's descriptions of the illness are folded into an entertaining story of contemporary personal events. Though lacking any major insights into the disease or medical care, the book popularized the illness perhaps even more than did the notorious swine flu epidemic. Baier[66] has also written a popular account of her ordeal with GBS, *Bed Number Ten*.

We hope that the material in this book—part review, part new data, and part carefully considered opinion—will be helpful to neurologists, intensivists, electrophysiologists, physiatrists, physical therapists, and all others who participate in the care of these patients.

ALLAN H. ROPPER, M.D.
EELCO F.M. WIJDICKS, M.D.
BRADLEY T. TRUAX, M.D.

Part I
BACKGROUND

Chapter 1

HISTORY OF LANDRY-GUILLAIN-BARRÉ-STROHL SYNDROME

Early Descriptions and Landry's Contribution
Guillain, Barré, and Strohl
Refinements after the Seminal Article
The "Guillain-Barré" Eponym
Pathologic Basis of the Syndrome
Modern Immunologic and Electrophysiologic Basis of the Syndrome
Treatments
Fisher's Syndrome and Variants
Personal Accounts

As with many other neurologic syndromes, the understanding of the Guillain-Barré syndrome (GBS) has been shaped by the historic sequence of its description and contemporary developments in medicine. Each contribution has led to "ascending knowledge" about the disease and there have been surprisingly few false steps.[320] The lineage of GBS has been traced by several previous authors[501,973,1203,1278] and in "la petite histoire" by Schott[1076] (Table 1–1). Excellent English translations are available of the original articles by Landry in 1859[669] and by Guillain, Barré, and Strohl in 1916.[467] The original clinical descriptions have not been exceeded in their accuracy or detail, and a recounting of certain features of these articles and the work surrounding them will enrich the physician interested in any aspect of GBS.

Table 1–1 HISTORY OF GUILLAIN-BARRÉ SYNDROME

1834–1837:	Wardrop and Ollivier describe cases of rapidly progressive paralysis and other features of GBS
1859:	Landry unifies clinical features in "acute ascending paralysis"
1876:	Term "Landry's (ascending) paralysis" first used
1916:	Guillain, Barré, and Strohl note albuminocytologic dissocation in CSF, new diagnostic feature in GBS
1920:	Guillain and Barré publish text, *Travaux Neurologiques de Guerre*, which links their names and briefly mentions GBS, distinguishing it from Landry's paralysis and from nerve gas poisoning
1937:	Brussels symposium cements exclusion of Strohl from eponym, adds many descriptive details of illness, and clarifies Guillain's definition of the syndrome
Late 1940s:	Development of respiratory ICUs and use of positive-pressure ventilation reduces mortality from GBS
1949:	Haymaker and Kernohan report clinical-pathologic correlations in series of 50 fatal cases of "Landry-Guillain-Barré syndrome"
1955:	Experimental autoimmune neuritis (EAN), a clinical and pathologic facsimile of human GBS, produced in animals by Waksman and Adams
1956:	Fisher's syndrome described
1969:	Pathologic study by Asbury and colleagues shows lymphocytic infiltration in spinal roots and nerves
1975:	Swine flu vaccination program spurs interest in GBS
1978:	Use of plasma exchange in treatment first reported by Brettle and co-workers
1981:	Symposium on GBS brings immune and pathologic features up to date and proposes modern diagnostic criteria

EARLY DESCRIPTIONS AND LANDRY'S CONTRIBUTION

Jean-Baptiste Octave Landry (Fig. 1–1), was the first to unify the major clinical features of the disease, distinguishing it from syphilis and the more common chronic neuropathies. In 1859 he coined the term "acute ascending paralysis" ("Note sur la paralysie ascendante aiguë").[668] Haymaker has written a synopsis of Landry's medical career,[500] and an extensive retrospective on Landry appeared in 1933.[979] He was an astute neurologist who published a "Traité complet des paralysies" (Paris, Masson). In addition to detailing his cases that set the stage for much classic late 19th century work on neuropathy and neuritis, he was among the first to point out the similarities between lower motor neuron nuclei for cranial nerves in the brainstem, which had not yet been defined anatomically, and the anterior horn cells of the spinal cord. He used this concept to explain the famous case of "crossed hemiplegia" presented by Foville.[667]

Landry, referring to prior similar descriptions of ascending paralysis by Ol-

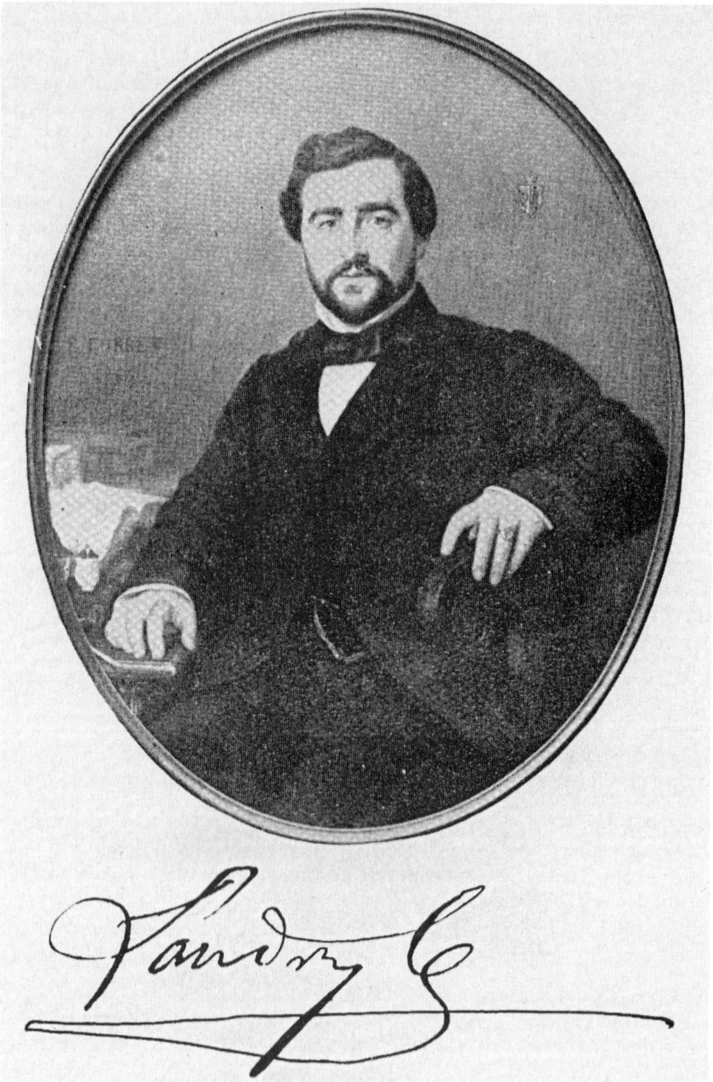

Figure 1–1. Photograph of Octave Landry taken approximately 1860. (From Haymaker,[500] p. 321, with permission.)

livier of Angers and Sandras, presented a patient with a new febrile illness on March 16, followed by sensory symptoms. The term used to describe the initial sensory symptoms that began on May 11 in the fingers and toes, "formillements," was translated by Hochberg as "formications"[669] but perhaps should be rendered as "tingling." On June 13 the patient's knees gave way when walking, and sensory symptoms had ascended; by June 17 he could no longer walk, and respiratory difficulty with paradoxical diaphragmatic movement led to death. Landry specifically noted sparing of bowel and bladder function, mild sensory signs, and preservation of electrical (faradic) muscle excitability. The autopsy failed to demonstrate the cause of illness after examination of some microscopic sections of the cerebrum, cerebellum, spinal cord (including "nerve origins"), and muscles. The peripheral nerves apparently were not examined. The original case therefore had a progression that was a bit long, more like chronic inflammatory polyneuropathy than acute GBS, but the respiratory failure and other features were consistent with acute GBS.

In the second part of the report, Landry reviewed four further cases of his own and five from the literature that were more like typical acute GBS. The notable absence of central nervous system (CNS) symptoms, the occasional fleeting cramps preceding paralysis, the possible relapses, and a relatively favorable outcome if the patient survived were highlighted and added to the previous descriptions. "Loss of reflexes" undoubtedly referred to several superficial-cutaneous reflexes that were being described at the time, many with eponymic self-attributions, rather than to tendon reflexes. Other new features included two cases that followed convalescence from an acute illness, two related to menstrual difficulties, one to childbirth, and one possibly to syphilis. Though Landry made little of the paresthesias, preferring to emphasize the paralysis, his formidable clinical descriptions of the daily progression of limb, trunk, and diaphragm weakness have only been embellished during the subsequent 125 years. All the signs and symptoms currently thought to be typical of GBS, except loss of tendon reflexes, appeared in the original rendering.

Prior to Landry's descriptions, "peripheral neuritis" served as an undifferentiated diagnosis akin to what is currently called "peripheral neuropathy." Graves (1884)[434] was credited with localizing neurologic disease to the peripheral nerves ("the nervous cords"), from casual observations of Chomel's (1828) during an epidemic of sensory neuritis at the Marie-Thérèse Infirmary, Paris. Pain in the feet and hands, probably painful paresthesias, were prominent in their patients, from Chomel's descriptions.[194] Many features suggested the disease was due to a toxin rather than to inflammation. Others have been retrospectively credited with first describing GBS 25 years or more before Landry—notably Ollivier, who presented two cases in 1837,[876] and Wardrop,[225,1251] who described patients with rapidly progressive paralysis in 1834. Landry remarked on the similarity of his cases to Ollivier's. None of these early clinical neurologists, including Landry, could have appreciated the significance of tendon areflexia, working 30 to 40 years before its relevance to peripheral neuropathy was established.[278] Through Landry's time, neurologists were uncertain whether the disease he described originated in the spinal cord or the nerves.

During the second half of the 19th century, many case reports of a similar illness appeared (the most extensive, a report of 18 patients by Pellegrino-Levi in 1865[907]), each emphasizing a different aspect or variation of the paralysis, such as an onset involving the cranial nerves with subsequent descent to the limbs;[907] pain;[98,1274] sensory symptoms;[326] and pronounced sensory signs.[581,1239] Most authors credited Landry in their work, and Westphal first used the term "Landry's ascending paralysis" in 1876.[1274] This apparently became a common eponym, perhaps leading to overdiagnosis of the illness during the late 19th century. Dejerine[262] and Leyden[695] wrote about further cases, accrediting the existence of the acute paralytic syndrome in the practice of European medicine. The connection between peripheral nerve damage and Landry's paralysis took several false turns on the basis of numerous incomplete or spurious pathologic reports, summarized by Bailey and Ewing in 1896,[67] who concluded that the entire cerebrospinal axis showed perivascular inflammation.

GUILLAIN, BARRÉ, AND STROHL

In 1916, 25 years after Quincke began examining the spinal fluid in neurologic diseases, Guillain, Barré, and Strohl fortuitously saw two soldiers who, within 2 weeks of each other, developed paralysis and tendon areflexia. They noted a new diagnostic feature, albuminocytologic dissociation in the cerebrospinal fluid (CSF)[466,467] (Fig. 1–2). No mention was made of Landry. The first paragraph of the article is a concise and classic description of the illness:[467]

> . . . characterized by motor difficulties, loss of the deep tendon reflexes with preservation of cutaneous reflexes, paresthesias with slight impairment of objective sensation, muscle tenderness, slight alteration in nerve conduction and electromyographic patterns, and a remarkable increase in cerebrospinal fluid albumin in the absence of a cellular reaction (albumino-cytologic dissociation.

Sur un syndrome de radiculo-névrite avec hyperalbuminose du liquide céphalo-rachidien sans réaction cellulaire. Remarques sur les caractères cliniques et graphiques des réflexes tendineux,

par MM. Georges Guillain, J.-A. Barré et A. Strohl.

Nous attirons l'attention, dans la présente note, sur un syndrome clinique que nous avons observé chez deux malades, syndrome caractérisé par des troubles moteurs, l'abolition des réflexes tendineux avec conservation des réflexes cutanés, des paresthésies avec troubles légers de la sensibilité objective, des douleurs à la pression des masses musculaires, des modifications peu accentuées des réactions électriques des nerfs et des muscles, de l'hyperalbuminose très notable du liquide céphalo-rachidien avec absence de réaction cytologique (dissociation albumino-cytologique). Ce syndrome nous a paru dépendre d'une atteinte concomitante des racines rachidiennes, des nerfs et des muscles, vraisemblablement de nature infectieuse ou toxique. Il doit être différencié des radiculites simples, des polynévrites pures et des polymyosites. Des recherches expérimentales par la méthode graphique sur la vitesse des réflexes et leur temps perdu, sur les modalités, la contractilité musculaire, montrent la réalité de la participation, dans ce syndrome, de tout l'appareil moteur neuro-musculaire périphérique. Nous insistons particulièrement aussi sur l'hyperalbuminose du liquide céphalo-rachidien sans réaction cytologique, fait qui, à notre connaissance, n'a pas été mentionné dans des cas semblables.

Figure 1–2. The original 1916 article (466) by Guillain, Barré, and Strohl from *Revue Neurologique*, with a concise introductory description of the disease that carries their names. The "dissociation albuminocytologique" is highlighted.

The first patient had a CSF albumin concentration of 2.5 g/L with 2 to 4 white blood cells per mm^3, and the second, 0.85 g/L with 3 to 4 white blood cells per mm^3. Second CSF examinations were performed in both patients with similar results, but the time of sampling was not given. Albuminocytologic dissociation (a term attributed by Guillain and the others to Siccard and Foix, who pointed it out in Pott's disease) was then considered characteristic of a new peripheral nerve disease and was distinguished from the same finding in cases of spinal cord compression. The observation of albuminocytologic dissociation had been made by others at about the same time in diphtheric polyneuritis[352,961,999] and in three cases of "idiopathic" polyneuropathy,[961] so the concept was not new but rather was applied to the diagnosis of a specific type of polyneuritis for the first time. We can only speculate why Guillain decided to perform a lumbar puncture in his Army patients. Could it have been to diagnose polio, or was it because the technique was becoming popular and widely applied in neurology?

Guillain, Barré, and Strohl were certainly aware of Landry's ascending paralysis and later seemed forced to defend differences between the two, based on a limited number of cases. One month after their major publication, Marie and Chatelin reported three similar cases with albuminocytologic dissociation,[745] and 1 year later Gordon Holmes, with the British Army in France, published the general features of 12 cases of "acute febrile polyneuritis" that were simply GBS.[531]

By this time, tendon areflexia was appreciated as a sign of polyneuropathy or posterior radiculopathy, based on experience with tabes dorsalis. Emphasis on the loss or preservation of various cutaneous reflexes continued, probably because it was an interest of Guillain's. In the only major discrepancy between the original work and modern understanding of neuropathy, the loss of deep tendon reflexes was attributed to a peculiar increase in muscle tone and tonic contraction of antagonist muscles. Increased limb tone remains a mystery in an otherwise archetypal description of the disease. Although the disease was ultimately explained as a radiculoneuropathy, at one point in the original article the authors suggested that there was combined polymyositis and polyneuritis, the distinction at times being "too fine for neurologists to make." In a striking electrophysiologic observation, the electrically recorded latency of deep tendon reflexes was prolonged, "almost double the normal," perhaps the first indication that the disease was demyelinating, though allusion is made to alterations in the "central part of the reflex." As in Landry's first case, direct mechanical excitability of muscle was preserved when the muscles were tapped with a reflex hammer, as were galvanic and faradic responses. The electrophysiologic contributions in the original article were probably entirely Strohl's.

REFINEMENTS AFTER THE SEMINAL ARTICLE

Various schemata of GBS were offered in the subsequent 30 years, most based on the topography of paralysis, including Guillain's ten new cases, four with ataxia,[459] but none was a major contribution to understanding. The absence or presence of sensory loss and a fatal outcome were points upon which many, including Guillain, made fine distinctions in classification. Guillain resisted identifying his cases with Landry's, preferring to believe that the one associated with his name was a benign disease incapable of direct fatal outcome. In a curious lapse, Guillain and Barré in 1919 reported a case of acute polyneuritis with albuminocytologic dissociation after typhoid vaccine,[463] and called it "paralysie ascendante aiguë de Landry," apparently because it was fatal. They failed to examine the nerves microscopically. In the United States, "Guillain-Barré syndrome" began being used in preference to "Landry's paralysis," while the latter remained in favor in Europe during the 1930s. It appeared often as an umbrella term for all types of rapidly spreading paralysis, including poliomyelitis. In 1902, Diller[277] stated, "The term Landry's paralysis cannot be dropped. It has been used too long to be erased from our nomenclature." As late as 1940, however, argument about the specificity of the term and its identity with GBS continued, and DeJong[264] suggested that the term should be used only descriptively for an ascending paralysis without poliomyelitis, rather than signifying a certain pathologic diagnosis.

Some confusion was caused by Guillain's later insistence that the CSF protein must be above 300 mg/dL for a case to be included as GBS.[459] He felt that the cause of protein elevation was leakage through damaged, or "paralyzed," leptomeningeal vessels. Subsequent work by Greenfield and Carmichael[439] suggested that local radicular factors caused elevated lumbar CSF protein and that cisternal protein was usually normal or only slightly elevated. Queckenstedt thought that venous obstruction around the spinal cord accounted for raised CSF protein.[961]

FISHER'S SYNDROME AND VARIANTS

Many clinical variations of GBS and associated illness have been described; a few contributions have been noteworthy because of their clinical utility. In 1956, Fisher[365] provided a clear descripton of a syndrome with ophthalmoplegia, ataxia, and areflexia, which had been in part reported before, leading to the retention of the eponym "Fisher's syndrome" after its use was introduced in 1957[1117] (see Chapter 8). Another likely variant of GBS, acquired dysautonomia, was described by Young and colleagues.[1309,1310] Others have emphasized unusual facets of GBS such as pseudotumor cerebri, ophthalmoplegia,[829] autonomic dysfunction, chronic and relapsing GBS,[310] and regional variants,[1008] adding to an appreciation of its clinical richness and variable nature. Each of these is addressed further in later chapters. Despite lingering uncertainty about the relationship, interest in the disease surged after the "swine flu" vaccination program. A major update guided by Dr. Arthur Asbury,[468] including a modern and useful set of diagnostic criteria,[51] appeared in 1981 and is comparable in historic impact to the 1937 Brussels symposium.

THE "GUILLAIN-BARRÉ" EPONYM

Guillain (Fig. 1–3) was most active in promoting the newly described disease, although he published numerous brief pieces on other neurologic subjects, particularly various reflexes. Several synopses of his contributions have appeared.[11,839] Barré collaborated with Guillain at the Hôpital Centre Neurologique de la VIe Armée in Amiens during the war, their previous military publications culminating in a well-received 1920 text, *Travaux Neurologiques de Guerre,*[464] (Fig. 1–4), which briefly mentions GBS, distinguishing it from Landry's paralysis after typhoid (see earlier) and from nerve gas poisoning. The latter diagnosis was apparently a consideration in the differential diagnosis of GBS in a combat setting. Strohl, as noted farther on, worked as a radiologist in the same Army Hospital.

Barré (Fig. 1–5) had an illustrious neurologic career,[1101] beginning as an intern with Maire and Babinski. He became the Professor of Neurology at Strasbourg, with more than 800 publications on numerous topics including postencephalitic parkinsonism, multiple sclerosis, and cerebellar abscess. He had an interest in cerebellar and vestibular syndromes that stimulated many subsequent theses by his students. His name is attached to a sign elicited by having the prone patient bend his knees and observing downward drift of the lower leg on the side of a subtle hemiparesis.

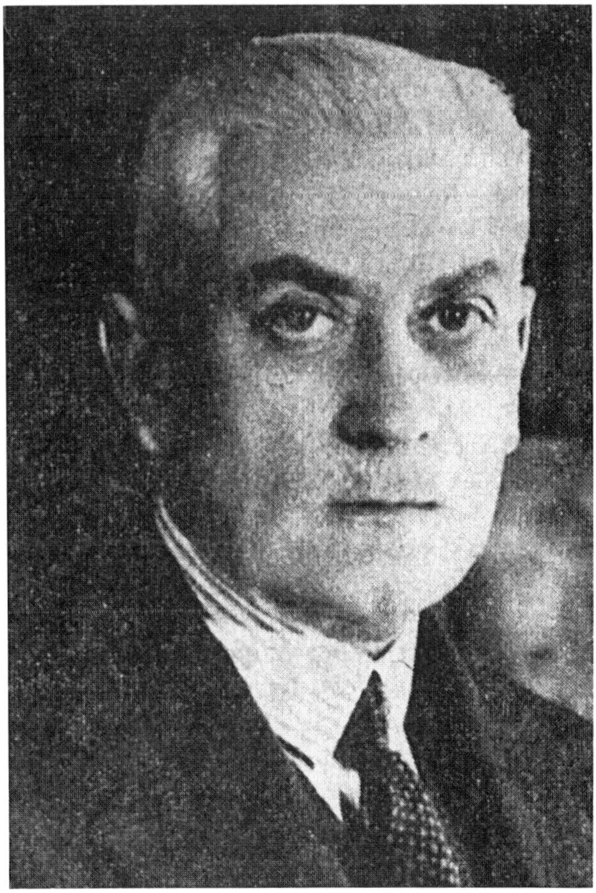

Figure 1–3. Photograph of Dr. G. Guillain from an obituary,[839] (Courtesy of Dr. Jean-Marie Leger, Hôpitaux de Paris.)

In the issue containing the original description, Guillain and Barré had three additional articles together and two with Strohl, and Strohl had one article alone, on his specialty, electrical recording of reflexes. The 1916 *Revue Neurologique* contained nine articles by Guillain and Barré jointly, without Strohl (Fig. 1–6). In 1917, the trio published five articles on the electrical ("graphiques") characteristics of several reflexes. From 1916 through the 1920s, Guillain's and Barré's names appear together far more frequently than with Strohl's, implicitly relegating Strohl's name to electrophysiologic contributions alone. Strohl wrote a number of books on electrophysiology, radiology, and physical medicine, but he infrequently published alone on clinical topics. For many years he was Professor of Physical Medicine at the University of Paris[271,996] (Fig. 1–7). Green[436] suggested that Strohl's omission from the eponym resulted from his broad-ranging medical interests, making him less credible as a neurologist. Petch[914] addressed the slight of Strohl's omission with an amusing response from a French physician that "Strohl was from Alsace." Schott[1076] suggested that Strohl was omitted either because he was a young (29-year-old) recent graduate or, more likely, because he was primarily involved with electrophysiology.

Our sense is that a generation of physicians, particularly French neurologists, associated the names of Guillain and Barré through the multitude of publications, books, and many follow-up articles that expanded on the original syndrome without Strohl. Guillain advanced the excommunication in 1925 with his first major article on GBS

GEORGES GUILLAIN J. A. BARRÉ

TRAVAUX NEUROLOGIQUES DE GUERRE

PREFACE DU PROFESSEUR PIERRE MARIE

MASSON ET Cie EDITEURS
LIBRAIRES DE L'ACADÉMIE DE MÉDECINE
120, BOULEVARD SAINT-GERMAIN, PARIS, VIe
1920

Figure 1–4. Title page from *Travaux Neurologiques de Guerre*, written by Guillain and Barré from their wartime experience at the Hôpital Centre Neurologique de la VIe Armée in Amiens.[464] Strohl was a radiologist there.

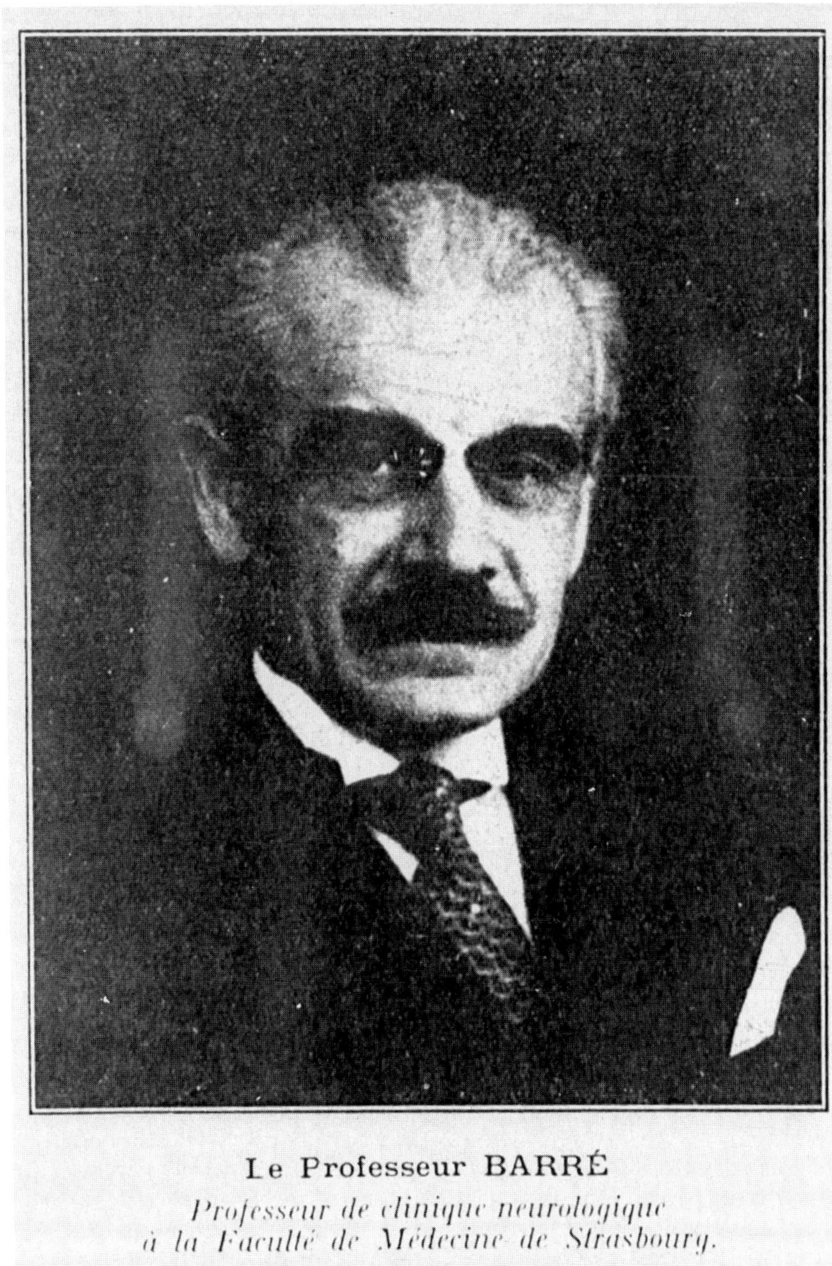
Le Professeur BARRÉ
Professeur de clinique neurologique
à la Faculté de Médecine de Strasbourg.

Figure 1–5. Photograph of Dr. J.A. Barré. (Courtesy of Dr. Jean-Marie Leger, Hôpitaux de Paris.)

SÉANCE DU 13 OCTOBRE 1916

Présidence de M. Gaucher.

SOMMAIRE

	Pages.
Correspondance.	
Allocution de M. le Président à propos du décès de M. Bourcy. . .	1437
PIERRE CAZAMIAN : Myélite « irradiée » du renflement lombo-sacré, consécutive à un traumatisme du gros orteil par projectile de guerre.	1437
P. AMEUILLE et P. TILLAYE : Hépatite amibienne suppurée autochtone et primitive.	1448
A. STROHL : Etude graphique de quelques réflexes tendineux. . . .	1452
GEORGES GUILLAIN, J.-A. BARRÉ et A. STROHL : Le réflexe médio-plantaire. Etude de ses caractères graphiques et de son temps perdu.	1459
GEORGES GUILLAIN, J.-A. BARRÉ et A. STROHL : Sur un syndrome de radiculo-névrite avec hyperalbuminose du liquide céphalo-rachidien sans réaction cellulaire. Remarques sur les caractères cliniques et graphiques des réflexes tendineux. .	1462
GEORGES GUILLAIN et J.-A. BARRÉ : Deux cas d'hémiplégie organique consécutive à la déflagration de fortes charges d'explosifs sans plaie extérieure.	1470
GEORGES GUILLAIN et J.-A. BARRÉ : Apoplexie tardive consécutive à une commotion par éclatement d'obus sans plaie extérieure . . .	1473
GEORGES GUILLAIN et J.-A. BARRÉ : Les réflexes de défense vrais au cours des syndromes méningés (hémorragies méningées, inflammations aiguës).	1474
G. BOURGUIGNON et CHIRAY : Libération des cicatrices adhérentes par l'ionisation d'iodure de po-	
M.-L. GIROUX : Hémiplégie consécutive à une intoxication par les gaz asphyxiants	1486
E. JOB et L. HIRTZMANN : Dysenterie amibienne et chlorhydrate d'émétine	1488
E. JOB et L. HIRTZMANN : Note sur quelques symptômes observés au cours de la dysenterie amibienne.	1500
FÉLIX RAMOND et B. DE LA GRANDIÈRE : Troubles de la sensibilité au cours de la diphtérie : l'hystérie diphtérique	1506
E. LENOBLE et R. INIZAN : Un cas de tumeur mélanique de la base du cerveau intéressant le facial droit, s'accompagnant de paraplégie flasque et d'irritation méningée de voisinage (sarcomatose de la pie-mère et paraplégie neurale)	1511
L. BABONNEIX : Hérédo-syphilis nerveuse probable	1516
P. NOBÉCOURT et E. PEYRE : Résultats des hémocultures pratiquées chez 128 malades du service des contagieux de F.., ...	1521
G. PAISSEAU et H. LEMAIRE : Accès pernicieux palustres et surrénalites aiguës	1530
PETZETAKIS : Réactions pleurales parabronchitiques. Réactions pleurales non tuberculeuses accompagnant les bronchites catarrhales aiguës. Rapports avec l'éosinophilie pleurale.	1545
CH. ACHARD et E. WELTER : Fractures claviculaires chez des syphilitiques (Discussion : M. GAUCHER).	1564
P. ARMAND-DELILLE, G. PAISSEAU et H. LEMAIRE : Le paludisme de	

Figure 1–6. One of many editions of *Revue Neurologique* with several articles by Guillain and Barré, without Strohl.

after the original. He introduced two cases by referring to the 1916 article written "en collaboration avec M. J.-A. Barré" (not Strohl) and remarkably cited the article in the footnote without Strohl's name.[462] The first two authors may also have encouraged the shortened eponym by presenting remarks ". . . sur *notre* Syndrome . . ." to the Société de Neurologie de Paris in 1936.[465] Strohl's omission was virtually sealed by the title and introduction of the widely distributed 1937 Brussels symposium in which the main title, the massive introductory article, and all but one of the 15 paper titles used "Guillain et Barré" or "Guillain-Barré." In that symposium, Barré refers to "le Prof. Guillain et notre ami Strohl . . . le syndrome qui naquit modestement à l'Hôpital d'Avalard à Amiens."[460] Considering the place of honor reserved at the symposium for Guillain (after Barré's comments on various clinical aspects of

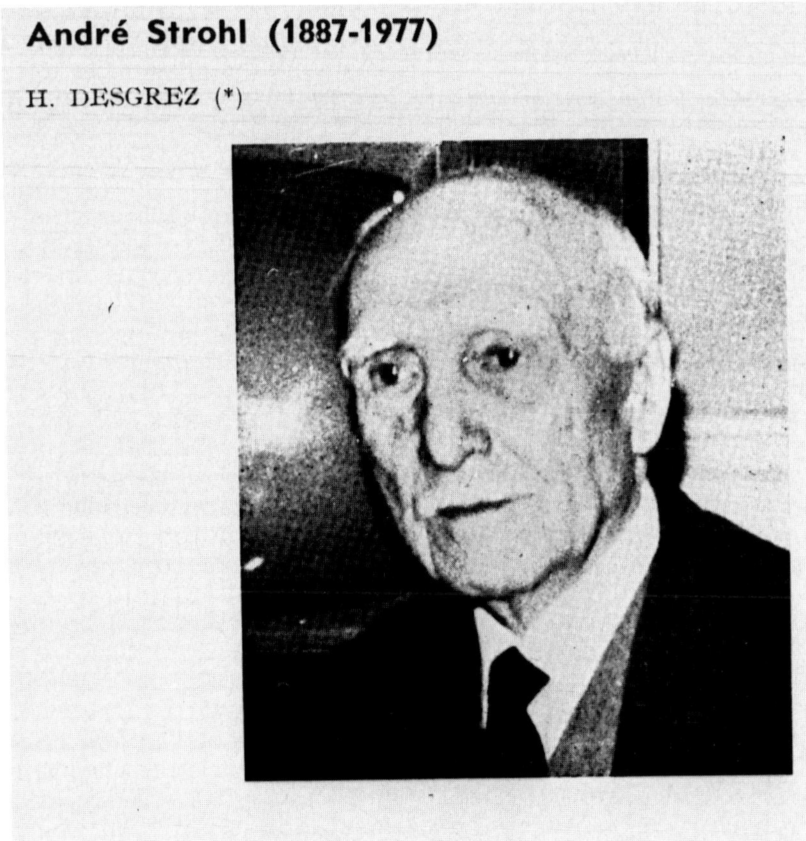

Figure 1–7. Photograph of Dr. André Strohl. (Courtesy of Dr. Jean-Marie Leger, Hôpitaux de Paris.)

the disease, Guillain summarized the symposium in the final paper), the influential professor must have acceded to the shortened eponym, not to mention the obvious exclusion of Strohl from the symposium. Whether Strohl simply could not attend or was not invited is unknown.

PATHOLOGIC BASIS OF THE SYNDROME

Some pathologic features of the disease were delineated early by Eichorst,[323] Mills and Spiller,[806] Walter,[1250] and others.[67,156,263,297] Neurologists appreciated, but before 1880 did not uniformly accept, that this was probably a disease of peripheral nerves. Most pathologists thought that the proximal peripheral nerves were not involved. Mills and Spiller[806] found degeneration of nerves and cell bodies in a case of "Landry's paralysis" and suggested a "neuronitis." Enough controversy was raised by the regular appearance of secondary chromatolysis of anterior horn cells that spinal cord disease was not consistently separated from neuropathy of any kind (except perhaps lead poisoning) until Leyden's work in 1880.[695] Dumeniul[297] is generally credited with showing nerve fiber loss without spinal cord abnormalities in a case of peripheral neuropathy in 1864; neither his nor Leyden's cases were likely to have been GBS. Ross and Bury,[1026,1137] on the basis of 90 cases of various types, concluded that Landry's paralysis was probably a disease of peripheral nerves. Schmaus,[1068] writing in 1904, first appreciated that GBS was a topographically selective, rather than a diffuse, pathologic process. Little attention was given to pathology in the 1937 Brussels symposium.

The first landmark in the pathologic description of GBS was an exhaustive series of 50 fatal cases reported in 1949 by Haymaker and Kernohan[501] (Fig. 1–8). In addition to using Landry's name to denote the syndrome, they preceded their original findings with an extensive historical review and a classification of the disorder based on clinical-topographic grounds. The clinical data in this series were apparently all gathered retrospectively; when no record was made of a particular finding, the authors generally noted this. It is interesting, as with Guillain, Barré, and Strohl, that the armed forces served as the collecting ground for their material. The clinical descriptions given by Haymaker and Kernohan are still most helpful to clinicians because they implicitly define the limits of the disease and give an extensive review of the neurologic findings in a large group of fatal cases (particularly their Table 10). They found that the incidence and severity of sensory symptoms were a function of the duration of disease, and cranial nerve paralysis was more frequent than previously appreciated. Details of recently preceding infectious diseases were reviewed and were likely to have been accurate, since most patients had been in the armed forces when their GBS began. The core of the paper gave the pathologic findings in great detail, with an attempt at clinical-pathologic correlation. For example, the purely paralytic syndrome showed disease predominantly in the anterior spinal roots.

Haymaker and Kernohan concluded that inflammatory cells were not present in peripheral nerves until the illness was relatively advanced; therefore, the term "polyradiculoneuropathy" was proposed, rather than the previously favored "polyradiculoneuritis." Edema of the proximal portion of the peripheral nervous system was the earliest and sole change during the first 4 days. Disintegration of myelin and swelling of axis cylinders appeared on the fifth day, and it was not until the ninth day or later that lymphocytes and phagocytes appeared. Secondary (retrograde) changes in anterior horn cells occurred later, presumably representing chromatolysis. The authors emphasized prominent damage to proximal (spinal) nerves, often at the junction of anterior and posterior roots, but they admitted that the paucity of distal nerve material precluded a definite comment on the distribution of pathologic change. They gave no sense of multifocal lesions, inflammatory or otherwise. There were no important primary CNS lesions, but almost one quarter of the cases had scanty perivascular lymphocytic collections in the spinal cord or brain. This classic paper established the clinical and pathologic unity of GBS and "Landry's paralysis," because sensory symptoms could be mild and the spinal fluid protein could be normal, or sensory symptoms and spinal fluid protein elevation could both be pronounced, all contrary to Guillain's excessively restrictive criteria. An attempt to yield virus from the body fluids in 17 cases

THE LANDRY-GUILLAIN-BARRÉ SYNDROME

A CLINICOPATHOLOGIC REPORT OF FIFTY FATAL CASES AND A CRITIQUE OF THE LITERATURE[1]

WEBB HAYMAKER, M.D. AND JAMES W. KERNOHAN, M.D.[2]

From the Army Institute of Pathology, Washington, D. C., and the Section of Pathologic Anatomy and Neuropathology, Mayo Clinic, Rochester, Minnesota

Figure 1–8. Title page from Haymaker and Kernohan's 1949 classic clinical-pathologic description of 50 fatal cases of GBS.[501]

was unsuccessful and no theory of pathogenesis was offered. This study has not been exceeded in breadth or detail of clinical material and is still an excellent reference for serious students of the clinical syndrome, although subsequent work has revised the pathologic outlook. Several extensive reviews, particularly one by Ravn,[973] followed, all largely subsidiary to the Haymaker and Kernohan opus but each adding refined points.

Asbury, Arnason, and Adams,[52] at the Massachusetts General Hospital, made a more detailed study of the pathologic features of the disease. Their experience was closely tied to the development in experimental pathology of an autoallergic or "experimental autoimmune neuritis" (EAN) that was produced by injecting peripheral nerve tissue with adjuvants into rabbits. Dr. Raymond D. Adams has indicated to the authors that his study of the human pathologic material, in which perivenous lymphocytes were prominent, suggested to him that an allergic phenomenon was responsible for GBS. He subsequently encouraged Dr. Byron Waksman to attempt nerve injections in rabbits. Used to produce a clinical and pathologic facsimile of the human disease, the EAN model has not changed appreciably during the subsequent 30 years.[1244] Because of the prevalance of protozoencephalitic disease in rabbit colonies, the significance of generalized paralysis was initially uncertain. The experiments were extended to guinea pigs with satisfactory and unsullied results. The experimental finding of early lymphocytic infiltration of peripheral nerves, however, was at odds with Haymaker and Kernohan's concept and directed the later pathologic study by Asbury, Arnason, and Adams[52] toward the primacy of inflammation in GBS.

The central finding in 19 patients studied by Asbury's group was a well-developed lymphocytic infiltration in the spinal roots and nerves in every patient examined, including those dying in the first few days. The descriptive and photographic detail of this work make it possible to determine that "the pathologic hallmark of idiopathic polyneuritis is a perivascular mononuclear inflammatory infiltrate."[52] Moreover, these infiltrates were adjacent to regions of segmental demyelination. The crucial feature of focal demyelination in inflamed regions of nerve had been alluded to in earlier works[650] but never captured as the germinal finding. A third feature was the widespread but spotty distribution of these infiltrates, involving not only roots, but also ganglia, cranial nerves, and regions of the whole length of nerve. Sympathetic nerves, and in some cases sensory ganglia, could also be inflamed. The proximal nerve roots were most prominently involved in only a few cases. This demonstrated the need for extensive sampling of pathologic material in GBS. No evidence of the previously emphasized early edema of nerves was found, and no significant lesions of the central nervous system occurred, although rare regions of perivascular inflammation were noted in the brainstem of one patient who had no corresponding clinical features. Persistent small foci of inflammation occurred in several recovered patients, leading to speculation about the source of relapsing or chronic GBS. This work, perhaps the fourth classic paper in GBS, turned from "polyneuropathy" confidently to "polyneuritis," and emphasized the role of lymphocytes in the pathogenesis of the disease (see Chapter 5). Experimental work that tested cellular hypersensitivity to peripheral nerve antigens later supported this hypothesis. Prineas[955,956] has been credited with pointing out the importance of macrophages in damage to Schwann cell processes that constitute the myelin sheath.

MODERN IMMUNOLOGIC AND ELECTROPHYSIOLOGIC BASIS OF THE SYNDROME

The immune origins of GBS have recently been re-examined. Circulating factors that fix complement have been found in EAN and in the blood of patients with GBS.[218] Some of these appear to be myelinotoxic antibodies and have been shown to cause segmental demyelination when injected into the psciatic nerve of rats or other animals. The possibility remains that these antibodies are a secondary phenomenon, occurring in response to neural damage. However, an early electrophysiologic conduction block has been produced by serum from patients with GBS, prior to evident morphologic change,[1163] suggesting that circulating factors, probably antibodies, play a role in the pathogenesis of GBS (see Chapters 5 and 13). The traditional concepts of the immune pathogenesis of GBS are therefore being revised; some of the early features of the illness may be related to humoral or other circulating factors, and the later anatomic nerve damage may be more closely related to inflammatory activity.

Electrophysiologic aspects of GBS were first alluded to in the original articles by Landry, and by Guillain, Barré, and Strohl, mainly through Strohl's graphic recordings. Several series of patients with GBS have reported various electrophysiologic patterns early in the illness, none specific and many normal. The description and clinical use of late responses added an important dimension to the accuracy and specificity of diagnosis in GBS[615,1088] and these tests began to supersede elevation of CSF protein as the most helpful early confirmatory laboratory test[14,781,1021] (see Chapter 13).

TREATMENTS

Specific treatment of GBS has been based on anecdotal experience, with most practitioners since the 1950s favoring some form of corticosteroid ther-

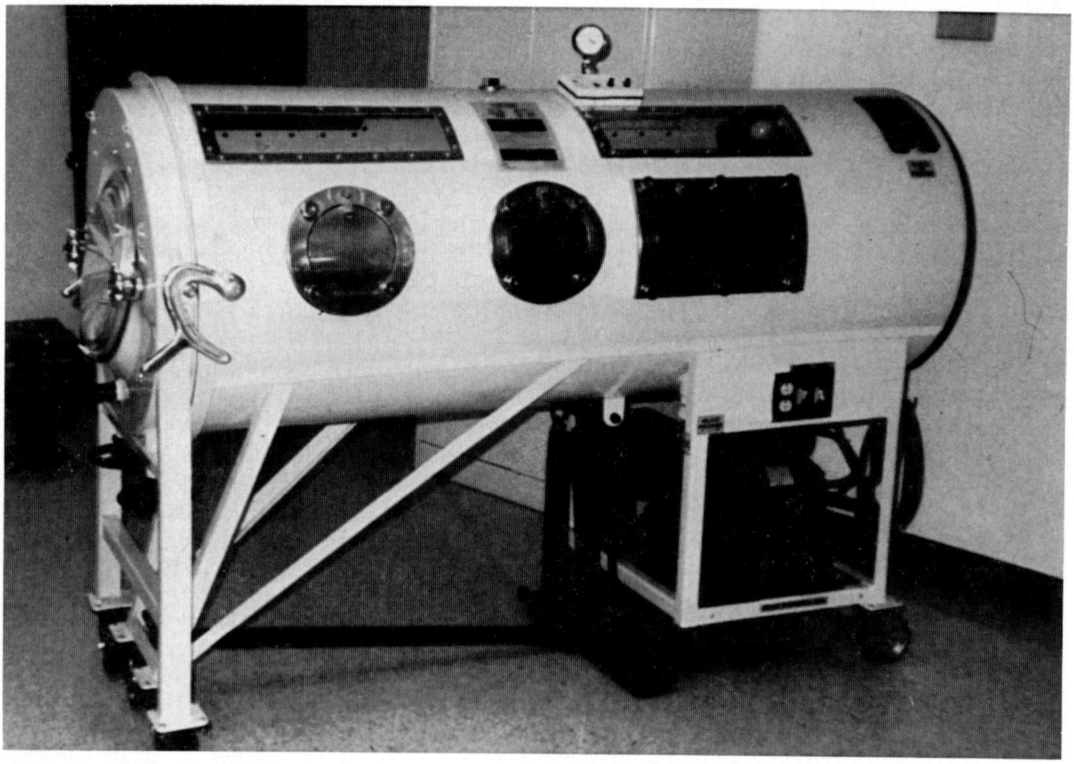

Figure 1–9. The negative-pressure "iron lung" used in the heyday of the polio epidemic and an early mainstay of GBS respiratory treatment. (Courtesy of Dr. John Spalding, Oxford.)

apy. Jackson's 1957 study[560] and others initially supported the effectiveness of steroids, but the majority of subsequent reports gave conflicting or equivocal results (see Chapter 15). A small trial carried out by Hughes and co-workers[547] suggested in 1978 that conventional-dose steroid treatment was not beneficial and perhaps detrimental. The use of plasma exchange, first reported in a single patient by Brettle and associates,[141] was in response to the study by Hughes and motivated by contemporary work in immunology. Brettle's report led to three formidable multicenter randomized trials that resolved that plasma exchange was beneficial (see Chapter 15).

More important than any of the specific therapies for GBS has been the inception, after World War II, of respiratory intensive care units (ICUs) and the routine use of positive-pressure ventilation.[431,1013] This change alone was responsible for a reduction in the mortality rate for GBS from approximately 20% to less than 5% (see Chapters 16 and 17). Negative-pressure ventilators such as the "iron lung" (Fig. 1–9) were the mainstay of respiratory support in the early 1950s but had limited use in patients with oropharyngeal weakness.

PERSONAL ACCOUNTS

Several personal accounts by physicians are reviewed in the introduction. A very peculiar historic event involves Harvey Cushing's wartime illness during World War I, Georges Guillain's obituary of Cushing, and their simultaneous presence at the Conference Chirurgicale Interalice in 1918, just after the war. Reich[977] has analyzed Cushing's illness retrospectively, giving journal entries that convincingly conclude that Cushing had GBS. The illness progressed through October 1918 with Cushing's legs being "asleep," "numb, wobbly," and "tabetic," with reflexes lost, marked rombergism, bilateral facial paresis, and later diplopia, unequal (and irregular) pupils, and eventually some muscular wasting. There was "soreness" and tenderness but no pain. Cushing performed an extensive neurologic self-examination that was quite consistent with GBS. In several letters, Cushing referred to a polyneuritis but not to Landry's paralysis or GBS, although it had been 2 years since the introduction of the concept of GBS in France, where Cushing was stationed.

Guillain, in an obituary on Cushing in 1939,[461] briefly mentions a polyneuropathy acquired during the war: "Les fatigues necessitées par un travail constant affecterent sa santé et quand il revint, en 1919, à Boston, il presentait des signes d'une polynevrite qui persista longtemps." No further analysis was made. He implied that the two met for the first time in Baltimore in 1919. Reich discovered that Guillain attended the surgical conference in 1918, from which Cushing had a guest list in his diary, but it is not entirely clear if Cushing was actually present. Reich surmises that Cushing's illness could have been correctly diagnosed had the two discussed it.

The history of GBS has a mainly clinical lineage, with clinicians of each epoch refining and building on previous work to produce an extensive body of material that is unlikely to change appreciably in the future. The next major advances will probably be in the detailed immunologic understanding of the disease and in new forms of therapy.

Chapter 2

DIAGNOSTIC CRITERIA

Proposed Evolution of Diagnostic Criteria

Twenty years after his original description, Guillain[459] proposed to "delineate the syndrome as exactly as possible." Many neurologists since that time have tried to define the clinical limits and nature of the disease with various diagnostic criteria,* but no single clinical finding or laboratory test enables one to make the diagnosis. Most "criteria" are therefore simply discursive descriptions. In clinical practice, the diagnosis can be, and usually is, made without fulfilling any rigid criteria. A committee of the National Institute of Neurological and Communicative Disorders and Stroke led by Dr. Arthur Asbury has established modern criteria for diagnosis.[51,53] Although these exemplary criteria have been criticized by some as being too restrictive,[943] they have greatly aided research in the field and clarified clinical thinking about the typical disease. An updated report in 1981[51] was expanded to include variants of the disease. Other variants and temporal courses, some modulated by treatment, have been described that do not strictly conform to the criteria. In modern practice, the most helpful criterion is not a clinical one; instead, the strongest evidence is provided by electrophysiologic changes that are consistent with a demyelinating neuropathy (see Chapter 13). Electrophysiologic testing is not required to make the diagnosis in the majority of cases, but clinically atypical cases can be best clarified by electrophysiologic resemblance to the typical illness. At times, the appearance of the full electrophysiologic picture is delayed, but without the typical pattern it is difficult to be certain that a process is related to GBS.

In their original descriptions, Guillain, Barré, and Strohl emphasized a specific syndrome that can be "easily recognized":[466,467]

> "We call attention to a clinical syndrome which we have observed in two cases, a syndrome characterized by motor disturbances, loss of tendon reflexes, with preservation of cutaneous reflexes, paresthesias with slight disturbance of objective sensibility, tenderness on pressure of the muscles, little change in the electrical reaction of the nerves or muscles, and noteworthy hyperalbuminosis of the cerebrospinal fluid in the absence of cytologic reaction (albuminocytologic dissociation). . . . The prognosis does not appear to be extremely serious, if we may judge from the course of the disease in our two patients; the first had almost recovered and the second was improving when they were discharged from the army."

In the landmark Brussels symposium of 1937,[460] Guillain proposed a clinical classification based on topographic considerations. He divided the syndrome into four types: (1) "la forme inferieure" involving the extremities only; (2) "la forme mixte spinale et mesocephalique" involving extremities and cranial nerves; (3) "la forme mesocephalique pure" limited to cranial nerves; and (4) "une forme de polyradiculonevrite avec troubles mentaux," polyradiculopathy with mental change.[459,460]

Numerous authors have attempted to refine this descriptive classification by

*See references 51, 53, 124, 777, 882, 943, and 945.

offering alternative diagnostic or exclusionary criteria. Brown and Baker[150] considered recurrences; symptoms of involvement of other organs; toxicity or fever; CSF protein concentration of 1 g/dL or more; meningeal symptoms; eosinophilia, anemia, hematuria, or albuminuria; or a progressive course as rare findings that cautioned against the diagnosis. Hand and Rudoy[483] questioned the generally held belief that once improvement began, it continued uninterrupted, and they reported a patient with an exacerbation of symptoms after partial recovery. Others[124] identified similar relapsing courses. These reports first separated acute GBS from an emerging new category of "chronic or relapsing GBS."

In 1960, Osler and Sidell[882] offered criteria and advised applying the original description with as much fidelity as possible. They were among those who favored, as did Guillain, severely restrictive criteria, considering many signs exclusionary that are now accepted as compatible with the diagnosis. The conservative nature of criteria of this type are understandable because they were drawn from personal experience with small series of patients.

Others have taken the opposite position,[945] suggesting that the GBS eponym be abandoned and replaced by the term "postinfectious radiculoneuropathy," based on cases showing a combination of central and peripheral nervous system involvement similar to postinfectious encephalomyelitis. Poser and Fowler[943] considered pure GBS "one end of a spectrum of conditions in which the nervous system is the site of an antigen-antibody reaction following a viral infection," an idea that has been recently revived.

Masucci and Kurtzke did much to broaden the definition of the syndrome in their report of 50 cases[761] by emphasizing the following findings as acceptable: pure motor variant; lower cranial nerve involvement; normal CSF, with "modest" elevation in the number of cells in the CSF; occasional Babinski signs; meningeal signs; papilledema; and fever. They also accepted relapses and recurrences and progression for 2 months or longer as consistent with the diagnosis.

Although his article "Diagnostic considerations in Guillain-Barré syndrome" began to be cited widely and used in studies of GBS, Asbury[51,53] concluded that the "precise diagnostic limits of GBS remain uncertain." These consensus criteria are nonetheless the best currently available. Our criteria clarify the ones currently used, drawing on our experience with complex cases that created diagnostic difficulty.

PROPOSED CRITERIA

Most neurologists are quickly able to identify typical cases and minor variations of the classic syndrome. Difficulty arises with atypical or fragmentary syndromes, which are discussed in Chapter 8. In order to avoid a discursive description of GBS that includes the limits of each typical feature simply and order to accommodate clinical variations, we have chosen to make separate criteria for typical GBS and for each variant. The criteria shown in Tables 2–1 through 2–6 allow the specific diagnosis of typical GBS, Fisher syndrome, and most variations encoun-

Table 2–1 DIAGNOSTIC CRITERIA—TYPICAL GUILLAIN-BARRÉ SYNDROME

Clinical Features:

1. Weakness that is approximately symmetric in all the limbs
2. Paresthesias in the feet and hands
3. Areflexia or hyporeflexia in all limbs by 1 week
4. Progression of the aforementioned three features over several days to 1 month

Laboratory Abnormalities that Confirm the Diagnosis:

5. Elevated CSF protein concentration (more than 45 mg/dL) within 3 weeks from onset
6. Abnormalities of F waves (absence, dispersion, impersistence) in at least two limbs, *or* motor nerve conduction block, or slowing (motor nerve conduction velocity below 80% of normal)

Table 2–2 DIAGNOSTIC CRITERIA—PURE MOTOR GBS*

Clinical Features:
1. Progressive, relatively symmetric weakness in all limbs
2. No paresthesias or sensory loss
3. Areflexia or hyporeflexia in all limbs by 1 week
4. Progression of weakness over 1 day to 3 weeks

Laboratory Abnormalities that Confirm the Diagnosis:
5. Elevated CSF protein concentration (>45 mg/dL) within 3 weeks of onset
6. Abnormalities of F waves in at least two limbs, *or* motor nerve conduction block, or slowing
7. Normal sensory nerve potentials

*See Chapter 8.

tered in practice. Each group of features is meant to be sensitive for a clinically recognizable illness, but their specificity depends on the previous exclusion of obvious imitators (eg, spinal cord disease). Electrophysiologic changes are included because they have become a central diagnostic feature of GBS, more sensitive and earlier than CSF protein elevation. Our experience at Massachusetts General Hospital (MGH) with puzzling cases has led us to the opinion that the germinal feature of GBS, besides the typical syndrome, is electrophysiologic evidence of a demye-

Table 2–3 DIAGNOSTIC CRITERIA—PURE SENSORY GBS*

Clinical Features:
1. Paresthesias in the feet and hands
2. No weakness or respiratory failure
3. Areflexia or hyporeflexia in all limbs by 1 week
4. Distally diminished sensation involving mainly vibration and joint position
5. Proximal progression of numbness and sensory loss on the limbs over several days to 1 month
6. Improvement in paresthesias and sensory loss by 2–4 months from onset

Laboratory Abnormalities that Confirm the Diagnosis:
7. Elevated CSF protein concentration (>45 mg/dL) within 3 weeks of onset
8. Severe sensory nerve conduction abnormalities
9. Minimal motor conduction and late response abnormalities

*See Chapter 8.

Table 2–4 DIAGNOSTIC CRITERIA—FISHER'S SYNDROME*

Clinical Features:
1. Bilateral, relatively symmetric weakness of several extraocular muscles, and ptosis
2. Limb and gait ataxia with cerebellar tremor
3. Areflexia in all limbs by 1 week
4. Progression of aforementioned three features over several days to 3 weeks
5. Minimal or no limb, facial, or oropharyngeal weakness, or paresthesias
6. Normal alertness; no cerebellar dysarthria except as a result of number 5; no Babinski signs

Laboratory Abnormalities that Confirm the Diagnosis:
5. Variable, usually slight, elevation of CSF protein concentration
6. Abnormal motor nerve conduction and late responses in the legs

*See Chapter 8.

Table 2–5 DIAGNOSTIC CRITERIA—REGIONAL VARIANTS OF GBS*

Pharyngeal-Cervical-Brachial Variant

Clinical Features:
1. Progressive weakness in the neck, shoulders, proximal arms, oropharyngeal muscles, and diaphragm over 1–3 weeks
2. Areflexia or hyporeflexia in the arms by 1 week of illness
3. Normal (or virtually normal) leg power and tendon reflexes
4. Minimal or no paresthesias or sensory loss

Laboratory Abnormalities that Confirm the Diagnosis:
5. Variable, usually slight, elevation of CSF protein concentration
6. Abnormal motor nerve conduction or late responses in the arms; no decrement or increment in compound muscle action potential with repetitive stimulation

Paraparetic Variant

Clinical Features:
1. Progressive leg weakness over 1–3 weeks
2. Areflexia or hyporeflexia in the legs by 1 week of illness
3. Normal (or virtually normal) power and reflexes in the arms and cranial nerve innervated muscles
4. Minimal or no paresthesias or sensory loss

Laboratory Abnormalities that Confirm the Diagnosis:
5. Variable, usually slight, elevation of CSF protein concentration
6. Abnormal motor nerve conduction and late responses in the legs

*See Chapter 8.

Table 2–6 DIAGNOSTIC CRITERIA—PURE PANDYSAUTONOMIA*

Clinical Features:
1. Progressive sympathetic and parasympathetic dysfunction over 1–3 weeks
2. No limb weakness, ophthalmoplegia, or ataxia
3. Areflexia or hyporeflexia by 1 week
4. Improvement of some autonomic dysfunction by 2–4 months

Laboratory Abnormalities that Confirm the Diagnosis:
5. Elevated CSF protein concentration
6. Normal (or virtually normal) motor nerve conduction studies, and abnormal sensory nerve conduction studies

*See Chapter 8.

linating neuropathy in clinically affected regions. This becomes important in interpreting unusual cases such as bifacial palsy with areflexia. The limits for several laboratory studies are taken from the extreme values in our prospective and retrospective series. The onset of illness is considered as the day on which the first symptom occurred, usually paresthesias or limb weakness. Criteria for chronic inflammatory demyelinating polyneuropathy (CIDP) are discussed in Chapter 10 and Table 10–5.

Chapter 3

EPIDEMIOLOGY

With the virtual disappearance of poliomyelitis, the Guillain-Barré syndrome has emerged as the most frequent cause of acute generalized neuromuscular paralysis. Epidemiologic data, despite many clinical shortcomings, are valuable in evaluating the frequency of GBS in various populations, studying changes in incidence over time, detecting outbreaks or clusters of unusual preceding illnesses, and possibly illuminating underlying causes.

GBS incidence rates in various series have been derived from population-based surveys or from hospitalized patients, and these groups are not always comparable. Many epidemiologic investigations after about 1980 differ from previous ones because of the use of contemporary and uniformly applied criteria for GBS that were commissioned by the National Institution of Neurological and Communicative Disorders and Stroke[51,53] (see Chapter 2).

DEMOGRAPHIC FEATURES

Incidence, Age, and Sex Distribution

The incidence rates among population-based studies of GBS in various countries and regions of the United States are remarkably similar, and these rates have not changed appreciably over the years (Table 3–1). The crude average yearly incidence rate of GBS is 0.6 to 1.9 cases per 100,000 population. A few recent studies in selected populations [588,687,1123] have shown slightly higher incidences, up to 4 cases per 100,000.

GBS occurs among all age groups, although reports of patients over 80 years old are infrequent.[400,552] A 95-year-old patient was mentioned in the 1978–1979 National Surveillance Study.[552] The youngest patient in a large series, 2 months old, was reported from India,[1053] and there has been a case report of a 1-month-old infant.[406] There are numerous other reports of older infants;[174] a convincing neonatal case has recently been reported.[24] These are discussed further in Chapter 9. The average age of onset of GBS, approximately 40 years, has been similar in most studies.

Various peaks of age incidence have been claimed.[88,1123] A relatively increased incidence of GBS in children was found in a study from Cape Town, South Africa,[611] based on an examination of hospital records. The yearly incidences for 1979 through 1981 were between 1.7 and 3.3 per 100,000 children under age 13, consistent with other surveys, but the incidence in children from birth to age 5 during this period was 5.4 per 100,000,[611] three times the incidence of Afro-Asian Jewish children from birth to age 4 in Israel[1123] and more than ten times the United States incidence for this age group.[552] One Michigan population survey suggested a slightly increasing incidence of GBS with age. High rates in individuals over age 45 were also found in unvaccinated patients during the National Immunization Program Survey, 1976–1977[1072] (see farther on). A predilection for patients from 16 to 25 years and from 45 to 60 years occurred in a hospital series of 776 patients in the New York–New

Table 3–1 POPULATION SURVEY INCIDENCES OF GBS

Author(s), Year	*Period*	*Population*	*No. of Patients*	*Incidence/ 100,000*	*M:F*
Kurland,[657] 1958	1945–1954	Rochester, MN	3	1.00	—
Brewis et al.,[142] 1966	1955–1961	Carlisle, England	3	0.60	—
Chen et al.,[188] 1968	1960–1966	Chamorros, Guam	5	1.90	1.5:1
Gudmundsson,[457] 1969	1954–1963	Iceland	13	0.75	—
Hogg et al.,[527] 1979	1972–1976	San Joaquin County, CA	18	1.20	1.6:1
Schonberger et al.,[1072] 1979	1976–1977	Unvaccinated US civilian population, excluding 7 states	332	0.97	1.3:1
D'Ambrosio et al.,[245] 1983	1971–1980	Campania (southern Italy)	76	0.16	1.5:1
Haberman et al.,[474] 1982	1978	North West Thames, England	39	1.10	1.1:1
Johnson,[568] 1982	1973–1975	US Army recruits	93	1.50	—
Bak,[68] 1985	1965–1982	Ringkobing County, Denmark	51	1.10	1.4:1
Breman and Hayner,[138] 1984	1976–1977	Michigan, unvaccinated	87	0.90	1.3:1
Soffer et al.,[1123]	1969–1972	Israel	89	0.75	—
Beghi et al.,[88] 1985*	1935–1980	Olmsted County, MN	48	1.70	1.5:1
Larsen et al.,[673] 1985	1957–1982	Western Norway	109	1.14	1.7:1
Kaplan et al.,[588] 1985†	1981–1983	Larimer County, CO	19	4.00	2.1:1
Hankey,[484] 1987	1980–1985	Western Australia	109	1.35	1.3:1

*Updated report; earlier reported by Lesser et al.,[687] 1973, and by Kennedy et al.,[606] 1978.
†Incidence 1975–1980; 1.2/100,000.

Jersey metropolitan area.[289] During the 39 months of the national surveillance program for GBS (third report),[589] from January 1978 to March 1981, increased incidences were noted in patients aged 15 to 35 and 50 to 74 years (more prominently in men), among 2,575 reported cases. The incidence in women fell progressively from age 25 to 44 but rose thereafter to baseline levels (Fig. 3–1).

The absence of concordance between studies suggests that there is no consistent age proclivity and that any apparent excess may have been due to selection bias. The age incidences in the Massachusetts General Hospital (MGH) retrospective and prospective series are shown in Figure 3–2. The mean age in the retrospective series was 39 years (range 8 months to 81 years), and in our prospective series, 45 years (range 13 to 84 years). The overall incidences of GBS remained virtually constant through the seventh decade although gender-related peaks were evident, as will be noted later.

Many major series of GBS show a slight but sometimes significant male preponderance (Table 3–1). In the MGH experience the male:female ratios were 1.1:1 in the retrospective series and 1.9:1 in the prospective series (Fig. 3–2). There was a modest peak among men aged 30 to 50. In the Centers for Disease Control (CDC) surveillance series (second report),[552] the age-adjusted attack rate for men was 0.52 per 100,000 and for women 0.40 per 100,000, among a total of 1,034 GBS cases. A slightly increased incidence among younger women in the MGH retrospective series (Fig. 3–2) has been highlighted in a study[992] of a population from West Virginia, and in the national surveillance program,[552,589] but was not reproduced in the MGH prospective series and does not have general support among other series. Moreover, if women who had a mononucleosis-like illness were omitted from analysis, the early peak in women no longer existed in the retrospective series.

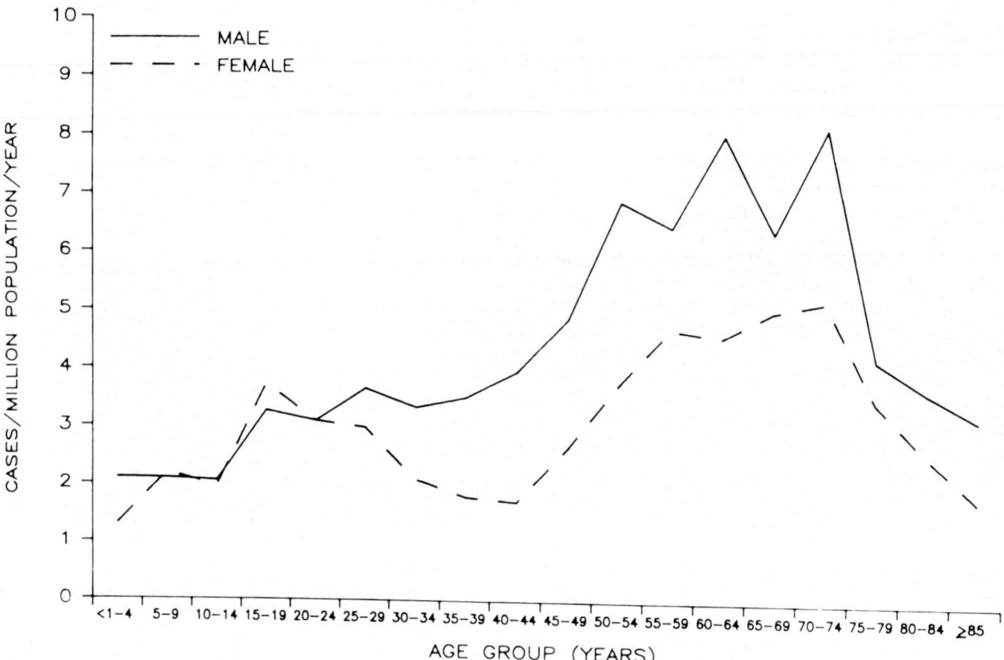

Figure 3–1. Incidence of GBS in the initial surveillance program 1978–1981, showing an apparent late peak in incidence with predominantly men. (From Kaplan et al.,[589] p. 634, with permission.)

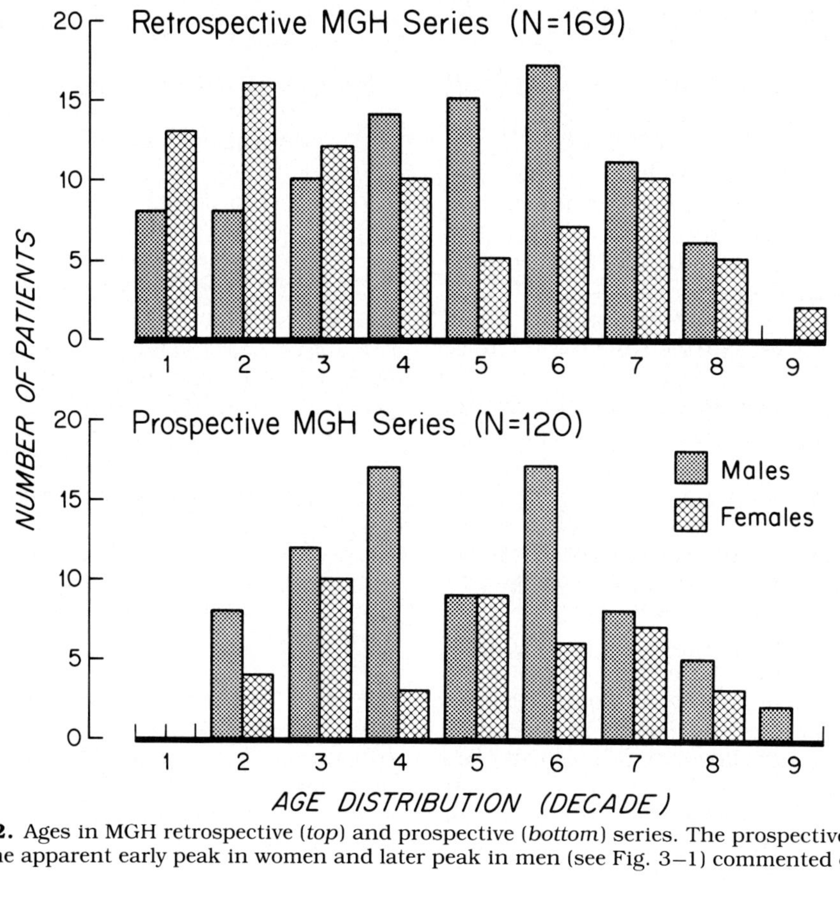

Figure 3–2. Ages in MGH retrospective (*top*) and prospective (*bottom*) series. The prospective series did not have the apparent early peak in women and later peak in men (see Fig. 3–1) commented on in other reports.

Geographic and Racial Distribution

GBS has been reported from all regions of the world, including the Third World countries, generally with attack rates similar to those of the United States. Separate reports have appeared from Australia,[484] Japan,[592,1177] Korea,[205] China,[1313] Iceland,[457] India,[199,1053] Israel,[1123] Kenya,[65] Singapore,[1193] South Africa,[611] Mexico,[422] Egypt,[475] Nigeria,[888] and virtually all European countries. An epidemiologic study[1313] of 156 cases admitted to the Capital Hospital in Beijing from 1949 through 1975 showed a predilection for children and adolescents, particularly in summer and fall, but there were otherwise no differences from American or European studies. A low incidence of 0.16 per 100,000 was found in southern Italy, in part attributable to the strict criteria used by the investigators.[245] No endemic areas of GBS have been identified.

The racial distribution in the national surveillance study (second study)[552] of 1,034 GBS patients was 83% white, 7% black, 5% Hispanic, 1% Asian, and others, 4% giving an annual age-adjusted attack rate for whites of 0.44 per 100,000 compared with 0.28 per 100,000 for blacks. Uncertainty about the true denominators for each race in the surveillance population makes these differences questionable. An impression that GBS was uncommon in blacks was not confirmed in one extensive study[761] that found 38% of the GBS population to be black, not significantly different from the 46% black general admissions rate to the hospital analyzed. There is no obvious racial difference in the clinical expresson of GBS, although one third of 34 Nigerian patients[888] had pure motor neuropathy (perhaps including cases of poliomyelitis). Outcomes in Nigeria were similar to those of European and North American series. A Kenyan report[65] had high incidences of cranial nerve palsies (more than 50%), respiratory insufficiency, and relatively poor outcome (9% mortality; 26% severe disability) among 54 GBS patients. One reason for the apparently poor outcome was that even a mild foot drop was considered a handicap because of the importance to rural inhabitants of walking.

A population-based study in Israel[1123] showed an apparently lower rate of GBS among Arabs (0.46 per 100,000) than in adjacent populations (Afro-Asian Jews 0.8, Israeli Jews 0.7, Euro-American Jews 0.8). This was explained by the investigators as possibly due to a reluctance of Arabs to be admitted to a hospital. A peak in children under age 5 was found among Sephardic Jews and Arabs with lower socioeconomic status, perhaps due to the earlier acquisition of childhood infections.

Outbreaks of GBS

GBS usually occurs sporadically, but clusters without an obvious source have been reported. Most older publications concerning outbreaks[1107,1216,1220] omitted patient descriptions or contained unusual cases that were probably not GBS. Several similar brief epidemics, including a report by Chomel[194] in 1828, before Landry's paper, were most likely due to toxic polyneuropathies (see Chapter 2). For example, a 5-month epidemic of flaccid tetraplegia in Spain caused a pure motor syndrome with repeatedly normal spinal fluid examinations; postmortem examination of peripheral nerve in three cases revealed no inflammation.[1216] All these features make the diagnosis of GBS suspect. Many other diseases that have been confused with GBS such as polio, botulism, Bannwarth's syndrome, paralytic rabies, and diphtheria may occur in outbreaks.

True common-origin clusters of GBS generally derive from an obvious precipitant, such as 16 cases in Colombia[1195] linked to antirabies vaccination with suckling mouse brain vaccine. Most of the Colombian patients had severe GBS with rapidly ascending weakness and respiratory failure, fatal in 6 individ-

Table 3–2 REPORTED "OUTBREAKS" OF GUILLAIN-BARRÉ

Author	Year	Population	Putative Cause
Van Bogaert et al.[1220]	1938	Belgium	Unknown
Singh and Jolly[1107]	1958	Patiala, India	Unknown
Lopez et al.[720]	1968	Antioquia, Colombia	Enterovirus
Valenciano et al.[1216]	1968	Albacete, Spain	Toxic?
Toro et al.[1195]	1977	Bogota, Colombia	Rabies vaccine
Cabrera et al.[163]	1982	Lima, Peru	Suckling mouse brain rabies, vaccine
Sliman[1115]	1978	El Sylt, Jordan	*E coli; Shigella*
Schonberger et al.[1072]	1977	US	A/New Jersey influenza vaccine
Kaplan et al.[588]	1983	Larimer County, CO	Unknown
Kashihara et al.[592]	1985	Kochi, Japan	Unknown

uals. Only 3 patients left the hospital without major sequelae. A reduced vaccine dose eliminated the associated GBS.[1195] In Lima, 6 severe cases occurred within 6 weeks, associated with two consecutive vaccine lots.[163] In 1976, 19 cases of GBS occurred in El Sylt, Jordan, allegedly associated with *Escherichia* contamination of the municipal water supply.[609,1115] Seventeen patients, mostly young adults, had gastrointestinal symptoms 2 to 21 days before the onset of neurologic symptoms. Several members of one family with diarrhea contracted GBS. An apparent increase in GBS incidence in Colorado over a 2-year period (Tables 3–1 and 3–2) remains unexplained.[588]

A simultaneous outbreak of Guillain-Barré syndrome in children and Bell's palsy in adults, with serologic evidence of recent cytomegalovirus (CMV) infection, has been reported in Hawaii.[587] One small Japanese series of 12 patients seen in 4 months included a disproportionate 10 patients with ophthalmoplegia.[592]

Seasonal Variation

Most population- or hospital-based studies have not shown a seasonal variation in the incidence of GBS. Notable exceptions included a 10-year epidemiologic study in New York and New Jersey[289] that found an increase during the 4 months of August through November. Seasonal clustering has also been reported during the autumn and winter months in Norway and Denmark,[673,973] associated with more upper respiratory infections and other antecedent illness during these months. Similar findings have been reported in a study from the Mayo Clinic[1278] and in Beijing.[1313]

No seasonal variation existed in our retrospective or prospective series, nor was there a difference in the proportion of patients who reported respiratory infections during each season (Table 3–3, 3–4 and Fig. 3–3).

Table 3–3 SEASONAL INCIDENCE

Season	MGH Retrospective	MGH Prospective
Spring	48 (29%)	31 (26%)
Summer	39 (23%)	24 (20%)
Autumn	41 (24%)	28 (23%)
Winter	41 (24%)	37 (31%)
Total number of patients	169	120

Table 3–4 RELATION OF SEASON AND UPPER RESPIRATORY INFECTION*

Season	Upper Respiratory Infection	
	Present	Absent
Spring	20 (34%)	11 (66%)
Summer	9 (16%)	15 (84%)
Autumn	12 (21%)	16 (79%)
Winter	17 (29%)	20 (71%)
Total patients	58	62

*MGH Prospective Series (number of patients).

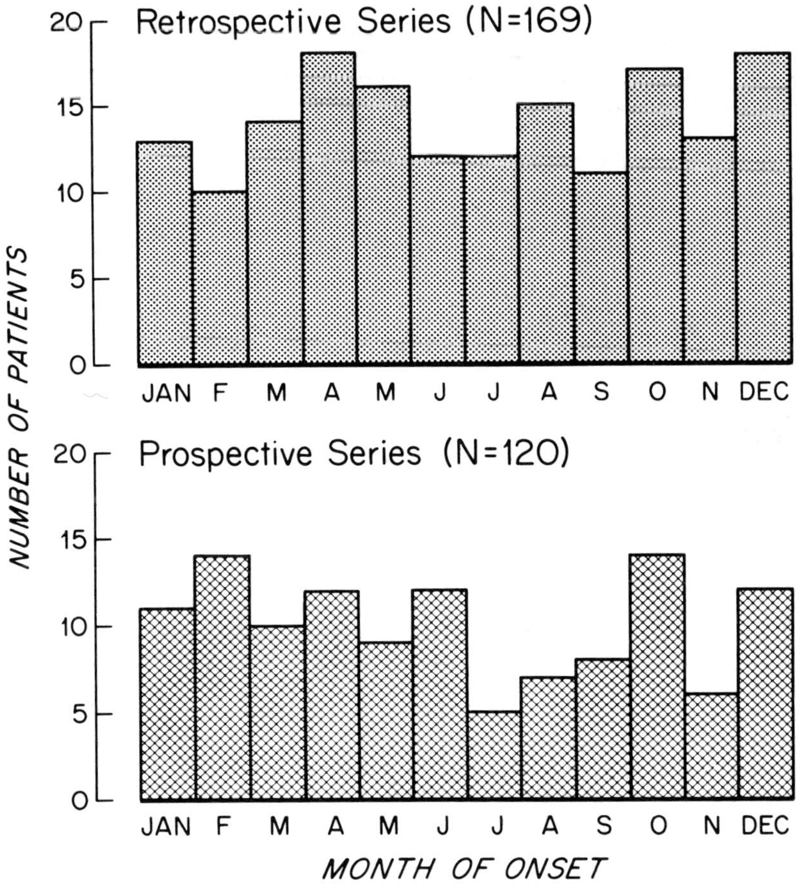

Figure 3–3. Monthly incidences of the onset of GBS in the MGH retrospective (*top*) and prospective (*bottom*) series.

Occupational Distribution

A few studies have retrospectively investigated the relationship between occupation and GBS. Ravn[973] compared occupations in his GBS patients with those in the population of Copenhagen but could not identify differences in distribution. No clustering among professions was found in the Mayo Clinic's Olmstead County population.[606] Two physicians, two dentists, and a veterinarian with GBS were among the population of 142 GBS patients admitted to the MGH between 1979 and 1988. In addition, however, three patients in the prospective study were hospital nurses, and we have seen two other nurses who had GBS. At least three of the five nurses had CMV infections with abnormal liver function test results. This may represent an occupational risk owing to the ubiquitous hazard of exposure to CMV and similar viruses that appear preferentially to precede GBS.

HLA Association

Genetic factors may influence susceptibility to GBS but there is no clear relationship between GBS and human leukocyte antigen (HLA). Mexican patients with GBS had an increased incidence of HLA-D3,[422] and Egyptian patients with GBS had increased frequencies of HLA-A3 and HLA-B8 compared with control subjects.[475] In larger United States studies, however, GBS patients have not differed in antigen frequencies at the HLA-A, -B, or -C loci compared with healthy control subjects.[4,5,593,678,1153] The results of a United Kingdom study[1287] were similar, except for a weak relationship between HLA-DR2 and severity of disease. One study[771] found a significant association between the protease inhibitor type M3 allele and GBS, as well as with chronic inflammatory demyelinating polyneuropathy (CIDP) and multiple sclerosis—all connections of uncertain significance.

THE "SWINE FLU"—GBS ISSUE

The "outbreak" of GBS associated with swine flu inoculation still generates a lively debate among neurologists and neuroepidemiologists.[658,944] In 1976, a national influenza immunization program sponsored by the United States government was intended to vaccinate a large part of the adult population with a vaccine manufactured against a 1976 New Jersey influenza A isolate (A/NJ-76). President Gerald Ford publicly advocated that "every man, woman and child" be vaccinated. The press premonitorily labeled the coming influenza outbreak as "killer flu," although its severity was ultimately less than anticipated. Two clusters of GBS and several individual case reports among 45 million vaccinated patients led to the program's suspension. The original *American Journal of Epidemiology* article[1072] purportedly showed a considerably higher risk of GBS in the vaccinated population than in the unvaccinated population for the 5 weeks after vaccination. In a surveillance program, more than 1100 cases of GBS were reported to the CDC by local health officers, of which all but two (excluded because more than 160 white blood cells (WBC) per mm^3 were found in the CSF) were "certified" by the CDC as valid GBS. The incidence time curve for 532 vaccinated cases showed an increase in GBS during the 6 to 8 weeks after vaccination, peaking in the third week, compared with level incidences in 543 unvaccinated cases. The relative risk of acquiring GBS after vaccination, approximately 1 case per 100,000 doses, led to a calculated relative risk ratio of 8.8 over the general population. A follow-up surveillance program failed to demonstrate any residual or ongoing risk of GBS after vaccination and even suggested a decreased risk of GBS in vaccinees from 1978 to 1981.[589] The data from a surveillance program cosponsored by the Centers for Disease Control and the American Academy of Neurology were reported sequentially in three papers[552,589,1072] mentioned earlier.

Other studies in Ohio[749] and Michigan[138] tentatively confirmed the association between this particular vaccine and GBS. Neurologic complications such as encephalopathy,[399] optic neuritis,[103] and myelitis,[1271] which had been reported with previous influenza vaccines, did not occur more frequently with A/NJ-76. One case of brainstem encephalitis, however, has followed swine flu inoculation.[190]

Concern about the validity of the initial results led to re-examination of the original data by a panel of experts consisting of two epidemiologists, a microbiologist, and a neurologist.[672] The relative risk was recomputed after 25% of the original data were discarded because essential clinical facts were missing in 3%, patients were under 18 years old (only two of whom had been vaccinated) in 11%, or there were insufficient or conflicting data after review in another 11%. The main conclusion, an association between A/NJ-76 vaccine and GBS, still could not be refuted. However, only patients with paresis of all extremities, the trunk, and/or cranial innervated muscles with respiratory "impairment" (coded as "extensive" cases) had an incubation curve consistent with a causal relationship to the vaccine (Fig. 3–4). "Limited" cases, defined as patients with only limb weakness, did not show such a relationship (Fig. 3–4). The estimated relative risk of acquiring "extensive" GBS ranged

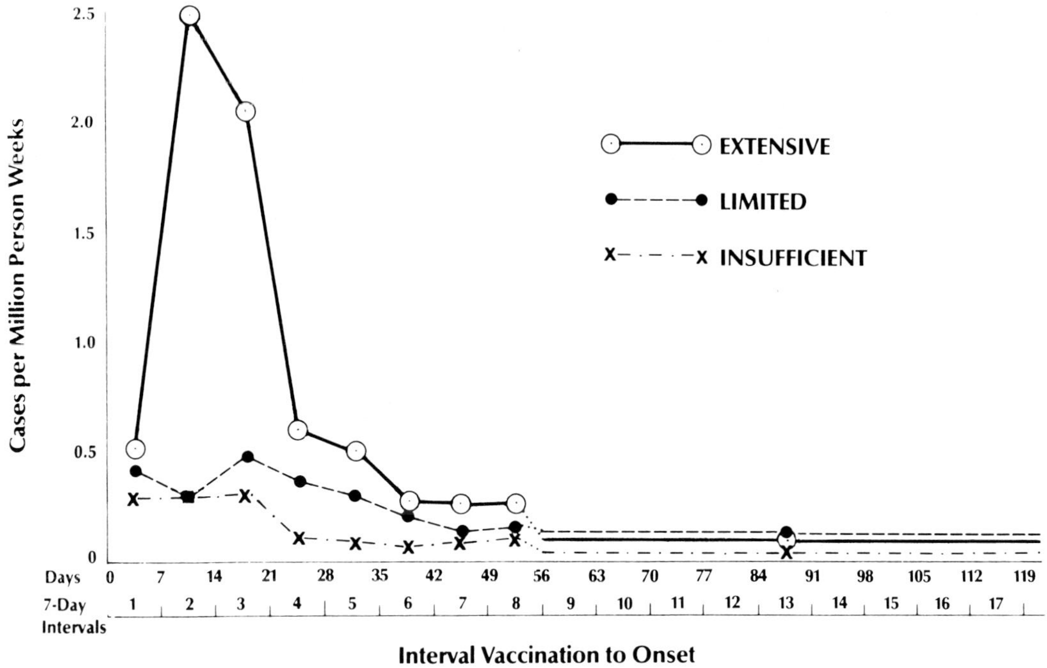

Figure 3–4. Epidemiologic evidence, with an incubation curve, for a causal relationship between the swine flu vaccination and only "extensive" (severe) cases of GBS. (From Langmuir et al.,[672] p. 855, with permission.)

from 4 to 8, depending on assumptions about baseline rates. The apparent duration of risk after vaccination was extended to 6 to 8 weeks in this paper.[672]

A further review of the situation was encouraged, perhaps generated by the number of legal suits against the United States government and by the impatience of responsible neurologists with some of the information used for litigation. The most important flaws in the original study after the first panel review were summarized by Dr. Kurland, one of the panel members:[658] medical and neurologic records were often unavailable for review, data were collected indirectly by health officers without clearly established criteria for diagnosis, unilateral limb weakness was present in approximately 8% of the cases, and definite lower motor signs were absent in many patients. All these inconsistencies, however, were approximately evenly distributed between vaccinated and unvaccinated patients. One source of bias that could not be excluded was the likelihood that the vaccinated group sought earlier attention and therefore may have been more likely to receive a diagnosis of GBS if a history of vaccination was given.

The evidence for an association may rest on deficient data, but the conclusion remains that there was an approximately five-fold increase in adult GBS associated with the A/NJ-76 vaccine. The risk was not increased, however, in the more than 1 million vaccinees under age 18 (Kurland, personal communication).

These findings contrast with an absence of an association in a large United States Army survey[568] with better data collection than the surveillance studies that included the period of swine flu vaccine use in the Armed Forces. Despite larger antigenic vaccine doses than used in civilians, no increase in the incidence of GBS was found among 1.7 million service personnel. A retrospective surveillance study in the Netherlands,[1298] with fewer cases than in the United States, also failed to support the association. Only one patient with GBS had received the vaccine during the epoch retrospective study and two in the prospective series had received it a decade earlier. No other influenza vaccine has been associated with GBS, but a recent study has suggested an increased incidence with a polio vaccination program (see Chapter 6).[619]

FAMILIAL GBS

There is no evidence that GBS is communicable (one of the most common questions asked by patients' families). In one report,[1056] two siblings developed GBS 4 years apart, each when they were approximately 70 years old. Both had bloody diarrhea and lumbar pain radiating to the buttocks, and each made a good recovery. One of the siblings, however, had a protracted course with wasting, somewhat uncommon in GBS. A 56-year-old man and his 24-year-old daughter had dissimilar courses of GBS 2 years apart.[737] Two patients in the MGH prospective series had first-order relatives (father and sister, respectively) with GBS many years previously. GBS in twins has not been recorded. Only one of our patients had a first-order relative with multiple sclerosis or other inflammatory nervous system disease.

OTHER POTENTIAL RISK FACTORS

A case-control study[594] sought possible risk factors for GBS, particularly in patients who contracted the disease after swine flu vaccination. In the small number sampled, previous vaccinations (including influenza vaccination) and a history of allergic itching, hives, or skin rash were less common in GBS patients. In a prospective study in the United Kingdom that specifically surveyed antecedent events,[1289] intrinsic risk factors such as these could not be identified.

Part II

NEUROBIOLOGIC BASIS OF GUILLAIN-BARRÉ SYNDROME

Chapter 4

PATHOLOGY

The history of the pathology of GBS, outlined in Chapter 1, has evolved through three stages. The first was a distinction between peripheral neuropathy and spinal cord disease in the 1860s through the 1880s. This was followed by an appreciation that GBS (then still "Landry's paralysis") was definitely a neuropathy.[1068] The third stage was the comprehension that it was primarily an inflammatory, demyelinating process.[52,650] The landmark light-microscopic study was performed by Asbury and colleagues[52] and complemented by electron-microscopic descriptions.[173,955] These studies have established the role of lymphocytes and macrophages in the destruction of peripheral myelin. Most of the details of the light-microscopic pathology described here are taken from seven recent Massachusetts General Hospital (MGH) autopsy cases; from Asbury and co-workers' article;[52] and from several older references.[12,501,650,917,1079] The insights gained from the pathology and immunology of EAN are discussed more fully in Chapter 5. The pathology of GBS should be considered in light of recent evidence that an IgM autoantibody may precipitate the inflammatory reaction, also discussed in Chapter 5.

THE INFLAMMATORY REACTION

There is no consistent macroscopic pathologic change in the nerves of patients who have had GBS. Arnason[40] has commented that he had not seen the gross (or microscopic) edema that was reported in earlier work. The main microscopic feature consists of inflammatory infiltrates with mononuclear and adjacent segmental demyelination. The cellular infiltrates consist mainly of small and medium-sized lymphocytes, macrophages, and a few polymorphonuclear cells early in the illness, with plasma cells and rare mast cells evident later. Some of the larger lymphocyte progeny are probably macrophages that play a role in myelin damage. More severely affected areas may have relatively more polymorphonuclear cells. The infiltrates tend to surround small endoneural vessels, particularly veins (Fig. 4–1), but clusters of cells may be seen apparently unassociated with vessels. Inflamed areas may surround small veins in all, or virtually all, cases. Some sheets of inflammatory cells are large enough to have a periphery quite distant from any vessel, but it is difficult to follow the full extent of a collection of lymphocytes without serial sectioning. In a few cases the infiltrates occur in separate sheets, with cells intercalated between fibers in a fascicle. Inflammatory lesions in roots do not surround epineural vessels, since these nerves lack an epineurium. Vesicular demyelination, appreciated by electron microscopy as discussed farther on, may represent a type of noncellular humorally mediated damage, possibly important in the genesis of neurologic signs and electrophysiologic abnormalities. Even in these cases, however, there is often cellular reaction near vessels.

Acute inflammatory lesions are seen within several days of the onset of symptoms. The earliest studied case[52] was autopsied less than 24 hours from

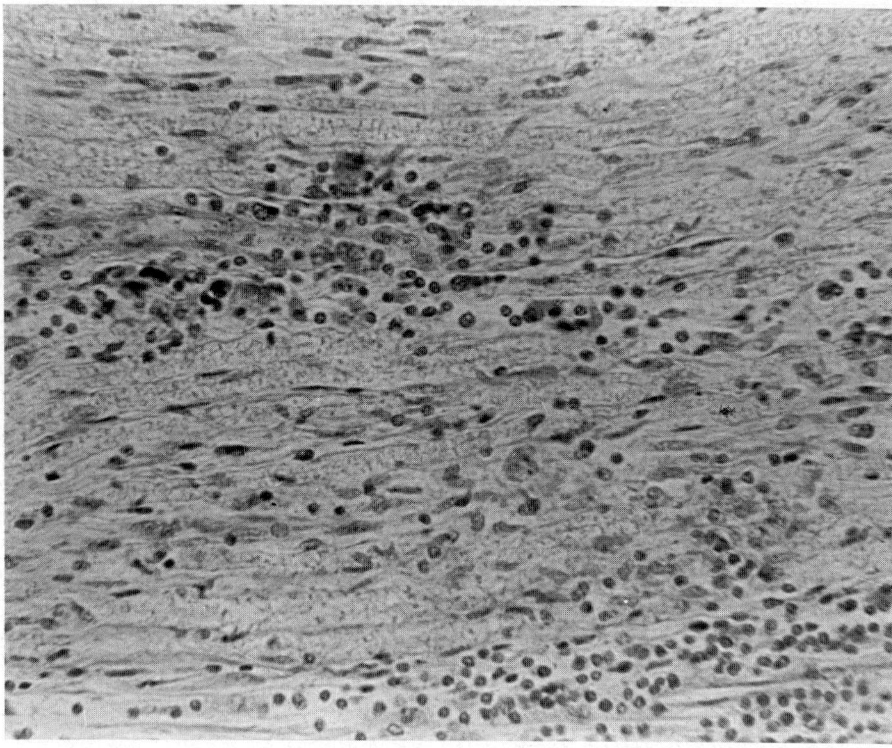

Figure 4–1. Median nerve from a case of fatal GBS showing the archetypal scattered collections of small lymphocytes with adjacent demyelination (*center*) and perivascular collections of lymphocytes (*lower right*). [Hematoxylin and eosin (H and E).]

the apparent (but uncertain) onset of symptoms. Clinically better documented cases have shown well-established inflammation 3 to 6 days after the onset of symptoms. Between 1 week and approximately 1 month after onset, depending on the severity of illness, inflammation becomes more widespread and often more severe. Plasma cells, though still rare, are more evident within inflammatory clusters. An interesting feature in cases of several weeks' duration has been the juxtaposition of acute evolving areas of inflammation with older lesions in other nerves, or rarely in adjacent areas of the same nerve.[52] Macrophages, which play an important part in myelin destruction, become prominent after the first several days and increase in number over the following 2 or 3 weeks. Small scattered foci of inflammation may be seen in the meninges adjacent to inflamed roots, perhaps explaining the small number of cells seen in the spinal fluid of some cases (see Chapter 12), but meningitis is not a component of the typical disease. When GBS is associated with human immunodeficiency virus (HIV) infection, Lyme disease, or mononucleosis, the meningitis seems independent of intraneural infiltrates. There is little information regarding the differences in inflammatory nerve reaction in cases of "symptomatic" GBS, such as the demyelinating neuropathy of systemic lupus or sarcoid, where epithelioid giant cells can appear in the nerve.

Cellular infiltrates seem identical in all cases of carefully examined postmortem material. Despite the general acceptance of perivenular inflammation as the core pathologic feature of GBS, this is probably not the only cause of peripheral nerve damage. Some cases seem to have disproportionately little inflammation for the extent of clinical

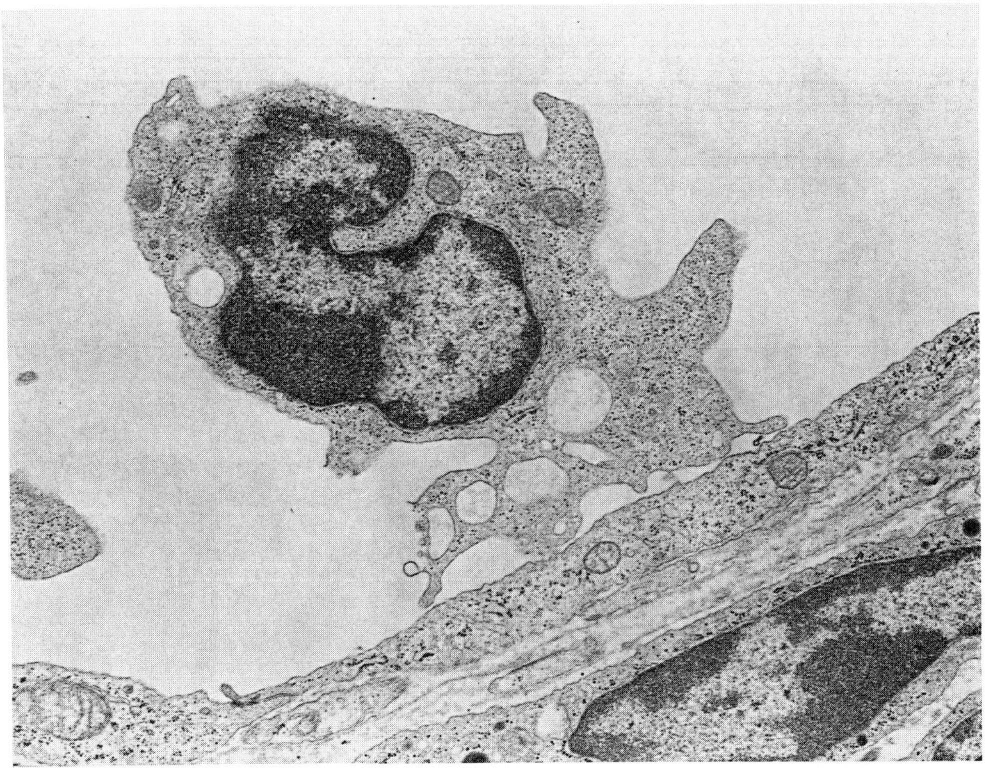

Figure 4–2. Electron micrograph of a lymphocyte process applied to the endothelial surface of an endoneural vessel, presumably just prior to entering the nerve.

or electrophysiologic findings. As alluded to earlier, limited sampling and long illness before autopsy may give the misleading impression of much nerve damage with limited or no inflammation. For this reason, few conclusions about the pathoanatomy of GBS can be drawn from nerve biopsies (see later).

The role and origin of activated lymphocytes in the demyelinative lesion remain unsettled. One view is that the macrophages are derived from monocytes or histiocytes as a response to myelin destruction, rather than causing it. Lymphocytes sensitized to peripheral myelin, after passing through endothelial cells surrounding venules, may elaborate antibodies that damage surrounding myelin and attract other cells. The role of capillary and venule endothelial cells is also unclear, but they probably participate in bringing sensitized lymphocytes to the nerve and reinforcing the local inflammatory reaction (see Chapter 5). Electron microscopy of areas with active inflammation in experimental autoimmune neuritis (EAN) and GBS may show lymphocytes attached to the endothelial surface of capillaries or venules (Fig. 4–2) (see farther on).

Scattered inflammatory infiltrates have been found[524,586,1038] infrequently in liver, heart, kidney, and other organs. Some of these cases were undoubtedly residua of preceding primary viral infections, but others may represent a more wide spread inflammatory reaction, occasionally with clinical manifestations as discussed in Chapter 11.

DISTRIBUTION OF INFLAMMATORY LESIONS

The loci of the inflammatory process in the peripheral nervous system have been a matter of confusion and debate, largely because their variable distribution requires extensive sampling to appreciate. The prevailing idea after Haymaker and Kernohan's series,[501] that spinal roots were maximally affected, was discounted by more comprehensive sampling.[52] While spinal roots were involved in most cases, they were the site of maximum inflammation in only a few.

Contiguous infiltrates may extend from the roots into the proximal spinal nerves, where the most severe inflammation is found in some cases. The plexuses and peripheral nerves are more often heterogeneously involved. Within a nerve, a single fascicle may have an inflammatory lesion while a neighboring one at the same level is spared. Infiltrates may be scattered anywhere along the extent of a nerve trunk, including in terminal myelinated muscular twigs. Instances of predominantly anterior or posterior radicular inflammation have occurred, rarely isolated to one or the other root at several levels. The existence of pure motor and virtually pure sensory syndromes, however, makes it likely that a fairly homogenous radicular pathologic localization exists (see Chapter 8).

The axial distribution of lesions also varies, with some cases showing differential involvement of adjacent spinal roots. There have been cases with preferential areas of involvement, probably explaining some of the functional and regional variants of the disease described in Chapter 8. For example, a case has been reported[253] with predominantly sensory features that showed extensive inflammation of posterior roots and nerve trunks, sparing ventral roots. There are, however, only a few careful clinicopathologic correlations of this type in GBS. The distribution of demyelinative lesions has been carefully analyzed[586] in a case that simulated "axonal GBS" with little inflammation and predominantly small myelinated fiber damage. The most proximal roots and the transition zone between peripheral and central myelin escaped damage, while changes occurred abruptly several millimeters beyond the transition zone. This case, however, was probably not representative of the more typical inflammatory pathology of GBS.

All the cranial nerves (except I and II) may be involved, occasionally as the most severely affected sites. The facial nerve in the temporal bone in a patient with facial myokymia, 17 days after onset, had swelling and multifocal disruption of myelin with myelin in macrophages, perhaps due to wallerian degeneration, but no inflammation.[1227] The pathology in Fisher's syndrome or cases of GBS with severe ophthalmoplegia[104,258,455] has been generally the same as in typical cases, with inflammatory infiltrates in the third, fourth, and sixth and peripheral nerves, and secondary chromatolytic change in cranial motor neuron cells. There has not been a systematic pathologic study of the eighth nerve (there are rare cases of acquired deafness). Such a study would be interesting because the transition from central to peripheral myelin outside the brainstem might show cessation of inflammation at the junction. Two of our cases had no demyelination or inflammation in the small portion of the acoustic nerve sampled. Sensory ganglia may be involved with inflammation (Fig. 4–3), at times simulating the pathologic appearance of the "sensory neuronopathy" that is usually associated with a systemic neoplasm.

The sympathetic nervous system may also contain typical inflammatory lesions in GBS. An unusual case[524] of a child who died approximately 3 weeks after the onset of severe dysautonomia and a GBS-like illness showed virtual elimination of dorsal root ganglion cells without inflammation. The celiac ganglion and vagal trunk were normal. Others[52,763] have found scattered inflammatory lesions in sympathetic and parasympathetic nerves and ganglia in patients with dysautonomia, usually with the ganglia less severely involved than somatic nerves and roots. Profound autonomic nerve inflammation

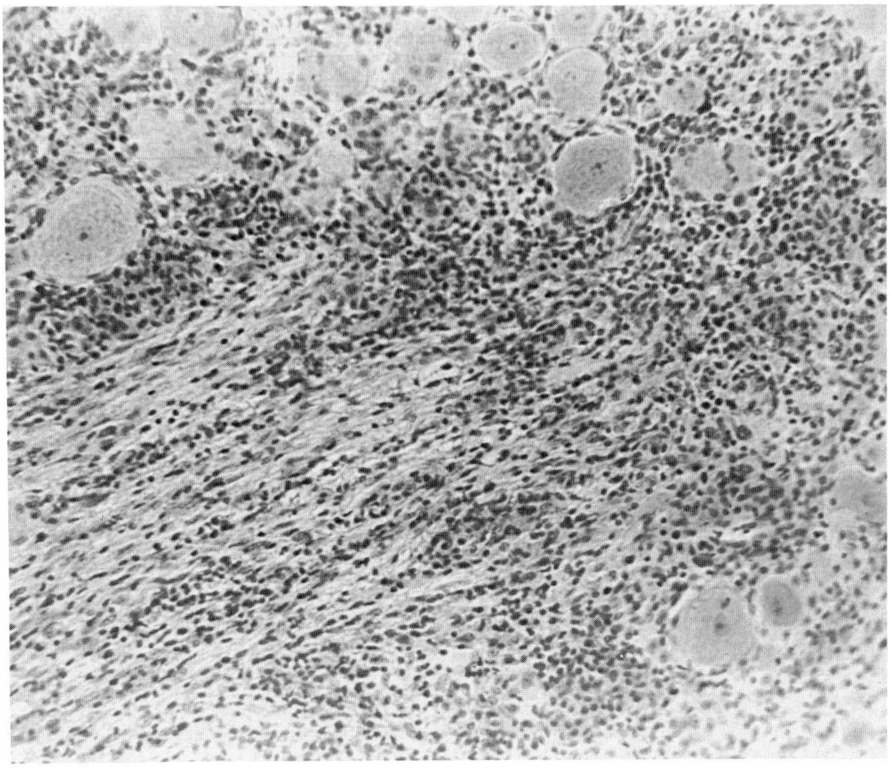

Figure 4–3. Sheets of lymphocytes in a posterior root ganglion in a fatal case of GBS. The myelin of exiting fibers (*lower left*) is damaged, but the cell bodies are spared. (H and E.)

has been reported[354] in a patient with sudden cardiac death.

Typical inflammatory lesions in autonomic nerves have been described in EAN by several investigators.[34,35,584] Sympathetic ganglia tended to be less involved than parasympathetic structures, and both were less involved than somatic ganglia and nerves.[584] Several authors[35,343] have made some clinicopathologic correlations in a virtually pure form of autonomic inflammatory neuropathy that is discussed more extensively in Chapter 8. A patient with noninflammatory demyelination in the vagus[586] died of an apparent autonomic catastrophe.

DEMYELINATION AND AXONAL LESIONS

The proximate cause of electrical conduction block and nerve dysfunction in GBS is likely to be the segmental demyelination that is regularly found adjacent to regions of inflammation. This is one of the strongest arguments for the primacy of lymphocytes in the pathogenesis of the disease. Myelin, rather than the Schwann cell, appears to be the target of the human immune response in GBS, as discussed in Chapter 5. This may be contrasted with an experimental neuropathy caused by an immune response to galactocerebroside in which Schwann cell necrosis results in secondary demyelination. In EAN, nodal retraction of myelin appears to be the earliest change, followed by myelin breakdown from the detached edge of the myelin loops. Macrophage processes separate myelin lamellae and ingest the detached membrane. The destruction of myelin then progresses toward the centrally located Schwann cell nucleus. Myelin breakdown, ovoid formation, and macrophages with ingested myelin debris become evident with light microscopy after several days.

"Vesicular" myelin change, discussed later, may be another mechanism of segmental demyelination. It apparently does not require the proximity of inflammatory cells. Cylinders of whole myelin, several lamellae thick, appear to be detached at interperiod lines and are ingested whole by macrophages. Other insights into the pathologic mechanisms of myelin destruction, derived mainly from electron microscopy, are discussed subsequently.

In all but the most intensely inflamed areas of nerve, axons stripped of myelin are themselves spared. Axons totally denuded of myelin have appeared within intact Schwann cell basement membranes. Secondary axonal damage does occur in severe cases, thought to be an "innocent bystander" effect of intense inflammation. Axonal section probably accounts for many instances of limited recovery, muscle atrophy, and electrophysiologic findings of denervation. There is no evidence for primary axonal destruction in GBS, but such a process is possible, perhaps on a similar basis to some of the paraproteinemic large-fiber axonal neuropathies. The clinical and electrophysiologic syndrome corresponding to widespread axonal lesions in GBS currently has not been studied extensively enough to determine if this is a specific attack on axons or the extreme of exudative reaction in nerve. Wallerian degeneration is found in many cases of GBS, presumably all distal to axonal section.

LATE LESIONS AND REPARATIVE PROCESSES

Older lesions show Schwann cell proliferation in areas of demyelination that is maximal in the second or third week. The new cells tend to be smaller than normal and their appearance probably precedes remyelination of a segment between nodes.[52,501] Each new segment of myelin is replaced by several shorter and thinner lengths that are the processes of new Schwann cells. There may also be secondary changes in axon diameter with demyelination. An intriguing finding in more mature cases, months after the onset of illness, has been residual inflammation, even in patients who have recovered clinically. Reactivation of these lesions has been offered as a possible explanation for chronic or relapsing inflammatory polyneuropathy (see Chapter 10).

LESIONS OF THE CENTRAL NERVOUS SYSTEM

Secondary chromatolysis of spinal or cranial motor nuclei is seen only in severe cases, rarely with microglial clusters surrounding degenerating neuronal bodies. The posterior columns may show degeneration due to cell loss in dorsal root ganglia or to destruction of axons in the posterior roots. The only primary lesions of the central nervous system have been rare clusters of perivascular lymphocytes in the brain or cord in otherwise clinically typical cases of GBS (Fig. 4–4). An ataxic case,[985] examined pathologically years after the acute illness, showed degeneration in Clarke's column that is difficult to explain as a direct result of sensory ganglion or root damage. No symptomatic or clinically important central lesions have been found in GBS, but, following the likely clinicopathologic correlations that exist for other features of GBS, Babinski signs, fleeting truncal sensory levels, or perhaps some "central" eye signs or optic neuritis may result from isolated focal inflammation in the central neuraxis.[1003] As a rule, however, it is probably best to consider GBS entirely a peripheral nervous disease. (See Chapter 8 for discussion of putative CNS lesions in Fisher syndrome and other forms of GBS.)

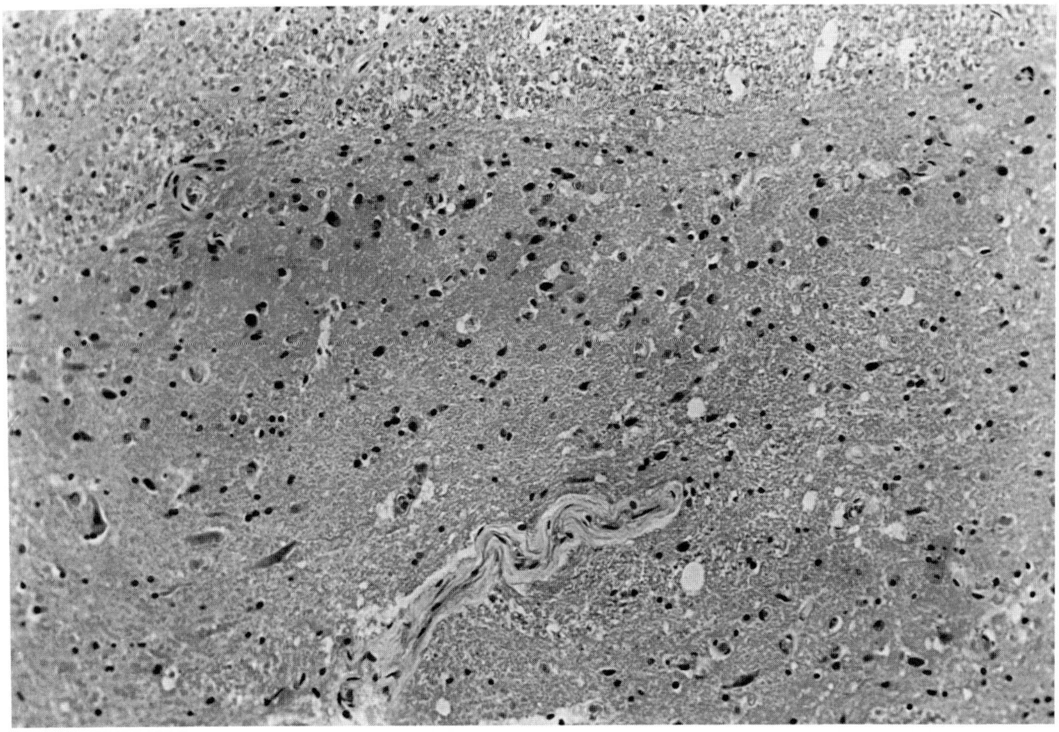

Figure 4–4. Rare clusters of small lymphocytes in the spinal cord of a fatal GBS case. (H and E.)

NERVE AND MUSCLE BIOPSY

Results of sural nerve biopsies are normal or show only minimal demyelination in most cases of GBS.[50,490,711,814] In the MGH prospective series, 4 of 7 patients with sural nerve biopsies had abnormalities, usually patchy demyelination with scant inflammation. If sural nerve potentials were normal, the results of the biopsy were normal as well. Teased fiber analysis has shown a variety of abnormal patterns, usually segmental demyelination. There is too little experience with motor fascicular biopsy to comment on its diagnostic usefulness in complex or pure motor cases.

Muscles show some degree of denervation and reinnervation in proportion to axonal disruption. The traditional notion that demyelination alone cannot cause denervation changes, or at least electrophysiologic evidence of denervation, has not been systematically tested in GBS. Fibrillations occur in many cases of GBS without subsequent atrophy. Small collections of inflammatory cells in muscle have been reported, apparently unassociated with inflammation in terminal nerve branches. The frequent early elevation of serum creatine phosphokinase (CPK) concentration has no obvious pathologic counterpart, except perhaps for this minor muscle inflammation. A case that has been cited in support of a primary muscle lesion in GBS did not have typical clinical features and the peripheral nerves were not examined pathologically.[497]

ELECTRON MICROSCOPIC FEATURES

Electron microscopy has illuminated the role of macrophages as the vehicle of a specific type of inflammatory myelin destruction.

Myelin Damage

Macrophages typically insinuate themselves between the basement membrane surrounding myelin lamellae and the outermost myelin sheath and peel the myelin off, (Fig. 4–5) similar to the way a roll of paper unravels from a cardboard tube. Cytoplasmic processes of the macrophage subsequently penetrate further along minor dense lines or through gaps in the sheath created by prior elevation.

Vesicular disruption of myelin is a second type of demyelinating lesion in GBS and EAN, initially attributed to postmortem autolytic degeneration, but seen also in biopsy specimens.[136,955,956] Vesiculation of myelin occurs by separation of whole segments of adjacent lamellae at major dense lines[136,173,956] (Fig. 4–6). The cylindrical vesicles, which may contain intact myelin, detach from adjacent normal myelin and are ingested virtually whole by phagocytes. The mechanisms of myelin destruction by organelle free macrophage pseudopods, or by freestanding vesicular detachment, are unknown. The initial descriptions did not make it clear

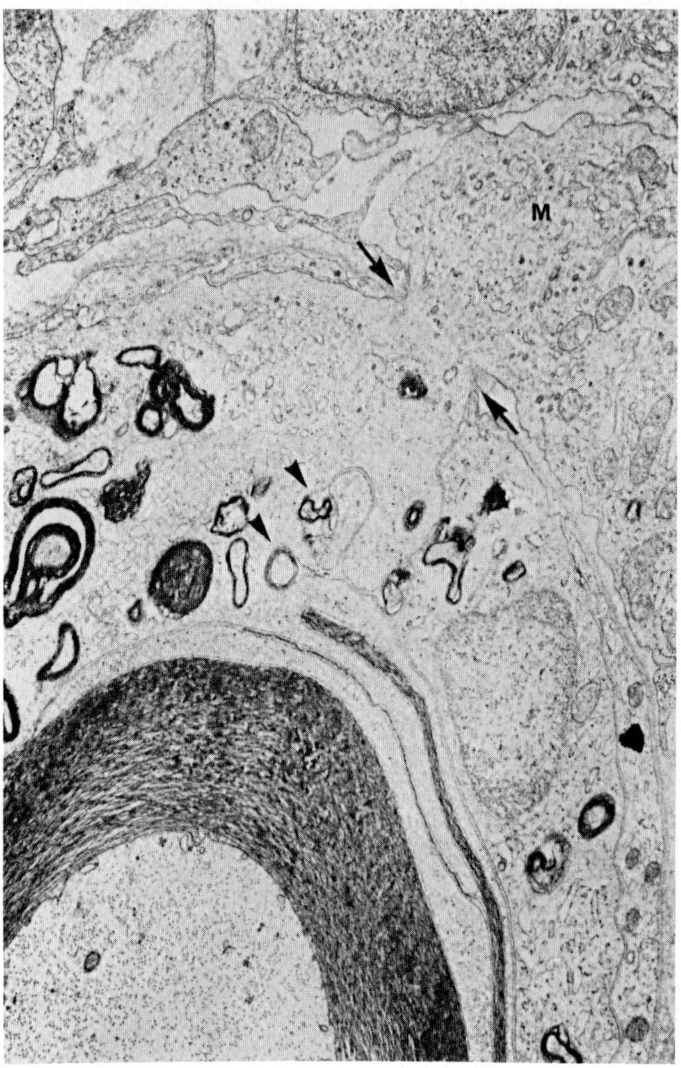

Figure 4–5. Macrophage (M) process insinuating itself through a gap in the basement membrane of a myelin sheath (*arrows*), and stripping the outer lamellae. Myelin that has undergone phagocytosis is shown by arrowheads. (From Prineas,[956] p. 10, with permission.)

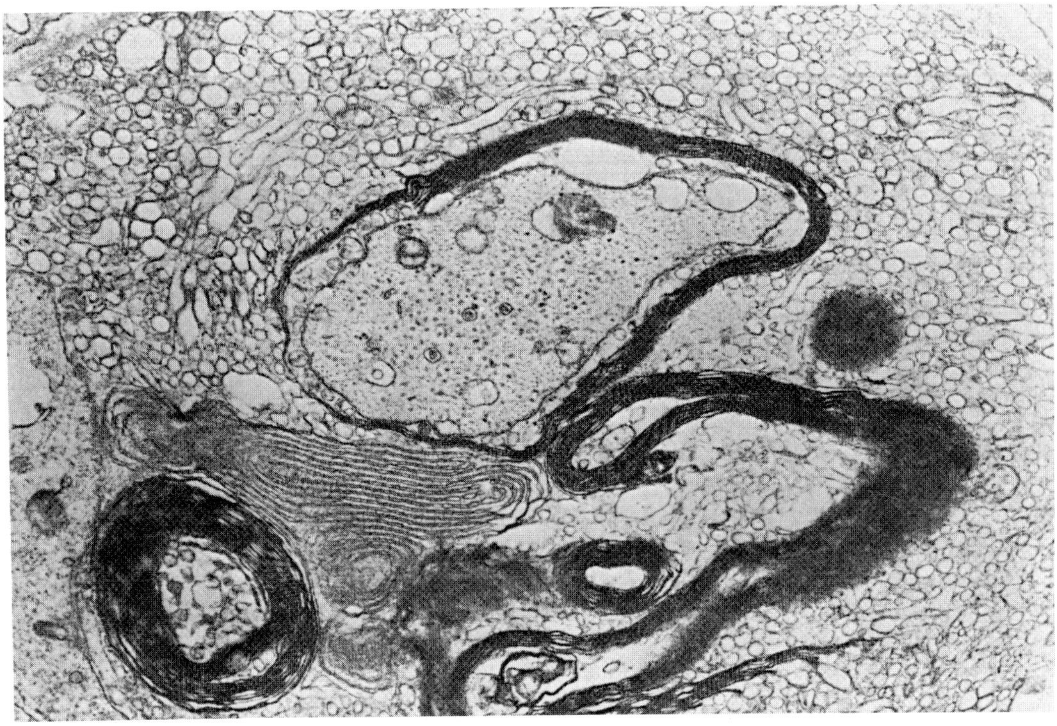

Figure 4–6. Vesicular demyelination in the superficial peroneal nerve of a patient with acute GBS and diabetes. The many small rounded structures and the skein of elongated material are apparently forms of noninflammatory myelin destruction seen in GBS as well as in other forms of neuropathy. (From Vital et al.,[1237] p. 838, with permission.)

(and it is still not entirely clarified) whether vesicular change requires the participation of lymphocytes.[1293]

Cross-sections of nerve may also show infrequent areas with sheaves of uncompacted or separated lamellae that maintain continuity. Noninflammatory myelin disruption, particularly uncompacted myelin, are more typical of chronic inflammatory demyelinating polyneuropathy (CIDP) and paraproteinemic neuropathies, although it seems to occur in the so-called acute axonal form of GBS.[586]

Vesicular demyelination occupies a provocative but somewhat uncertain position in our understanding of the clinical symptoms and electrophysiologic abnormalities in GBS. Several laboratories have demonstrated that sera from GBS patients produce in vivo noninflammatory demyelination of rat sciatic nerve.* The important observation is that early serum-induced segmental demyelination may be vesicular with secondary myelin ingestion, rather than by lymphocytic infiltration and direct macrophage-induced destruction. Several authors[151,1047,1163] have postulated that serum-induced demyelination contributes to the pathogenesis of early GBS and EAN, perhaps at sites of damaged blood-nerve barrier. If so, vesicular change could be a pathologic substrate of many symptoms and signs in GBS, in particular, weakness that results from conduction block across demyelinated segments as early as 30 minutes after intraneural injection of GBS serum (see Chapter 12).

One problem with attributing important features of GBS to vesicular demye-

*See references 151, 350, 488, 1047, and 1163.

lination is its infrequency in pathologic material. One researcher[955] found it in 2 of 9 biopsies, and another,[136] in only 8 of 65 biopsies and in less than 1% of myelinated fibers. The late sampling in these series, however, may have skewed the pathologic appearance. Another discrepancy between the pathologic and electrophysiologic findings may be that the smallest myelinated fibers are blocked earliest. Vesicular demyelination is not unique to GBS and has been reported with diphtheria, lead intoxication, and irradiation injury. Prominent vesicular demyelination has also been reported[1237] in a nerve biopsy specimen taken from a diabetic patient with GBS. Phagocytes, evident in GBS and EAN but not in these other conditions, have been thought necessary for the initial vesicular breakdown.[173] The implication is that inflammatory cells or their progenitors may still somehow be involved in the noninflammatory demyelination.

Viral Particles

Only scant evidence favors viral particles within nerves or Schwann cells in typical GBS;[107] most electron microscopic studies have specifically failed to detect them. Reports of cytomegalovirus (CMV) inclusions in Schwann cells contained within areas of severe inflammation in two patients with acquired immunodeficiency syndrome (AIDS) must be interpreted cautiously because Cowdry type A inclusions were present in virtually all tissue sampled,[107,824] and AIDS has been associated with CMV inclusions in nerve in the absence of peripheral neuropathy.[456]

Chapter 5

IMMUNOLOGY

Since the early 1960s research has focused on the cellular immune response in GBS, based mainly on compelling pathologic findings and on the transfer of experimental allergic neuritis (EAN) with sensitized lymphocytes. The presence of antibodies to whole nerve antigens was, until recently, considered secondary to myelin damage. Attention has recently shifted to the role of the humoral immune system in GBS because of the presence of circulating antibodies to several elements of myelin, favorable experience with plasma exchange, and the production of experimental conduction block and demyelination by serum from patients with GBS. In all likelihood, both the cellular and the humoral elements of the immune system interact and participate in myelin damage. This chapter reviews the most pertinent aspects of research in this field.

ANIMAL DISEASES THAT SIMULATE GBS

Three naturally occurring animal diseases simulate GBS to varying degrees and offer some immunologic and pathologic insights into the human disease: coonhound paralysis of dogs, Marek's disease of chickens, and cauda equina neuritis of horses. None, except possibly coonhound paralysis, is close enough to GBS clinically or pathologically to make it a naturally occurring animal equivalent of the human disease.

Coonhound Paralysis

An acute polyneuritis in dogs with clinical, cerebrospinal fluid (CSF), and electrophysiologic features of GBS has been reported, possibly representing a naturally occurring acute inflammatory polyneuropathy.[862] Kingma and Catcott[618] described coonhound paralysis, a different acute polyradiculoneuritis in hunting dogs that were exposed to raccoons. Experimental allergic neuritis has also been produced in dogs, but the pathologic features, more similar to those of GBS, have also been more severe and widespread than in coonhound paralysis.[529]

The characteristic clinical features of coonhound paralysis are hind limb weakness that ascends to produce flaccid quadriplegia, jaw droop, loss of tendon reflexes, and in some animals, respiratory failure. The bark becomes weak or changes in quality, but the dog remains alert and afebrile. Weakness improves after 3 to 8 weeks. A raccoon bite or scratch typically precedes the neurologic syndrome by 7 to 21 days. Several members of a hunting pack may be bitten but only one, or a few, may develop acute polyneuritis, and there is a tendency for geographic clusters.[233,525,530] Up to 5% relapse with subsequent exposures to raccoons. CSF protein values are usually elevated and electrophysiologic features are similar to those of GBS, except perhaps for more frequent denervation.[234]

Light microscopic examination of nerve has demonstrated segmental demyelination adjacent to focal perivascular mononuclear inflammatory infiltrates and small aggregates of plasma cells, in most ways identical to GBS. Lumbar and sacral nerve roots are commonly affected, with more profound changes in the ventral than in the posterior roots.[234,529] One electron microscopic (EM) study has suggested that axonal damage is more severe in this condition than in GBS.[234] In some areas of nerve, edema and myelin splitting have preceded macrophage infiltration,[234] similar to galactocerebroside-induced demyelination.[1044,1046,1048]

Marek's Disease

Marek's disease, an inflammatory paralytic disorder of chickens caused by a herpesvirus, has limited similarity to GBS but may offer some insights into pathogenesis. Lesions are generally restricted to the peripheral nervous system, but may be found in the uveal tract, brain, and other viscera.[743] Clinical signs in chickens occur in less than half of affected birds 5 to 6 weeks after exposure to Marek's disease virus. Infected chickens have progressive drooping of their wings and an abnormal gait, and ultimately die. The illness can spread to other birds and become endemic.

Two major types of EM abnormalities have been described: macrophages stripping normal myelin after the appearance of invading mononuclear cells, or total destruction of axons and myelin surrounded by massive lymphoblastic infiltrates that simulate neoplastic infiltration.[958] Viral capsids can be demonstrated in peripheral nerves, root ganglia, and lymphocytes.[1150]

Marek's disease probably results from direct infection of nerve by a group B herpesvirus.[197] It is unlikely that a similar process causes GBS in human cytomegalovirus (CMV), Ebstein-Barr virus (EBV), or human immunodeficiency virus (HIV) infection because the pathologic details differ and virus particles are not seen in EM studies of GBS nerve (wth a few rare and sporadic exceptions) (see Chapter 4). Marek's disease, however, resembles GBS immunologically and may offer insights into viral-induced T-cell myelin damage. T cells are believed to cause demyelination because ablating the bursa of Fabricius, the main source of B cells, does not alter the disease.[903] Serum IgG antibodies against myelin have been demonstrated by an indirect immunofluorescence test 5 to 7 weeks after Marek's infection, but this is probably too late to represent a primary humoral response.[1150]

Cauda Equina Neuritis of Horses

This disease is characterized by a subacute polyneuritis of sacral and coccygeal nerves. It occurs predominantly in continental Europe. The clinical picture includes sphincter paralysis, perianal hyperesthesia, hind leg flaccidity, and occasional cranial nerve involvement—particularly ptosis, drooping of the lower lip, and atrophy of the masseter and temporal muscles.[441,752]

Inflammatory and demyelinating lesions are most prominent in the cauda equina, but abnormalities may be found in the trigeminal, facial, and acoustic-vestibular nerves. Nerves show swelling of myelin sheaths, large infiltrates of mononuclear cells, and, following myelin destruction, fibrous thickening of the epineurium separating nerve fibers. Trauma and previous respiratory infections have been suggested as potential causes of the neuritis, but numerous attempts to isolate bacteria or viruses have been unsuccessful. Significant titers of serum antibodies against bovine P2 have been demonstrated in four horses with cranial nerve deficits.[579]

These animal models demonstrate several potential mechanisms of demyelination: direct attack on or viral destruction of Schwann's cells, humoral or cellular myelin damage, or an allergic response with perivascular inflammatory lesions that simulate acute GBS. Models may be exploited to understand inflammatory demyelination, but none precisely reflects the immunopathology of GBS.

EXPERIMENTAL ALLERGIC NEURITIS (EAN)

Waksman and Adams' landmark experiment[1244] created the first animal model of a noninfectious inflammatory neuritis, experimental allergic neuritis. Allergic (or autoimmune) neuritis was produced by injecting rabbit nerve or ganglia, and Freund's adjuvant, intradermally into a rabbit's footpads. Approximately 2 weeks after inoculation, rabbits became clumsy, had difficulty hopping and righting, and eventually became quadriplegic. Respiratory failure occurred in advanced stages. Animals reached their maximum neurologic disability within 3 days, usually followed by recovery. The CSF protein concentration has usually been elevated without cells in all EAN models, but normal CSF protein, as well as marked pleocytosis, has occurred. EAN is species specific, as shown by the ability of bovine P2, but not rabbit P2, to induce EAN in rats.[238,578,1168] There are also species differences in clinical presentation.

In the original model, inflammatory lesions were located predominantly in dorsal roots, spinal ganglia, and peripheral nerves. Cellular infiltrates were occasionally found in muscle, liver, and myocardium but not in the central nervous system.[1244] The sequence of pathologic events during the first week has been elucidated further by several groups.[56,478,664,950,1244] Electron microscopy 12 to 16 days after inoculation shows mononuclear cells attached to or between endothelial cells, followed by migration of lymphocytes to myelin and separation of myelin from adjacent axon cylinders. Demyelination, starting with "bubbly" dissolution of the outer lamella, has been observed only in the presence of mononuclear cell infiltrates. The mechanism of this type of myelin damage has not been clarified.[644] The "bubbles" are bounded by pieces of major dense lines of myelin. After dissolution of myelin lamellae, macrophages remove the myelin debris or remaining intact myelin sheets. Axonal damage may be seen in severe cases, but Schwann cells remain intact. Others[950] have emphasized additional features of early endoneural edema and degranulation of mast cells. This raises the provocative possibilty that mast cells may be involved in demyelination because their proteases damage myelin in vitro.[569] Degranulating mast cells are found in EAN sciatic nerve,[146] and local secretion of vasoactive amines may recruit T cells and open the blood-nerve barrier to inflammatory cells.[478]

Myelin Antigens in EAN

The target of activated T cells in EAN is still uncertain. Most studies have implicated one of the basic myelin proteins, P2, as the most important antigen in EAN, but P0, another major peripheral myelin protein, can induce EAN as well.

P2 is located predominantly in the area of Schmidt-Lanterman clefts, although some investigators have found it more widely distributed in myelin; it does not appear on axons.[1198] There may be neuritogenic fragments of P2 that can be derived by cleavage of bovine P2 protein, in particular residue 66 (leu) – 78 (arg).[1212,1269] A synthetic peptide, SP26 (corresponding to amino acids 53 through 78) of bovine P2 protein, and a cyanogen bromide–derived peptide from the P2 protein, CiT4, are also capable of causing extensive root and sciatic nerve demyelination when used to elicit EAN.[1028]

Experimental allergic neuritis is probably exclusively (or at least predominantly) a cell-mediated disease, since it can be passively transferred to naive rats by lymphocytes from sensitized animals. It cannot be induced in T cell–depleted rats.[149] Furthermore, the number of T cells in sciatic nerves has been tentatively correlated with the appearance and disappearance of clinical deficits in EAN.[1157]

Effects of Immunosuppression in EAN

Immunomodulation of the cell-mediated response in EAN has been studied in great detail (Table 5–1). Many studies elucidate the mechanisms of EAN, but few can be extrapolated to GBS. Some early work suggested that previous exposure to peripheral nerve antigens protected against the development of EAN.[148,235,684] Suppression or amelioration of EAN has been reported,[617] by means of prophylactic or later 12- to 21-day administration of cyclosporin A, an agent that inhibits T-cell response by interfering with macrophage activators and T-cell growth factors. Several studies[32,450,496] have also reported a reduction in the severity of EAN after plasma exchange, similar to the experience in GBS. Benefit was demonstrated after membrane plasma exchange with removal of 50% to 60% of circulating antimyelin IgG and IgM antibodies, but there was a rapid rebound to preexchange antibody levels.[496] This may correspond to the clinical response and limited relapse seen in approximately 10% of GBS patients who receive plasma exchanges (see Chapter 15). A number of other manipulations have been shown to effect the expression of EAN, including depletion of complement, alpha prostaglandin administration, interleukin-2 receptor blockade, and various macrophage inhibitors.

Table 5–1 EFFECT OF IMMUNOMODULATORS IN EAN

Author, Year	*Agent*	*Possible Mechanism*	*Effect on EAN Given before/after Expression*
Lehrich and Arnason,[684] 1971 Cunningham et al.,[235] 1983 Brosnan et al.,[148] 1984	Nerve-saline suspension	Anti-idiotypic antibodies	+/NS
Antony et al.,[32] 1981 Gross et al.,[450] 1983 Harvey et al.,[496] 1988	Plasma exchange	Elimination of IgM or other serum factor?	NS/+
King et al.,[617] 1983	Cyclosporin A	Inhibition of T-helper cells	+/+
Craggs et al.,[228] 1984 Hartung et al.,[493] 1988	Silica	Inactivation of macrophages	+/NS
Brosnan and Tansey,[147] 1984 Seeldrayers et al.,[1080] 1988	Reserpine Nedocromil	Inhibition of degranulation of mast cells	+/NS
Holmdahl et al.,[528] 1985 Strigard et al.,[1158] 1988	Monoclonal anti–T cell antibodies	Blocking of T-cell subsets (CD 4, CD 8, Anti Ia)	+/− or W
King et al.,[616] 1985	Corticosteroids	Reduce capacity of APC;* inhibit IL-1 release; interfere with arachidonic acid metabolism	+/+
Feasby et al.,[349] 1987	Cobravenom	Complement depletion	+/NS
Hartung et al.,[493] 1988 Hartung et al.,[494] 1988	Oxygen radical scavengers	Inactivation of hydrolytic enzymes of macrophages	+/+
	Indomethacin	Cyclo-oxygenase inhibitor	+/+
	Monoclonal antibodies to IL-2 receptor of T cell and to gamma interferon	Blockade of T-cell antigen expression	+/NS
		Reduction of T-cell growth and macrophage deactivation	+/+

*APC = antigen presenting cell; IL = Interleukin; NS = Not studied; W = Worsening clinical expression; + = Blocks or enhances recovery; − = No effect.

There are conflicting reports on the effects of corticosteroids on EAN. Prednisolone, 1 mg/kg per day, did not cause improvement in guinea pigs, but in rats, disease severity and recovery were slightly improved.[616] High-dose dexamethasone, 4 mg/kg twice daily, has recently been demonstrated to block the clinicopathologic manifestations of EAN in rats.[493] The influence of corticosteroids on macrophages is still not completely understood, but inhibition of interleukin-2 production,[491] as well as interference with macrophage arachidonic acid metabolism by blocking phospholipase A, have been suggested as ameliorating mechanisms.[493]

The appearance of mast cells in sural nerve biopsy specimens of GBS patients[867] and degranulating mast cells in EAN[950] (as mentioned previously) have prompted some investigators to study the amines contained in these cells. Reserpine delayed the onset of EAN in one experiment,[147] similar to results achieved by the administration of a sodium chromoglycate derivate that depletes histamine.[1080]

Monoclonal antibodies directed against T-helper cell antigens[1158] and an antibody against the beta chain of the T-cell interleukin-2 receptor have protected animals against EAN.[491] An effect could not be demonstrated when these antibodies were given after the onset of EAN. One type of monoclonal anti–T cell antibody (OX19) paradoxically exaggerated EAN when administered after inoculation.[1158] Monoclonal antibodies to gamma interferon (a lymphokine necessary for the activation of macrophages, migration of lymphocytes and perhaps increase in vascular permeability) result in markedly less demyelination.[492]

The studies just described suggest that the T cell–mediated myelin damage in EAN is subject to modulation at several levels. Most, however, require pretreatment or intervention very early in the disease (which evolves more rapidly than GBS), making clinical application difficult.

GALACTOCEREBROSIDE-INDUCED DEMYELINATION

Saida and co-workers induced demyelination by intramuscular injection of bovine brain galactocerebroside and Freund's adjuvant in rabbits.[1046] The clinical features are similar to EAN: rabbits lose weight and have an ataxic gait, postural tremor of the limbs, and predominantly distal limb weakness, eventually progressing to quadriplegia. The signs usually remit within a few months.[1155] A related model has been produced by direct intraneural injection of rabbit antigalactocerebroside (anti-GC) in rat sciatic nerves, thus bypassing the in vivo sensitization and induction of antibody. The EM features of this type of neuropathy are summarized in Table 5–2. The most promi-

Table 5–2 ELECTRON MICROSCOPIC SEQUENCE; INJECTION OF RABBIT ANTI-GALACTOCEREBROSIDE SERUM INTO RAT SCIATIC NERVES*

Time After Injection	*EM Findings*
20 min	Schwann's cells with plasma outfoldings and swollen mitochondria and dilated endoplasmic reticulum
1–5 hr	Irregular, swollen, split myelin fibers and vesiculation of outer and inner myelin lamellae; numerous polymorphonuclear cells within endoneurium
8 hr	Extensive myelin vesiculation; some macrophages, *not attached to myelin*
15 hr–3 days	Pronounced subneural, perineural, and endoneural edema, large mononuclear cells and macrophages, *attached to demyelinated fibers*
After 5 days	Most fibers completely demyelinated, asssociated with debris-filled macrophages

*Adapted from Saida et al.,[1044] p. 103–104.

Table 5–3 OBSERVATIONS SUPPORTING CELL- AND ANTIBODY-MEDIATED RESPONSES

Cell-Mediated Response	*Antibody-Mediated Response*
MHC class II antigen expression on Schwann cells	Demyelination by GBS serum injected endoneurally and in tissue culture
Suppressor T-cell decrease relative to T-helper cells	Circulating IgM antibodies closely related to disease activity
Myelin destruction in tissue culture by elements of buffy coat lymphocytes from GBS patients	Complement complexes in serum and CSF
Macrophage inhibitory factor generation after lymphocyte exposure to P2	Complement and immunoglobulin deposits on nerve
Macrophage stripping of normal myelin	

nent findings are early myelin splitting and vesiculation, followed by macrophage infiltration and peeling of disrupted myelin. Perivenular lymphocytes are not prominent at any stage of the disease.[1044,1046,1048,1155] The demyelinating activity of anti-GC serum is complement-dependent, as it is lost after heating. (The potential but controversial role of vesicular demyelination seen in this model is discussed in Chapter 4.)

Galactocerebroside models of demyelination are most interesting as contrasts to the T cell–mediated damage in EAN. They demonstrate that virtually identical demyelination to EAN and GBS can be produced by purely antibody-mediated, noninflammatory damage. The primary target of antigalactocerebroside damage may, however, be the Schwann cell rather than the myelin sheath.

IMMUNE MECHANISMS IN GBS

The presumed immunopathologic mechanisms of GBS are based on the following observations: (1) ultrastructual studies demonstrate perivascular inflammatory cells and macrophages within normal myelin sheaths in GBS and EAN; (2) there are circulating and nerve-bound IgM antibodies to myelin antigens; and (3) demyelination is caused by intraneural injection of EAN and GBS sera or by antigalactocerebroside antibody. The relative contribution of cellular and humoral demyelination remains uncertain, but the predominant evidence still favors a primarily T-cellular mechanism.[495a] There are many links between the humoral and cellular immune systems that need further clarification, leaving open the possibility that a primarily antibody-mediated form of GBS exists (Table 5–3) or that antibodies contribute to myelin damage or dysfunction.

Cell-Mediated Immune Response

IN VITRO STUDIES

Most studies of T-cell transformation after antigen exposure have been concerned with the peripheral nerve target antigens in GBS. The reported responses of lymphocytes from GBS patients to P2 (or its neuritogenic fragment P66–78) have been conflicting. In several earlier studies,[3,90,237,785,873] lymphocytes transformed to P2 (or one of its fragments) only during the progressive phase of acute GBS. The best work to date, however, has shown circulating activated T-cells in patients with acute GBS, as demonstrated by expression of several key receptors on peripheral blood T-cells and by increased serum concentrations of interleukin-2 and its soluble receptor.[495a] Some studies,[544,554,1316] however, have failed to corroborate the findings of lymphocyte transformation to a P2 challenge. One study[1094] found that lymphocytes from

26 of 34 GBS patients inhibited macrophage migration when exposed to peripheral nerve antigens.[89] This inhibiting activity was no longer present months later. Others,[178] however, found persistent leukocyte activity after exposure to antigens several years after GBS. Macrophage inhibition, however, has also been demonstrated to a lesser degree in patients with stroke, suggesting that it may be a secondary event resulting from nervous tissue damage.[997] A specific cell-mediated response to P2, that was not present in healthy subjects or patients with other neuropathies, has been found in the majority of GBS patients tested in one study.[397] Serum antibodies to P2, however, were similar in the GBS patients and controls. Cell-mediated responses to rat trigeminal ganglion cultures have been examined.[42] Buffy coat lymphocytes, but not sera, from 7 of 9 GBS patients destroyed myelin in culture. Since humans and rats are not major histocompatibility (MHC) matched (see farther on), an alternative interpretation of these findings is that the destruction resulted from natural killer cells or antibodies secreted by B lymphocytes. In summary, T cells from patients with GBS appear to be sensitized to the P2 antigen, but the specificity of this response and its relation to myelin destruction are unclear.

The role of MHC antigens in GBS has been studied in nerve biopsy specimens from two GBS patients. MHC class II antigens, essential for T cell–antigen recognition and induction of the immune response, are expressed by endothelial, perineural, and Schwann cells in GBS.[935] The specificity of this finding was recently challenged in a brief report[811] showing no differences in class II antigen expression between patients with chronic inflammatory demyelinating polyneuropathy (CIDP) and those with other noninflammatory neuropathies. Most evidence suggests that the myelin, rather than the Schwann cell, is the immunologic target in GBS. The appearance of MHC antigens on Schwann cells, however, raises the possibility that the antigens participate in the presentation of the antigen to T cells.

T-CELL SUBSETS

Results of T-cell subset analysis and of T-helper:T-suppressor ratio studies have been conflicting: reduced T-suppressor cells,[430] no change in ratio,[498] and variable results have all been reported. For example, one study[708] found 3 of 13 GBS patients with relatively decreased T-helper cells, 3 with relatively increased suppressor cells, and 2 with decreased suppressor cells. Decreased T-suppressor cells in the largest immunologic study[1288] were found only in the acute phase of GBS, but there was considerable overlap with controls. Depression of T-suppressor cells and an enhanced humoral response to peripheral nerve antigens has been suggested as a possible explanation of the paradoxical occurrence of GBS in immunosuppressed patients, incuding those receiving steroids[291,433,707,1147] (see Chapter 3). Patients have developed GBS when high-dose methylprednisolone, used for severe asthma or other immunologic diseases, has been tapered.

Antibody-Mediated Immune Response

Humoral demyelinating factors have been demonstrated in GBS by various techniques but their primary role in GBS remains uncertain.

DEMYELINATION AND CONDUCTION BLOCK BY ENDONEURAL INJECTION

The findings of conduction block (see Chapter 15) and demyelination after intraneural injection of EAN sera into rat sciatic nerves[1163] has led several investigators to study the morphology and electrophysiology of rat intraneural injection with sera from GBS patients (Table 5–4). Feasby and colleagues[350]

Table 5–4 ENDONEURAL INJECTION OF GBS SERUM IN RATS

	Proportion with Histologic Verification of Demyelination	
Author, Year	***GBS Serum***	***Control Serum***
Cook and Dowling,[217] 1981	0/21	0/48
Tandon et al.,[1179] 1980*	0/11	ND
Hansen et al.,[485] 1982	5/5	0/6
Saida et al.,[1047] 1982	11/27	3/40
Feasby et al.,[350] 1982	13/17	2/30
Brown et al.,[151] 1987	5/6	0/7
Winer et al.,[1288] 1988	0/5	0/5

*Includes patients with chronic inflammatory demyelinating polyneuropathy (CIDP); ND = not done.

have demonstrated demyelination after injection of serum from all but a few of their patients. Myelin breakdown was sometimes present without apparent macrophage participation. The demyelinating factor was heat labile. Intraneural injection of lymphocytes from the same GBS patients did not produce endoneural damage. Others[488] have demonstrated conduction block in rat nerve after injection of fresh acute GBS serum, an effect that was not demonstrable after storage or injection of serum from recovered GBS patients, but demyelination was not histologically verified. Vesicular disruption of myelin without mononuclear cells or macrophages may occur after intraneural injection of GBS serum, while control sera has not produced these changes.[151,1047]

Other investigators[217,725,726,1288] have been unable to confirm that GBS serum produces demyelination or a consistent conduction block compared with controls. The absence of histologic confirmation of injection or differences in technique may explain some conflicting results, as serum-induced demyelination depends on precise needle manipulation, needle size, volume of injected serum, and the use of fresh GBS serum.[309,488]

TISSUE CULTURE DEMYELINATION

Virtually all acute sera from the GBS patients in one series[218] demyelinated mouse dorsal root ganglia and cerebellar tissue cultures. Myelinotoxic activity was complement dependent. However, similar effects occurred in tissue culture from one-third of patients with other acute neurologic disorders and from 1 of 11 normal sera. Several other studies[296,519] have confirmed these observations with tissue cultures of dorsal root ganglia, but the specificity of demyelination of tissue cultures has been appropriately challenged[1102] because complement-dependent demyelinating activity can be demonstrated from normal sera applied to mouse cerebellar cultures. Trigeminal ganglion culture experiments,[42] the interpretation of which was discussed earlier, demonstrated demyelination of cultures by lymphocytes, but not by sera, from GBS patients. No certain conclusions can be drawn from the experiments summarized here.

IMMUNE COMPLEXES

Circulating immune complexes have been infrequently identified in acute or convalescent GBS serum (Table 5–5). Only 3 of 100 GBS patients had immune complexes in a large series,[1288] all 3 with recent CMV infections. Except for two French Studies,[430,681] other smaller series have had similar low inci-

Table 5–5 INCIDENCE OF CIRCULATING IMMUNE COMPLEXES IN GBS C1q ASSAY

Author, Year	***No. Positive/ No. Tested***
Tachovsky et al.,[1176] 1976	5/11
Goust et al.,[430] 1978	15/16
Laville et al.,[681] 1981	21/27
Glikmann et al.,[411] 1980*	3/4
Winer et al.,[1288] 1988	3/100
van Doorn et al.,[1224] 1988	1/17

*CSF

dences of immune complexes. Clinical improvement after plasma exchange with a decrease in immune complex titers has been reported,[1215] but in another larger series[681] no relation was found between immune complex concentrations and plasma exchange. Most evidence favors only a minor role for immune complexes in the pathogenesis of GBS.

SERUM AUTOANTIBODIES IN GBS

The role of antineural antibodies in GBS has been reconsidered since a beneficial response to plasma exchange has been demonstrated. The often rapid response to plasma exchange in (antibody-mediated) myasthenia gravis is, however, seldom seen in GBS. Factors other than antibodies are likely to be removed by exchange, and may influence T cell–macrophage interactions at the site of inflammation (interleukin 1 and 2; gamma interferon), macrophage mediators involved in myelin breakdown (eicosanoids and oxygen-free radicals), and perhaps complement. Antibody removal from the circulation may also have an effect on T-cell responses but it is difficult to conceive that the local inflammatory process would be substantially altered by systemic removal.

Extensive work to identify the putative antigen in GBS has been inconclusive, as previously noted. Autoantibodies to a number of peripheral nerve antigens have been sought with variable success (Table 5–6). In a study of 100 consecutive GBS patients,[1288] a few had detectable antigalactocerebroside antibodies and none had antibodies against human P2, but most serum samples were taken after the acute illness. Using a modified antihuman peripheral nerve myelin complement fixation assay, Koski and co-workers, in contrast, have demonstrated markedly elevated serum IgM antibodies against peripheral nerve myelin in all 27 GBS patients tested early in their illness.[644] Patients with GBS had titers up to 40-fold higher than those of most normal individuals or patients with other peripheral nerve disorders. The antibodies detected in this assay appeared to be directed against a neutral glycolipid of peripheral nerve that cross-reacted with Forssman antigen, a common nonspecific viral and bacterial antigen.[644] In seven serially tested patients, antibody titers declined in all, becoming undetectable 3 to 4 weeks after admission.[643] IgM antibody titers corresponded well with the overall clinical course and the need for respiratory support. In support of pathogenetic IgM antibody, relapses of antibody titers have been found[1238] correlating with recurrent clinical symptoms and worsening electrophysiologic abnormalities in five patients.

Another group[887] could not completely confirm these results using less specific assays. In this study, 19 of 36 GBS patients had antibodies against peripheral nerve tissue in a mixed hemagglutination test, and 30 to 36 patients had IgM antibodies against lumbar nerve root by a complement fixation test. Another researcher[1037] found circulating IgG but not IgM antibodies, restricted to the IgG3 subclass, in 4 of 10 patients tested early in the disease.

In conclusion, some careful but preliminary work suggests that antineural IgM antibodies are present in many GBS patients early in the disease. Their inconsistent demonstration by some groups leaves their pathogenetic role unclear.

A few GBS patients have had anticardiolipin antibodies,[376,487,897] probably as nonspecific acute phase reactants. One large study[376] showed significantly elevated IgA anticardiolipin (but not IgG or IgM) antibodies in GBS, compared with control subjects. These antibodies were unrelated to antecedent infections but they may be present in normal subjects. They may be directed against myelin phospholipids.[376] Many other circulating antibodies, such as cold agglutinins, have been described inconsistently in GBS patients.[287]

Table 5–6 SERUM ANTIBODIES IN GBS

			No. Positive/No. Tested	
Author, Year	***Antigen***	***Method***	***GBS***	***Source Control or Other Neurologic Disease***
Melnick,[791] 1963	Human spinal cord	Compliment fixation	19/38	20/467
Cook et al.,[218] 1971	Dorsal root ganglion	Tissue culture	26/31	23/73
Tse et al.,[1204] 1971	Myelin, spinal cord, and PNS	Immunofluorescence	4/6	1/45
Nyland and Aarli,[866] 1978	PNS	Antiglobulin consumption	15/30	4/40
Tindall et al.,[1192] 1980	Neuroblastoma	Cytotoxicity	8/10	5/166
Latov et al.,[676] 1981	PNS	Complement fixation	3/11	6/93
Zweiman et al.,[1316] 1983	Bovine P2	ELISA	1/19	0/32
Luijten et al.,[730] 1984	Human P2	Direct plaque-forming cell assay	5/5	0/3
Hughes et al.,[544] 1984	Human myelin, rabbit myelin, galactocerebroside	Complement fixation	2/17 5/17 2/17	1/34 0/34 1/34
Epstein et al.,[332] 1987	HIV core protein	Particle agglutination assay and immunoblot	0/14	0/37
Winer et al.,[1288] 1988	Human optic nerve, human sciatic nerve galactocerebroside	Complement fixation	11/100 7/100 0/100	2/100 0/100 0/100
Frampton et al.,[376] 1988	Cardiolipin	ELISA	21/92	3/82
Palosuo et al.,[897] 1985	Cardiolipin	ELISA	4/9	4/380
Osterman et al.,[887] 1988	Lumbar nerve root	Complement fixation, mixed hemagglutination	30/36	0/50
van Doorn et al.,[1223] 1987	Sciatic nerve	Mixed hemagglutination, immunofluorescence	11/16	4/91
van Doorn et al.,[1224] 1988	Neuroblastoma cell line		20/48	7/138
Negishi et al.,[841] 1988	Bovine P2	ELISA	6/11	3/32
Ilyas et al.,[555] 1988	Gangliosides	ELISA	5/26	0/29
Koski,[642] 1988	PNM	C1 fixation and transfer	27/27	0/38
Koski et al.,[644] 1988	Forssman	C1 fixation and transfer	12/12	0/36

PNS = peripheral nerve; ELISA = enzyme-linked immunosorbent assay; PNM = polymorphonuclear leukocyte; HIV = Human immunodeficiency virus

COMPLEMENT ACTIVATION

Possible roles of complement, none definitively shown in GBS, include activation and chemotaxis of macrophages, increasing vascular permeability, and degranulation of mast cells. Complement factor C3 and the terminal activation complex, C5b9, have been found on sural nerve, bound to IgG and IgM in nerve from GBS patients.[645,729,956] Myelin can activate the classic complement pathway in vitro, potentially enhancing damage that is incited by any of the mechanisms discussed above. Although a direct role in myelin destruction has not been demonstrated,[1225] the early appearance of terminal complement complexes, mentioned earlier,[645] has been closely related to the appearance of IgM antibodies. Others[495,1054] have found activated complement C3a and C5a in CSF without a similar elevation in serum.

SUMMARY OF THE IMMUNOPATHOGENESIS OF GBS

A simplified synopsis of the possible sequence of immune damage to myelin in GBS is illustrated in Figure 5–1. The ability of cell-free preparations to produce both demyelination and conduction block in some experiments, and the variable presence of antineural antibodies in GBS, are reasons to balance the traditional view of a purely cell-mediated illness. Both arms of the immune system may participate in GBS to varying degrees, and it is unlikely that the two are separable.

A wide spectrum of triggering events has been incriminated in GBS (see Chapter 7), suggesting that the immune system may be responding to an antigen that cross-reacts with myelin. The frequent association with preceding viral infections suggests either a mainly cell-mediated response or simply the ubiquity of viral infection compared with bacterial. The pathology of GBS, T-cell perivenular inflammation, supports a cell-mediated pathogenesis. A "dual antigen" hypothesis has been suggested[1273] in which a second antigen is required, in addition to the infectious agent, to trigger the immune damage. The high incidence of wound infections in patients with postoperative GBS in our series (see Chapter 6) may support this hypothesis in a limited number of cases.

The cell-mediated response begins with presentation of a specific antigen and associated major histocompatibility complex antigens. Recent preliminary work has shown that Schwann cells are capable of expressing MHC class II molecules in GBS, suggesting that Schwann cells may act as antigen-presenting cells for the T-cell response.[935] T cells will not proliferate or activate macrophages without these antigens ("MHC restriction"). Macro-

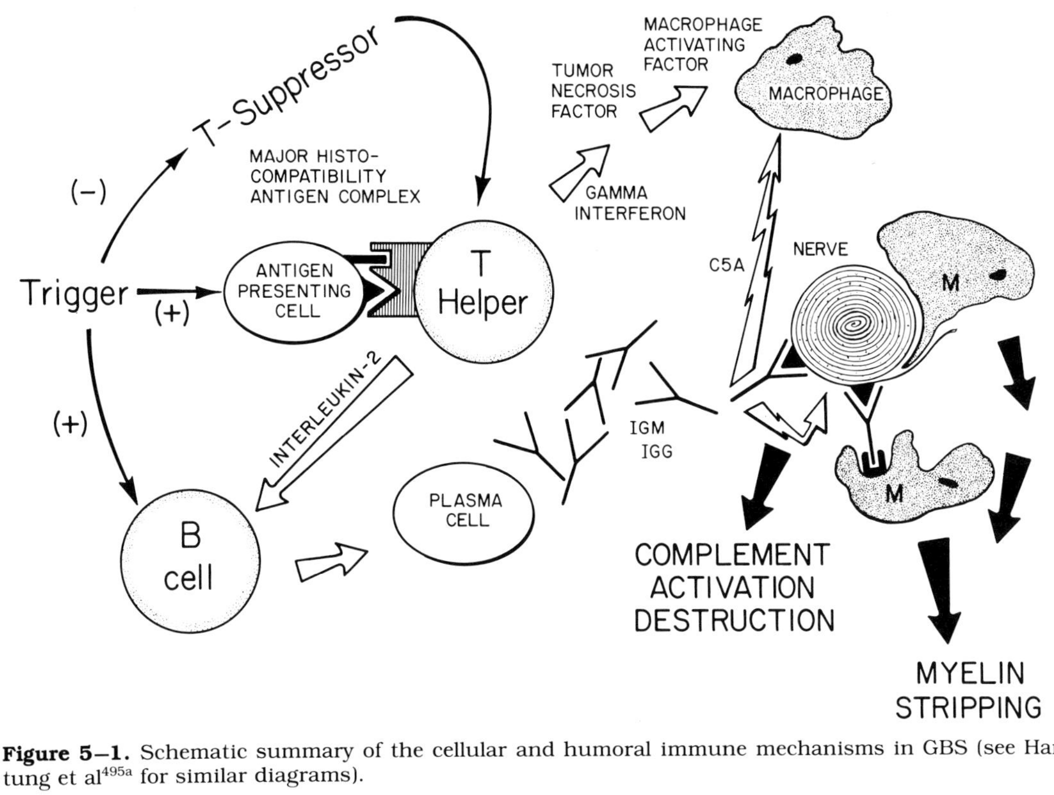

Figure 5–1. Schematic summary of the cellular and humoral immune mechanisms in GBS (see Hartung et al[495a] for similar diagrams).

phages are probably also involved both in initiation of responses as antigen-presenting cells and in the effector phase as myelin destructive cells. They may be activated by a number of lymphokines (macrophage activating factor, gamma interferon). For example, a recent report[1082] suggested that "tumor necrosis factor" could demyelinate mouse spinal cord.

B cells, although not essential in cell-mediated responses, may also be stimulated by activated T-helper cells (through interleukin 2), resulting in antibody-producing plasma cells that are scattered within GBS inflammatory lesions. Antibodies may participate directly in myelin destruction or activate the complement cascade, which in turn attracts macrophages (through C3a and C5a) or causes damage directly. This series of interactions may be enhanced by the decrease of T-suppressor cells found in the acute stage of GBS in some patients.[1288]

A parallel humoral mechanism with a primary IgM antibody response seems likely. Damage to the blood-nerve barrier allows large molecules such as IgM and C1, which do not normally penetrate the barrier, to cause or activate demyelination. One appeal of the finding of IgN directed against a glycolipid of PMNs that cross reacts with ubiquitous Forssman antigen, is the ability to explain GBS after a wide variety of inciting events. The observations of vesicular disruption in studies with endoneural injection of GBS serum, and the ability to induce EAN with galactocerebroside, tentatively support this idea.[151] In an antibody-induced model of GBS, macrophages later remove myelin, probably in part by their ability to recognize Fc and C3b receptors.

Factors that mute the immune response or abort the inflammation in GBS and EAN are not understood. Anti-idiotypic antibodies (antibodies directed against the variable portion of the antibody) could limit the damage or turn off the immune response to make GBS a self-limited illness.[732] This is tentatively supported by the cessation of disease with gammaglobulin infusion in some patients. A recent study[731] could not demonstrate anti-idiotypic antibodies against P2 antibodies in the sera of GBS patients, but this may not be relevant because P2 is not a surface determinant and therefore may not be involved in demyelination.

In conclusion, many of the mechanisms of antigen presentation and of demyelination have not yet been clarified. The mechanisms that open the blood-nerve barrier are particularly interesting because large IgM antibodies, present very early in GBS, do not normally cross this barrier. This may also be the explanation for the absence of neonatal GBS, since IgM, in contrast to IgG, does not cross the placenta. Characterizing the initial humoral response, B- and T-cell interactions, and in particular identifying the neural antigens, will allow a better understanding of the immune triggers in GBS and may lead to new therapies.

Part III

CLINICAL FEATURES OF GUILLAIN-BARRÉ SYNDROME

Chapter 6

ANTECEDENT AND ASSOCIATED ILLNESS

Viral Infections
Bacterial Infections
Vaccination
Symptomatic GBS
Endocrine Disorders
GBS and Pregnancy
Surgery and Spinal Epidural Anesthesia
Uncertain Associations

Acute illnesses are associated with or occur soon before GBS in approximately two-thirds of patients. The interval between the prior illness and the onset of first symptoms of GBS is generally 1 to 3 weeks; some cases have a longer interval, but the relation to GBS after 5 or 6 weeks becomes problematic. In the "swine flu" surveillance studies, in which the index event (vaccination) and onset of illness were well documented, "incubation" curves suggested that the latency could be as long as 6 to 8 weeks, with a peak during the third week (see Chapter 3). There was an average interval of 11 days (range 3 to 36 days) between a reported preceding event and the onset of symptoms of GBS in our retrospective series.

A remarkable diversity of infectious agents, usually viral in nature, has been described preceding an episode of GBS. Most cases in large series follow a mundane upper respiratory infection, presumably viral, that has often been difficult to characterize further. Published reports concerning preceding illnesses have been anecdotal; a few have been case-control studies and even fewer, cohort studies. An extensive retrospective survey of 1100 cases of GBS from 1949 to 1966,[686] listed more than 700 possible associations; however, many were probably fortuitous, diagnosed by laboratory tests only, and in other cases the neurologic disease was probably not GBS. Nevertheless, this survey is the only one of its size.

Herpes group viruses have been the most frequently identified preceding pathogen,[286] but serologic studies[583] (unconfirmed and not comparable to the herpes studies) have suggested that *Campylobacter jejuni* may be almost as common. An association between GBS and the human immunodeficiency virus (HIV) is also being recognized increasingly. The MGH experience with preceding acute illness is summarized in Figure 6–1.

VIRAL INFECTIONS

Influenza

A panoply of mundane viral infections, usually with upper respiratory symptoms, have appeared in case reports of GBS.[40,100,1001] Several agents have been reported more frequently, partly because they are serologically identifiable, particularly if systematic serologic testing was performed during brief epochs. For example, during the pandemic of influenza in the fall of 1957, sporadic cases of GBS occurred in South Wales owing to the Asian strain of type A influenza virus; serology confirmed a recent infection in two patients with fatal outcome.[1272] Type A, B, or C influenza was identified as frequently in GBS patients as in control subjects in another serologic study (6 of 29 GBS and 239 of 1817 controls), lead-

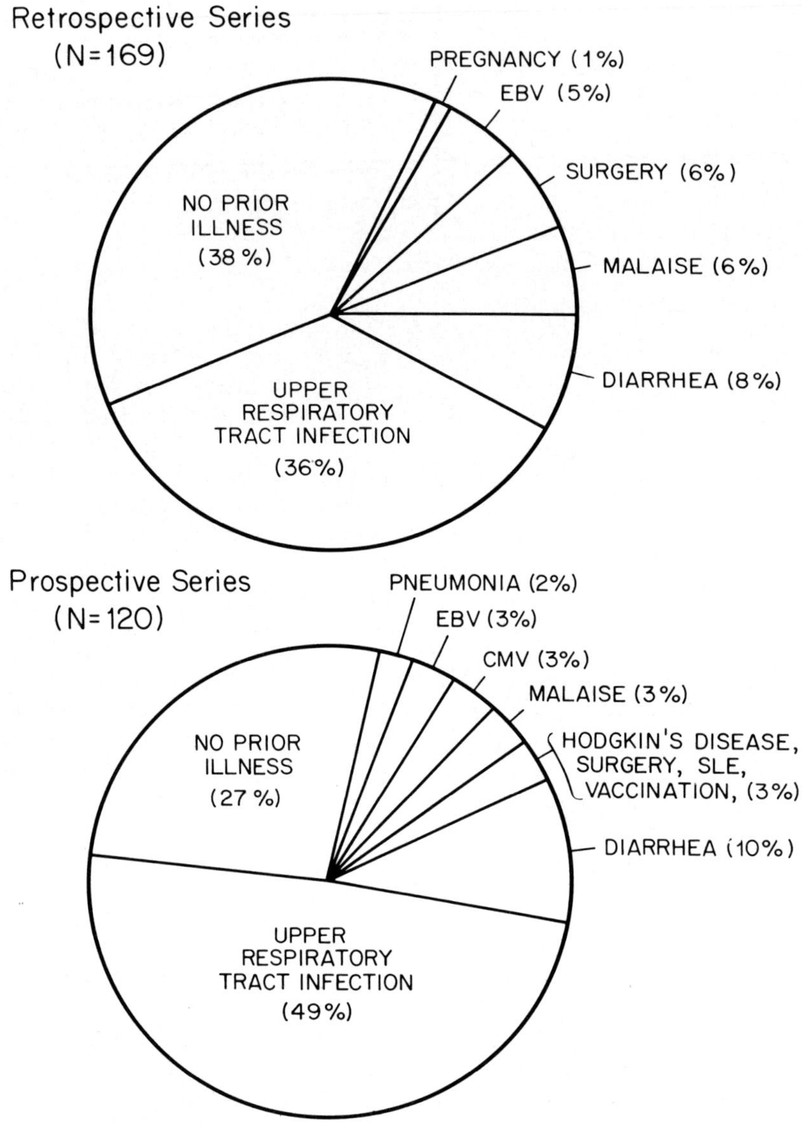

Figure 6–1. Relative frequencies of antecedent illnesses in MGH retrospective (*top*) and prospective series (*bottom*). In the retrospective series the large number lacking a clear prior illness may reflect the way in which data were collected.

ing one group[792] to conclude that influenza virus infection played no special role in precipitating GBS. Other viruses (eg, coxsackie virus, parainfluenza virus) have been identified serologically in relation to GBS (see farther on), but their prevalence in any series and in the general population was probably similar.[324,559,1211,1272]

Herpes Virus

A "glandular fever" or mononucleosis syndrome caused by cytomegalovirus (CMV) or Epstein-Barr virus (EBV) has been described preceding GBS in numerous case reports, and a special, frequent association between GBS and serologic evidence of infection has been shown.* The clinical features of the preceding illness caused by EBV and CMV have been similar: an upper respiratory tract infection, pharyngitis, headache, and, less often, gastrointestinal complaints. One study[286,288] found 15% of 220 GBS patients had high titers of IgM antibodies against CMV antigen in tissue culture, often without a mononucleosis syndrome, whereas none of 40 control sera had high titers. CMV was isolated from urine in some patients. There was a correlation between CMV titers and the course of acute GBS, in that elevated titers occurred persistently in severe and protracted cases and rapidly declining titers occurred in more benign cases. Half of these patients had atypical lymphocytes, immunoblasts, cold agglutinins, and liver enzyme abnormalities. In the MGH experience, GBS has occurred slightly less frequently after EBV than after CMV infection, and health care workers with GBS after CMV have often had asymptomatic abnormalities of liver function.

Infectious mononucleosis has been considered a mild disease with a few neurologic complications, but severe and sometimes fatal GBS is well known as a sequelae.[988] No cases of typical GBS were found in a retrospective series of 109 hospitalized patients with mononucleosis,[395] whereas encephalomyelitis, mononeuritis, or lymphocytic meningitis occurred in 7%. After an episode of severe headache, one patient developed bilateral ophthalmoplegia and ptosis, bilateral facial weakness, tongue weakness, and paresthesias in both extremities, but the deep tendon reflexes remained present, probably representing an atypical GBS case. A systematic study of EBV serology and GBS[286] found that eight of 100 GBS patients had EBV-specific IgM antibodies and positive heterophil test results, compared with only 2 of 109 control subjects. In another study,[447] 7 of 24 patients with GBS and 3 of 16 patients with facial palsy, meningoencephalitis, or transverse myelitis had antibodies to EBV-related antigens but not to CMV; an additional 5 had suggestive serologic evidence.

GBS after segmental herpes zoster has been reported rarely.[254,631] A rather long interval between dermatologic and neurologic illness in several cases suggests that the two conditions may, at times, be unrelated.[254,631] GBS has followed the dermatologic eruption by 2 days to 2 months. Most reported GBS cases have been in patients with thoracic shingles; in one, polyradiculitis followed ophthalmic herpes zoster.[631] Many patients have become quadriplegic, but some milder cases have followed a longer latent period. The distinction from a necrotic myelitis caused by direct infection with herpes zoster has been difficult to make at times.

Several reports have appeared of GBS after herpes simplex labialis or vaginalis[795,875] and two after herpes simplex meningitis.[99,1081a] Dowling[286] found that only 1 of 74 routinely tested patients with GBS had herpes simplex virus IgM–specific antibodies. A case report[402] has shown herpes simplex IgM–specific antibodies (without an eruption) that fluctuated with the clinical course of GBS. All of the herpesvirus associations with GBS would have been more convincing if a convalescent rise in antibody titer had been shown.

Hepatitis

Up to 10% of patients have abnormal liver function tests on admission to the hospital for acute GBS. Asymptomatic cases of hepatitis may be due to several agents, including, in order of frequency, CMV, EBV, and hepatitis A, B or non-A, non-B, especially if blood products have been given. Several hepatitic GBS cases have had no serologic evidence for any of these agents.

The first symptoms of GBS after hepatitis A infection have occurred 3 days

*See references 43, 226, 286, 316, 336, 409, 489, 577, 623, 826, 923, 1069, 1243, and 1264.

to 2 weeks after headache, fatigue, myalgia, and jaundice.[454,573,744] Recovery has generally been good, with residual facial palsy, ataxia, and areflexia or no residua in patients with adequate follow-up. In a consecutive series of 167 GBS patients, only two had high titers of hepatitis A virus–specific IgM antibody and abnormal liver function test results,[123] suggesting that the association is rare. After an epidemic of hepatitis A in Shanghai, there was not thought to be a subsequent rise in the incidence of GBS.[1303]

A few cases linking hepatitis B with GBS have been reported.* Hepatitis B surface antigen has been found in high titers in the serum and cerebrospinal fluid (CSF) of one patient with GBS, with clearance of the virus antigen paralleling clinical recovery.[540,908] Recently, a provocative report[738] suggested that non-A, non-B hepatitis may be a sporadic cause of GBS after surgery. The lack of a serologic test for non-A, non-B hepatitis until recently has made it difficult to determine how common these cases are.

HIV and AIDS

Peripheral neuropathies in patients with HIV infection are being increasingly recognized, now reportedly accounting for 20% of neurologic complications.[214a,221,242a,266,477,802,960] HIV-infected patients characteristically have a distal sensory neuropathy, often with painful, burning dysesthesias in the feet. Weakness is usually mild, and areflexia may be limited to the ankle jerk. Other neuropathies associated with HIV have included mononeuropathy multiplex, sometimes involving cranial nerves, and a more profound distal symmetrical polyneuropathy. There have been, in addition, at least eight well-documented cases of acute GBS in association with HIV (Table 6–1). A series from Johns Hopkins University[221] found 3 of 39 patients (8%) with acute GBS and HIV in a 4-year experience, but this high frequency may be related to the population tested. We are familiar with a case of Fisher's syndrome associated with HIV. Several cases of chronic inflammatory neuropathy have also been associated with HIV infection.[221,960] Seroconversion for anti-HIV antibody after the course of acute GBS has been reported.[926]

The clinical symptoms of HIV-associated GBS are similar to those of other cases (Table 6–1). Rapidly evolving flaccid paralysis progressing to respiratory failure occurs, but milder cases have also been described. Electrodiagnostic studies have revealed a variety of demyelinative and axonal changes, although F-wave and somatosensory evoked potential abnormalities have occurred less frequently than expected for typical GBS.

A common feature in patients with HIV infection is a tendency toward CSF pleocytosis, up to 40 cells per mm^3 (see Chapter 12); follow-up lumbar puncture results have often been normal. Asymptomatic HIV-seropositive patients may also have a CSF pleocytosis, suggesting that the aseptic meningitis may be a separate phenomenon from the neuropathy.[242a] Sural nerve biopsy specimens have features typical of GBS with demyelination and phagocytic ingestion of myelin. One patient had extensively vacuolated perineurium and prominent subperineural edema. Others[221] have shown extensive endoneural mononuclear cell infiltrates and perivascular inflammatory cells.

HIV has been isolated from sural nerves in several patients, most with chronic inflammatory demyelinating polyneuropathy (CIDP). Therefore, direct neural infection remains a possible cause of GBS in these patients. Alternatively, altered T-lymphocyte function disrupting immune regulation may lead to immune responses against Schwann cells or myelin. Other, better-known coinfections such as CMV, EBV, herpesvirus, and hepatitis B virus must also be considered as potential triggers

*See references 97, 362, 540, 853, 908, 942, and 1246.

Table 6–1 GUILLAIN-BARRÉ SYNDROME IN HIV-POSITIVE PATIENTS

Author	Age/Sex	Clinical Picture	Antecedent Illness	CSF Cells/ Protein	Outcome
Mishra et al.,[809] 1985	23/M	Progressive quadriparesis, bifacial weakness	*Pneumocystis, Candida*	N/A	Gradual recovery, outcome not stated
Hagberg et al.,[477] 1986	56/M	Numbness		38/83	Grade 1
	69/M	Ascending paralysis, cranial nerve involvement assisted ventilation	Diarrhea, fever	2/85	Grade 1
Piette et al.,[927] 1986	53/M	Slow progressive quadriparesis, rash	Fever, diarrhea	100/40	Grade 2
Vendrell et al.,[1230] 1987	42/M	Progressive quadriparesis to complete paralysis, bilateral facial weakness	None	NA/72	Moderate quadriparesis at 2 months (grade 3 or 4)
Cornblath et al.,[221]* 1987	18/M	Rapid flaccid paralysis and assisted ventilation	None	24/210	Grade 2
	27/M	Same as above	None	40/25	Grade 4
	26/M	Same as above	None	25/28NA	Grade 3

*Hepatitis B serology positive in two cases.
NA = not available.

to the illness. Typical CMV inclusions have been demonstrated in lumbar dorsal roots in a patient with HIV-GBS.[107]

Other Viruses

Many other serologically identifiable viruses have been linked to GBS in single case reports, including rubella,[1040] measles,[295,698] chickenpox,[125,251] mumps,[211] coxsackievirus,[335,1211] and types A and B influenza.[295,324,370,1040]

BACTERIAL INFECTIONS

No estimate of the incidence of bacterial infections preceding GBS can be made, but they are clearly less common preceding agents than viruses, perhaps because bacterial infections generally occur less frequently than viral infections.

Campylobacter Jejuni

The discovery of serologic evidence of *Campylobacter* in many GBS patients has directed interest to this agent. After the first report in 1982[981] a number of cases have appeared over the last several years (Table 6–2), some with only serologic evidence of infection.* Individual cases of *Campylobacter* enteritis and GBS have been alluded to in other series but without many details.[385,1289] The clinical features of *Campylobacter jejuni* enteritis are identical to those of other bacterial enteritides: abdominal cramping, fever, bloody or watery diarrhea, tenesmus, and often abnormal sigmoidoscopic findings. Stool specimens containing erythrocytes or leukocytes are likely to yield the pathogenic microorganism.[113] The median duration of fecal excretion is 2 or 3 weeks but may be up to 3 months in untreated patients. The overall isolation rate is 8.8% from stool cultures and 5.8% from rectal swabs.[114] The sensitivity rises to 22% in patients with grossly bloody stool. The summer season and patient age of 10 to 30 years are factors that are also associated with an increased rate of isolation of the organism.

The clinical signs of GBS in symptomatic *Campylobacter* infection have reflected the spectrum of GBS variants, including Fisher's syndrome,[204,638,959] with a delay between the enteritis and the onset of GBS of 6 to 21 days (mean 10 days) (Table 6–2). The CSF in patients with positive stool cultures has generally had fewer than 3 WBC per mm^3, and most have had elevated protein concentrations.

Serologic and western blot studies by a group with a wide experience with the pathogen[583,1135] have suggested the possibility that *Campylobacter* is the most common infection preceding GBS. Serologic evidence of *Campylobacter* was found in 38% of a retrospective study of 56 GBS patients, as opposed to none in control subjects.[583] Only half of the patients with antibodies recalled a recent episode of diarrhea. The outcome appeared to be worse in patients with preceding *Campylobacter* in a prospective study of 100 GBS patients,[1289] although the incidence of a positive serologic test was low (14%).

The best estimate of the incidence of *Campylobacter* preceding GBS is approximately 15%.[1289] There was serologic evidence of recent *Campylobacter* in only 3 of 17 (18%) consecutive prospectively studied patients from the MGH series who were tested for serotypes 1 and 12.* Both patients had severe diarrhea and cramping preceding GBS; one had the organism isolated from stool culture. None of the serologically negative patients had preceding gastrointestinal symptoms. In the MGH prospective series,[1009] 12 patients (10%) had diarrhea, four with positive cultures for *Campylobacter;* their outcomes varied. Antibiotic treatment did

*See references 204, 215, 1289, 583, 638, 639, 816, 959, 1009, 1131, 1135, and 1300.

*Courtesy of Dr. Reuben Gruenewald, New York City Department of Public Health.

Table 6–2 CAMPYLOBACTER PRECEDING GBS: CASES IN THE LITERATURE*

Source/Year	Age/Sex	Interval (days)	Neurologic Signs	EMG	Stool Culture/Serologic Findings	Treatment	Outcome
Rhodes and Tattersfield,[981] 1982	45/M	15	Quadriplegia	Slow MNCV and SNCV; denervation	+/+	E	Poor
Molnar et al.,[816] 1982	42/M	13	Quadriparesis	Normal MNCV and SNCV; denervation	+/ND	None	Not stated
Constant et al.,[215] 1983	34/F	10	Fisher's syndrome and respiratory failure	—	+/−CSF	E	Diplopia and arm weakness at 3 mo
Speed et al.,[1135] 1984	16/M	10	"Severe"	—	+/+	—	Good
Pryor et al.,[959] 1984	34/M	21(?)	Mild weakness	Dispersed CMAP; normal SNCV	+/ND	E	Good
Kaldor and Speed,[583] 1986	2/F	9	Quadriplegia, bulbar palsy, ventilation (6 wk)	—	+/+	—	Good
Wroe and Blumhardt,[1300] 1985	27/M	7	Ophthalmoplegia facial and palatal weakness	Normal MNCV; dispersed or absent SNAP or SNCV	+/ND	ND	Good
DeBont et al.,[256] 1986	2/F	9	Quadriplegia, bulbar palsy, ventilation (6 wk)	Slow MNCV; prolonged distal latency; normal SNCV	+/+CSF	ND	Good

Table 6–2 CAMPYLOBACTER PRECEDING GBS: CASES IN THE LITERATURE*

Source/Year	Age/ Sex	Interval (days)	Neurologic Signs	EMG	Stool Culture/ Serologic Findings	Treat- ment	Outcome
Kohler and Goldblatt,[639] 1987	69/M	3	Quadriparesis	—	+/ND	E	Good (slight weakness, arms)
Kohler et al.,[638] 1988	19/M	13	Fisher's syndrome	—	ND/+ and +CSF	—	Good
Sovilla et al.,[1131] 1988	38/M	6	Quadriparesis	Slow MNCV; denervation	+/−	—	Good
	81/M	8	Mild quadriparesis	Slow MNCV; denervation	+/ND	E	Good
	60/M	12	Severe quadriparesis	Extensive denervation	ND/+	C	Good
Clavelou et al.,[204] 1989	30/M	12	Distal weakness, no sensory symptom or signs	Inexcitable nerves, legs; distal denervation	ND/+	ND	Good
	62/M	10	Distal weakness, no sensory symptoms or signs	Slow MNCV; distal denervation	ND/+	ND	Good
	74/M	15	Distal weakness, no sensory symptoms or signs	Slow MNCV; absent F-responses; distal denervation	−/+	ND	Not stated

*C = clioquinol; E = erythromycin; ND = Not done; MNCV = motor nerve conduction velocity; SNCV = sensory nerve conduction velocity; SNAP = sensory nerve action potential; CMAP = compound muscle action potential.

Table 6–3 GBS FOLLOWING *CAMPYLOBACTER JEJUNI* DIARRHEA (MGH CASES)

Age/Sex	Gastroenteritis	GBS	Outcome	Electrophysiology	CSF
63/F	Profuse nonbloody diarrhea and fever for 5–7 days before and during early GBS; + stool culture, not treated	Weakness beginning in one arm, progressing to quadriplegia and respiratory failure in one day; no paresthesias or ocular palsies	Wheelchair-bound at 2 yr	Severe distal block with only single units on day 3, mostly normal NCVs, later denervation; sural nerve biopsy specimen normal	Protein 34 mg/dL WBC 3/mm^3
74/F	Cramping abdominal pain and diarrhea for 3 days; 8 days before GBS; + stool culture, treated with erythromycin	Bilateral hand weakness, unable to walk without assistance on day 2, and acral paresthesias, urinary incontinence day 3, bifacial weakness day 5	Good at 6 mo	Normal NCV with absent late responses on day 4	Protein mg/dL WBC 1/mm^3
32/M	Abdominal pain and diarrhea 1 week before GBS; + stool culture, treated with erythromycin	Progressive mild weakness and areflexia without sensory signs or symptoms	Good at 6 mo	Normal NCV with prolonged late responses on day 11	Protein 160 mg/dL WBC 1/mm^3
19/M	Bloody diarrhea 10 days before GBS; + stool culture treated with trimethoprim-sulfamethoxazole	Distal paresthesias and mild leg weakness with normal reflexes except ankle	Good at 2 mo	Normal NCV with dispersed, prolonged muscle action potentials	Protein 0.42 g/L (42 mg/dL) 0 WBC
76/M	Watery diarrhea 2 days before GBS; + stool culture	Left arm numbness, facial weakness, bilateral ptosis, progressive quadriparesis marked dysautonomia	Poor at 6 mo	Normal NCV; decreased distal CMAP; absent F responses;	Protein 10 mg/dL 0 WBC

*NCV = nerve conduction velocity; CSF = cerebrospinal fluid; and WBC = white blood cells.
†Adapted from Ropper,[1009] p. 656.

not prevent the subsequent development of GBS in five patients treated (Table 6–3). A recent study[910] to determine the diagnostic value of assays to measure serum antibodies to *Campylobacter pylori,* implicated in antritis, is interesting because it shows an age-related rise in the serologic prevalence of positive ELISA test results, reaching 50% after the fifth decade. Some of the serologic evidence of *Campylobacter* infection in GBS therefore may be similarly nonspecific, especially in older patients. *Campylobacter jejuni,* nonetheless, appears to be a frequent preceding infection for GBS, and should be suspected if there has been enteritis.

Mycoplasma

Mycoplasma pneumoniae remains an important preceding bacterial pathogen in GBS, although it probably does not occur as frequent as previously thought.[330,331,369,523] Most affected patients are children or young adults. The diagnosis may be suspected when polyneuropathy follows fever, severe headache, pharyngitis, and a dry cough, when no clear abnormalities appear upon physical examination but an interstitial infiltrate is seen on chest x-ray examination. *Mycoplasma* may be identified by fluorescent or complement-fixing antibody tests. The presence of cold agglutinins, common with *Mycoplasma,* can be a helpful sign, but their presence is nonspecific; they may occur with other respiratory infections and mononucleosis syndromes. Five of 100 GBS cases had serologic evidence for *Mycoplasma,* as detected with counterimmunoelectrophoresis and complement fixation.[416] The severity of GBS after *Mycoplasma* varies widely. Cranial nerve abnormalities were frequent in a literature review,[523] and 2 of the 7 patients described in one series[416] developed papilledema. Respiratory failure does not appear to be more common than in GBS related to other infectious agents.[416,523]

Spirochetal Infections

Neurologic involvement occurs in approximately 10% of patients with Lyme disease, which is caused by tick-borne *Borrelia burgdorferi* but many cases of alleged GBS remain poorly documented and difficult to interpret. A meningoradiculitis syndrome with facial palsy, severe radicular and back pain, sensory loss, weakness, areflexia, and a mononuclear CSF pleocytosis, termed *Bannwarth's syndrome,* is well known in Europe and may simulate acute GBS.* The peripheral neuropathy in this syndrome and its variants is generally not ascending and is typically asymmetric or monoparetic, but two cases with many characteristics of GBS have been reported.[892,1148] Ascending limb weakness and symmetric mild bifacial palsy occurred in both cases, but the CSF had markedly elevated cell counts (many of the CSF cells in Lyme disease are immunoblasts or plasmacytes). Electrophysiologic examination was consistent with a demyelinating neuropathy. Many patients with Lyme disease develop a subacute mild sensory neuropathy with paresthesias and ankle areflexia, often without CSF pleocytosis, but it is our impression that typical GBS is only rarely associated with Lyme disease. The distinction between GBS and Lyme disease neuropathy can sometimes be made by persistent pleocytosis and atypical clinical features. It would not be surprising, however, to encounter rare cases that so closely mimic GBS that the clinical and electrophysiologic differences are too subtle to be useful. Patients with GBS with serum IgG antibodies against the Lyme disease pathogen have been reported from the Auvergne,[203] an area with endemic Bannwarth syndrome.

Another pathogen rarely associated with GBS, *Leptospira icterohaemorrhagiae,* occurred in one patient with a

*See references 43, 44, 481, 482, 892, and 1302.

pure motor ascending neuropathy that progressed to a flaccid quadriplegia, followed by recovery in 4 months.[820]

Other Bacteria

Salmonella infections have been reported in a few cases of GBS, often during an epidemic. In three large series of *Salmonella* enteritis, totaling 1,105 patients, however, none fulfilled the established criteria for GBS, suggesting that the association is rare.[184,608,889] GBS may occur concurrently with the enteritis or during convalescence.[96,284] An instance of ataxic GBS has been reported.[284] Clinical recovery in these cases was good.

GBS has been reported sporadically after *Yersinia enterocolitica* arthritis,[345] *Pasteurella tularensis*,[834] *Listeriosis*,[1060] *Brucellosis*,[18,1252] *Shigella*,[609] *Legionella*,[753] and tuberculosis.[906,1240] Some of these associations are unconvincing.

A polyneuropathy following recurrent bacterial sepsis in an intensive care unit (ICU) setting, distinguishable from GBS as discussed in Chapter 14, has been highlighted by Bolton and coworkers[118] and other researchers.[733,878,1315]

VACCINATION

Neurologic allergic reactions characterized by acute monophasic demyelinative processes may occur after immunization in less than 1 per 100,000 vaccine recipients.[359] Numerous cases of vaccine-induced GBS have been reported; the most celebrated are those from the "swine flu" incident (see Chapter 3). Vaccination is generally considered to be a safe procedure, but patients have been reported with GBS after vaccination for rabies[37,510] and more sporadically after bacille Calmette Guérin (BCG),[596] tetanus (toxoid),[851] smallpox,[703] type A Asian influenza, measles,[448] mumps, rubella,[612] and hepatitis B[982,1092] and polio vaccines. A recent study from Finland has suggested that the use of line attenuated oral polio vaccine in 1985 was associated with an increase in GBS cases.[619] A study of 850,000 hepatitis B vaccinations[1092] concluded that the risk of GBS was only slightly, if at all, elevated (9 cases in 3 years following this vaccine). In a series of 1,100 cases of GBS[686] only one case was associated with an influenza vaccination. The clinical features of postvaccination GBS are similar to those in sporadic cases, but fever and systemic symptoms (from the vaccination) may occur more frequently. We have seen a patient with severe, predominantly sensory and ataxic GBS after rubella vaccination. Sera from patients with GBS after rabies vaccines have had antibodies to myelin basic protein, but no detectable antibodies to P2 protein or to Schwann cells were found, suggesting in this particular situation that cellular antigens may not be important immunogens.[509]

In 1976, the potential influenza epidemic due to a "swine flu" strain of virus led to a nationwide immunization program in the United States. An apparent increase in GBS cases during the 8 weeks after vaccination led to several epidemiologic studies and editorials. (This controversy is discussed in greater detail in Chapter 3.) It was suggested that the vaccine was the specific cause of GBS for the following reasons: (1) clustered distribution of intervals between vaccination and the onset of GBS in the first 4 weeks; (2) a lower than expected frequency of other acute illness in the 4 weeks before GBS (33% in the vaccinated versus 62% in the concurrently collected unvaccinated cases); and (3) comparable severity of the disease in vaccinated and unvaccinated patients during this epoch, suggesting that vaccinated cases were not over-reported.[1072] In a later review of these data, however, it was found that the claimed "incubation" curves were observed only in those GBS patients with extensive motor deficits, not in milder cases. The entire issue is still debated. The most recent evidence, summarized in Chapter 3, still suggests that this particular vaccine was associated with a slightly increased risk of GBS, similar to some of the other vaccines listed here.

The question frequently arises of the safety of various vaccinations in patients who have recovered from GBS. No systematic study has been performed, but on the anecdotal basis of a relapse in two patients in our series and a report of relapses after tetanus toxoid[937] and after BCG revaccination,[596] it seems prudent to avoid all but necessary vaccinations.

SYMPTOMATIC GBS

Several systemic diseases have repeatedly been associated with acute (and sometimes chronic or relapsing) GBS (Table 6–4). All of the diseases listed in Table 6–4 more often cause a subacute progressive neuropathy, but a GBS-like illness is indistinguishable from the typical acute syndrome. Most of these diseases may also be associated with other subacute or chronic noninflammatory neuropathies. Though the association is infrequent, minor aberrations from the typical GBS syndrome should lead to consideration of an underlying systemic disease. Specific points that distinguish the disease-specific neuropathy from acute GBS are discussed here, as well as in Chapter 14.

Cancer and Lymphoma

Peripheral nerve disorders that resemble acute GBS are common in patients with malignancies and paraneoplastic or paraproteinemic neuropathies (see Chapter 14). Typical acute GBS, however, has been linked regularly only to Hodgkin's disease.[27,167,480,576] The association with acute GBS though definite, is probably rare, since in two series[236,553] 370 patients with continuing neurologic complications of Hodgkin's disease and neurologic complications, no definite cases were found. The clinical features in Hodgkin's-related GBS have been identical to those of the idiopathic variety and inconsistent with other neuropathies, for example vincristine neuropathy. Some patients have developed progressive and fatal oropharyngeal weakness and respiratory failure.[626] One reported patient recovered after prednisone treatment with marked residual weakness after 18 months;[707] another relapsed 2 months after initial improvement. Two MGH patients with Hodgkin's disease and typical GBS improved with plasma exchange, and other researchers refer to similar cases.[512] One of our patients, and another who did not respond well to exchanges, had a peculiar temporal course with initial improvement followed by rapid deterioration. One patient also had features of Castleman's disease, an association previously reported with GBS.[281]

An exceptional patient has been described[626] with leg pain, paresthesias, and progressive areflexic quadriparesis as the first expression of an oat cell carcinoma. Postmortem examination showed demyelination and axonal changes thought to be consistent with GBS. The description and figures, however, do not allow a distinction from paraneoplastic neuropathy. Another case has been associated with adenocarcinoma of the lung.[480] A recent study[30] has demonstrated antineural antibodies in a variety of neurologic disorders associated with small-cell lung cancer, including two cases of GBS. These two patients developed a progressive lower motor neuron weakness,

Table 6–4 MOST COMMON SYSTEMIC ILLNESSES ASSOCIATED WITH TYPICAL AND ATYPICAL GBS

Sarcoidosis
Systemic lupus erythematosus
Lymphoma (particularly Hodgkin's disease)
HIV infection (pleocytosis common)
Lyme disease (pleocytosis common)
Solid tumors (particularly lung cancer)

painful dysesthesias, severe joint position sense loss, and autonomic signs 2 months before the discovery of the tumor. Plasma exchange did not influence the course, and both died within 4 months. Postmortem examination in one patient showed perivascular lymphocytic infiltrates in the medulla, spinal cord, dorsal root ganglia, and spinal roots, consistent with GBS. It is difficult to be certain that the infrequent association between solid tumors and GBS is anything more than chance. Many reported cases have not been clearly distinguished from more typical paraneoplastic neuropathies.

Several authors[782,951] have described GBS in association with chronic lymphocytic leukemia. A patient with acute myelomonoblastic leukemia, a polyneuropathy, and optic neuropathy has also been reported.[919] This 18-year-old patient had progressive facial weakness, ptosis, diplopia, and blurring of vision and subsequently developed progressive dysphagia and generalized weakness with repeatedly normal CSF cytology. Postmortem examination showed focal fragmentation of myelin in all cranial nerves, spinal nerves, and cauda equina. A patient of ours, not in the series, has been reported with complex relapsing central and peripheral demyelinating lesions, beginning with an illness that simulated Fisher's syndrome, associated with hairy cell leukemia.[265]

Autoimmune and Collagen-Vascular Disease

A number of autoimmune diseases have occurred concurrently with acute GBS, although there is a more frequent association between these diseases and chronic-relapsing inflammatory neuropathy (CIDP) (see Chapters 10, 11, and 14). These associations are probably more than fortuitous, leading several investigators to seek a common immunopathogenesis by studying the humoral and cellular systems in patients with GBS and CIDP.[641]

Approximately 10% of patients with systemic lupus erythematosus (SLE) have a peripheral neuropathy, often a mononeuritis multiplex or relapsing demyelinating polyneuropathy.[572,641,691,1065] The typical neuropathy in SLE does not simulate GBS; rather, the onset is gradual, the weakness is more distal, and the course is more prolonged. When acute progressive ascending weakness does occur ("idiopathic polyneuritis"),[572,804] the pathologic findings resemble those in GBS. Other signs of SLE are usually well established when acute GBS becomes evident, but chronic inflammatory neuropathy has preceded signs of SLE in several cases. A patient has been described[415] with one episode of pure motor paralysis and total recovery in 3 months, followed by a second episode with both motor and sensory signs. During the second episode other symptoms of SLE were evident. Other similar cases have appeared in the literature.[641]

The MGH prospective series had one patient with definite, but inactive, SLE and another with possible disease at the time of GBS symptoms. In one patient, proximal weakness in the arms and legs progressed to quadriplegia with bifacial palsy and respiratory difficulty. There was axonal degeneration and proximal conduction block. She improved slightly after plasmapheresis, then virtually completely over 6 weeks with steroid therapy. Five similar cases have not been included in the MGH prospective series.

Definite acute GBS has not yet been described well in other collagen disorders such as polyarteritis nodosa, Wegener's granulomatosis, rheumatoid arthritis, and idiopathic thrombocytopenic purpura although anecdotal cases of the latter can be found.[641] Mononeuritis multiplex is more typical of these disorders (see Chapter 14). Cases of GBS with temporal arteritis,[223] Hashimoto's thyroiditis,[948] and Graves' disease,[641] as well as an interesting case with myasthenia gravis, have been described.[976a]

Sarcoidosis

There is a complex relationship between GBS and the many neuropathies caused by sarcoidosis. Typical cases of GBS have been reported infrequently.[685,1077] Some have a meningeal reaction, occasionally with hypoglycorrhea.[412a] Several reports describe a GBS-like[803a] illness with paresthesias, pain, and rapid limb weakness. There was excellent recovery after corticosteroid treatment in most patients.[1156] Other patients have had spontaneous neurologic improvement while the systemic manifestations of sarcoidosis progressed.[685] Other similar cases have been alluded to, but these usually showed signs of superimposed mononeuropathy. More often, patients have a subacute or chronic sensorimotor neuropathy with demyelinating features or bifacial palsy with a mild polyneuropathy. Vocal cord paralysis is probably more frequent in this disorder than in typical GBS where it is rare. Like Hodgkin's-associated GBS, the initial temporal course of sarcoidosis and GBS may fluctuate.

ENDOCRINE DISORDERS

GBS has been rarely linked to endocrine disorders, leading to speculation about an analogous immune mechanism for both, but it is not clear whether the two are related or just associated. Hyperthyroidism occurred at the same time as GBS in a patient who recovered spontaneously from both disorders.[106] In other patients, GBS has occurred during or after treatment of hyperthyroidism and did not recur with re-emergence of the thyroid disorder.[145] Hashimoto's thyroiditis with typical GBS,[948] Graves' disease,[641] hypothyroidism,[898] Cushing's syndrome,[140,300,315] and two cases of Addison's disease with rapidly ascending tetraplegia and remarkable improvement after treatment with steroids have all been anecdotally reported.[1,1133]

GBS AND PREGNANCY

More than 35 cases of patients having GBS during pregnancy have been described, mostly in the third trimester.* In a summary of 27 of these,[1160] half had a preceding respiratory infection. Most patients improved before delivery and the infant was not adversely affected. Several cases have had relapses in successive pregnancies. Recently, two cases with a rapidly progressive course have been described, with improvement after plasmapheresis.[334] Late pregnancy that is complicated by GBS has a perinatal infant mortality rate approaching 10% because of the increased likelihood of premature labor and delivery. Close attention to respiratory function is required, particularly in view of already diminished lung volumes from an elevated diaphragm. Furthermore, increased respiratory demands during labor may cause diaphragmatic decompensation. An important facet of management is adequate ventilation of the mother when respiratory failure occurs. Labor can occur spontaneously in convalescing patients, but forceps assistance is often needed. No cases of fetal malformation have been reported. Unlike the situation with transient neonatal myasthenia, the fetus does not acquire GBS from an affected mother (see Chapter 5).

Two patients in the MGH series developed GBS 2 weeks postpartum. Further details of management of GBS in pregnancy are discussed in Chapter 16.

SURGERY AND SPINAL EPIDURAL ANESTHESIA

Surgery was emphasized as a trigger for GBS in an initial report of six patients.[41] Large GBS series usually include 5% to 10% of cases that occur after surgery.* Although urinary tract or

---

*See references 9, 78, 135, 244, 679, 899, 962, 1033, and 1160.

*See references 469, 686, 1123, 1138a, 1278, and 1289.

respiratory infections had occurred in some, surgery was a more apparent precipitant. Type of operation, duration of surgery, mode of anesthesia, postoperative wound infection, or blood transfusion was not consistently associated with GBS. In a series of more than 700 postoperative patients examined for carotid bruits and stroke at MGH, however, no cases of GBS were encountered, indicating the rarity of this complication.[1019] In the retrospective MGH series, 10 patients were identified with GBS 1 to 3 weeks (average 14 days) after various types of surgery (6 abdominal explorations, 2 craniotomies, 1 arm amputation, and 1 vein stripping). Postoperative wound infections among these patients were common, and half the cases received blood transfusions. One was followed by a possible CMV infection, and one patient had an acute relapse 6 years later, following a swine flu vaccination. When blood transfusion or cardiac pump bypass is a part of the surgery, the infectious hepatitis viruses may be the precipitant for GBS. A pump-related case of GBS has been traced to a CMV infection.[226] Non-A, non-B hepatitis, undetectable until recently, has also been proposed as a trigger in postsurgical GBS, but studies of large series have not been undertaken. We are familiar with an unusual case of bifacial palsy, areflexia, and elevated CSF protein concentration (with cells) after multiple orthopedic surgeries for a leg injury. A case of ascending paralysis 8 days after coronary bypass surgery with good recovery after plasma exchange has been described.[980]

Two cases of GBS have been reported[1146] 1 to 2 weeks after spinal epidural anesthesia. Both patients' illnesses began with leg weakness and areflexia, progressing to severe quadriparesis and bulbar weakness in one patient. Nerve conduction studies and CSF findings were compatible with those of GBS. In an extensive series of 10,440 patients who had received epidural anesthesia,[922] however, only 38 experienced weakness and sensory symptoms; these disappeared after 5 days in most and therefore were unlikely to represent GBS. A case report[1205] of a patient with severe loss of fibers in the posterior roots and loss of cells in sensory ganglia 4 years after spinal anesthesia is possibly representative of GBS after spinal anesthesia.

GBS is not a recognized complication of other types of anesthesia. A patient having a relapse of GBS after nerve biopsy[121] seems to have been a sporadic exception or a coincidence in a case of relapsing neuropathy.

The pathogenesis of postsurgical GBS (that is not the result of infection with a virus) is unknown. Local damage to peripheral nerves and release of nerve antigen leading to a vigorous immunologic response has been suggested.[41] Virtually nothing is known about the risk of subsequent surgery. Approximately 10 patients in the MGH prospective series had major surgical procedures (coronary bypass, tracheal repair, hysterectomy) 1 to 4 years after GBS without any signs of relapse; at least 20 patients had minor procedures, including nerve biopsy. Tracheostomy seems to be tolerated regularly without worsening of the neuropathy. The relation of nonsurgical trauma to GBS is discussed later.

UNCERTAIN OR RARE ASSOCIATIONS

Four reported cases of GBS have occurred 10 to 13 days following streptokinase therapy;[48,201,319,682] two had typical CSF and electrophysiologic features. This seems more than coincidental. Captopril has reportedly caused reversible paresthesias and peripheral neuropathy that improves on withdrawal of the drug, but there also have been at least two cases of GBS with excellent recovery.[57,183] Other drugs have been tentatively associated with GBS in single reports, including gold therapy,[276] penicillamine,[627] danazol,[535] zimelidine,[340] and an amitriptyline overdose,[696] but all require further confirmation. A few cases of acute polyneuropathy resembling GBS have occurred after intravenous heroin abuse.[716,986,1119] In one patient this occurred after re-exposure following a 4-year abstinence. Possible mechanisms that have been proposed for drug-related GBS include a direct toxic effect, hypersensitivity reaction, or the introduction of subacute infection. Three cases of GBS with cranial nerve involvement and severe limb weakness have been reported after insect stings (bee and red fire ants);[63] however, two of the patients had upper respiratory tract infections. Other anecdotal associations have involved hyperthermia,[394,994] cholera,[1078] Brucellosis,[389a] tularemia,[1175] toxoplasmosis,[128] metrizamide myelography,[410] urethritis,[750] and malaria.[61,893] One of our patients had a recurrence of GBS after a bout of malaria. A unique case of GBS has been associated with myasthenia gravis.

Trauma without surgery has not emerged as a precipitant to GBS, although one patient in the MGH prospective cases had no other apparent preceding illness and developed GBS while recovering from an automobile accident and several fractures. A case has been reported after head injury.[299] We have been made aware of several other similar anecdotal instances after injury.

No specific unifying features explain the wide variety of infections, systemic illnesses, and other immunologic perturbations that may precede GBS. It does not seem plausible that both GBS and the preceding illness are manifestations of a common underlying immune dysfunction. This mechanism seems likely, however, in patients with systemic diseases such as Hodgkin's or sarcoidosis that disturb cellular immune function. Some activation of the immune system is necessary, and certain precipitants—particularly the herpesvirus family—are involved more often than their incidence in the population would explain. Re-exposure to an initial precipitant only occasionally causes an acute relapse, making the primacy of any particular agent questionable. On the other hand, re-exposure relapse in some patients suggests that there may be a specific host-agent interaction in rare individuals. Further immunologic research with organisms such as *Campylobacter jejuni*, CMV, and EBV to look for immune relationships in patients who have had GBS, as discussed in chapter 5, may elucidate this issue.

Chapter 7

CLINICAL FEATURES OF THE TYPICAL SYNDROME

In a comment on 10 unpublished cases of GBS,[459] Guillain stated, "The recognition of the disease is usually easy." Munsat and Barnes[829] added, "The Guillain-Barré syndrome is easy to diagnose but impossible to define." Despite easy recognition in most cases, the difficulty in establishing useful clinical criteria for the diagnosis of typical GBS and its variants is reviewed in Chapter 2. Certain characteristic clinical features stand out in relief to the variable pattern and distribution of signs and symptoms in GBS and to the absence of pathognomonic features: weakness in all limbs, progressing over several days to weeks; distal paresthesias; and diminished or absent deep tendon reflexes. Other frequent but not invariable features include facial, oculomotor, oropharyngeal, or diaphragmatic weakness; distal sensory loss; pain; and an extremely rapid, relapsing, or slowly worsening illness. This chapter details the limits and variations of each of these features. In order to preserve the idea of an easily recognizable typical syndrome, the major variant patterns of GBS are discussed separately in Chapter 8.

FREQUENCY OF THE MAJOR FEATURES IN TYPICAL GBS

Major series have reported similar frequencies of the principal clinical features of GBS (Table 7–1). Most studies are retrospective, not personally examined cases, but they probably give an accurate aggregate representation of the illness. Some differences in the frequency of signs are due to difficulty separating initial symptoms reported by the patient, or those at the admission examination, from the cumulative features as the illness progresses. For example, weakness and areflexia have been present on first examination in most patients in some series as a result of definitions that equate onset of illness with hospital admission. Other series exclude variants, making the typical signs appear more ubiquitous.

A realistic estimate of the incidence of major features at the onset or early in the illness is weakness in all limbs, 60%; paresthesias, 80%; both, 30%; areflexia, 70%; and hyporeflexia, 30%* (Table 7–1). As the illness progresses, weakness in all limbs occurs in every patient with typical GBS, paresthesias in approximately 95%, and areflexia in 98% (Table 7–2). A study that accumulated the features in eight previous papers[548] gives 32% with weakness at presentation, 46% with sensory symp-

*See references 714, 973, 1053, 1278, and 1291.

Table 7–1 NEUROLOGIC FINDINGS AT INITIAL EXAMINATION IN LARGE SERIES*

Series, Year	No. of Patients	Cranial Nerve Abnormalities III-VI (%)	V (%)	VII (%)	IX-X (%)	XII (%)	Distribution of Weakness L	A	L&A	N	Sensory Loss (%)	Areflexia (All Limbs) (%)	Pain (%)
Wiederholt et al.,[1278] 1964	97	5	0	29	1	1	8	2	85	5	38	52	14
McFarland and Heller,[777] 1966	100	6	15	55	48	10	24	1	74	1	70	NA	15
Andersson and Siden,[31] 1982	60	2	8	25	6	0	2	10	83	5	50	85	3
Winer et al.,[1291] 1988	100	13	31	53	46	13	0	0	100	0	59	83	50

*Percent of patients.

Table 7–2 CUMULATIVE NEUROLOGIC FINDINGS IN LARGE SERIES

Series, Year	No. of Patients	Cranial Nerve Abnormalities III-VI (%)	V (%)	VII (%)	IX-X (%)	XII (%)	Distribution of Weakness (%) L	A	L&A	N	Sensory Loss (%)	Areflexia/ Hyporeflexia (%)
Haymaker and Kernohan,[501] 1949	50	18	28.0	50	94	20	44	14	42	0	38	NA
Marshall,[751] 1963	35	28	23.0	60	54	54	3	0	97	0	47	100
Ravn,[973] 1967	127	18	3.0	36	31	6	6	2	86	6	NA	NA
Loffel et al,[714] 1977	123	7	0.8	29	23	5	14	2	80	4	83	100
Soffer et al,[1122] 1978	89	7	0	24	13	1	38	0	60	2	37	24
Samantray et al.,[1053] 1977	302	2	7.0	46	13	0	94	1	4	1	0	NA

NA = Not available.

Table 7–3 NEUROLOGIC FINDINGS IN RETROSPECTIVE MGH SERIES (N = 169)

Initial Symptoms				
Weakness + paresthesias				26%
Weakness + pain				14%
Weakness alone				12%
Weakness + pain + paresthesias				12%
Pattern of weakness				
Legs>Arms				54%
Arms>Legs				14%
Approximately equal				32%
Cumulative Symptoms after Progression (Includes Variants)				
Weakness				98%
Numbness/Paresthesias				72%
Pain				71%
Cranial nerve symptoms (except face)				40%
Ataxia				22%
Sphincter symptoms				18%
Tendon Reflexes on Admission (168 Patients)				
Reflex*	2+	1+	0	Asymmetric
Biceps	20%	23%	57%	4%
Brachioradialis	13%	19%	68%	2%
Triceps	16%	22%	62%	6%
Quadriceps	8%	13%	59%	5%
Gastrocsoleus	4%	8%	88%	0%

*2+ = normal; 1+ = reduced; 0 = absent.

toms, and 21% with both. The distribution of the major features encountered in the Massachusetts General Hospital (MGH) retrospective series is similar (Table 7–3). Facial weakness occurs at some time in the illness in half of patients; ophthalmoplegia in 15%, oropharyngeal weakness in approximately 40%; pain in more than half; and distal sensory loss demonstrable at the bedside with numbness in somewhat less than half early in the illness, and in almost three-quarters if the examination is performed later.

PATTERN OF WEAKNESS

Patients typically notice weakness in the legs before the arms and shoulders, although all limbs become weak differentially as the illness progresses. Bilateral facial weakness appears early, but rarely as the first sign (see farther on). Larger series usually report a predominance of early leg weakness over arm weakness.[1122] The study with the most skewed results [1053] had leg weakness in 94% of 302 patients early in the illness. Haymaker and Kernohan's 50 fatal cases[501] may have been more representative, with the legs predominantly weak in 22, the arms in 7, and muscles supplied by cranial nerves in 7. The remainder of their cases had weakness that was similar in several regions. In the MGH retrospective series 54% had greater leg than arm weakness with an "ascending" progression, in 14% the weakness "descended" from the cranial nerves or arms to later involve the legs, and 32% had approximately equal weakness in arms and legs (see Table 7–3). Approximately 5% in both the retrospective and prospective MGH series had cranial nerve involvement before any limb weakness, sometimes as a component of one of the variants discussed in Chapter 8, but as often descending to involve the limbs in a mirror image of the typical pattern. One careful analysis of the mode of progression[31] showed that 43% had weakness that ascended from legs to arms, 28% spread from all four limbs to the trunk and cranial nerves, and 5% descended from the cranial nerves or arms. In another large series,[973] weakness ascended in 37% and descended in only 4%.

The hips and shoulders tend to be involved earlier and more profoundly than the feet and hands,[1291] although proximal and distal weakness progress equally in one third of patients, and unlike the pattern more typical of neuromuscular junction disease, the proximal muscles are rarely involved alone for very long. As weakness increases, particularly toward the end of 2 weeks of illness, distal weakness becomes more prominent. Patients notice difficulty climbing stairs or arising from a chair for several hours or a day before they realize they are ill. This has led to the proposal that the "large muscles of the thigh or the upper portion of the arm" are affected first,[1190] to which Haymaker and Kernohan[501] rejoined that these areas are more likely to be noticed because they are used in daily physical activities. Weakness was more pronounced proximally in 58% and distally in 26%, and was approximately equally distributed in 16% of the MGH retrospective series; similar proportions were found in the prospective series. Only one patient in the retrospective series and three in the prospective series had variant illnesses with persistent and virtually isolated leg weakness (discussed in Chapter 8), although many more had this pattern at the onset of illness.

Guillain and Barré emphasized a predilection for weakness in the flexor muscles in the legs and extensors in the arms,[465] similar to the dissociation between hamstring and quadriceps weakness noted by others.[762] In the MGH experience, this flexor leg weakness predominance has occurred, but not nearly as prevalently, and the extensor and flexor arm muscle groups have not shown a consistent differential weakness.

Limb weakness is said to be symmetric but is almost never precisely so. Often one foot or leg can be raised from the bed whereas the other cannot. The asymmetry is more frequently subtle but still evident to the patient. Both limbs on one side may be weaker, or there may be a crossed or "alternating" pattern, but we are unaware of a truly hemiparetic onset in which one side has normal power and the other is weak. Only two patients in the prospective series had a virtual monoplegia of the arm at the onset, probably the smallest region affected by weakness in isolation. The other limbs became severely weak in 2 days, though they remained stronger than the originally affected arm. The earliest and most severly affected limb generally retains its prominence. This "slight tendency for . . . further functions in the limbs to be affected before spreading to other parts" has been noted by others.[751]

Weakness referable to a single motor root, or isolated weakness of a single muscle group or finger, has not occurred in the MGH experience despite surveillance for this sign; nor has there been a relationship between the patient's dominant side and the weakest limbs. There were, however, three patients whose first and most severely affected limb had been used heavily in the hours before the onset of symptoms. For example, a man who had been hammering in his workshop developed severe right arm weakness that night; another who had been climbing up and down stairs all morning had severe leg weakness and areflexia with arms spared. This use-related paresis, alluded to in polio and lead neuropathy, has been reported before[501] in three GBS cases, the most convincing being a soldier with arm weakness on the rifle range, followed by leg weakness after the return march. Other similar instances more likely represent notice taken of an active limb, rather than a direct result of its use. A few patients have rapid and uniform paralysis of all limbs, usually associated with respiratory failure within a few days. A useful Medical Research Council grading system for limb weakness, used in British and American treatment trials and elsewhere in this book, is shown in Table 7–4.

Diplopia occurs in 10% to 20% of cases, about 3% to 5% at the onset. Because some of the ocular features of GBS are complex and relate to arguments concerning central nervous system lesions, they are discussed separately later on. Incomplete, asymmetric lateral rectus weakness is the most common cause of diplopia. Ptosis

Table 7–4 MEDICAL RESEARCH COUNCIL (MRC) MUSCLE POWER GRADING SCALE*

0	No movement
1	Muscle contracts, flicker of movement
2	Joint moves with gravity eliminated
3	Resists gravity
4	Offers resistance, but not normal
5	Normal power

*Adapted from Hughes et al.,[547] p. 751.

unassociated with other signs of third nerve involvement occurs in approximately 5% to 10% of cases of typical GBS, usually with partial facial weakness[1006, 1008] (see Chapter 8 and subsequently). Lid elevation and other ocular signs often improve briefly with the administration of intramuscular neostigmine,[275] but the ptosis does not fatigue, fluctuate, or display a lid twitch sign as in myasthenia. Ptosis may be due to terminal nerve conduction block in a neuromuscular system with a low threshold for failure of transmission of rapid volleys.

Oropharyngeal weakness is eventually present in half or less than half of typical GBS cases, usually appearing after all limbs have been affected or at least lagging in progression. There is probably a relationship between impaired swallowing and the overall severity of illness since all but three of 50 fatal cases in one series had 9th and 10th nerve palsies.[501] Difficulty swallowing solid food and, later, secretions and saliva, are the usual presenting symptoms. In mild cases, patients may complain of a slight fullness in the back of the throat. Nasal regurgitation and a velopalatine nasal-sounding dysphonia, as occur in myasthenia gravis, have been uncommon. Neck flexion and facial weakness are almost always present in typical cases when swallowing is impaired. A "brassy" cough indicating vocal cord paralysis, though rare, suggests that the vagus can be differentially affected.[765] The frequency of tongue weakness referable to the 12th nerve varies widely among reports in the literature: half of patients in one series,[751] and 6% to 20% of patients in others.[501,777,973,1291] Tongue weakness is not selective or isolated and parallels other oropharyngeal weaknesses, but there were three patients with an almost purely lingual dysarthria in the MGH series (see Table 7–1). The issues relating to airway protection and anticipation of oropharyngeal failure are discussed in Chapter 17.

A useful and fairly consistent rule is that weakness of shoulder elevation and neck flexion parallels diaphragmatic weakness and respiratory failure. Other features of mechanical "bellows" respiratory failure are also taken up in Chapter 17. The forced expiratory vital capacities on admission in the MGH retrospective series are shown in Table 7–5. (In practice, it is useful to express these as milliliters per kilogram.) Patients with vital capacity (VC) under 1000 ml were all unable to stand or lift their arms off the bed; we have not seen selective or disproportionate diaphragmatic and intercostal weakness without approximately commensurate limb and trunk weakness. A patient with respiratory failure as the first sign of GBS is alluded to in a series of 30 patients.[444] Early and predominant respiratory weakness is more typical of neuromuscular junction disease (see Chapter 14).

Considering all reports, the seventh nerve is the most frequently affected cranial nerve. Facial weakness occurs in more than half of patients, usually early and particularly when limb weakness is severe. Virtual quadriplegia without facial weakness should cause reconsideration of the diagnosis, though there are exceptions. Facial weakness most often becomes evident after a few days of limb weakness but then may progress with little further worsening of limb weakness. Several of the MGH patients who have acquired facial paresis relatively late (during the second or third weeks of illness) have had a longer than usual progression of limb weakness, sometimes fluctuating

Table 7–5 VITAL CAPACITY (VC) ON ADMISSION—MGH RETROSPECTIVE SERIES*

VC	*No. of Cases (%)*
0–1000 mL	16 (17)
1000–2000 mL	31 (32)
2000–3000 mL	23 (24)
3000–4000 mL	17 (18)
4000–5000 mL	6 (6)
>5000 mL	3 (3)

*Adults only.

before reaching a plateau. There are no convincing data that establish a purely facial form of GBS, despite some cases of bifacial palsy with abnormal CSF[187] and a postoperative case not included in the MGH series (see Chapter 8).

Facial weakness affects the upper and lower facial muscles inhomogeneously in a neuropathic pattern. The upper lip and upper perioral muscles are initially usually weaker than the lower lip, buccinator, and mentalis. In addition to flattening of the nasolabial fold, facial weakness is often first evident in the periorbital muscles. A subtle delay or lack of force in blinking may be an early sign. We have only rarely seen incomplete eyelid closure while lip closure and nasolabial movement were normal. As with limb weakness, facial diplegia (paresis) is usually slightly asymmetric and rarely purely unilateral, the side first affected remaining the worse side. A few patients have had impaired taste sensation.* Facial weakness does not necessarily herald other cranial nerve involvement or respiratory failure, though such a relationship has been proposed.[373] In the MGH retrospective and prospective series, approximately 60% of patients had facial weakness at some time in their course; in 12% it was markedly asymmetric but not purely unilateral (see Table 7–3).

The typical facial weakness of GBS is probably due to multifocal conduction block, as in peripheral motor nerves (see later), and it correspondingly differs from Bell's palsy and the facial weakness of sarcoidosis. Bilateral but incomplete involvement, slower evolution, and the rarity of several features such as loss of taste,[1129] hyperacusis, retroparotid pain, and subjective sensory change over the face, all distinguish GBS facial paresis from Bell's palsy, but rare exceptions to each of these distinctions were found in the MGH series (see Chapter 14). Corneal exposure and signs derived from efforts to keep the lids closed are discussed subsequently.

Although some series report jaw closure weakness referable to the fifth nerve, this has been mild and generally uncommon (only 1 of 50 patients in one series).[501] Jaw closure is usually disproportionately spared compared with jaw opening.[1004] The "hanging jaw" or "slack jaw" appearance in myasthenia gravis and myopathies is therefore unusual. Weakness of jaw opening was present in almost one third of the patients in one series.[1291]

Muscle tone is most often normal until the limb can no longer resist gravity. Flaccidity supervenes with further weakness. The increased limb tone referred to in the original articles[466,467] has not been commented on subsequently. With persistent paralysis the feet assume plantarflexion, and the fingers, a passively flexed posture that may lead to pseudocontractures. "Fibrillations" in the acute stage have been noted[8] but must be rare.

When limbs, eye movements, eyelids, and oropharyngeal muscles have become severely weak, the patient's state may simulate a "locked-in" syndrome.[176,646] Careful examination, however, will demonstrate that, unlike those with brainstem damage, severely affected GBS patients cannot breathe at all or move their eyes vertically. Because GBS patients progress to this condition under observation, there is no practical difficulty in distinguishing the clinical states.

In the past decade, several laboratories have made a convincing, though inferential, case that conduction block is the proximate cause of limb and cranial musculature weakness in early GBS (see Chapters 5 and 13). The efferent volley in the motor nerve is presumably blocked or attenuated as it traverses a series of demyelinated regions (Table 7–6). A diminished neural impulse excites fewer motor units, resulting in a smaller action potential and a weaker muscle contraction. Conduction block is believed to result from loss of saltatory conduction in demyelinated

*See references 377, 1023, 1167, 1242, and 1250.

Table 7–6 PROBABLE PHYSIOLOGIC MECHANISMS OF MAJOR FEATURES OF GBS

Weakness	Conduction block at critical sites or in series
Paresthesias	Ectopic impulse generation along entire nerve; fibers from Meissner's, Merkel's, and Pacinian's organs
Areflexia	Dispersion and desynchronization due to heterogeneous slowing in afferent large fibers
Sensory loss	Cumulative conduction block from demyelinating lesions in series
Pain	Ectopic impulse generation along entire nerve; fibers from deep pain-pressure organ (? ephaptic transmission)

segments. In addition, conduction may be impeded by (1) the exposure of internodal segments of axon that have too few sodium channels to support normal conduction, (2) the exposure of potassium channels that tend to keep the membrane close to resting potential, and possibly (3) by impedance mismatching between demyelinated and normal axonal segments. (All but the loss of saltatory conduction are theoretical.) A critical failure of conduction could theoretically occur at a single site rather than through the cumulative effects of multiple demyelinating lesions in series, but some models suggest that multifocal demyelination is responsible.[1221,1261] Later in the illness, axonal damage with attendant denervation may play a role in some patients' weakness. Neurologic functions that require impulses to arrive in a strict temporal sequence, or within a brief epoch, are adversely affected by heterogeneous demyelination in large fibers that desynchronizes electrical volleys. This may apply to deep tendon reflexes and to lid and extraocular muscles, which require rapid coherent signals. Slowed conduction velocity, until profound, is unlikely to contribute to weakness.[232]

The most limited region of the peripheral nervous system that may display conduction block and weakness is a single limb, in a few patients in the early stages of GBS. In contrast, early paresthesias affect a considerably larger distribution—usually bilateral—suggesting the two major characteristics of GBS have different electrophysiologic mechanisms (see later and Table 7–6). Models of demyelination[1261] are more successful in explaining distal paresthesias (see farther on) than the variable regional distribution of weakness. Regional weakness is presumably due to areas of demyelination and block corresponding to regions of more intense inflammation in certain roots, trunks, or nerves. Some regional biases could be due to a lower threshold for neuromuscular failure in certain motor units.

PARESTHESIAS AND SENSORY LOSS

Paresthesias in the fingers and toes are the initial symptom in more than half of patients with GBS, specifically a "pins-and-needles" or "prickling" sensation. Symptoms progress proximally over several days or weeks but generally remain distal to the wrists and ankles. Paresthesias were eventually present in 72% of patients in the MGH retrospective series (see Table 7–3) and in more than 90% of other series.[501] Sensory symptoms often precede weakness by 1 or 2 days, and, more than weakness, paresthesias truly ascend (though Landry used the term to denote motor progression). Despite difficulty articulating the quality of paresthesias, patients are very definite about their presence or absence; for example, patients with a purely motor form of GBS emphatically deny paresthesias. Even complete immobilization from quadriplegia is not associated with positive sensory complaints. The relationship between the distribution of paresthesias and the pattern of limb weakness is inconsistent, and many cases in the MGH experience have had initially crossed or alternating motor and sensory features.

The paresthesias of GBS most frequently begin as a vague pins-and-needles feeling—a tingling—akin to sensation in a limb that is beginning to "awaken" after "falling asleep" from pressure. Other descriptions from our patients include the following: "like there's no circulation," "like being out on a cold day without gloves," "tight skin" (common), "shoes too tight," "a light numbness," "the very end when your leg wakes up from falling asleep." Occasionally there is a transitional "electric buzzing" or stinging sensation. Within several days or during recovery, the tingling may be replaced by stronger, coarser, or more discrete pins and needles, a prickling feeling, momentary punctate sensations, distinct in time and separated by more distance than the finer paresthesias. At this point individual descriptions diverge as a vaguer sense of numbness or a velvety sensation appears, associated with diminished touch intensity. Some patients have described "burning" when the sensory symptoms are fully developed or during recovery from numbness. Later in the course, touch may be dysesthetic or uncommonly painful or burning.[1017] True paresthesias, with a few exceptions, remain distal to the wrists and ankles and are more intense on the palms and soles than on the ventral surfaces. More proximal sensations are usually a numbness or perverted sensation corresponding to sensory loss. As paresthesias progress and sensory loss becomes pronounced, the hands or feet may be described as "dead" or "numb" with less spontaneous tingling, but some positive sensory phenomenon often persists distally, sometimes elicited by stroking the limb. A few patients become averse to bedsheets touching the legs. Formications, a sensation of crawling in the skin, have been described, but only as a transitional sensation in a few MGH patients. Others experience a "wave" of paresthesias that spreads from regions that have been stroked. Spontaneous cold or warm sensations, or the reversal of hot and cold—more typical of marine toxin poisoning—have been reported[591] but must be uncommon. A separate stiffness, not related to immobility and weakness, can be distinguished from paresthesias by a few patients.

Paresthesias are intensified by hyperventilation and occasionally by hypocalcemia induced by the citrate used in plasma exchange. Other maneuvers that often exacerbate the prickling sensation include passive or active limb motion, such as vigorously waving the hand, which produces symptoms distal to the manipulated joint (including the finger joints), or constant pressure on a finger or portion of the hand, which produces coarse paresthesias only in the region under pressure (see farther on for similarities to and differences from postischemic paresthesias). Tinel's sign has been found infrequently. Two patients in the prospective series reported a tight "band" or "belt" circumferentially around one calf, late in the illness.

Compared with symptoms of weakness, sensory symptoms tend to be more symmetric and can be far more focal. The proximal or leading edge of paresthesias may be slightly higher on one side, and we have seen a few exceptional instances of paresthesias well established only in one foot or hand at the onset. Paresthesias are often noticed in one region for hours before spreading. The feet may be symptomatic for several days before the hands. In contradiction to the classic neuropathic pattern of sensory loss predicated on fiber length,[1039] the fingertips usually have paresthesias soon after the feet are affected (i.e., well before symptoms reach the knees).

A few patients have had initial paresthesias in a single finger, most often the third, fourth, or fifth on one side, up to the middle interphalangeal joint, before involving the other fingertips, and then migrating more proximally in tandem. One MGH patient had lateral hypothenar numbness on the first day, without distal fifth finger paresthesias. Patients have occasionally been able to differentiate isolated paresthesias of the great toe before appreciating it in the other toes. A few begin with paresthesias of the sole and ball of the foot rather than the toes.

Facial paresthesias, an uncommon symptom, were reported by single patients each in some series[501,973] and as an eventual symptom in 8% to 29% in other studies.[31,501] These figures are higher than those found in the MGH experience (2%–4%). Paresthesias have usually involved the lips, tip of the nose, and tip of the tongue, but it is not clear if published reports are actually referring to numbness. In advanced cases with profound sensory signs in the limbs, numbness (less often paresthesias) may occur in the earlobes, gums, inner and outer surfaces of the cheeks, and, in only one of the MGH patients, the vertex scalp in a "beanie cap" pattern (C-2 dermatome). Some of these regions are not in distal sensory nerve territories, contrary to the length-dependent relationship of sensory loss in the trigeminal distribution. Pharyngeal paresthesias have not occurred. Occasionally patients have a sensation of the teeth "floating" or feeling mushy. Some have facial stiffness, particularly on the cheek, analogous to Bell's palsy, perhaps because of diminished muscle tone resulting in altered proprioceptive input.

Paresthesias on the trunk, slightly more frequent than facial paresthesias, are still uncommon, particularly at the onset. Some patients with severe limb paresthesias have sensory symptoms on the anterior chest, over the acromion, scapula, breasts, or occasionally the abdomen, near the umbilicus, but not, in the MGH experience, in a typical teardrop-shaped distribution, corresponding to the longest truncal nerves. The back is rarely involved and the symptoms on the anterior trunk, though bilateral, may be patchy and asymmetric. Hypesthesia is usually present in these regions. We have not encountered a truly suspended syringomyelic sensory loss over a large portion of the trunk or a lepromatous type of patchy numbness and sensory loss, but two patients have had a large band of truncal paresthesias.

During the first few days of illness, sensory loss demonstrable by bedside testing has been reported in a small number to approximately half of patients, depending on the time of examination. Dissociation between pronounced sensory symptoms and little or no sensory loss, often commented on in the literature, tends to be an early phenomenon. At the end of a week of illness, most patients except those with a purely motor variant, have diminished distal sensation with careful testing. Extremely high incidences of objective sensory loss have been reported—up to 70%[777]—but this finding has been absent in other series.[1053] A synopsis of a large series[548] found that two thirds of patients eventually had sensory loss, half of these proprioceptive. Definite pallanesthesia in the feet has been reported in approximately 15% of patients on first examination. Sixty-two percent of patients in the MGH retrospective series eventually had definite sensory loss, mostly a raised threshold for vibration perception. At least two-thirds of prospectively studied MGH patients had sensory loss when carefully tested in the first week. Most patients have a graded diminution of vibration sense in the feet and legs, in severe cases extending to the hips.[751] Severe sensory loss in the legs only rarely coexists with normal sensation in the hands, though milder cases may show this pattern.

Sensation associated with large fiber conduction is most affected, but thermal and pinprick sensation are often diminished distally if vibration and joint position sense are severely affected. One third of retrospective and prospective patients had loss of pinprick sensation distally, but only 2% without associated pallanesthesia.

Analgesia on the limbs and trunk with a discrete sensory level simulating spinal cord disease has been reported.[501, 898a, 973] Three patients in the prospective MGH series had a transient sensory level on the trunk, but the upper level, rather than being sharply demarcated, delimited a more ambiguous change in the perception of pinprick. Patients were unaware of the level until it was elicited by examination. A well studied case report had a perivenular lymphocytic infiltrate at the upper thoracic spinal cord corresonding to hypalgesia below the nipples.[898a] (see Chapter 8.) Infrequent "band" tightness around the thorax is traditionally associated with demyelination of the posterior columns and may be due to the same type of lesion in GBS. However, these patients invariably have severe sensory signs and symptoms attributable to their GBS, suggesting that a bandlike sensation might also result from neuropathy.

Notable differences between the distribution of paresthesias and the centripetal sensory loss in GBS suggest that they result from different mechanisms. First, paresthesias appear in the fingers before they reach the knees. Second, as noted above, the truncal and facial paresthesias do not occur in the end territories of corresponding nerves. Finally, paresthesias occur earlier than sensory loss and may persist without sensory loss in a few patients; they are not simply a manifestation of mild sensory loss. Associated vibration sensory loss may be absent or profound; there is no relation to the severity or distribution of paresthesias.

Induced paresthesias from ischemia may be useful in understanding GBS paresthesias. The physiology of postischemic paresthesias has been investigated by microneurographic recording from nerves after tourniquet release.[870] Earlier classic reports[420,796] demonstrated spontaneous sensory nerve fiber discharges that correspond to pins-and-needles sensations. Larger myelinated fibers apparently participated in ectopic impulse generation all along the sensory nerve (see Table 7–6). Ectopic discharges correlated temporally with the subjects' report of a burning sensation after release of ischemia with the recording of prolonged high-frequency discharges, and of prickling or tingling (more typical of GBS) with shorter repetitive electrical bursts. Another, less well-defined sensation, *pseudocramp*, a feeling of tension or of the fingers or toes being strongly flexed, may result from discharges in large fibers originating in Golgi's tendon or other sensory organs.[693] The various paresthesias have been postulated to result from ectopic discharges in fibers originating in different peripheral receptor organs.[870] The sensory end organs themselves are not essential for postischemic paresthesias.[870]

Demyelination in sensory fibers may cause similar spontaneous firing along the sensory unit. Some experimental models of peripheral demyelination[165] and the ventral roots of dysmyelinated mice[970] show ectopic activity at isolated sites. GBS patients describe a feeling of the hand "awakening" after "falling asleep," suggesting a relationship to tourniquet-induced ischemic paresthesias. The spectrum of tingling, prickling, buzzing, and tightness located beyond the wrist and ankle, and a predilection for the palm and soles, are all reported both in GBS and in tourniquet experiments. Hyperventilation and motion enhancement of paresthesias in GBS may be nonspecific phenomena, but they match the experimentally induced variety. However, one clinical feature suggesting that the paresthesias of GBS differ from the postischemic variety is the infrequency of Tinel's sign in GBS (the sign indicates a lowered threshold for mechanical excitability).

If ectopic activity causes the paresthetic sensations of GBS, there should be a correspondence between paresthesias and specific sensory end organs that supply large IA afferent fibers. One possible scheme would connect tingling with fibers from Merkel's disks or Meissner's corpuscles subserving fine touch, tightness with pacinian and Golgi-Mazzoni organs subserving pressure, prickling with firing from individual Meissner's corpuscles that localize touch, and buzzing with vibration sense receptors, not yet fully defined. Complex paresthesias might be a combination of several fundamental ones. Only two of the MGH patients have complained of the sensation of spontaneous motion of a limb and two have expressed a feeling that movement would induce pain (pseudocramp). These similarities allow only the speculation that paresthesias of GBS are due to increased spontaneous firing along the sensory nerve (see Table 7–6).

To test this hypothesis, a tourniquet was applied to the upper arm for 10 minutes in several GBS patients in the MGH series. This brief period does not usually induce a feeling of being "asleep," but with release of the tourniquet most patients develop the expected sequence of thermal paresthesias (6 to 10 seconds after release), followed by brief "buzzing," then spontaneous "prickling" or tingling, beginning 2 to 3½ minutes after release and persisting for 3 to 6 minutes (Fig. 7–1). The most informative results have been (1) persistence of spontaneous GBS paresthesias during ischemia and (2) a consistent reduction in GBS paresthesias for several minutes after the postischemic prickling ceases. The ectopic activity associated with release of nerve ischemia may have interfered (collided) with the spontaneous ectopic activity derived from demyelination, as occurs in a electrophysiologic collision study. An alternative explanation, that the ischemia created a temporary nerve block in sensory fibers, seems unlikely because the nerve was able to conduct ectopic impulses in the postischemic period and the spontaneous paresthesias persisted through most of ischemia.

Sensory loss in GBS generally follows a neuropathic "glove-and-stocking" pat-

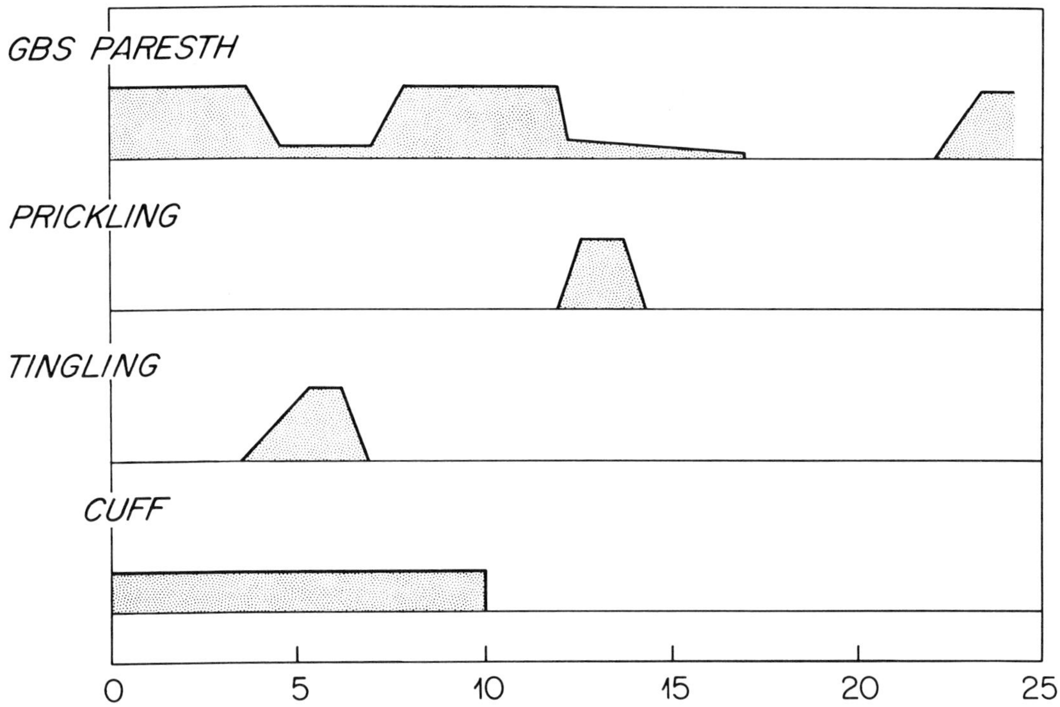

Figure 7–1. Pattern of postischemic paresthesias in a patient with GBS. Spontaneous paresthesias from the illness, shown in the top panel, are muted after release of the brachial cuff.

tern probably due to cumulative conduction blocks in sensory fibers[1039] (see Table 7–6). Sensory conduction block is by nature more difficult than motor block to demonstrate by clinical electrophysiologic techniques. The preferential disruption of large fiber sensation corresponds to early large and intermediate fiber block from demyelination. Those few patients with analgesia presumably have demyelination of pain fibers or axonal disruption in small fibers.

DIMINISHED TENDON REFLEXES

Areflexia, a core feature of GBS, may sometimes be delayed until weakness and paresthesias are well developed (see Tables 7–1 and 7–2). When the legs are weaker than the arms, the leg reflexes tend to be lost first. Reflexes are almost always lost by the time the limbs are too weak to resist gravity. A closer concordance existed between early areflexia and severe sensory symptoms than with weakness in the MGH patients, although other researchers have proposed the opposite. There are undoubtedly patients whose reflexes, though muted, persist for much of the initial illness, but retention of all reflexes throughout the course is very uncommon. The major importance of early reflex loss is emphasized by the frequency with which young patients with acral paresthesias are discharged from an emergency room with a diagnosis of anxiety, only to return with generalized weakness and respiratory failure. Attention to the depressed reflexes prevent this error.

In both the retrospective and prospective MGH series, approximately 65% of patients were entirely areflexic on admission and 10% lost reflexes only in the weakest limbs; however, 90% had at least absent ankle reflexes and 80%, absent knee reflexes (see Table 7–3). In one large series,[1122] complete areflexia was reported early in the illness in only approximately 25%, absent reflexes in the legs with normal or diminshed arm reflexes in 44%, reduced but present reflexes in all limbs in 10%, and other combinations in the remainder. The biceps reflex has been most commonly spared in the MGH patients. A subacute peripheral neuropathy with persistently spared reflexes should direct attention to sarcoidosis, paraproteinemic neuropathy, or carcinomatous meningitis, all of which may otherwise mimic GBS (see Chapter 14). The jaw (masseter) reflex has not been studied systematically, but it is lost early in most patients and is eventually unobtainable whether or not there is facial or masseter weakness.

"Reflex loss" in many of the early papers on Landry's paralysis (and some on GBS) referred to numerous eponymic superficial reflex signs. Superficial reflexes are typically absent once GBS is fully developed. Half of the 48 patients with information recorded in the retrospective series had absent abdominal reflexes, similar to other reports.[1291] Babinski's sign has been reported in very few patients in most large series; an extreme incidence of 5 of 100 patients (in one patient explained by Friedreich's ataxia) occurred in one series.[1291] The interpretation of central nervous system signs in GBS is discussed in Chapter 8.

The electrophysiologic cause of reflex loss is uncertain but evidence supports dispersion and desynchronization of the high-frequency synchronized afferent volley necessary to trigger the monosynaptic arc (see Table 7–6). Heterogeneous slowing or block in some large IA afferents would mute reflexes before producing almost any other signs. Slowing of nerve conduction appears too late to alone explain areflexia, and in any case must be profound to desynchronize an afferent volley. Preservation of normal power in areflexic limbs belies a lesion in efferent fibers as the cause of areflexia. Areflexia in the pure motor GBS variant, and loss of the jaw reflex, however, are not easily explained (since facial paresthesias or numbness are rare). Reflexes are often lost when electrophysiologic tests show isolated proximal motor conduction block (see Chapter 13).

In contrast to tendon areflexia, almost all patients with arm weakness have a preserved or exaggerated fascicular muscle contraction in response to direct percussion (Fig. 7–2). This response, also present in many healthy individuals, is most easily elicited by a

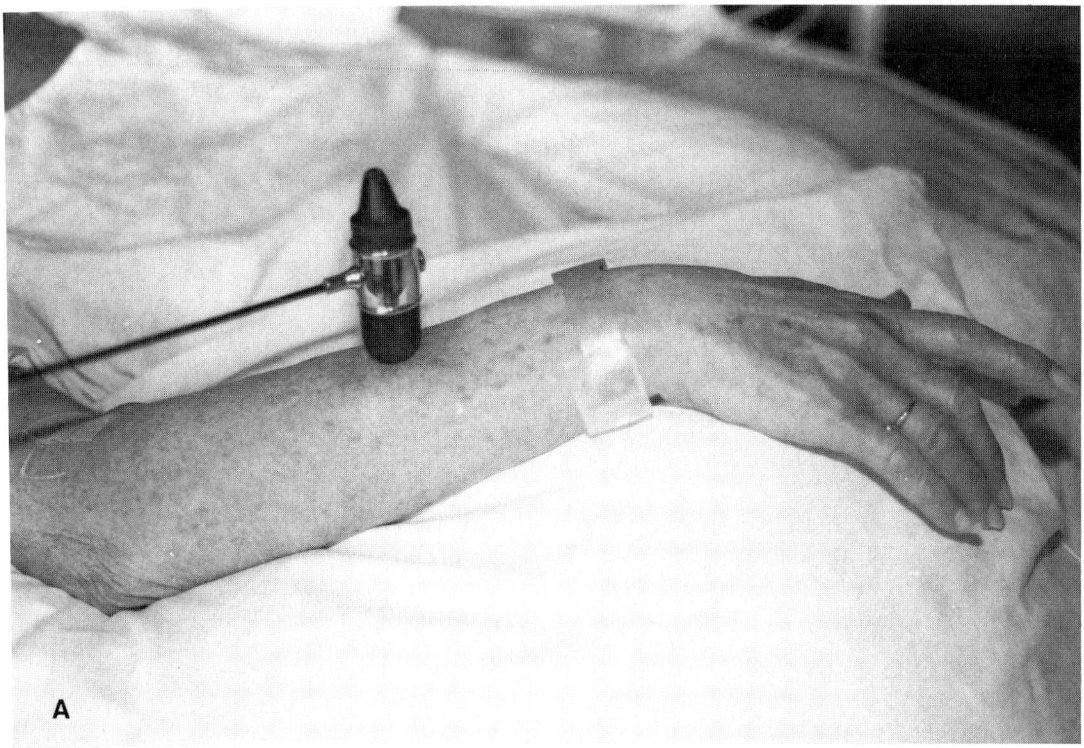

A

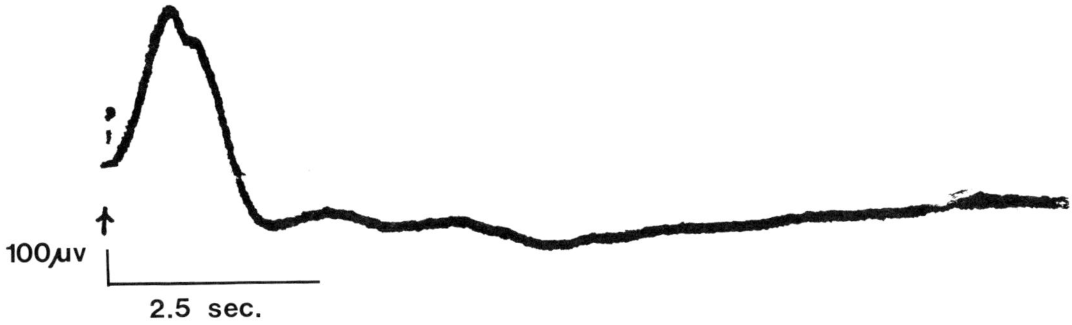

B

Figure 7–2. *A*, Method of eliciting a direct fascicular contraction by striking the long finger extensors in the forearm. Each finger can be made to extend. This mechanical response contrasts with tendon areflexia. *B*, Electrical recording of *A* tendon. The arrow and stimulus artifact are followed in 1 to 3 milliseconds by muscle contraction, too fast for a reflex response.

rapid forceful tap using a small-headed hammer, over the middle of the relaxed brachioradialis muscle, with the patient's forearm pronated. This produces contraction of a fascicle under the percussion or extension of a single finger. A similar direct muscular response can be obtained, albeit less consistently, in the anterior tibialis or quadriceps femoris. The latency of contraction is approximately 3 to 5 milliseconds, far too fast to represent a tendon reflex (see Fig. 7–2). This response has not been present as consistently in other neuropathies or in myasthenia gravis. It is occasionally mistaken for a preserved brachioradialis tendon reflex in GBS. The "reactive myotonia" described in early papers[1299] may have connoted this direct-percussion response. The reaction is probably not pathologic, but rather represents the exposure of the fascicular contraction in the absence of reflex muscle contraction.

PAIN

Pain was prominently recorded in early descriptions by Landry,[668,669] Guillain and co-workers,[466,467] and Haymaker and Kernohan,[501] but it has been relatively neglected subsequently. Some textbooks claim it is rare in GBS and suggests another type of neuropathy. Most major series report pain in 15% to 50% of patients but do not further differentiate it (see Tables 7–1 and 7–2). In contrast, 60% to 70% of MGH patients had pain in one of three forms, in order of frequency: (1) symmetric deep aching in the large muscles of the hips, upper legs, and back; (2) asymmetric sciatica with Lasègue's sign; and (3) foot or hand pain associated with intense paresthesias or burning.[1008] Acute, excruciating mid-line thoracic back pain at the onset of illness ("le coup de poignard"), a rare phenomenon more typical of spinal subarachnoid-subdural hemorrhages, occurred in two patients in the prospective series.[1008]

Patients describe the most common pain as a "charley horse," or use similar terms suggesting an internal muscular discomfort after strain or exercise, at times coupled with stiffness ("like I bowled all day"; "as if I moved all the furniture in my house"; "like I hadn't exercised in a long time"). The buttocks, quadriceps, lower back, hamstrings, and less often trapezeii, deltoids, posterior neck, and gastrocnemius regions are affected. We have seen four patients with intense muscular pain and two whose sciatica preceded weakness by several days to a week, leading to hospitilization for presumed disc or rheumatologic disease. The pain may be initially more intense in one limb, but is otherwise relatively symmetric in the axial muscles, and worse in the evening, usually from 10 PM to 2 AM. Motion does not have a consistent effect on the pain (see Chapter 16 for details of pain management).

Radicular pain, usually in the form of sciatica, can coexist with the aching pain in large proximal muscles or may occur independently. Patients usually become aware of it when bending over. It can be elicited by straight leg raising in some patients who do not have spontaneous pain. One MGH patient had radicular pain originating in the lower neck and radiating into the arms and another had pain in the distribution of the femoral nerve, but the discomfort was less severe and briefer than seen in patients with sciatica. Patients have rarely reported radicular pain in the thorax or abdomen, more typically associated with diabetes or herpes zoster.[501] One MGH patient was thought to have acute abdominal processes on the basis of transient truncal radicular pain, and a similar patient has been reported.[1297]

Painful dysesthesias, discussed earlier, are more prominent later in the course of the disease and are not often a management problem. Immobilized patients also develop periarticular stiffness that is relieved by massage or slow passive movement. Three MGH patients had this type of pain precipitated by steroid withdrawal. Lancinating limb pain, though commented on by a few patients, has been rare. A tight "band" or circumferential tightness around the low calf or forearm, more typical of spinal cord lesions in multiple sclerosis, has occurred as a late phenomenon in a few patients. It may be a form of paresthesia (see earlier). We have not encountered facial, ocular, or head pain as a direct result of GBS.

The common muscular GBS pain has not been related to other neuropathic signs or specific features of the illness, except perhaps that most affected patients become bedridden and many have an elevated serum creatine phosphokinase (CPK) concentration.[1017] There is no unifying electrophysiologic explanation for the muscular pain. It is unlike true paresthesia or pseudocramp; nevertheless, it may derive from spontaneous ectopic firing of intermediate-sized fibers originating from receptors for deep pain.

PROGRESSION OF GBS

Advancing weakness and paresthesias are requisites for the diagnosis of GBS but the acceptable time limits of progression are somewhat arbitrary. Table 7–7 and Figure 7–3 summarize the intervals from onset of symptoms to stabilization or plateau in several series (including that of the MGH). Most patients worsen over 1 to 2 weeks, some for up to 4 weeks, and a few are quadriplegic within a day or two; anything but several hours of progression is then difficult to appreciate. In a few patients, there is a temporary halt in progression, sometimes followed by rapid worsening over several days. Transient spontaneous improvement in power or paresthesias followed by further worsening does not occur, except in relation to plasma exchange or steroid treatment (see Chapter 15). Progression therefore usually continues steadily until a plateau is reached. The subsequent courses of many patients with halting or other unusual temporal courses have been most consistent with chronic inflammatory demyelinating polyneuropathy (CIDP) or a paraneoplastic neuropathy. Patients who continue to worsen

Table 7–8 MAXIMUM MOTOR DEFICIT* (N = 169)

Deficit	*No. of Cases (%)*
Quadriplegic	53 (31)
Bed- or chair-bound	53 (31)
Has difficulty walking	19 (11)
Walks unassisted	44 (26)

*Retrospective MGH Series.

Table 7–7 INTERVAL TO MAXIMAL WEAKNESS (PLATEAU)

Series, Year	*No. of Patients*	*Interval*	*Range*	*Duration of Plateau*
Marshall,[751] 1963	35	74% within 7 days	1–42 days (mean 5.6 days)	—
Wiederholt et al.,[1278] 1964	97	79% 1–25 days	—	69% 2–17 days
Ravn,[973] 1967	127	95% <25 days	1–46 days (mean 12 days)	1–69 days (mean 9 days)
Loffel et al.,[714] 1977	123	—	Mean 12 days	—
Andersson and Siden,[31] 1982	60	87% <20 days	2–42 days	2–60 days
Winer et al.,[1291] 1988	100	34% 7 days 70% 14 days 84% 21 days 92% 28 days	Few hr–44 days	48% >21 days 52% <21 days
Retrospective MGH, Series, 1962–1979	169	38% 7 days 77% 14 days 92% 21 days 95% 28 days	1–49 days (mean 12 days)	1–90 days (mean 15 days) 71% <2 wk 85% <4 wk

after 4 weeks will usually, but not invariably, have a chronic progressive or relapsing course (see Chapter 10). Steroids may cause fluctuations and prolonged duration of worsening, also making distinctions between acute GBS and CIDP difficult.

Peak disability in the MGH series, shown in Table 7–8, is discussed further in Chapter 18. Improvement in strength usually begins after a latent or plateau period of several days to 2 weeks, but sometimes of only 1 or 2 days—too brief to be appreciated (see Table 7–7). The overall period from onset to the end of the plateau phase, shown in Figure 7–4 (time to improvement), correlates with the frequency of residual deficits as discussed in Chapter 18.

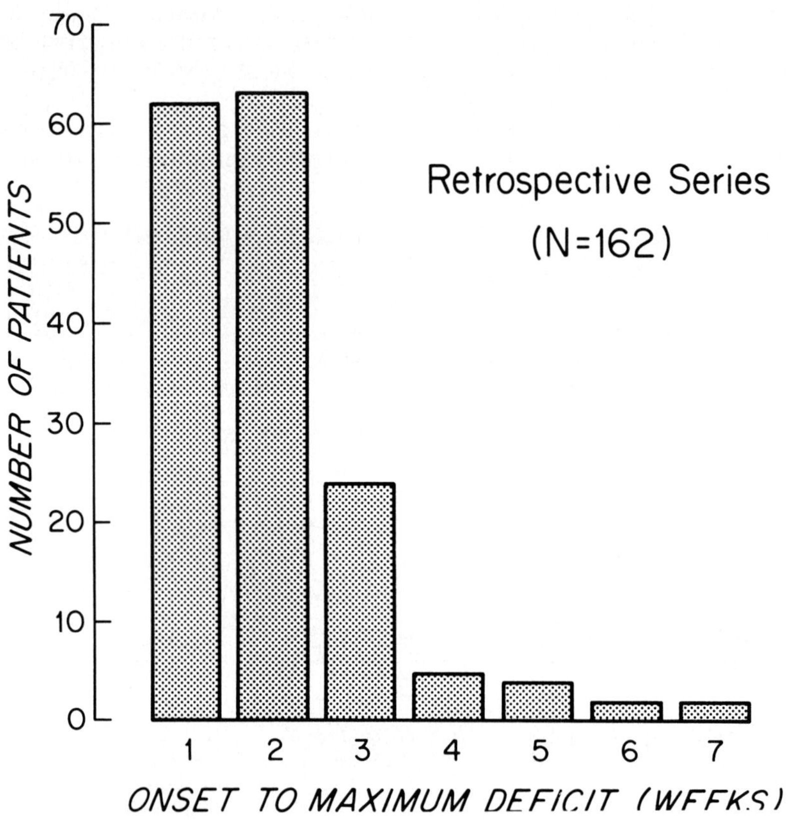

Figure 7–3. Time from first symptoms of GBS to cessation of clinical worsening (onset of plateau phase) in the MGH retrospective series.

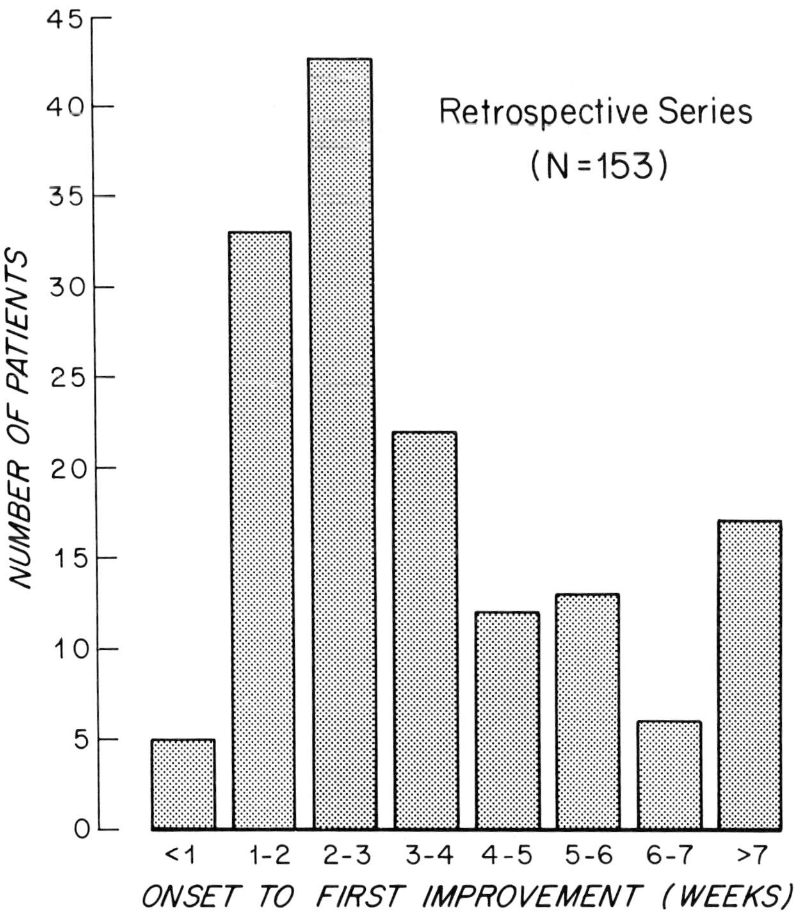

Figure 7–4. Time from onset of illness to onset of improvement (end of plateau phase) in the MGH retrospective series.

UNUSUAL CLINICAL FEATURES IN OTHERWISE TYPICAL CASES

Table 7–9 lists some unusual features of GBS not discussed in other sections. Some occur sporadically in otherwise typical cases and must be considered idiosyncratic rather than signs of a consistent area or type of inflammatory demyelination. Others are anecdotal, mentioned once in the literature without detail, and may be spurious. Gait or limb ataxia, present in approximately 5% of cases, is discussed in relation to Fisher's syndrome in Chapter 8.

Table 7–9 UNUSUAL FEATURES IN TYPICAL GBS

Rare	*Unexplained*
Facial myokymia	Dystonia and action myoclonus
Hearing loss	Muscular fasciculations
Meningeal signs	Mental changes
Headache	Convulsions
Priapism	Limb edema
Vocal cord paralysis	

Several patients with facial palsy have had myokymia beginning early in the illness, most often bilaterally[246,580,1227,1258] but occasionally unilaterally.[511] One patient[1227] had no central lesions at autopsy. Hearing loss, rare in GBS, has occurred acutely in patients with other severe cranial nerve deficits.[842] In the MGH patients, deafness occurred more frequently as a result of serous otitis due to an endotracheal tube. Meningismus and headache have been described in approximately 10% of patients in some large series,[501,714,777] generally without a CSF cellular reaction. One MGH patient in the prospective series had minimal neck stiffness; other patients described muscular neck achiness typical of GBS but had no true flexion-induced pain or limitation. Priapism has been reported once,[501] and vocal cord paralysis without other cranial nerve abnormalities has been mentioned several times in the literature.[765,1291] Dystonia has been reported in two patients,[714] and "action myoclonus" in one.[714] None of these was seen in the MGH series. Fasciculations occurred in seven patients in one series[1299] who had a rapid onset of quadriparesis, but the interval from onset was not clear; fasciculations are not mentioned prominently in other series.

Drowsiness, stupor, convulsions, or electroencephalogram (EEG) abnormalities have been listed in many older series, implying that they resulted directly from GBS; alternative explanations, however, were not explored. A recent prospective series[1291] did not mention changes in levels of consciousness. In the MGH retrospective series, 14% of patients experienced diminished consciousness at some time in the course of their disease, but all were hyponatremic, hypercarbic, or medicated with sedative drugs at the time. One patient in the retrospective series had an unexplained convulsion with normal EEG and computed tomography (CT) examinations. Subsequent EEGs on nine typical patients revealed no abnormality. Limb edema, mentioned in an older series,[501] did not occur in the MGH experience, although some patients complained of a "swollen" sensation in regions with paresthesias.

OPHTHALMOPLEGIA AND OTHER OCULAR SIGNS

The varied and intriguing neuro-ophthalmologic signs in GBS occur less frequently than limb weakness but nonetheless are important features of the typical illness. Ophthalmoplegia as a component of GBS was first pointed out in 1902 by Culbertson[231] in Landry's paralysis, and was discussed specifically by others more recently.* Ophthalmoplegia occurs in one of two forms: as complete or virtually complete external ophthalmoplegia as a major feature of Fisher's syndrome (see Chapter 8), or as a prominent sign in some cases of typical, usually severe, GBS (and perhaps as an isolated postinfectious oculomotor neuropathy, see later). The clinical features of ophthalmoplegia alone do not distinguish the syndromes. In a few cases of generalized GBS, eye movement abnormalities have preceded limb weakness by one to several days. More often, however, the limb weakness evolves simultaneously or before diplopia.

Eye Movement Abnormalities

The reported incidences of eye movement abnormalities in several large series of GBS is shown in Table 7–10. A few patients with mild or moderate generalized GBS will have incomplete ophthalmoparesis. Approximately 10% to 20% of patients will have oculomotor paresis at some time in their course. In retrospective and prospective series, 13% and 28% of patients with GBS had ophthalmoparesis and 3% and 5% had ophthalmoplegia, respectively. The

*See references 45, 54, 175, 185, 211a, 404, 405, 437, 479, 563, 751, 759, 829, 843, 925, and 1219.

Table 7–10 NEURO-OPHTHALMIC SIGNS IN LARGE SERIES OF ACUTE GBS

Series, Year	*No. of Patients*	*III, IV, VI Paresis (%)*	*Papilledema (%)*	*Optic Neuritis*	*Nystagmus (%)*
Haymaker and Kernohan,[501] 1949	50 (fatal)	12 (24)	2 (4)	0	3 (6)
Marshall,[751] 1963	35	6 (17)	0	0	0
Wiederholt et al.,[1278] 1964	97	5 (5)	0	0	0
Castaigne et al.,[179] 1966	457	45 (10)	0	0	5 (1)
McFarland and Heller,[777] 1966	100	13 (13)	0	0	7 (7)
Ravn,[973] 1967	127	9 (7)	0	0	0
Samantray et al.,[1053] 1977	302	5 (2)	4 (1)	0	0
GBS Study Group,[469] 1985	239	40 (17)	2 (1)	0	0
Winer et al.,[1291] 1988	100	13 (13)	1 (1)	0	0
Retrospective MGH Series, 1962–1979	169	21 (13) (5 complete)	5 (3)	0	0
Prospective MGH Series, 1979–1988	120	32 (28)	2 (2)	0	2 (2)

most common limitation of eye movement early in the illness was an a symmetric sixth nerve paresis, sometimes simulating "divergence paresis," with horizontal diplopia at a distance. Most often, when horizontal eye movement is affected on one side, there is similar but unequal weakness on the other side. Pure and complete unilateral third or sixth nerve paresis with generalized limb weakness was not seen in the MGH series. Once apparent, ophthalmoplegia tends to evolve to its worst point over several days, a shorter period of progression than for limb weakness.

As complete ophthalmoplegia improves, vertical gaze commonly begins to recover before horizontal gaze. Complete loss or recovery of versions in one direction (horizontal or vertical) alone has been alluded to but rarely well documented.[211a,829] The section on Fisher's syndrome discusses a (pseudo) internuculear ophthalmoplegia with adductor paresis and abducting nystagmus,[58,1170,1266,1312] rebound nystagmus,[790] preserved Bell's phenomenon wth absent upgaze,[563] and other apparent CNS signs. Careful examination during evolution and recovery discloses that ophthalmoparesis is usually dissociated between the globes, though on casual observation versions may appear conjugate. Better elevation of the globes with forced eye closure (Bell's phenomenon) than with voluntary attempts at upgaze[563,1312] was common in MGH patients. Nystagmus has been reported rarely, sometimes during recovery from complete ophthalmoplegia.[501,777] The few instances of nystagmus in MGH patients have been at end-points of gaze, or in the context of CNS depressant medications, rather than with other ocular or cerebellar signs.

Isolated third nerve palsy has been mentioned.[413,659] There are other rare cases of areflexia without weakness, and islated ophthalmoplegia or single oculomotor nerve dysfunction, most often involving the third nerve.* There may be similar cases involving only the sixth nerve.[630] None of the reported cases were associated with ataxia, but they may nevertheless have been similar to Fisher's syndrome. These virtually isolated palsies have been attributed to a postinfectious inflammatory process and may represent an extreme of the spectrum of ophthalmoplegia due to GBS, but too few cases have been studied to establish the clinical bound-

*See references 104, 185, 479, 1114, and 1166.

aries of a purely ophthalmoplegic form of GBS.

Several cases of relapsing ophthalmoplegia with a chronic demyelinating neuropathy have been reported.[280,590] Some of these cases represent a relapsing form of Fisher syndrome.

Eye movement recordings in patients with ophthalmoplegia and GBS have shown a variety of complex saccadic "fatigue" phenomena, interpreted as the result of intermittent peripheral conduction block.[358] In Fisher's syndrome, certain electro-oculographic findings have been attributed to combinations of central and peripheral lesions.[790,1312] Because the interpretation of the oculographic findings has not been validated, the electrophysiologic evidence for brainstem disease is uncertain (see Chapter 8).

Pupillary Abnormalities

Most patients with pupillary abnormalities have had severe ophthalmoparesis with ptosis. Some have described light-fixed, dilated pupils in GBS.[79,928] In contrast, fewer than half of the patients reported in the literature with ophthalmoplegia have had associated pupillary abnormalities. Abnormal pupils in patients with ophthalmoplegia are usually assymetrically dilated, round, and unreactive to light. Light-near dissociation during recovery of dilated and fixed pupils has been reported, persisting years after Fisher's syndrome. Rare patients have been reported with light and near paralysis of the pupils in association with areflexia but with normal ocular movements.[1282] One patient,[1266] in an intriguing case similar to Fisher's syndrome, had reversible ataxia, areflexia, and fixed pupillary dilation but no ophthalmoplegia. During recovery there was slight accommodation and absent light response. Pharmacologic testing suggested combined postganglionic parasympathetic and sympathetic lesions. A patient has also been described with bilateral Argyll Robertson–type pupils.[890] The pupils are generally normal in patients with dysautonomia as a component of generalized GBS. One MGH patient, however, had tonic pupils and generalized autonomic neuropathy from GBS. In contrast, pupillary abnormalities occur frequently in pure pandysautonomia (see Chapter 8). This disparity may reflect, in part, a lack of attention to the pupils in GBS cases without ophthalmoplegia.

Lid Abnormalities

Almost all patients with severe restriction of eye movements have ptosis, sometimes complete. (Rare exceptions without ptosis have been suggested as evidence of a central lesion.) At times, concomitant facial weakness minimizes the appearance of ptosis. A common, though trivial, eye finding is widening of the palpebral fissure due to incomplete lid closure from facial weakness, present in 60% to 85% of typical cases. Ptosis has occurred in virtually all patients with complete ophthalmoplegia.

Approximately 8% of patients with generalized weakness in the MGH prospective series had incomplete ptosis without ophthalmoparesis or pupillary abnormalities (Fig. 7–5).[1008] Ptosis may rarely precede generalized weakness.[700] We have observed several instances where brief but definite improvement of ptosis has occurred with the intramuscular administration of 1.5 mg neostigmine methylsulfate. Ptosis has been particularly common in patients with isolated cervico-brachial-pharyngeal weakness and upper limb areflexia (see Chapter 8).[1008]

Lid lag, noted in a few cases of GBS, has been attributed indirectly to facial weakness. Several authors have hypothesized that corneal exposure produces constant attempts at blinking, resulting in lid elevation from the associated Bell's phenomenon.[598,840] So-called "upper lid jerks" noted in Fisher's syndrome may have a similar mechanism to lid lag.[1052]

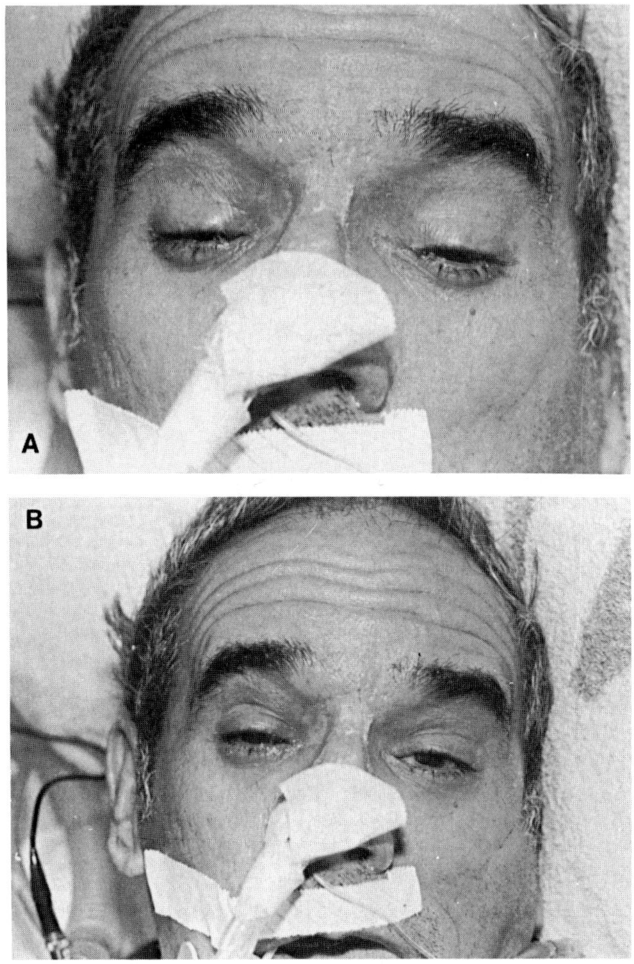

Figure 7–5. Ptosis in GBS is more frequent than commonly appreciated. It may be profound, as in this patient who can barely elevate his eyelids by lifting his forehead and eyebrows, in the absence of much facial weakness or any ophthalmoplegia. (From Ropper,[1008] p. 1151, with permission.)

Pathology in Cases with Ophthalmoplegia

Dehaene and associates[258] reported the definitive autopsy study of a patient with ophthalmoplegia and Fisher's syndrome, ptosis, and unreactive pupils. They found demyelination and inflammation of oculomotor nerves; there were no primary central nervous system lesions. Other cases with ophthalmoplegia have had similar findings, with only secondary chromatolytic changes in oculomotor neurons.[104,455,921]

Optic Neuritis

Several instances of bilateral, and less often unilateral, retrobulbar optic neuritis have accompanied typical GBS* and Fisher's syndrome.[801] A case of bilateral optic nerve swelling also was reported.[91] One of the most interesting instances of optic neuropathy, confirmed by prolonged latencies of visual evoked potentials, occurred with

*See references 298, 659, 755, 825, 855, 898a, 1208, and 1294.

an illness simulating Fisher's syndrome.[1196] Electrophysiologic testing demonstrated a predominantly sensory peripheral neuropathy, but bilateral Babinski's signs and hypoactive (not absent) reflexes complicate interpretation of this case. A case of GBS with 2 days of resolving visual loss[1036] and a case of "encephalomyelitis" with amblyopia[1281] must be classified as of uncertain cause. Optic neuritis did not occur in the MGH retrospective or prospective series and has not been reported in other large series of GBS (see Table 7–6), but it remains the only consistent, albeit very uncommon, evidence of inflammation of CNS myelin in GBS.

Papilledema and Pseudotumor Cerebri

Papilledema with pseudotumor cerebri has been reported in adults and children as an uncommon complication of GBS.† It generally becomes evident after the third week of illness in approximately 1% to 3% of cases in large series of acute GBS (see Table 7–10). The highest reported incidence has been 6% of 126 patients.[968] Papilledema may be relatively more common in children than adults,[735] in patients with lupus erythematosus and GBS, and in those with CIDP (see Chapter 12). Many of the infections that typically precede GBS, including *Mycoplasma*,[416] have been represented among these cases.

Greatly elevated cerebrospinal fluid (CSF) protein level (above 200 mg/dL) usually accompanies the raised CSF pressure and pseudotumor syndrome, particularly in patients with slowly progressive or chronic-relapsing GBS. Elevated CSF protein concentration has been proposed as a unifying hypothesis for pseudotumor in patients with small cranial or spinal tumors and in those with GBS. In contrast, an exceptional case with normal lumbar CSF protein concentration has been reported,[1161] making the role of protein in the pathogenesis of pseudotumor uncertain. Another patient with pseudotumor and CIDP[159] also had a CSF protein level of less than 100 mg/dL. Moreover, protein concentrations in the cervical and ventricular fluid are considerably lower than in lumbar CSF.

One review of the general state of neurology in the early 1950s[267] alluded to a case of pseudotumor, neuropathy, and systemic lupus erythematosus with proteinaceous material in the arachnoid villi. Another report[575] found edema in a brain biopsy specimen and suggested this was the proximate cause of pseudotumor in GBS. Several careful CSF dynamic studies[565,1110] have demonstrated an increased absorptive resistance in CSF pathways, but others,[247,822,1014] using several types of CSF infusion techniques, have failed to demonstrate an increase in resistance large enough to explain the elevation in CSF pressure. The oncotic pressure of CSF protein is not great enough to cause an elevation in CSF pressure. Thus, the mechanism of pseudotumor in GBS is uncertain.

The retrospective MGH series had five cases (3%) with papilledema, most with severe GBS (four of the five had respiratory failure), and CSF pressures well above 200 mm H_2O. In all but one, CSF protein concentration was above 200 mg/dL. Two patients in the prospective series[1014] had papilledema and pseudotumor; the lumbar CSF protein in one was 727 mg/dL early in the course, and CSF pressure was above 500 mm H_2O for 3 weeks. With the exceptions just noted, CSF protein concentration is either causal, or at least a relatively consistent marker, for pseudotumor in GBS. Patients with headache or visual blurring after the third week of illness should be examined for papilledema and perhaps should have CSF pressure measured.

In most patients the pseudotumor subsides as the GBS improves. The problem may be more recalcitrant when a chronic demyelinating neuropathy occurs with persistent and marked ele-

†See references 159, 247, 293, 346, 371, 392, 408, 564, 575, 808, 822, 902, 915, and 1014.

vations of CSF protein. Visual loss can result from the papilledema in GBS, making sequential visual field and evoked response testing helpful. Repeated lumbar punctures or administration of corticosteroids, as in idiopathic pseudotumor, have been useful in reducing CSF pressure.

DYSAUTONOMIA

A wide variety of interesting autonomic nervous system disturbances occur in GBS, most without serious consequences. Dysautonomia is more frequent in patients with severe motor deficits and respiratory failure, but some autonomic disturbances occur in less severe, otherwise commonplace cases. Several authors have addressed the problem of autonomic dysfunction in case studies or selected patient populations, particularly intensive care unit (ICU) patients. Few large unselected series provide enough details to estimate the overall incidence of the various types of autonomic dysfunction;[1108,1200] 65% of patients with typical GBS in our retrospective series had some dysautonomia. Autonomic dysfunction occurs infrequently in Fisher's syndrome or CIDP but is common in predominantly sensory GBS. Severe dysautonomia was reported in all five patients with an axonal form of GBS,[348] although most of MGH patients with similar clinical and electrophysiologic features have not had prominent autonomic abnormalities.

It is advisable to assume that cardiovascular disturbances in GBS are not due to autonomic dysfunction until secondary causes have been excluded, including hypoxia, pulmonary embolus, gastrointestinal bleeding, or fluid-electrolyte disturbances. Numerous cases of sudden death in GBS have been attributed to dysautonomia,* but these probably over-represent the frequency of this drastic complication. In some of these cases, postmortem examinations failed to show an obvious cause of death, leading to an assumption that autonomic cardiovascular failure was responsible. Dysautonomia may have contributed to death in one case in the MGH retrospective series, but no connection could be found in the prospective series. Dysautonomia usually resolves as other features of GBS improve, but blood pressure lability may persist for several weeks or longer.

*See references 52, 75, 105, 122, 137, 143, 199, 209, 354, 501, 515, 524, 600, 655, 751, 761, 830, 888, 968, 1165, and 1291.

Hypertension

The incidence of hypertension in GBS varies from 5% to 61% in various series,[697] partly depending on the criteria for diagnosis (Table 7–11). In the retrospective MGH series, excluding patients with preexisting hypertension, 24% had intermittent or paroxysmal hypertension and 3% had sustained hypertension (diastolic pressures greater than 90 mm Hg and systolic pressures greater than 140 mm Hg on at least five occasions, or continuously). Paroxysmal hypertension was almost always associated with quadriplegia and respiratory failure and often occurs in combination with orthostatic hypotension (12 of 40 patients in the retrospective series).

Hypertension in GBS has occasionally been so severe or paroxysmal that pheochromocytoma has been suspected.[168,812,984] Extremes of blood pressure (BP) elevation in patients with GBS have been tentatively associated with subarachnoid hemorrhage,[137,250] seizures, increased intracranial pressure and papilledema,[247] and, possibly, neurogenic pulmonary edema,[137] all in single or sporadic cases. One of the best-documented cases[784] demonstrated a brief hypertensive encephalopathy and seizures in a 4-year-old boy.

One study of hemodynamic abnormalities in dysautonomia[303] showed a slightly elevated peripheral vascular resistance, cardiac output, and stroke index during hypertension in a GBS pa-

Table 7–11 BLOOD PRESSURE CHANGES IN LARGE GBS SERIES

Series, Year	*No. of Patients*	*Hypotension (%)*	*Hypertension (%)*
Chuttani et al.,[199] 1968	63	0	37
Gecow and Pawela,[396] 1971	83	0	12
Goulon et al.,[426] 1975	172	2	14
Raphael et al.,[968] 1986	223	0	43
GBS Study Group,[469] 1985	245	13	9
de Jager,[260] 1988	57	26	79
Retrospective MGH Series, 1962–1979	169	19	27
Prospective MGH Series, 1979–1988	120	3	5

tient. CSF levels of 5-HIAA and HVA were high, suggesting that sympathetic overactivity led to an elevated peripheral vascular resistance.[1231] In another report,[243] a patient with mild hypertension between episodes of profound hypotension had parallel elevation of systemic vascular resistance (SVR) and blood pressure. An MGH patient, detailed later,[1020] had simultaneous marked elevations in SVR and cardiac output with minimal, if any, tachycardia during hypertension.

The precise mechanisms of disordered blood pressure control are not known, but some evidence favors an afferent baroreflex abnormality as the cause of hypertension. A number of physiologic observations in GBS have been compatible with disinhibition of central cardiopressor systems, owing to reduction of afferent input from baroreceptors. One study[968] has correlated cardiac dysautonomia and disturbed deep sensibility, suggesting a role for afferent dysfunction. Baroreceptor sensitivity has also been shown to be reduced, probably on the basis of an afferent lesion.[247,812,1206] Microneurographic techniques have demonstrated increased muscle sympathetic activity with maintenance of the normal fluctuations of sympathetic bursts that are coupled to the cardiac rhythm.[341] Similar increases in muscle sympathetic activity occurred in normal subjects with bilateral lidocaine blockade of the vagus and glossopharyngeal nerves, but, unlike the situation in GBS, the cardiac rhythmicity of sympathetic impulses was lost.[342]

The autonomic baroreflexes play an insignificant role in long-term blood pressure regulation but are the major buffers for acute pressure changes. In animals, baroreceptor denervation does not change the summated average daily BP, but it does allow wide pressure deviations with alternating hypotension and hypertension. The most dramatic cardiovascular dysautonomias, precipitous hypertension alternating with periods of hypotension, are probably due, in part, to loss of this baroreflex buffering. An abnormal BP rise in response to pressor agents in patients with GBS[105,137,688,1267] may reflect loss of the normal buffering capacity of the baroreflexes rather than true denervation hypersensitivity (see farther on). Impaired vasodilatation in response to heating in GBS patients[36] reflect an inappropriately raised systemic vascular resistance, but this does not explain hypertension in the presence of intact baroreflexes.

Another mechanism that could potentially cause hypertension in GBS patients is an elevated venous renin level, reported with[984,1306] and without abnormalities of circulating catecholamines.[680,1141] Several investigators* have reported elevated levels of plasma catecholamines or their urinary metabolites in patients with GBS and hypertension; however, others[680,697,1141] have reported normal urinary catecholamine metabolites. One patient, discussed later, had greatly elevated plasma ca-

*See references 10, 168, 247, 250, 303, 426, 812, 984, 1231, and 1306.

techolamine concentrations during periods of both hypertension and hypotension. Dysfunction of afferent input from atrial stretch receptors that normally inhibit renin release could elevate renin and perhaps catecholamine output. Similar abnormalities could account for reported elevations of atrial natriuretic factor,[1058] a finding confirmed in three GBS patients with dysautonomia.[1280]

Because hypertension in GBS patients is usually short-lived, it requires treatment only if severe, or if it is accompanied by certain conditions such as angina. Beta-adrenergic blocking drugs seem to be well tolerated, but sometimes they have an inconsistent effect on blood pressure and generally do not lower pulse rate. Drugs that cause orthostatic hypotension should be avoided. If immediate blood pressure reduction is necessary, short-acting titratable agents such as nitroprusside should be used. Clonidine, dihydralazine, nitroprusside, and nifedipine have been used with varying results.[652]

Hypotension and Orthostatic Hypotension

In several small prospective series of GBS patients, the frequency of orthostatic hypotension has been from 5% to 10%[1108] to 57%.[1206] Three selective series[250,812,1206] reported orthostatic hypotension in 100%, 57%, and 29% of patients, respectively. In the MGH retrospective series, 19% of patients had a reduction in systolic pressure of greater than 20 mm Hg, a drop in diastolic pressure of greater than 10 mm Hg from supine to standing, or a similar drop when the patient was attached to a positive pressure respirator. Quadriplegia, respiratory failure, and involvement of cranial nerves IX and X were associated with orthostatic hypotension. Several mechanical factors including paralysis of calf and abdominal muscles and impaired venous return to the heart may contribute to hypotension. Dehydration or positive pressure ventilation may also cause symptomatic orthostatic hypotension even when baroreflexes are intact. Orthostatic hypotension is probably due to an effective partial sympathectomy, causing failure of reflex arteriolar and venous constriction,[1259] accentuated by the inability of many dysautonomic patients to increase heart rate.

Supine hypotension (see Table 7–11) may be profound and paroxysmal, and may alternate with episodes of hypertension, then giving rise to the most dramatic form of dysautonomia in GBS. A 76-year-old patient with severe GBS became quadriplegic during the course of 3 days. He had increasingly severe episodes of labile blood pressure over the following days. At the height of his dysautonomia up to 20 episodes of severe hyperhypotension occurred daily. He was unresponsive during some episodes of low BP. Trend monitoring (Fig. 7–6) showed precipitous drops in mean BP, at times below 50 mm Hg, associated with a slight decrease in heart rate. Pulmonary artery pressures declined in parallel with BP but usually followed hypotension. Hypotension was treated with fluid infusion and, occasionally, phenylephrine. Severe hypertension, above 150 mm Hg mean BP, was treated with nitroprusside. Cardiac output was measured 14 times over several days, using a thermodilution technique, and SVR was calculated (Fig. 7–7). BP was most closely related to SVR over a wide range of pressures. Cardiac output changed in parallel with heart rate. As expected from the Starling mechanism, cardiac output varied with filling pressure (pulmonary artery diastolic or wedge) only during hypotension.[1020]

Studies employing Swan-Ganz catheters[243,303,898a,1020,1267] have demonstrated a parallel and virtually simultaneous reduction in cardiac output, central venous or wedge pressures, and SVR during hypotension. An important feature accompanying each episode of hypotension has been a slight bradycardia relative to a usually fixed heart rate (see Fig. 7–6).[243,1020] Although an inap-

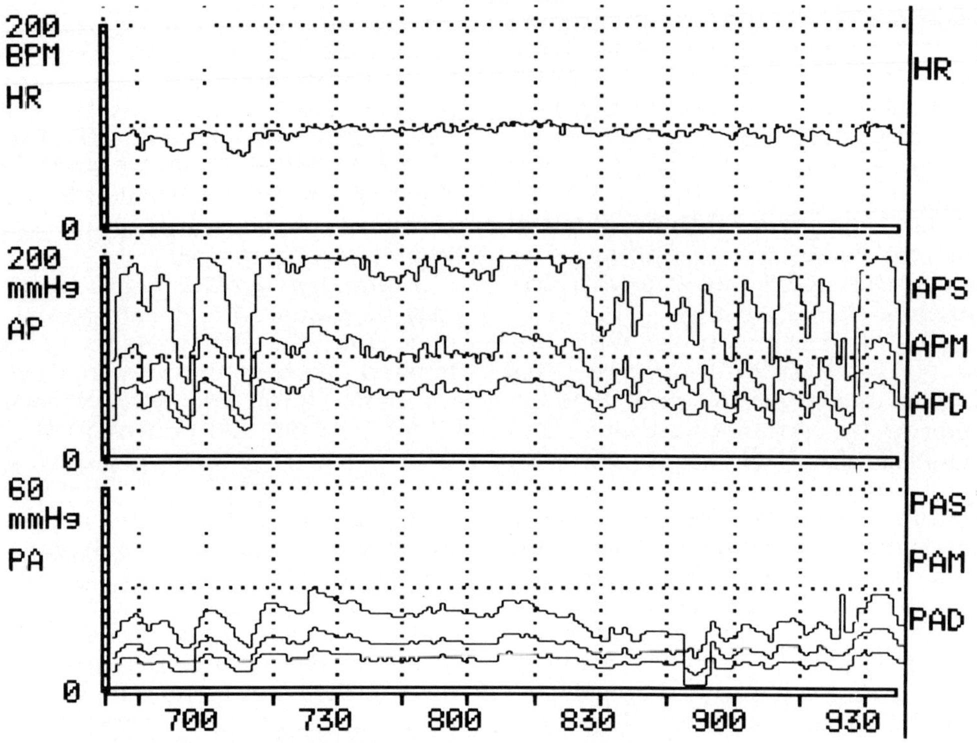

Figure 7–6. Trend recording from the patient described in the text with profound cardiovascular dysautonomia. Pulse (BPM)—*top panel*; blood pressure (AP; systolic, mean, and diastolic)—*center panel*; pulmonary artery pressure—*bottom panel*. Blood pressures above 200 mm Hg are truncated. The relatively invariant pulse with slight slowing during hypotension suggests a vasodepressor response as the cause of hypotension. (From Ropper,[1020] p. 707, with permission.)

propriate bradycardia accounted for only a small portion of the reduced cardiac output, the low heart rate suggested that hypotension was precipitated by a vasodepressor response. Some hypotensive episodes have been preceded by "vagotonic" stimuli such as intubation, tracheal suctioning, or medications, but others have been spontaneous. Any of the stimuli capable of producing reflex vagal syncope, such as gagging, tracheal stimulation, or distention of a hollow viscus, may trigger vasodepressor episodes at some times, and not at others. The inability to mute the vasodepressor response, and alternating episodes of severe hypertension, suggest that one component of the blood pressure swings is due to an afferent lesion from baroreceptors, as discussed earlier. Measurements of cardiac output and pulmonary artery diastolic pressure (see earlier) have suggested that changes in SVR were the major determinant of blood pressure, with central filling pressures playing a lesser role.[1020]

Orthostatic hypotension is seldom a management problem, as it has usually resolved by the time the patient is able to walk. Its presence should nevertheless be appreciated before ambulation or sitting are attempted. Management of supine paroxsymal hypotension is complex; simple volume expansion sometimes sufficies. The benefits of using a Swan-Ganz catheter to guide volume expansion must be weighed against the risks in each patient. Pressors such as phenylephrine (Neo-Synephrine) are required for symptomatic hypotension (patients may lose consciousness), but patients with impaired baroreflexes may become excessively hy-

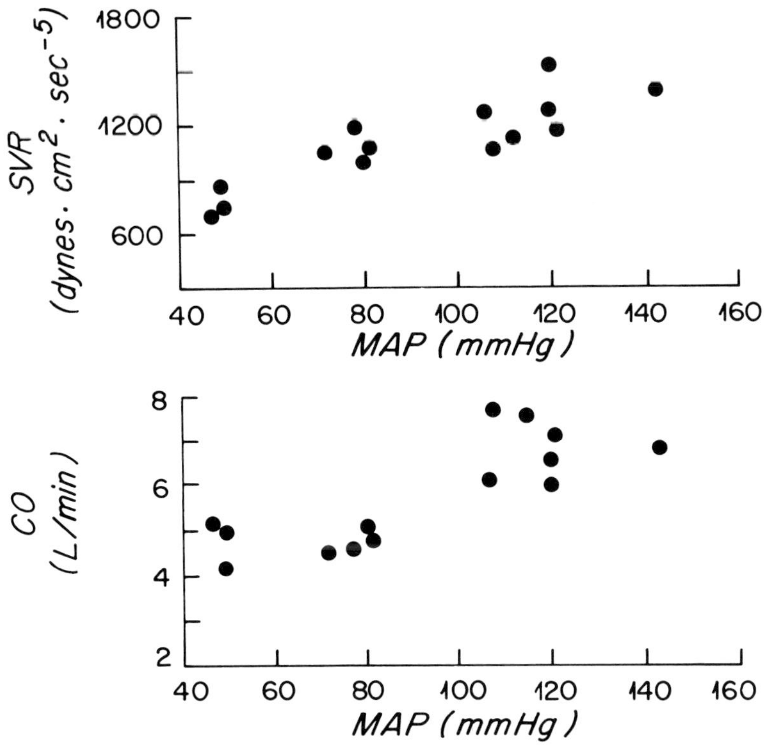

Figure 7–7. Relationship between mean arterial pressure (MAP) and systemic vascular resistance (SVR; $r = .86$), and cardiac output (CO; $r = .85$) in the patient described in Figure 7–6. (From p. 708, with permission.)

pertensive during pressor infusion. There is often a delay of several minutes in blood pressure response to pressors.

Sinus Tachycardia

Sustained sinus tachycardia is probably the most common, though usually harmless, abnormality of the autonomic nervous system in GBS. In the MGH retrospective series, 37% (at some time during the illness) had sustained sinus tachycardia (heart rate greater than 100 beats per minute) in the absence of fever. Table 7–12 lists the incidence of sustained sinus tachycardia in several GBS series. The wide range, 8% to 80% of patients, probably reflects differences in attention to this finding. A persistent sinus tachycardia has been more common in ICU and respirator patients. In the retrospective series, sinus tachycardia, present in almost one third of patients on admission, was associated with later quadriplegia, respiratory failure, and oropharyngeal paralysis. Many patients had sinus tachycardia early in their course when they were still ambulatory, but it ceased by the time weakness was maximal. Several patients with postsurgical GBS, who were hospitalized before the onset of GBS, developed sinus tachycardia just prior to the onset of neurologic symptoms. Sinus tachycardia may therefore be a helpful diagnostic sign in early GBS. In most cases tachycardia has persisted for several days to 1 to 3 weeks.

Diminished R-R interval variation is common in GBS and experimental autoimmune neuritis (EAN),* even when corrected for heart rate.[1050,1124] One study has found that reduced R-R inter-

---

*See references 321, 383, 506, 869, 911, 1108, and 1118.

Table 7–12 ARRHYTHMIAS IN LARGE GBS SERIES*

Series, Year	*No. of Patients*	*Sinus Tachycardia*	*Sinus Bradycardia*	*Asystole*	*Pacemaker*
Kunst and Grosser,[655] 1974	58	36	0	0	0
Goulon et al,[426] 1975	172	13	13	2	0
Soffer et al.,[1122] 1978	89	8	0	0	0
Sunderrajan and Davenport,[1165] 1985	40	0	5	6	3
Lambregts and Op de Coul,[663] 1985	47	28	30	0	6
Raphael et al.,[968] 1986	223	39	24	0	0
French Cooperative Group,[380] 1987	220	0	34	0	0
de Jager,[259] 1980	61	79	11	—	—
Winer and Hughes,[1288a] 1988	100	62	1	6	—
Retrospective MGH Series, 1962–1979	161	37	8	0	0
Prospective MGH Series, 1979–1988	120	1	2	1	1

*Percent of patients.

val variation was associated with a risk of serious arrhythmias.[1288a] Approximately half of MGH patients tested prospectively had abnormal R-R interval variation (see Chapter 13).[1085a] Lack of atropine-induced tachycardia is also common.[75,1108] Both are probably the result of loss of vagal efferent innervation.

Sinus tachycardia cannot be explained easily by a vagal efferent lesion alone,[1200,1201] because adaptation occurs in response to vagotomy. Adaptation is complete in hours or days at most, whereas sinus tachycardia persists longer. Incomplete lesions of the afferent baroreflex fibers alone, however, could produce sinus tachycardia and orthostatic hypotension. One potential mechanism is selective demyelination of low-threshold A fibers that carry information about dynamic blood pressure changes, sparing the higher-threshold static C fibers. Stimulation of baroreceptor afferents or vagal efferents produces different degrees of cardiodeceleration when the stimuli are applied at different points during the cardiac cycle. The timing of afferent volleys of impulses determines the extent of cardiodeceleration. Demyelination in either the afferent or vagal efferent fibers of the baroreceptors could slow the afferent volley triggered by each ventricular contraction, causing impulses to arrive at the sinus node during a relatively refractory state. Because phasic activity continues at both baroreceptor and CNS levels, adaptation would not occur. Further increases in the latency of the volleys as demyelination worsens would result in impulses reaching the sinus node during a nonrefractory period of the next cardiac cycle, causing appropriate deceleration. This may explain the disappearance of sinus tachycardia in some GBS patients whose illness progresses and becomes more severe. This partial deafferentation hypothesis is compatible with diminished R-R interval variation during deep breathing, lack of change in heart rate after intravenous atropine, absence of orthostatic hypotension, and perhaps with retained cardiodeceleration to carotid sinus massage in most patients, but it requires an ideal phase shift of signals in baroreceptor afferents. In a complex case of severe GBS with constant tachycardia, fever and low systemic vascular resistance, autopsy showed inflammatory demyelination of ventral rami.[898a]

Treatment of sinus tachycardia is unnecessary unless it causes myocardial ischemia. Resolution of severe tachycardia has been reported with verapamil or pindolol administration.[652]

Lability of heart rate, mainly transient episodes of sinus tachycardia, occurred in 8% of patients in the MGH series. The lability usually represented a normal autonomic response to a variety of stimuli, as there was no correlation between labile heart rate and other types of cardiovascular autonomic dysfunction.

Vagal Spells

Vagally mediated arrhythmias are among the most ominous cardiac complications in GBS. Various degrees of bradycardia have been reported in up to 35% of some selected series (see Table 7–12). Vagal spells are episodes of bradycardia, sinus arrest, or asystole that may occur with or without an obvious vagotonic stimulus. Atrioventricular block and other arrhythmias may also occur in response to a direct vagotonic maneuver (eg, ventricular tachycardia precipitated by carotid sinus massage). In our retrospective series, 8% of patients had multiple vagal spells, typically sinus bradycardia or asystole, during tracheal suctioning or Valsalva-like maneuvers. Vagal spells generally appeared during the period of peak motor disabilty but have been reported also during convalescence.[458] In the MGH series, vagal spells were transient, ending spontaneously or after intravenous atropine administration. None of the MGH patients died or required a cardiac pacemaker solely for intermittent bradyarrhythmias, although numerous cases requiring pacemakers have been reported.*

The role of transient hypoxemia in causing bradycardia during tracheal suctioning has been demonstrated in other (non-GBS) ICU patients.[891,1095] Bradycardia, however, occurs even with optimal respiratory care techniques in GBS patients, suggesting that it is a vasodepressor vagal response. Abnormal oculocardiac reflexes[112,303,426,428] or pathologic carotid sinus massage responses[649] may be present in GBS patients with vagal spells. Atrioventricular block (but not other arrhythmias) was associated with evidence of autonomic dysfunction in one study.[440] Other phenomena have been ascribed to parasympathetic overactivity in GBS, including episodes of facial flushing, a tightening sensation in the chest and abdomen, generalized warmth, and profound weakness, often after a Valsalva-like maneuver.[697] Episodes have lasted up to 30 minutes and some were followed by a deep sleep. In one patient, intravenous edrophonium duplicated the episodes. Facial flushing has been noted by others.[202,426] Failure of sympathetic reflexes to counteract vagally mediated bradycardia is unlikely to explain vagal spells entirely; their mechanism, perhaps the result of an afferent autonomic lesion, remains obscure.

Other Arrhythmias

Arrhythmias other than sinus tachycardia or vagal spells occurred in only 4% of patients in the MGH retrospective series. They included premature ventricular contractions (PVCs) (3 cases, 1 with bigeminy), premature atrial contractions (PACs) (1 case), paroxysmal atrial tachycardia (PAT) (2 cases), and ventricular fibrillation (1 case) (see Table 7–12). All but one had other signs of autonomic dysfunction, but there also were other potential causes of arrhythmias in each case (hypoxemia, electrolyte disturbance, or intrinsic heart disease). Of 16 ICU patients with GBS in one report,[440] 6 had atrial fibrillation or atrial flutter, 5 had PAT, and 4 had nonfatal ventricular tachycardia. A prospective survey of 100 patients[1288a] identified serious arrhythmias in 11 patients—7 fatal—and all in patients requiring mechanical ventilation. Systolic hypertension and reduced R-R interval variation were more common in patients with subsequent serious arrhythmias. One patient in the prospective series acquired complete heart block while in the ICU and has continued to require a pacemaker despite complete recovery from GBS. Morphologic ECG changes and other cardiovascular fea-

*See references 52, 77, 112, 328, 347, 354, 428, 440, 458, 649, 652, 663, 688, and 1165.

tures are discussed in Chapter 11 and sudden death attributed to ventricular arrhythmias are detailed above.

Bladder Dysfunction

Several large GBS series have reported frequent bladder involvement, a sign more typical of spinal cord disease (Table 7–13). In the MGH retrospective series early urinary retention occurred in 27%, and in the prospective series, in 14%. In contrast, urinary incontinence, discussed below occurred in only 2%. None of the patients with retention could walk at the time, and 83% eventually required mechanical ventilation, thus making the sign an early predictor of severe disease. Bladder involvement, often present at the time of maximum motor deficit, usually persists for several days to less than 2 weeks.

The few reports of urodynamic studies in GBS patients with urinary retention suggest a paralytic bladder with detrussor paralysis. Bethanechol supersensitivity testing was negative in one patient, but another had denervation of the external urethral sphincter.[637] Cystometrograms in three MGH patients with urinary retention or incontinence also demonstrated flaccid, paralytic bladders. One also had slightly impaired bladder sensation.

Although most GBS patients are almost quadriplegic at the time of their urinary disturbance, abdominal muscle paralysis probably plays a minor role in urinary retention. With partial outflow obstruction, abdominal wall paralysis may contribute to urinary retention, but internal sphincter abnormalities have not been found in GBS.

Urinary incontinence, much less common than retention, is usually an overflow phenomenon. Even with dysfunction of the external (striated) sphincter, continence is maintained by the internal (smooth muscle) sphincter. Frequent urinary incontinence, especially in the absence of significant residual volume or urinary tract infection, suggests a myelopathy. In reviewing patients for the retrospective series, several putative GBS cases with early bladder dysfunction or bladder dysfunction disproportionate to limb weakness all ultimately had transverse myelitis. One report[778] notes protracted and incomplete recovery of bladder function in GBS, but only one MGH patient had incomplete recovery, probably due to vesicular overdistension.

Urinary retention in GBS is best treated by intermittent catheterization, which prevents vesicular overdistension and reduces the risk of urinary tract infection. Almost 85% of MGH patients with indwelling Foley catheters developed urinary tract infections. In acute GBS drugs such as urecholine, that may have detrimental cardiovascular effects in the setting of the other autonomic dysfunction, have little use.

Gastrointestinal Dysfunction

Fourteen percent of patients in the MGH retrospective series had constipa-

Table 7–13 BLADDER AND BOWEL DYSFUNCTION IN LARGE GBS SERIES

Series, Year	*No. of Patients*	*Urinary Retention (%)*	*Ileus (%)*
Ravn,[973] 1967	127	22	NA*
Chuttani et al.,[199] 1968	63	24	0
Gecow and Pawela,[396] 1971	83	6	0
Winer et al.,[1291] 1988	100	32	NA
de Jager,[260] 1988	57	75	2
Retrospective MGH Series, 1962–1979	169	27	9
Prospective MGH Series, 1979–1988	120	14	3

*NA = not available.

tion; 9% had ileus or gastric distension; 3% had diarrhea, and 1% fecal incontinence (excluding gastroenteritis or abdominal surgery as antecedent illnesses). There was other evidence of autonomic dysfunction in 23 patients with constipation, but immobilization alone may have accounted for many cases. Other authors have commented on constipation in GBS in 3 of 89 patients;[1122] and 6 of 35;[751] 1 patient was reported with fecal impaction.[888] Ileus or gastric dilatation have also been mentioned* (Table 7–13). Gastric dilatation, which occurred in several MGH patients, responded partially to metoclopramide. In a child with GBS, hypertension, and ileus, surgical exploration revealed only edema and petechial hemorrhages of the ileum.[521] Abdominal pain has been highlighted as the presenting symptom in a case of GBS.[1297] Six patients in the MGH prospective series had severe ileus, one progressing to colonic perforation. In other patients, the condition occurred with painful and impeded nasogastric feeding (see Chapter 16).

Fecal incontinence occurred in only two patients in the MGH series, neither with urinary incontinence. Other cases are mentioned in several series.* Persistent diarrhea in five of our retrospectively studied MGH patients was adequately explained by causes other than GBS. Antibiotic-induced enterocolitis (usually caused by *Clostridium difficile*) or intolerance of tube-feeding formulas were the most common causes. Prominent preceding diarrhea may be a clue to *Campylobacter jejuni* or another enteritis as a precipitating illness for GBS (see Chapter 6).

The smooth muscle of the gut has intrinsic rhythmicity and should continue to contract and relax even if its neural innervation is ablated. The autonomic nervous system may, however, affect intestino-intestinal reflexes indirectly. Ileus, unlike most cases of constipation in GBS, is probably dysautonomic.

Abnormal Drug Responses

Abnormal responses to various drugs have been reported in patients with GBS. In the MGH retrospective series, one patient became hypotensive, without bradycardia, after injection of 10 ml of edrophonium, but at least 10 other GBS patients tolerated it without complications. Severe hypotension has been reported with phentolamine,[697,812] nitroglycerin,[105] thiopental, and morphine.[243] Phenylephrine,[105] ephedrine, dopamine, and isoproterenol[137] reportedly have caused excessive hypertension,[243] but most instances have been poorly documented. No true denervation hypersensitivity has been established, and impaired reflex buffering of blood pressure changes is more likely.

The risk of cardiovascular autonomic dysfunction during general anesthesia has not been defined, but many severely ill patients have tolerated inhalation agents for tracheostomy or gastrostomy. One MGH patient with severe orthostatic hypotension had a cardiac arrest during general anesthesia. Suxamethonium may cause severe hyperkalemia and cardiac arrest in immobilized and denervated GBS patients.[360] In general, if minor procedures can be performed with local anesthesia, it may be preferable.

Neurogenic Pulmonary Edema

A GBS patient has been described with alternating episodes of severe hypotension and hypertension, who became severely hypoxic and died.[137] Pulmonary congestion, edema, intrapulmonary hemorrhages, and moderate left ventricular hypertrophy were found at autopsy, but the myocardium was histologically normal. This may represent a rare case of neurogenic pulmonary edema from dysautonomia, but a

*See references 83, 122, 230, 426, 513, 521, 524, 649, 697, 1167, and 1263.

*See references 322, 761, 813, 888, 973, and 1122.

causal relationship is uncertain without hemodynamic measurements. Another patient with severe dysautonomia and an axonal form of GBS developed pulmonary edema while severely hypertensive.[348] This and other reports of pulmonary edema[112] appear more likely to have been cardiogenic than dysautonomic, but they have not been studied well enough to determine if there was a relationship to autonomic innervation of lung vessels.

Lacrimal and Salivary Function

In the MGH experience, reduced lacrimation did not occur even in patients with severe facial palsy but a systematic study with Schirmer's test has not been performed. Corneal abrasions or conjunctivitis occur as complications of incomplete eyelid closure rather than of impaired lacrimation. One patient in the MGH retrospective series had an unexplained dry mouth (without Sjögren's syndrome). Several authors have commented on hypersalivation in GBS* but have not quantified the abnormality.

Pupillary and Accommodation Abnormalities

As discussed in the section on ophthalmoplegia, many patients with MGH oculomotor abnormalities have pupillary abnormalities, but pupillary changes have not generally been a component of generalized dysautonomia. Rare cases of isolated pupillary abnormalities without ophthalmoplegia are believed to reflect local inflammation of autonomic nerves.[1282]

Sexual Dysfunction

Erectile dysfunction was reported during recovery by two men in the retrospective series, but a systematic survey has not been conducted. One man, aged 19, had other autonomic abnormalities (urinary retention, orthostatic hypotension, dry mouth). The other, aged 30, had difficulty sustaining an erection but no other evidence of autonomic dysfunction. Both patients had only moderate weakness and minimal sensory loss, and were able to walk. Other authors[459,778] have mentioned sexual dysfunction in GBS patients without giving details. One patient[1129] had transient erectile and ejaculatory dysfunction. Decreased libido was reported in 9 of 26 GBS patients,[199] mostly male, but erectile or ejaculatory impotence were not mentioned.

Premature labor occurs in patients with GBS, and the initial stages of labor are often precipitous and painless. The expulsive stages of labor may be protracted, sometimes requiring instrumentation for delivery (see Chapter 17).

Temperature, Sweating, and Vasomotor Regulation

Disordered thermoregulation has been studied in GBS patients[77,426] and fever has been ascribed to the inability to dissipate heat. Fever in GBS should nevertheless be assumed to be due to infection. An exceptional case with fever 41.5°C and tachycardia had a moderate perivenular lymphatic infiltrate in the hypothalamus and through the brainstem, but apparently without tissue destruction.[898a]

Cutaneous vasomotor instability with skin erythema or pallor was said to have occurred in almost all the children in one series;[396] 21% had persistently cold extremities that were susceptible to frostbite, even years later. These observations are unconfirmed. A number of MGH patients have had prominent dermatographia, often during anxiety or with vagal stimuli.

Episodic diaphoresis occurs in a few GBS patients with cardiovascular dysautonomia, probably as a general sympathetic response rather than a true

*See references 122, 259, 426, 428, 649, and 860.

disturbance of thermoregulatory sweating. Of 41 GBS patients questioned about perceptions of their own sweating patterns, 2 felt they had excessive sweating, 6 had reduced sweating, and the remainder perceived no sweating abnormalities. Reports of hyperhidrosis or sweating crises in GBS have not quantified sweat production.[77,122,259,396,860] In very selective series, 12% to 56% of patients have noted excessive sweating,[259,396,1108] probably over-representing this abnormality.

Sweat testing in six GBS patients using alizarin red powder and a heat cradle[1206] showed that five had reduced leg sweating, four had areas of impaired sweating on the trunk, and one had normal sweating except for a patch of anhidrosis on one foot and leg. Occasionally GBS patients have had an impaired sweating response to increased body temperature,[571] but a normal sweating response to elevated core body temperature was found in most GBS patients in whom circulatory reflexes were impaired. Indirect electrophysiologic evidence of preserved sudomotor function has been reported in GBS.[36,341] The conflicting evidence in the literature matches the anecdotal MGH experience that thermoregulatory sweating abnormalities are infrequent and probably not clinically important in GBS.

Bronchial Smooth Muscle Dysfunction

Bronchoconstriction and dilation are mediated in part by vagal and sympathetic innervation. One series[396] observed paresis of bronchial smooth muscle during bronchoscopy in 15% of cases with respiratory failure. This report emphasized impaired constriction and dilatation of bronchial smooth muscle in failure of bronchial clearing of secretions, and implied that bronchial paresis could contribute to atelectasis and pneumonia and persist longer than paresis of respiratory muscles. Recommendations that bronchoscopy be performed immediately before removal of a tracheotomy cannula, to be certain that the bronchial smooth muscle paresis has regressed, has not been widely adopted. Other authors[122,259,860] have commented on increased tracheobronchial and salivary secretions in GBS.

Chapter 8

VARIANT SYNDROMES

Pure Motor GBS
Sensory GBS
Pure Pandysautonomia
Pharyngeal-Cervical-Brachial Weakness
Paraparetic Weakness
Fisher's Syndrome

Several clinical variants of GBS merit separate description because they simulate other diseases and because they may illuminate the pathophysiology of the typical illness. There are variants that maintain their atypical pattern throughout the illness, but more commonly GBS begins with a variant pattern before progressing to the generalized weakness and areflexia that obscure the original syndrome and make the diagnosis obvious. The connection between these syndromes and GBS is based on (1) a close resemblance to portions of the typical disease; (2) overlap cases between typical GBS and variant syndromes; (3) laboratory findings that confirm the diagnosis of GBS, particularly raised cerebrospinal fluid (CSF) protein concentration and electrophysiologic abnormalities; and (4) exclusion of other more common causes of the variant syndrome. Atypical variants of GBS are usually more common than typical presentations of the rarer diseases these variants simulate, such as botulism or diphtheria. Chapter 2 lists separately diagnostic criteria for each of the variants that has a bias toward one modality (pure motor GBS, sensory GBS, pure pandysautonomia), the regional variants (pharyngeal-cervical-brachial, paraparetic, or oculomotor weakness), and Fisher's syndrome, which has elements of both regional and cerebellar abnormalities. Separate criteria are preferable to numerous inclusionary and exclusionary modifications of the criteria for typical GBS.

The relative frequencies of the variants are given in Table 8–1, from the prospective Massachusetts General Hospital (MGH) series of 120 patients. Fisher's syndrome occurred most commonly, followed by pure motor GBS, pharyngeal-cervical-brachial weakness (without and with ophthalmoplegia), a paraparetic pattern, and, occurring least frequently, a predominantly ataxic form. Fifteen percent of the patient's in this series, therefore, had "atypical GBS." During the years of the prospective study, an additional 10 patients were examined at other hospitals and brought to our attention, four with acute pure sensory GBS, (two of these ultimately were found to have underlying malignancies), one with pandysautonomia, two with pharyngeal-cervical-brachial variant, and three with Fisher's syndrome. Variations in the temporal course of GBS, particularly relapsing and chronic forms, are discussed in Chapter 10.

Few variant cases are truly "pure"; instead they have elements of the classic syndrome or share minor parts with variants. Several variants also have a proclivity to share common features

Table 8–1 FREQUENCY OF CLINICAL VARIANTS IN PROSPECTIVE MGH SERIES*

Fisher's syndrome	7	(6%)
Pure motor GBS	4	(3%)
Pharyngeal-cervical-brachial weakness	4	(3%)
Without ophthalmoplegia	3	
With ophthalmoplegia	1	
Paraparetic pattern	2	(2%)
Ataxic form	1	(1%)

*120 consecutive patients.

with each other, particularly the pure sensory and dysautonomic syndromes, the pharyngeal-cervical-brachial variant and ptosis, and, perhaps the best example of features that segregate together, the ataxia and ophthalmoplegia of Fisher's syndrome.

The taxonomic place of a purely axonal form of GBS is still uncertain, as it is currently based largely on electrophysiologic evidence of multiple inexcitable nerves (see Chapter 13). More complete pathologic studies may demonstrate that this is truly an axonal disease, not simply a very severe form of GBS with secondary axonal damage (see Chapters 4 and 13).

The question of the existence of purely facial or oculomotor forms of GBS is also unresolved, as discussed in Chapter 7. We have seen examples of each (not included in the prospective MGH series), with areflexia and mildly elevated CSF protein concentration, after surgery and viral infections. Purely facial GBS with diminished blink reflexer exists but must be rare, and bifacial palsy is more often caused by diseases other than GBS. Cases in the literature claiming to represent these variants have not made a convincing connection between these syndromes and GBS because tendon reflexes or CSF have often been normal and other diseases such as Lyme disease or sarcoidosis were not excluded.[186] Areflexia, distal paresthesias, raised CSF protein level, and typical electrophysiologic findings, at least with blink reflex abnormalities suggesting demyelination, would all need to be present to be confident that a neuropathy restricted to the facial or oculomotor nerves was an inflammatory and demyelinating variant of GBS.

PURE MOTOR GBS

Four of Haymaker and Kernohan's 50 cases with otherwise typical GBS[510] had no sensory signs or symptoms. Similar cases are alluded to in many other series, usually without clinical details. The unity with GBS rested on areflexia, raised CSF protein level, conduction block, and a course of recovery that was similar to typical cases. Another brief report[1132] describes abnormal motor and normal sensory nerve conduction studies in three young men with pure motor GBS. Four MGH cases with pure motor GBS were similar to each other and to those in the literature, with progressive, relatively symmetric limb weakness, incomplete facial weakness, areflexia, and raised CSF protein concentration in some (see Chapter 2 and Table 12–4), as well as early proximal conduction block (see Chapter 13 and Table 13–5)—all in the absence of paresthesias, sensory loss, or abnormalities of sensory nerve conduction. The vital capacities of these patients were diminished but none required ventilatory support. Two patients had lateral rectus paresis; otherwise, ophthalmoplegia was not a prominent feature. Recovery took several weeks to 4 months. Patients who have no paresthesias at the end of a week or 10 days of GBS usually will have a persistent pure motor syndrome. In a few cases, sensory nerve potentials become abnormal after several weeks, but in most of the MGH patients with pure motor variant GBS, sensory nerve electrical studies have been normal 1 month after the onset of weakness. The axonal form of GBS, clinically more severe than these cases, can be a pure motor syndrome.

Illustrative Case 8–1 Pure Motor GBS

A 34-year-old dentist had coryza, malaise, headache, and fever, and 2 days later, diarrhea, from which he recovered completely. Several days later his calves ached and he had difficulty climbing stairs. By that afternoon he had finger and hand weakness that caused him to cut his work short. He fell while carrying garbage the following day. There were no paresthesias. He had slight weakness in the deltoids, triceps, and finger extensors, and could barely overcome gravity with foot movements, but no definite facial weakness. He walked with a slightly wide-based gait but had no ataxia or Romberg's sign. The biceps and triceps jerks were 1+, knee jerks 2+, one ankle jerk absent and the other 1+. Sensation in response to vibration, light hair pulling, and joint movement were normal. Vital capacity was initially 5 L. Two days after admission, the patient could no longer stand unassisted, and by the sixth day he could barely move his feet. CSF protein concentration was 58 mg/dL, without cells, 2 days after admission. The patient improved over 3 weeks and was able to walk when discharged. There were no subsequent sensory symptoms or sensory loss at bedside testing. Peroneal and median nerve sensory evoked potentials were normal 2 weeks after onset, and conventional electrophysiologic testing showed only proximal conduction block.

Preferential inflammation of ventral roots probably accounts for pure motor GBS. Restricted lesions of this nature have been demonstrated in several autopsied cases of GBS at autopsy, although a complete clinical pathologic correlation has not yet been made. The severe weakness juxtaposed on normal sensory function makes it less likely that peripheral motor nerves alone are involved (see Chapter 4). The differential diagnosis of acute, predominantly motor neuropathy is restricted to rare diseases such as porphyria, poliomyelitis, toxins, tick paralysis, and a few other infrequently occurring diseases discussed in Chapter 14.

SENSORY GBS

Early GBS is occasionally characterized by severe early distal paresthesias followed by numbness during the first or second week but little weakness until the second week. Even fewer cases retain the purely or predominantly sensory quality, with areflexia but little or no weakness for the duration of the illness. Paresthesias in the pure sensory variant are no more prominent than in typical GBS. A graduated, large fiber sensory loss evolves with minimal or moderate loss of pain and thermal sensibility. Most patients will have varying, but usually mild, dysautonomic features, particularly loss of normal variation of the R-R interval variation. Many cases reported as pure pandysautonomia (see farther on) have more consequential sensory loss than autonomic dysfunction. Several others have had ataxia or tremor (discussed later), but this often seems to be a function of the length of illness. Most have raised CSF protein concentrations by the second or third week (see Chapter 2 and Table 12–4) and the MGH cases have had absent or severely abnormal sensory action potentials. There are invariably minor electrophysiologic abnormalities of motor nerves (possibly indicating a higher threshold for clinically evident dysfunction from sensory than for motor nerve demyelination). Severe cases may have sensory loss on the trunk or distal trigeminal territories (see Chapter 7), thereby suggesting a sensory neuronopathy. Pure sensory cases, like pandysautonomia, generally have a longer evolution than typical GBS; a distinction from chronic inflammatory demyelinating polyneuropathy (CIDP), on clinical grounds alone, may then become difficult.

Illustrative Case 8–2 Pure Sensory GBS

Two weeks after a rubella vaccination, a 26-year-old woman experienced paresthesias in her right hand, then in her left, progressing later to her ankles and wrists. She had minimal proximal leg weakness but could walk unassisted. She later developed gait ataxia and some asymmetric clumsiness of her hands. Examination 1 week after onset showed areflexia and greatly reduced vibration, joint position, and 2-point discrimination in her hands and feet. There was slight proximal weakness and ataxia. A first lumbar puncture showed a CSF protein concentration of 45 mg/dL; a week later the concentration was 475 mg/dL, without cells. The patient slowly recovered but still has paresthesias, dysesthesias, areflexia, and mild ataxia.

Pure sensory cases in the literature have often followed an acute infectious illness, with minimal or no proximal weakness, and often dysautonomia. The most instructive autopsy case of this type[253] showed a multifocal lymphocytic infiltrate surrounding endoneural vessels, archetypal for GBS. The sensory ganglia had mild inflammatory changes, but the most salient findings were infiltrates and patchy demyelination of posterior roots, contrasted with entirely normal anterior roots. The prominent CSF pleocytosis may have suggested human immunodeficiency virus (HIV) infection in that case. A sural nerve biopsy in another case[1041] with prominent autonomic features had a noninflammatory degeneration of sensory fibers, but limited biopsy sampling may have been misleading. A case attributed to a preceding spinal anesthetic[1205] showed severe fiber loss in posterior roots and degenerated sensory and sympathetic ganglia 4 years after the acute illness. The long interval between illness and autopsy explains the absence of active inflammation, and this case was therefore not identified as GBS.

The differential diagnosis in these cases includes paraneoplastic sensory neuropathy or neuronopathy that appear acutely, both of which are probably more common than pure sensory GBS variant[534] (see Chapter 14). With the exception of a higher incidence of confusion or dementia and the infrequency of spontaneous improvement in the paraneoplastic group, the clinical course, raised CSF protein level, and electrophysiologic features of rapidly evolving paracarcinomatous cases may be similar to those of acute GBS. The underlying malignancy may be discovered months or longer after the onset of neuropathy (or at autopsy), making a GBS-related condition virtually a diagnosis of exclusion. Hodgkin's disease and other lymphomas have been the most common associated illnesses in our experience, but solid tumors, and cases apparently associated with antibiotics,[1149] have also been reported. Nonetheless, GBS and inflammatory paraneoplastic sensory neuropathy are distinct entities.[1217] Several patients with an acute peripheral sensory syndrome have had predominantly acral, truncal, and facial paresthesias evolving over a week, with normal electrophysiologic study results at the outset. All ultimately evolved to have severe ganglionopathies (neuronopathies) with malignancy. Two additional helpful distinctions between inflammatory sensory neuropathy and neuronopathy may be the relative sparing of pain and thermal sensation, and the tendency for diminished sensory nerve action potentials to become abnormal earlier in sensory GBS.

Other conditions confused with sensory GBS, because of prominent paresthesia or sensory loss, are ciguatera or other neurotoxic marine poisonings, early myelopathies with distal paresthesias, delayed organophosphate polyneuropathy, and other conditions discussed in Chapter 14.

PURE PANDYSAUTONOMIA

Young and associates[1309,1310] first reported a syndrome that resembles, in pure form, the autonomic component of severe acute GBS. Approximately 15 similar patients have been described, not all conforming to the originally described illness. A disproportionate number have been children.* The relationship of pandysautonomia to GBS is the most tenuous of all the variants, but the two are probably related on the basis of (1) similarities to the autonomic failure of typical severe GBS; (2) cross-over syndromes with varying degrees of neuropathic sensory loss; (3) elevated CSF protein levels in many cases; (4) absent or diminished reflexes in most cases (Table 8–2); (5) absent intermediolateral column spinal cord lesions, which would explain autonomic failure on a central basis;[343] (6) patho-

*See references 28, 33, 35, 208, 427, 532, 620, 874, 1189, 1292, and 1305.

Table 8–2 ACUTE DYSAUTONOMIA

Reference No.	***Type***	***Sensory Symptoms or Signs***	***Reflexes Reduced or Absent***	***Residua (>9 mo Follow-up)***	***CSF Protein Elevated***	***Abnormal EMG/NCV***	***Antecedent or Associated Illness***
28	Cholinergic	–		+		–	
35	Mixed	–	+	–	–	–	
193	Mixed					–	Oat cell cancer
208	Mixed	+	+	+	+	+	Headache, fever
318	Mixed	+	+, Asymm	+	–	–	+ANA, hyperthyroidism
343	Mixed	+	+	+	+	+	Upper respiratory infection and testicular cancer
427	Mixed	–	+		–		
486	Cholinergic	–	–	+	–	–	
532	Mixed	–	–	–	–	–	Diarrhea
532	Mixed	–	–	+	–	–	
533	Cholinergic	–	–	+	–	–	Fever
620	Cholinergic			+			
620	Mixed			+			
724	Mixed	+	–	+	–	–	
724	Mixed	+	–		+	–	Influenza and Pancytopenia
838	Mixed	+	–		+	+	
838	Mixed	+	–		–	–	
838	Mixed	+	–	–	–	+	Upper respiratory infection
874	Mixed	–	–	+	–		
874	Mixed	–	–	–	–		
949	Mixed	+			+	–	
1162	Mixed	–	–	+	+	–	Rubella
1187	Mixed					–	Pancreatic cancer
1189	Cholinergic	–	–	+	–	–	Pharyngitis, fever
1305	Mixed	–	+		+		Infectious mononucleosis
1307	Mixed			+			Hypothyroidism
1310	Mixed	–	–	–	+	–	

*ANA = anti-nuclear antibody, Asymm = Asymmetrical.

logic evidence of peripheral neuropathy including typical lymphocytic infiltration in cases with concomitant sensory loss;[343] and (7) the existence of an experimental autonomic immune neuropathy.[34] Suggested criteria for diagnosis of this variant are given in Chapter 2. A few cases have followed a well-delineated preceding infection such as mononucleosis,[1305] rubella,[1162] or herpes zoster. Others have had a nondescript, febrile preceding illness. A virtually identical paracarcinomatous acquired dysautonomia has also been described.[193,1187]

In the typical case, fatigue, gastrointestinal dysfunction, or orthostatic dizziness are the initial symptoms. Vomiting, abdominal pain, and constipation, occasionally (inexplicably) alternating with diarrhea, have been reported frequently at the onset, though in a few cases these may have been part of a preceding acute enteritis. Several patients have had laparotomies because of severe gastrointestinal symptoms, particularly ileus and abdominal pain. A spectrum of orthostatic hypotension occurs, from mild upright dizziness to definite syncope. Most patients have diminished or absent tendon reflexes within several weeks of the onset. Additional dysautonomic features in many patients have included an atonic bladder with urinary retention; diminished sweating, salivation, and lacrimation; impotence; and an invariant heart rate. Gastric achlorhydria has been mentioned. Pupillary abnormalities have varied, incuding light-near unreactive pupils with blurred vision, and enlarged or oval pupils.

The illness usually evolves over several weeks. The literature suggests that the full syndrome is slower than typical GBS to reach a plateau. Cases with longer progression or the abrupt appearance of new features over several months have an uncertain relation to the acute cases.[28,1307] There are no other neurologic findings in typical cases, though several instances of an associated sensory neuropathy have been reported, as cited farther on.[873a] Ophthalmoplegia, ataxia, pure motor neuropathy, or the types of pain typical of GBS have not been reported with pure pandysautonomia. The CSF protein concentration has been elevated in most cases but there have been exceptions. Conventional motor and sensory electrophysiologic test results are normal.

Several patients have had partial failure of sympathetic or, more commonly, parasympathetic function, as opposed to the ubiquitous autonomic failure of the original cases. Predominantly cholinergic dysfunction has been described, with internal ophthalmoplegia, dry mouth, ileus, atonic bladder, and tachycardia.[28,486,532,533,1189] Young and colleagues have distinguished these cases from theirs.[1310] Other variations have included cases with aseptic meningitis, an associated severe sensory neuropathy typical of dorsal root ganglion involvement;[208,838,873a] lesser degrees of sensory involvment,[343,838] or an association with connective tissue disease.[318] Subclinical sensory involvement has been shown in a case of pandysautonomia.[949] The features of published cases with predominantly pandysautonomic or mainly cholinergic abnormalities have been summarized.[620]

Recovery is complete in about half of cases and incomplete in the others after one to several years. Disabling residual symptoms are rare but a few patients have had persistent bowel and bladder dysfunction. Nerve biopsies performed in several patients, often months or years after the onset of symptoms, have been normal or have shown an increased number of small unmyelinated axons, interpreted by some authors[35,1310] as evidence of reactive sprouting. A few sampled autonomic ganglia and nerves in one report[343] were normal or had unconvincing changes. Pathologic changes in an animal model and in GBS patients with dysautonomia (see Chapter 4) indicate that the same inflammatory process that affects roots, nerves, and somatic ganglia occurs in autonomic ganglia and nerves.

No evidence of centrally mediated autonomic failure has been presented, nor have there been central signs.

The differential diagnosis in these cases includes botulism, ciguatera (neurotoxic fish poisoning), organophosphate or atropinic drug poisoning, and primary cardiovascular failure. Idiopathic orthostatic hypotension or Shy-Drager syndrome has similar features when considered as a static illness, but the slow evolution, preserved reflexes, normal spinal fluid, and parkinsonian signs allow a distinction from pure pandysautonomia. Treatment varies and is largely symptomatic, but, if the patient has symptoms of orthostatic hypotension a mineralocorticoid may be administered.

PHARYNGEAL-CERVICAL-BRACHIAL WEAKNESS

A number of patients will have prominent pharyngeal, facial, and neck-flexion weakness at the onset of GBS, which descends to involve the arms, and soon after, the legs. The unusual distribution of weakness, preservation of leg reflexes, and usual absence of paresthesias directs diagnostic attention toward myasthenia, botulism, or diphtheria. In a few such patients the illness halts when it has caused severe oropharyngeal, neck, shoulder, and proximal arm weakness, completely sparing power and reflexes in the legs.[1008]

Other, more typical features of GBS that have occurred variably include incomplete (or in one case complete) ophthalmoplegia, facial weakness, mild hand weakness, and diaphragmatic weakness. Ptosis has been prominent in five of seven of our cases and two patients have had accommodation paralysis. Most have required intubation to prevent aspiration. In these patients, the CSF protein concentration is often elevated but usually less so than in typical cases sampled at a similar time (see Table 12–4). Conventional electrophysiologic study results tend to be normal or to show late response abnormalities in the arms only. Results of blink reflex studies are abnormal, consistent with the degree of facial weakness. In two patients, single-fiber recording showed mildly increased "jitter" of paired motor fibers but no blocking. The ptosis has been slightly improved by neostigmine or endrophonium, whereas other testing for botulism and myasthenia have had normal results.

Illustrative Case 8–3 Pharyngeal-brachial-cervical GBS

A 19-year-old man began to have trouble swallowing and blurred vision, 10 days after a cough and fever. Three days later he had facial and pharyngeal weakness, 5-mm light-reactive pupils with sluggish near reaction, blurred monocular vision, incomplete ocular abduction, and symmetric ptosis. Versions were normal by the fifth day. The patient was unable to lift his head from the bed or raise his arms when sitting. He could barely resist gravity when bending his elbows. There was slight hip flexion weakness but otherwise normal leg and foot power. Reflexes were absent in his arms and 2+ at the knees and ankles. There was a left-sided Babinski's sign. Vital capacity was 500 mL at its worst. There was no change in ptosis or weakness with edrophonium or neostigmine administration. The CSF had no cells and a protein concentration of 33 mg/dL. Late responses, nerve conduction velocities, and repetitive stimulation were initially normal, but 2 days later there was dispersion and delay in median and ulnar F waves; late responses in the legs remained normal. There were fibrillations in the deltoid and facial muscles at 1 month. The patient never had paresthesias or sensory loss. His leg power was normal by the third week but he required a tracheostomy for 3 months before recovering completely. His serum had no effect on a mouse bioassay for botulinum toxin.

Two possible disparate anatomic explanations for this syndrome are (1) a truly regional distribution of inflammatory lesions in cranial nerves, particularly the lower ones, and in the cervical roots or nerves in the arms; and (2) a distal axonopathy that affects parts of the neuromuscular system prone to failure when high-frequency volleys are blocked. The latter is an appealing explanation for a syndrome that simulates the pattern of weakness seen in diseases of the neuromuscular junction, but electrophysiologic studies in these cases suggest a more proximal lesion. With frequent ptosis and ophthalmoplegia, response to anticholinesterase drugs, and minimal single-fiber recordings of "jitter."

All but one of the MGH patients with the pharyneal-cervical-brachial variant have had slow recoveries over several months, but two were discharged from the hospital, walking, with a tracheostomy and feeding tube in place.

PARAPARETIC WEAKNESS

More prominent leg than arm weakness is common at the onset of GBS, but three MGH cases had persistent, isolated leg weakness and areflexia that simulated a spinal cord or cauda equina lesion. The arms and cranial nerves were unaffected. Back, leg, or sciatic pain have preceded weakness in all cases, but paresthesias and sensory loss in the legs have been variable. There has been minimal bladder involvement and CSF protein concentration has been elevated, generally 40 to 100 mg/dL (see Table 12–4). Results of electrophysiologic studies in the legs have been typical of GBS (see Chapter 13). Hyponatremia may occur, as in typical GBS. The rarity of this variant relative to spinal cord compression and myelitis, requires radiologic confirmation of a normal spinal canal.

Illustrative Case 8–4

A 74-year-old woman had buttock and low back pain for a week, followed by progressive leg weakness that made her unable to walk. She could not raise her legs from the bed; foot movements were stronger than hip movements. Reflexes were absent in the legs and normal in the arms. The toes were flexed. There was a graduated loss of vibration and pin sensation in the distal legs. CSF was acellular with protein concentrations 78 mg/dL and 133 mg/dL on sequential spinal taps, 3 weeks apart. The face and arms were normal. A myelogram and a magnetic resonance imaging (MRI) scan of the thoracic and lumbar spine were normal. Late responses were absent or prolonged in the legs and normal in the arms. The patient was treated with corticosteroids for 3 weeks and recovered over 3 months. Power and reflexes in the arms were never affected.

FISHER'S SYNDROME

Numerous cases of ophthalmoplegia (reviewed in Chapter 7) or ataxia as major features of GBS have been discussed in the literature.[466,467,985,993] The juxtaposition of these two signs has also been alluded to previously in case descriptions, but Fisher's extensive discussion[365] in 1956 brought the syndrome into focus as an interesting variant. He discerned "an easily recognizable syndrome . . . characterized among other features by total external ophthalmoplegia, severe ataxia and loss of the tendon reflexes." Smith and Walsh introduced the eponym "Fisher's syndrome" in the title of a case report.[1117] Fisher's name paradoxically became attached to an illness outside his major field of interest, stroke, but his refined clinical analysis of the syndrome was consistent with his detailed descriptions of cerebrovascular cases. Subsequently, more than 50 adult cases have appeared in small series; approximatley another 50 cases individually, including many in which ophthalmoplegia is highlighted and ataxia mentioned incidentally; and more than 20 cases in children[85,748,953] (see Chapter 9). The incidence of Fisher's syndrome among typical acute GBS cases is approximately 5% (7 of 120 patients in the prospective MGH series began with the syndrome). Rare cases have relapsed, often showing only fragments of the complete syndrome with subsequent episodes.[280,590]

The relation of Fisher's clinical triad to GBS was originally inferred from the elevated CSF protein level in some cases, reflex loss, similarity to the ophthalmoparesis of typical GBS, and by cross-over cases that had progressed to typical GBS. More recently, numerous abnormal results of electrophysiologic studies consistent with those of acute GBS have been found in patients with Fisher's syndrome. Much of the interest in the syndrome, as discussed originally by Fisher[365] and others,[1219] has been in the "cerebellar" appearance of the ataxia and other signs putatively of central origin. This spawned a debate over the origin of the clinical features, and the possible relationship to brainstem encephalitis,[19,20] as well as cross-over cases in which the central and peripheral nervous systems may be simultaneously involved (see later).

The Clinical Syndrome

The initial symptom is usually diplopia (5 of 7 cases in the prospective MGH series) with limb and gait ataxia appearing 3 or 4 days later, or at times concurrently with diplopia. Patients may complain of mild dizziness without vertigo. Normal or diminished reflexes persist for several days, but invariably the reflexes are absent in completely developed cases by the end of a week (all 7 of our prospective cases became areflexic). There is a paucity of other symptoms, except paresthesias in approximately half of patients and mild proximal weakness in approximately a third.

Some latitude in the diagnosis seems acceptable in including cases with mild oropharyngeal or facial weakness (present in 2 of 7 of the MGH series patients) if the core triad of findings is present. Proposed criteria for the diagnosis of Fisher's syndrome appear in Chapter 2. Some cases are transitional between pure Fisher's syndrome and typical GBS. Limb weakness may be initially insufficient to obscure the ataxia, or there may be paresthesias and distal sensory loss. Ataxia frequently reappears as weakness improves. The initial impression that Fisher's syndrome is benign has been supplanted by vigilance for the approximately one third of cases that progress to profound weakness and respiratory failure.[115] One patient[582] had a relapse with generalized polyneuritis about 2 months after Fisher's syndrome.

Ophthalmoplegia usually advances over several days from relatively symmetric, incomplete eye movements in all directions to complete or virtually complete immobility of the globes. Uniocular movements demonstrate subtle asymmetries, even when binocular movements seem conjugate. Ptosis occurs in most patients, but associated pupillary paralysis has been reported in only a minority. Isolated pupillary light and near paralysis without other third nerve oculomotor abnormalities or ptosis is rare.[1282]

The usual early ocular findings are unilateral or asymmetric bilateral abducens paralysis (as with oculomotor paresis in typical GBS). There are sporadic reports of upward gaze paralysis,[599] pupil-sparing oculomotor palsy, a simulated internuclear ophthalmoplegia,[58,275,1170,1266] or divergence paresis, but these progress to more evident bilateral ophthalmoplegia within 2 or 3 days in most cases. Less severe restriction of eye movement may be seen in a few patients with the fully developed illness, most often persistent bilateral abducens paresis. Detailed aspects of the ophthalmoplegia, eye movement recordings, and pupillary and lid abnormalities are discussed in the section on ophthalmoplegia in Chapter 7.

The ataxia of Fisher's syndrome has the dysmetric qualities of cerebellar intention tremor, usually involves all the limbs, and is often slightly asymmetric, but it lacks components of a static "rubral" type tremor, or asterixis or the pseudoathetoid movements of a deafferented limb. If some cases have differences from classic cerebellar tremor, they consist of less finger incoordination compared with arm tremor, and a tendency for less decomposition of rapid alternating movements—but even these features are not consistently present. Varying degrees of gait ataxia accompany the limb abnormalities, and the two do not necessarily parallel each other. Unsteadiness, lightheadedness, or dysequilibrium sometimes occur early, but cerebellar dysarthria, vertigo, and nystagmus are not part of the syndrome. Mentioned rarely in case reports, dysarthria has not, in the MGH experience, had a cerebellar quality and has had alternative explanations in facial or oropharyngeal weakness. Approximately one half of patients have acral paresthesias; some also complain of facial paresthesias. Mild superimposed proximal limb weakness may diminish the tremor. An instance of aggravation of preexisting blepharospasm has been reported,[390] probably owing to the patient's futile attempts to move the eyes.

Of the 7 patients (6%), strictly defined by the criteria in Chapter 2, who had Fisher's syndrome in the MGH prospective study, 3 progressed to have generalized weakness in 1 to 4 days. Diplopia was the initial symptom; external ophthalmoplegia was complete, with ptosis in 6 and pupillary paralysis in 3. All but 2 had some paresthesias, and 2 had oropharyngeal weakness. Limb ataxia was mild in 2 and severe in 5. Three patients complained of some aching muscular pain characteristic of typical GBS.

Illustrative Case 8–4 Typical Fisher's Syndrome

A 43-year-old man awoke with horizontal diplopia several days after a viral syndrome with fever, nausea, and diarrhea. The following day the diplopia worsened, and he began to stagger when walking; he also noticed incoordination of his arms and mild acral paresthesias. On the third day he had bilateral incomplete abducens paralysis, 7-mm unreactive pupils, mild ptosis, areflexia, and mild proximal leg weakness. Sensory testing was normal. Gait was wide-based and ataxic, but the patient could walk with assistance. There was a severe ataxic tremor in his arms—more on the left side—and in the legs. Fine finger and toe movements were normal. Vital capacity was 75% of that predicted. CSF protein level concentration was 43 mg/dL with 2 white blood cells (WBC) per mm^3. The next day, ophthalmoplegia was complete, ptosis was worse, and the cerebellar tremor in the arms, legs, and gait ataxia had worsened; the patient could no longer walk. The head and trunk were unsteady with slight titubation when he sat with eyes closed. At the end of the week there was mild but definite distal vibration and joint position sense loss with only mild proximal weakness. Electrophysiologic testing (Table 8–3, patient No. 1) showed a predominantly sensory neuropathy. Eye movements began to improve in the second week with a 2-mm voluntary upward gaze, improved with Bell's maneuver. Cool water caloric testing did not elicit eye movements. In the third week, 2 mm of ocular abduction could be obtained with the oculocephalic maneuver. Forearm and triceps aching pain developed. By the end of the fourth week, incomplete dysconjugate eye movements returned in all directions and the pupils were light-reactive; ptosis was improved. The patient was discharged, able to walk unassisted with mild ataxia. There was no dysarthria, nystagmus, vertigo, Babinski's sign, or diminished level of consciousness.

Illustrative Case 8–5 Fisher's Syndrome with Ataxia before Ophthalmoplegia, Progressing to Typical GBS

A 57-year-old woman had light-headedness, dysequilibrium, and acral paresthesias. The following day her unsteadiness increased and she had circumoral paresthesias with brief, intermittent horizontal diplopia. There was slight right ptosis, markedly diminished and apparently conjugate upward gaze, and a slightly diminished downward gaze. Left eye adduction was slightly limited, with nystagmus of the right eye on abduction. Limb power was normal, reflexes were absent, there was no Babinski's sign, and the gait was ataxic. There was mild cer-

Table 8–3 EARLY ELECTROPHYSIOLOGIC FINDINGS IN FISHER'S SYNDROME*

	Median Motor			Peroneal/Tibial Motor			Median/Ulnar Sensory			Sural Sensory			
Pt No/Day	***NCV (m/s)***	***Ampl (μV)***	***Lat (m/s)***	***NCV (m/s)***	***Ampl (μV)***	***Lat (m/s)***	***NCV (m/s)***	***Ampl (μV)***	***Lat (m/s)***	***NCV (m/s)***	***Ampl (μV)***	***Lat (m/s)***	***F waves***
1/6	54	7500	4.4	51	6000	5.0		Absent			Absent		Prolonged
2/9	61	800	3.8	54	8000	5.2	54	10	2.8	45	21	3.3	Dispersed
3/10	48	2400	3.4	46	3000	3.8	50	7	2.4	54	5	2.8	Prolonged
4/10	58	5000	2.7	46	3500	4.4		Absent			—		Absent
5/8	42	7000	4.7	35	1500	6.0		Absent			Absent		Prolonged
6/7	52	9800	5.5	43	2600	5.2		Absent			Absent		Prolonged

*Prospective MGH Series.

ebellar-appearing, ataxic limb tremor. CSF protein concentration was 46 mg/dL without cells. Vibration sense was slightly diminished in the patient's toes. The following day her ophthalmoplegia became virtually complete, with normal pupillary light reaction. The ataxia worsened, and her limb, oropharyngeal, and facial muscles were weak. By the fifth day, weakness obscured the ataxia; she could not lift her limbs from the bed and intubation was required for airway protection. Vital capacity was normal. An MRI of the brainstem was normal. Electrophysiologic studies (see Table 8–3, patient No. 6) showed a predominantly sensory neuropathy. The patient received plasma exchanges and recovered first power and then eye movements. Cerebellar-like limb ataxia was evident during improvement. Six months after onset she was normal except for mild bifacial weakness and areflexia.

The eponymic syndrome as originally described is useful because it allows differentiation from other diseases. Therefore, ophthalmoplegia alone or with generalized weakness, ataxia alone with severely abnormal joint position and vibration sense, or isolated supranuclear eye movement abnormalities are best considered different from Fisher's syndrome (see later).

CSF protein concentration is elevated in most cases if sampled late enough in the course,[327] although the proportion with persistently normal or minimally elevated concentrations is higher than in typical GBS (see Table 12–3). The CSF protein concentration measured in the first week was above 40 mg/dL in 5 of 7 MGH patients. Three had from 2 to 10 WBC per mm^3 in the CSF.

The syndrome follows the same mundane infections as typical GBS (see Chapter 6), including Epstein-Barr virus[1113] and *Campylobacter* infection.[385] At least one case has been associated with HIV infection; it was distinguished by CSF pleocytosis, as are many other GBS cases associated with the virus. Patients with the illness have been brought to our attention with systemic lupus erythematosus and lymphoma. Even without an underlying systemic illness, Fisher's syndrome may recur.[160,582,1061]

Once the triad is fully developed, the limited differential diagnosis obviates further laboratory evaluation such as angiography, but there may be initial difficulty in excluding brainstem ischemia. Vertigo, not a feature of Fisher's syndrome, is a strong indication of basilar artery occlusion, but it also occurs with brainstem encephalitis. When the ataxia is minimal, several diagnostic considerations arise (superficially) for the ophthalmoplegia, such as botulism, myasthenia gravis, tick paralysis, hypophosphatemia,[1304] or pituitary apoplexy. Treatment is usually similar to that for typical GBS, including the use of plasma exchange as discussed below and in Chapter 15.

Cerebellar Ataxia without Ophthalmoplegia

Occasional patients have severe cerebellar-like ataxia at the onset of GBS, without ophthalmoplegia or severe loss of proprioceptive sense. Distal paresthesias, areflexia or hyporeflexia, raised CSF protein level, and a sensory neuropathy suggest the disease is a variant of GBS. Most such patients have some weakness and may progress to typical GBS, whereupon the ataxia becomes obscured. Two such patients were seen in the MGH prospective series. Electrophysiologic studies show a sensory neuropathy.

Illustrative Case 8–7 Ataxic GBS

Two weeks after receiving a Pneumovax vaccine, a 69-year-old man noted a "pinching" sensation in his toes and fingertips. Several days later he had minimal limb weakness, disproportionate limb incoordination with cerebellar tremor, and prominent gait ataxia. There was mild distal decrease in vibration sense and areflexia. CSF protein concentration with 49 mg/dL. Electrophysiologic studies showed normal motor nerve conduction except for slight prolongation of distal latencies in one median nerve, absent sensory potentials in the median and sural nerves, prolonged F responses, and normal electromyography. One month after onset, he could walk ataxically, had slight limb ataxia, normal limb strength, and distal paresthesias.

Similar cases have been reported or alluded to in the literature. Richter's cases[985] are commonly cited because one had pathologic examination. His first patient had staggering gait, arm ataxia, less leg ataxia, areflexia, right abducens palsy, and moderate reduction of vibratory sensation in the hands, without Romberg's sign. The second had profound gait and limb ataxia and areflexia without ophthalmoplegia reported. Sensory loss in the limbs appeared later. She improved, though some gait and limb ataxia persisted. Breast cancer and cirrhosis led to death 4 years later. An autopsy showed extensive degeneration of the posterior columns, root entry zones, and sensory roots, all consistent with a polyneuropathy. Clarke's columns were demyelinated but the cells within these zones were normal in number and appearance. Richter concluded that the ataxia resulted from loss of afferent fibers to Clarke's column. The obvious similarities to tabes dorsalis were noted. No other primary lesions of the central nervous system could be demonstrated. Other autopsied cases with prominent ataxia but no sensory loss have also failed to show lesions in the cerebellum.[754,1075]

Isolated ataxia in GBS, as in Fisher's syndrome, is apparently the result of selective dysfunction of spinocerebellar afferent fibers, most likely in peripheral nerves, with secondary tract degeneration in the spinal cord in severe or protracted cases. This may be a remarkable example of the functional separation of fiber type damage that may be caused by inflammatory polyneuropathy. A physiologic explanation for the ataxia has been proposed based on the finding of abnormal conduction in IA spinocerebellar afferent fibers originating in muscle spindles, as reflected in abnormalities of silent periods.[1016]

Ataxic GBS should be distinguished from cases in which a neuropathy causes incoordination or clumsiness of the limbs due to severe loss of proprioceptive sense without cerebellar tremor.[1090,1121] Sensory ataxia is accompanied by small athetoid movements (pseudoathetosis) or rapid tremor of the outstretched fingers and some dysmetria, but not the intention tremor of cerebellar disease.

Electrophysiology in Fisher's Syndrome

Virtually all conventional electrophysiologic studies of Fisher's syndrome have shown a peripheral neuropathy.* Most case reports with incidental descriptions of electrophysiologic studies have shown similar abnormalities. Chapter 13 details the various electrophysiologic patterns in typical GBS. The most extensive study[385] of 10 patients with Fisher's syndrome found normal motor nerve conduction velocity in 4 and only mild slowing in the others. Distal motor latencies were generally normal and conduction block was minimal or absent. Late responses were mildly abnormal, similar to those of typical GBS. The major abnormalities were prominently reduced sensory nerve action potential amplitudes, disproportionate to the degree of slowing. The sensory nerve abnormalities worsened for a period of time, despite clinical recovery. This was interpreted as reflecting a predominantly sensory axonal neuropathy. Others[1057] have found similar electrophysiologic sensory abnormalities, with prolonged latencies or reduced amplitude in 8 of 10 patients. Serial studies of patients with Fisher's syndrome[561,987] have shown initially normal motor conduction studies that became abnormal after several weeks.

*See references 385, 470, 561, 562, 987, and 1057.

Sensory potential amplitudes were reduced and latencies prolonged, both improving over several months. Late responses were abnormal in all patients. Electromyogram (EMG) needle examinations have been normal or have shown mild neuropathic changes. In the two best-studied pathologic cases of Fisher's syndrome, motor nerve conduction velocities were slow in one[921] but normal in the other.[258]

Blink responses have been inconsistently abnormal, generally paralleling reduced facial compound muscle action potential amplitudes in various studies (4 of 7 abnormal;[385] none of 4;[1057] and 2 of 3[561]). With a few exceptions, blink response abnormalities reported in the literature could be accounted for on the basis of peripheral facial nerve disease. In the MGH prospective series, a predominantly sensory neuropathy occurred in 3 patients with Fisher's syndrome who did not progress to generalized weakness, and in one who did progress but was studied early (see Table 8–3). Two patients without progression (patient Nos. 2 and 3) had normal sensory studies. One initially had absent H reflexes with no other motor abnormalities, but later developed proximal motor conduction block. The other had a mild motor neuropathy, with axonal features. Blink responses were absent in 1, prolonged in parallel with slowed facial nerve conduction in 1, and normal in 4.

Evoked potential abnormalities, when present, have generally suggested solely peripheral conduction delays. Three patients in a recent study[561] had peripheral conduction delay in median nerve somatosensory potentials and normal brainstem auditory evoked responses and visual evoked responses. Three previously reported MGH patients had normal brainstem auditory evoked responses and peripheral delay in median nerve and lower extremity somatosensory evoked responses.[1012] In contrast, there are several reports[927,1034,1301] of patients with central conduction delays in brainstem or visual evoked potentials. In a well-studied autopsy case of Fisher's syndrome,[258] brainstem auditory and visual evoked responses were normal on the 10th day of illness.

Central Versus Peripheral Origin of Signs in Fisher's Syndrome and Autopsy Pathology

Several authors[20,789] have proposed that Fisher's syndrome is the result of a brainstem encephalitis. They have cited the cerebellar appearance of ataxia, apparent supranuclear ophthalmoparesis in a few patients (including recovery of vertical before horizontal versions), upper eyelid jerks,[1052] rebound nystagmus,[790] other eye movement abnormalities (discussed in the section on ophthalmoplegia), occasional electrophysiologic studies suggesting a central lesion, and mid-brain lesions on computed tomography (CT) scans in several cases.[81,268,709,864,1312] The inconsistency of any group of findings of brainstem involvement in Fisher's syndrome, however, makes the hypothesis tenuous that brainstem lesions account for the findings. Other clinical points against mid-brain or cerebellar involvement include the absence of dysarthria or cerebellar oculomotor abnormalities, preserved consciousness, areflexia, the dysconjugate oculomotor abnormalities, absence of Babinski's signs, and cases that cross over with typical GBS. The central nervous system hypothesis requires two lesions—one central and the other peripheral. Moreover, an extensive brainstem lesion would be required to explain ataxia and complete ophthalmoplegia. It is unclear how this proposed tegmental mid-brain and pontine lesion could consistently produce complete ophthalmoplegia and leave consciousness unaffected. There are mid-brain syndromes that may simulate Fisher's syndrome, but clinical scrutiny virtually always allows a distinction based on the presence or absence of other regional brainstem signs. The similarity between cases of brainstem encephalitis and cases of Fisher's syndrome is usually superficial.

Alternate explanations for ataxia, based on peripheral mechanisms, have been proposed[1016] and numerous pathologic examinations have demonstrated an adequate peripheral explanation for ophthalmoplegia. Thus, cases with incomplete ophthalmoparesis, vertigo, unilateral limb ataxia, and hyporeflexia should not be considered Fisher's syndrome, particularly if there are Babinski's signs or stupor. All the cases in the literature with CT abnormalities in the brainstem have had obvious signs of a brainstem lesion, not the clinical triad characteristic of Fisher's syndrome.[1010]

Two recent reviews[19,1196] have presented excellent summaries and citations concerning a central origin for Fisher's syndrome, and the proposal of a "spectrum hypothesis." They propose that the syndrome is part of a spectrum of central and peripheral inflammation. Two reported cases with ophthalmoplegia, ataxia, and areflexia had, in addition, undoubted profound brainstem signs such as coma, dysarthria, and apnea, and both had evidence of a neuropathy. Another patient had bilateral optic neuropathy, ophthalmoplegia, ataxia, and Babinski's signs. The reflexes were hypoactive, but electrophysiologic testing showed a severe sensory and moderate motor neuropathy. These are posited as representing the middle of a spectrum of a postinfectious central and peripheral nervous system inflammation. These cases with brainstem pathology that happen to have ophthalmoplegia and ataxia as components of their illness do not explain the typical Fisher's syndrome. We believe that the syndrome is diagnostically useful when it is not confused with various incomplete mid-brain lesions.[1006]

The proponents of a central hypothesis are correct that rare cross-over cases that do not conform precisely to Fisher's syndrome, but resemble it, occur as a result of both central and peripheral pathology.[134,895] The only well studied acute GBS case with pathological examination that showed widespread lymphocytic infiltrates in the brainstem had no corresponding neurological signs,[898a] but it suggests that some central signs could occur. (It is important to point out that the brain tissue has not been shown to be damaged in regions with perivascular infiltrates.) Most cases with combined central and peripheral features have been subacute or relapsing. One such unusual patient had a relapsing brainstem encephalitis and severe peripheral neuropathy.[265] A related situation of multiple sclerosis with polyneuropathy, the latter often asymptomatic, has been discussed in the literature.[372,675,938] Cases of chronic inflammatory polyneuropathy with MRI lesions, but no corresponding clinical signs, have been reported.[794] In contrast, there are numerous cases of patients who had Fisher's syndrome and a normal MRI[385,666,739,1010] (Fig. 8–1).

The most compelling evidence for a peripheral origin of Fisher's syndrome remains well-studied pathologic cases. Two groups have failed to find brainstem lesions except secondary chromatolytic neurons in oculomotor areas[258,921] (as also found in cases with ophthalmoplegia[104,455]). The extra-axial oculomotor nerves were demyelinated. An MGH patient with Fisher's syndrome who died from aspiration pneumonia after 7 months of illness, showed peripheral nerve demyelination, including in the oculomotor nerves, but no brainstem lesions. A further perspective on central signs in GBS is given in Chapter 7.

Perhaps the most interesting feature of Fisher's syndrome is that the peculiar combination of signs occurs consistently, accounting for approximately 5% of GBS cases. The frequent juxtaposition of ataxia, from peripheral nerve dysfunction, and motor dysfunction of cranial nerves III, IV, and VI suggests these nerves have some property in common, perhaps an antigenic similarity between spinocerebellar IA afferent and oculomotor fibers.[1006,1016]

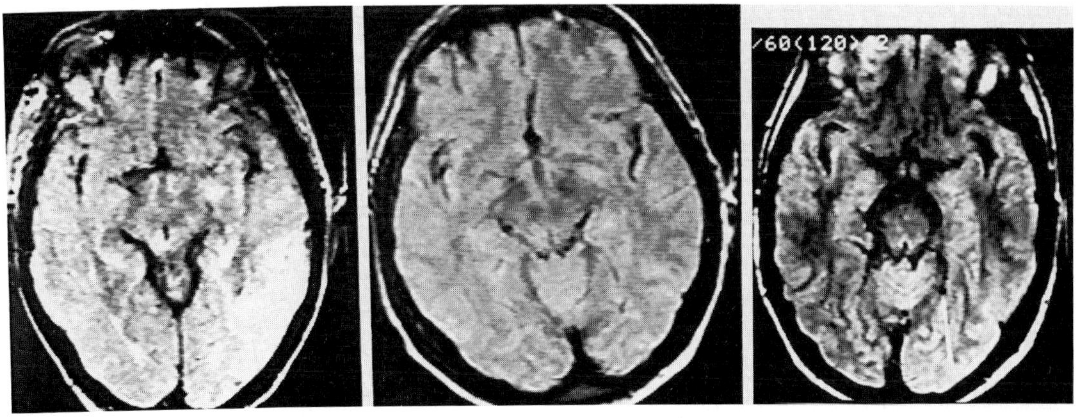

Figure 8–1. Axial MRI of the mid-brain from three patients with Fisher's syndrome. T2 weighted (TR 2000/TE 60). No brainstem lesions were seen in these sections or elsewhere in the brainstem or with other image sequences. Studies were made 6 days (*left*), 7 days (*center*), and 5 weeks (*right*) after onset, when patients had typical symptoms.

Treatment of Fisher's Syndrome

Numerous patients with Fisher's syndrome have been treated by plasma exchange,[557,709,1308] most with apparent improvement. The underlying mechanism of disease and response to treatment are presumably the same as for typical GBS, but this would be difficult to prove without a trial (see Chapter 15). It seems prudent to treat with plasma exchange patients who can no longer walk because of severe ataxia or superimposed weakness. Steroids have also been used, but, as in typical GBS, their effect is difficult to judge. Alternate eye patching, corneal care, and physical therapy to assist gait have been useful in our experience.

Chapter 9

Guillain-Barré Syndrome in Children

Preceding Infection
Clinical Features
Differential Diagnosis
Laboratory and Electrophysiologic Findings
Prognosis
Management

The Guillain-Barré syndrome may affect any age group, including children. The epidemiology of childhood GBS is discussed in Chapter 3. In 24 (15%) of 162 cases of neuropathy evaluated in the Children's Hospital of Philadelphia, GBS was thought to be the most likely etiology.[1111] Most reports of pediatric GBS have concerned patients older than 2 years, but a few case reports have called attention to GBS in the very young, including two probable cases in neonates.[24,406] A 2-month-old patient[1053] was mentioned in a series of 302 cases. Approximately two thirds of pediatric cases occurred in children under age 8 in one series,[62] and half of 95 cases were under age 6 in another.[1185] The ages of patients in other series have ranged from 16 months to 15 years. The proportion of boys to girls, approaching 2:1 in some reports, has been equal in most others. In general, the clinical findings, progression, and outcome have been similar in children and adults, but management and the differential diagnosis, especially of the ataxic child, of pediatric GBS is subtly different.

PRECEDING INFECTION

The preceding illnesses that have been reported in approximately 50% to 70% of GBS in children are listed in Table 9–1. Although *Campylobacter* is common in children, only a few anecdotal reports of GBS have appeared.[981,1308] Most often, a nonspecific upper respiratory tract infection has occurred within 4 weeks before neurologic symptoms. Various exanthems associated with GBS have been emphasized in the literature, but the association is rare. In a large retrospective series,[686] only 1% of 1100 cases occurred after an exanthem. Numerous children have developed typical GBS during or after chickenpox.[227,1270] Complicated cases of chickenpox have been reported with ataxia, abducens palsy,[665] loss of reflexes in the legs, or coarse tremor in the hands.[901] The relationship of these cases to cases of GBS is sometimes uncertain, but most share enough features to consider them postinfectious polyneuropathies. Extreme ataxia in the absence of other cerebellar signs—but with areflexia and loss of kinesthetic and vibration sense—suggests that occasional cases of childhood idiopathic ataxias associated with an exanthem may represent a sensory neuropathy due to GBS rather than cerebellitis. GBS has been described in a child with

Table 9–1 PRECEDING ILLNESS REPORTED IN CHILDHOOD GBS

Upper respiratory infection	Mumps-Rubella vaccination
Campylobacter	Coxsackie virus
Otitis media	Herpes simplex virus
Measles	Echovirus 7
Rubella	Pertussis
Chickenpox	Epstein-Barr virus (usually in adolescence)
Smallpox vaccination	
Measles vaccination	

echovirus 7 isolated from stool and CSF.[1210] In a study of 24 children and young adults, definite serologic evidence of acute Epstein-Barr virus infection was found in 7.[447]

There are only a few reports of childhood GBS after vaccination, suggesting the incidence of this complication is extremely low. Two children (aged 10 months and 19 months) developed GBS within a week after receiving measles-rubella and live measles vaccines.[448] A 20-month-old boy had GBS that progressed to complete flaccid paralysis of all extremities 10 days after receiving a combined mumps-rubella vaccine;[471] the patient recovered over 3 months. A case with predominantly ataxic findings following rubella vaccine was mentioned in the same report.

CLINICAL FEATURES

Although the clinical features of childhood GBS are similar to those in adult GBS, some important differences have been reported (Table 9–2). Thieffry and associates' large series of 95 children is summarized separately in Table 9–3.[1185] Signs of meningeal irritation, including mild neck stiffness or limitation on Lasègue's maneuver, are sometimes present early in the childhood illness. In most children the distribution of weakness has been equally proximal and distal, but distal weakness can predominate. Progressive leg weakness with relative sparing of the arms may occur more commonly in children than in adults. Flaccid quadriplegia has been reported in 6 of 26 cases from the Mayo Clinic.[915]

Special presentations of GBS in infants include a 4½-month-old girl with GBS presenting as a "floppy infant."[174] The patient had mild hypotonia, normal deep tendon reflexes, and failure to thrive. After an episode of diarrhea, the weakness progressed to marked hypotonia (worse distally), abduction paralysis of eye movements, bilateral facial palsy, and loss of deep tendon reflexes. The cerebrospinal fluid (CSF) protein concentration was elevated, and nerve conduction velocities were markedly slowed. Improvement began 9 weeks after the onset of hypotonia and areflexia. A neonatal patient with GBS presented with a weak cry, shallow breathing, and feeding difficulties during the first days of life. The pregnancy had been uneventful except for decreased fetal movement, and a cesarean section had been done because of breech presentation. The tendon reflexes were absent at birth, CSF protein was 40 mg/dL, and motor nerve conduction velocities were 7 m/s in the legs and 16 m/s in the arms, very slow even for a neonate. The child improved clinically, and electrophysiologic tests normalized. The provocative immunologic implications of this case were discussed by the authors.[24]

Paresthesias are common, frequently painful, and tend to appear early in the course of the illness in children. One case report[799] described a 3-year-old girl with low back, buttock, and hip pain, who refused to walk; 19 days later she developed areflexia and slowly progressive weakness. A 5-year-old in another report[735] had severe neck, back, and radiating arm and leg pain with pseudotumor cerebri and probably GBS. In children, presenting clinical symptoms are rarely restricted to painful dysesthesias and sustained hypertension resembling pure pandysautonomia.[838]

Cranial nerve involvement, particularly bilateral facial weakness, has occurred in about 50% of reported cases. In the study by Thieffry and co-workers,[1185] half of the patients had swallowing difficulty and a quarter had facial weakness (see Table 9–3). Fisher's syndrome has been reported in children; a review of the literature reveals at least 20 well-documented cases in patients under 18 years[85,748,953] (see Chapter 8). Oculomotor abnormalities have occurred approximatley as frequently as in adults.[700] Papilledema and pseudotumor have evolved in approximately 5% of children with GBS, including in a 1-month-old infant with a very high CSF protein level associated with hy-

Table 9–2 MAJOR SERIES OF PEDIATRIC GBS CASES

Series, Year	***No. of Patients***	***Age Range***	***Ventilator (Tracheostomy)***	***Autonomic Failure***	***Outcome***
Low et al.,[723] 1958	30	17 mo–16 yr	2 (2)	Bowel dysfunction in 1; hypotension in 1	1 died 1 residual weakness
Peterman et al.,[915] 1959	26	16 mo–15 yr	0 (0)	Bowel dysfunction in 2	1 died 17 complete recovery 7 persistent weakness 2 relapsed 1 lost to follow-up
Debre and Thieffry,[257] 1951	32	2½ yr–4 yr	—	—	2 died All others good recovery
Markland and Riley,[746] 1967	19	18 mo–16 yr	1 (—)	Transient bowel dysfunction in some	0 died 14 complete recovery 1 significant weakness 2 lost to follow-up 2 residual weakness
Paulson,[902] 1970	46	4 mo–19 yr	11 (8)	Blood pressure changes in 6	4 died "A few" residual weakness
Gecow and Pawela,[396] 1971	83	13 mo–13 yr	40 (—)	46%, emphasized bronchial smooth muscle dysfunction	5 died 5 relapsed
Eberle et al.,[317] 1975	47	Under 18 yr	—	—	36 complete recovery 11 mild residual weakness 2 relapsed
Rossi et al.,[1027] 1976	38	2 yr–12 yr	—	5 (not specified)	0 died 11 residual weakness 27 complete recovery
Briscoe et al.,[143] 1987	23	19 mo–13 yr	1 (—)	4 blood pressure changes, 3 cardiac arrythmias, 2 sphincter abnormalities	1 died 19 complete recovery 3 relapsed
Total patients	344				14 died 143 complete recovery

Table 9–3 CLINICAL FEATURES IN 95 PEDIATRIC GBS PATIENTS‡

Characteristics	*No. of Patients (%)*
Age (years) 1–5	45 (47)
6–10	36 (38)
11–15	14 (15)
Sex (M:F)	1.4:1
Antecedent Illness*	38 (40)
Clinical Features at Onset	
Weakness in all limbs	73 (77)
Weakness in legs only	21 (22)
Cranial nerves	1 (1)
Cranial Nerve Involvement	
Oculomotor	7 (7)
Abducens	13 (14)
Facial	26 (27)
Swallowing	51 (54)
Tongue	8 (8)
Respiratory Failure	22 (23)
Tracheostomy	2 (2)
Outcome	
Death†	9 (10)
Residual weakness	5 (5)
Good recovery	81 (85)

*Variety of antecedent infections: gastroenteritis, tonsillitis, pertussis, measles, mumps, chickenpox, hepatitis (2 patients).

†Causes of death: no available respiratory support, before 1954 (3 patients); pulmonary edema (1); postanoxic coma (1); hemorrhage from tracheostoma scan (1); duodenal perforation (1); acidosis, hyponatremia cardiac failure (1).

‡Adapted from Thieffry and co-workers.[1185]

drocephalus,[406,723] and a 5-year-old with pseudotumor, hyporeflexia, cranial nerve abnormalities, and ataxia, who probably had GBS.[735] The incidence of respiratory failure has been 5% to 10% in large series, generally lower than in adults (see Table 9–2) (see Chapter 17). Several large series, however, have reported high numbers of children requiring ventilators.[396,902,1185] Recovery has usually been excellent within 6 months of onset, but areflexia and mild ocular deficits have persisted.[93]

Autonomic disturbances are seen frequently in children, or perhaps are reported more frequently than in adults (see Table 9–2). One article focusing on this complication in childhood GBS[396] cited dysautonomia in 46% of 83 cases and emphasized apparent paralysis of bronchial smooth muscle in 15%.

The case of a 7-year-old child included prominent "postural guarding" due to orthostatic hypotension. Cardiac arrhythmias and blood pressure fluctuations can bc life threatening and led to death in 2 of 16 patients admitted to a pediatric intensive care unit in one series.[122] Severe myocarditis with destruction of dorsal root gangion cells was found in a 12-year-old boy with GBS who died of intractable cardiac arrhythmias.[524] Extremely labile blood pressure, severe and rapid enough to cause a temporary hypertensive encephalopathy with seizures, was noted in a 4-year-old boy.[784]

DIFFERENTIAL DIAGNOSIS

Several differential diagnostic considerations are more relevant in childhood GBS than in adults with GBS (see Chapter 14). Since the advent of polio immunization, poliomyelitis is extremely rare in industrial countries and can be readily distinguished from GBS by the presence of fever, rapid onset of muscle weakness, elevated CSF cell count, and normal electrophysiologic test results.

Botulism shares many features with GBS (see Table 14–37), particularly in infants, but early onset of constipation, pupillary changes, and preserved reflexes and sensation suggest the correct diagnosis. Cases of botulism usually occur in clusters, but the diagnosis should be considered in any infant with acute weakness, because GBS is rare in children under 1 year of age (see Chapter 14 for a more detailed discussion of childhood botulism).

Differentiation of GBS from acute cerebellar ataxia can be difficult in a child. Slight muscle weakness is often manifest as gait incoordination in this age group, particularly if cooperation is limited. An important differentiating point is that the ataxic child can generally rise from sitting on the floor without difficulty if supported, but those with limb weakness cannot. Poisoning by organophosphates and other toxins such as heavy metals causes weakness, autonomic dysfunction, and, more often, encephalopathy. A diphtheric polyneuropathy may be observed after diphtheria immunization, but this is rare. Most other childhood causes of weakness can be distinguished from GBS by their slower onset.

LABORATORY AND ELECTROPHYSIOLOGIC FINDINGS

CSF protein concentration may be elevated more frequently in children with GBS than in adults with the syndrome. In one series,[915] all children had elevated CSF protein levels, up to 800 mg/100 mL. Most series, however, show a distribution of CSF protein similar to that in adults.

Electrodiagnostic testing can be used to confirm the clinical diagnosis and need not be traumatic or uncomfortable for children if each step is clearly explained. The findings in children have been similar to those in adults in most studies,[71,902,915,932] although two reports[784,1027] suggested that severe slowing of motor nerve conduction is more pronounced in children. The mean motor nerve conduction velocity in 19 children was 17 m/s, compared with 40 m/s in adults at comparable times in the illness.[784] Several infants have had particularly slowed nerve conduction, even compared with the expected norms for age. One group[71] found a complete motor block in 3 of 4 of their patients. The prognostic value of electromyogram (EMG) in childhood GBS has not been evaluated systematically in large series.

PROGNOSIS

In a review of 94 published cases of childhood GBS from 1925 to 1951,[62] now outdated, there was an overall mortality rate of 7%, many associated with pulmonary infarction, mostly in children who had difficulty swallowing or respiratory failure. Thieffry's series[1185] had 9 deaths among 95 children, but 3 occurred prior to the routine use of ventilators (see Table 9–3). In more recent series, mortality in pediatric GBS was lower than in adults (see Table 9–2). Most deaths are from early respiratory failure or severe dysautonomia.[122]

In a study of 47 children admitted to a rehabilitation facility after GBS,[317] the most significant early predictor of incomplete recovery was the interval between the plateau phase and the beginning of improvement. Plateau periods longer than 10 days were associated with incomplete recovery. CSF protein concentration was lower, and severe weakness in distal muscles more frequent, in the group that did not recover completely. Less than 5% of Thieffry's patients had residual deficits.[1185] In a study of 23 children,[143] 19 recovered completely after 7 years of follow up; 1 patient died, 2 had a chronic relapsing course, and 1 had a protracted chronic course. In another series,[421] 10 of 12 children who were contacted several years after GBS had subtle residual deficits; 6 had undergone orthopedic surgical procedures, apparently in an attempt to improve function. Outcome in children has tentatively been associated with early fibrillation potentials in a limited retrospective study.[235a]

MANAGEMENT

General care of the pediatric patient with GBS is similar to that of the adult (see Chapter 16). Secondary pressure neuropathy seems to account for some of the residual weakness in children and deserves proper attention. Autonomic lability occurs frequently in children, especially when there are breathing and swallowing difficulties.[122] The temporary use of a pacemaker may be required in selected cases with heart block.[766a]

Plasma exchange in children with GBS has not been studied systematically in large trials. Children were excluded in the British and North American studies (see Chapter 15). The treatment has been well tolerated, however, and anecdotally successful.[1030,1155a] Seven children in one report,[607] aged 2 through 16, received 55 exchanges without complication; all were able to walk again at 6 months' follow-up. Three of four children in another series[1308] had a rapid increase in muscle strength and return of all deep tendon reflexes after the third exchange, although ophthalmoplegia and difficulty swallowing recovered more slowly. Plasmapheresis was apparently successful in a 14-year-old boy with Fisher's syndrome, who had dramatic improvement of vital capacity after the first session.[709] Exchange transfusion was reportedly successful in an infant with respiratory failure from GBS.[1108a] The potential benefits and risks of steroid treatment have not been evaluated in children, except perhaps in a series of 38 personally observed cases,[1027] which had inconclusive results. Others have anecdotally reported no beneficial effect of steroids in children with GBS.[143,723,746,973] Gamma globulin infusions have been tried[1041a] with anecdotal success in children.

Chapter 10

RELAPSING AND CHRONIC INFLAMMATORY POLYNEUROPATHY

Early Relapses Without Chronic Progression (Biphasic Acute GBS)
Relapsing Acute GBS Separated by Long Asymptomatic Intervals
Chronic Inflammatory Demyelinating Polyneuropathy (CIDP)

The Guillain-Barré syndrome is usually a monophasic illness, with a rapid initial onset, progressive weakness over 1 to 4 weeks, and recovery over subsequent months. The majority of patients recover completely or have mild residual deficits 6 to 12 months after onset. A few patients with an otherwise typical episode of acute GBS relapse, have a protracted onset, or slowly improve and then worsen again over weeks or months. Some have a chronic course that presents special problems in diagnosis and treatment. Austin[60] first highlighted the chronic and relapsing form of GBS, defining it largely by steroid responsiveness. For many years, the term "chronic GBS" was used for these patients because of similarities in signs, symptoms, and elevated CSF protein level to acute GBS.[1186] The acute and chronic forms are both inflammatory and demyelinating, but chronic inflammatory demyelinating polyneuropathy (CIDP) is now regarded (rightly or wrongly) as a different clinical entity from acute GBS, with diagnostic criteria proposed by Dyck and co-workers[310] among others.[80,240,1164] Enough experience has been gathered to characterize "typical" patients with CIDP and define differences from typical acute GBS, including (1) a longer progression (2 to 3 months) before plateau, (2) a tendency for the illness to be less severe by comparison with the typical acute disease, (3) fluctuations in the severity of symptoms over many years, (4) greater elevations in CSF protein concentration, (5) more profoundly slowed motor nerve conduction velocities (NCV), and (6) a frequent association with systemic diseases such as lupus erythematosus and Hodgkin's disease. The clinical features alone do not allow a distinction between CIDP and demyelinating neuropathies associated with paraproteinemias and some neoplasms (see later). Most reviews[80] have included demyelinating neuropathies associated with various systemic diseases within the category of CIDP.

Many different clinical courses of CIDP have been reported. This chapter focuses mainly on patients whose initial illnesses are indistinguishable from acute GBS. Among our own patients with acute GBS, we have discerned several temporal courses (Fig. 10–1): (1) early limited acute relapses; (2) relapsing acute GBS separated by asymptomatic intervals; (3) CIDP beginning as acute GBS; and (4) more typical CIDP with a protracted fluctuating course. These distinctions are useful clinically, but they may simply represent a different time-evolution of a similar underlying immune mechanism. On the basis of clinical, laboratory, and pathologic similarities, there is a fundamental relationship between the acute and chronic inflammatory demyelinating polyneuropathies. Profoundly slowed nerve conduction velocities and raised CSF protein concentration may simply reflect the length of illness rather than

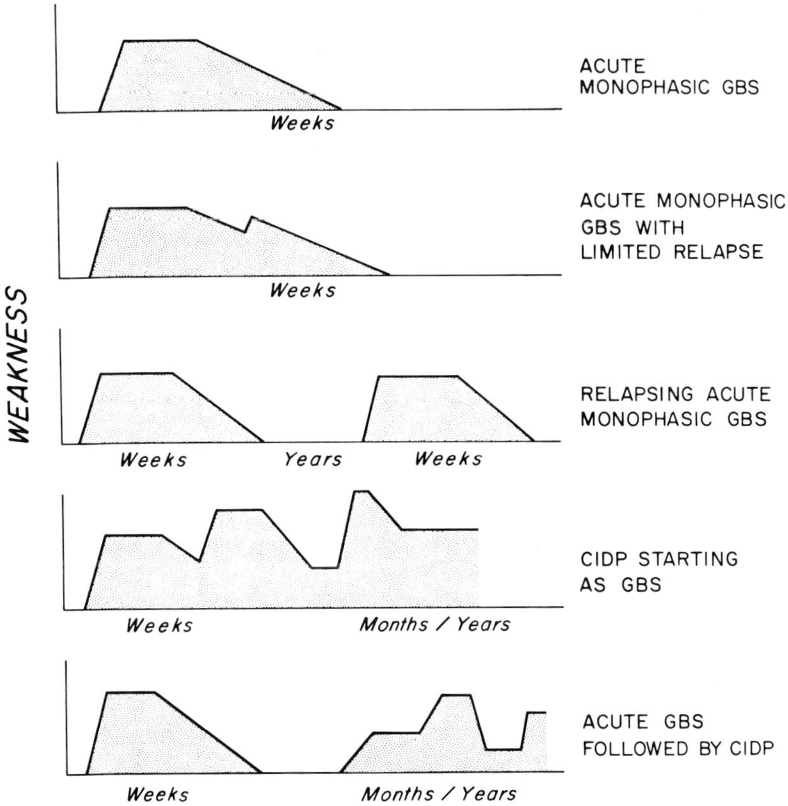

Figure 10–1. Possible temporal courses following acute GBS (see Fig. 10–3).

an important underlying pathologic or immunologic difference from acute GBS.

EARLY RELAPSES WITHOUT CHRONIC PROGRESSION (BIPHASIC ACUTE GBS)

Minor daily fluctuations in muscle strength, rarely more than a grade on the Medical Research Council[547] (see Table 7–4) scale, are common in GBS patients who have reached the plateau of illness or have started improving. Temporary, brief worsening of limb or diaphragmatic weakness may occur immediately after plasma exchange, after strenuous physiotherapy, or with acute respiratory infections. The insignificant degree of worsening with most acute infections is surprising. Reinstitution of the ventilator is sometimes required after successful weaning, but this is more often the result of premature extubation or a new pulmonic process. None of these circumstances is likely to represent a worsening of the inflammation in nerves.

True biphasic courses after plasma exchange have been reported in up to a quarter of patients[885] 2 to 4 weeks after initial improvement, and in 10% of Massachusetts General Hospital (MGH) patients receiving plasma exchange[1011] (from the MGH and the University of Michigan, Ann Arbor, courtesy of Dr. J. Albers). After a second course of plasma exchange, most of our patients have improved even more rapidly than after the first series. Patients in the MGH series with this type of limited relapse have had (1) an intercurrent upper respiratory tract infection, (2) ongoing cytomegalovirus (CMV) pharyngitis, and (3) a persistent pharyngitis with nega-

Table 10–1 PATIENTS WITH RELAPSES AFTER PLASMA EXCHANGE[§]

Patient No./Age (yr)/Sex	*Days from Onset to First Plasma Exchange*	*Days to Relapse**	*Clinical Worsening†*	*Second Course‡*	*Follow-Up*
1/34/M	8	8	Inability to lift legs from bed	3/14/15	Paresthesias
2/21/M	10	14	Grade II-III	3/11.5/6	Third course 30 days after last; normal by 14 mo
3/20/M	19	42	Slowly worsening gait and paresthesias	3/12/7	Normal by 9 mo
4/28/M	22	20	Pain and increasing leg weakness	3/13/5	Normal by 10 mo
5/24/M	10	7	New facial weakness, worsening gait	4/12/10	Facial weakness
6/31/F	7	10	Grade II-III worsening paresthesias, new pharyngeal weakness	5/12/8	Third course 16 days after last; normal by 2 mo; prophylactic immunosuppression
7/17/F	12	20	Grade III-IV, inability to lift legs	5/12/9	Improved 5 days later; normal at 15 mo
8/77/M	12	25	Increasing leg weakness; inability to lift legs from bed	No	Improved beginning 3 wk later
9/63/M	3	5	Increasing limb weakness; inability to lift arms from bed	4/14/5	Improved 7 days later; walking unassisted at 4 mo
10/30/M	4	11	Decreasing respiratory function; increasing arm weakness	No	Improved beginning 13 days later

*From end of last plasma exchange.
†Grading system: II, Minor signs and symptoms; III, Able to walk 5 m with assistance; IV, Bed-bound; V, On respirator.
‡Course of plasma exchange: number of treatments/total volume-exchanged (L)/days.
§Adapted from Ropper et al.,[1011] p. 315.

tive cultures for CMV but most have not had an obvious precipitant for relapse. Limited relapses have been characterized by worsening gait, often with new facial or pharyngeal weakness, and decreased limb strength or vital capacity, usually insufficient to cause a decrease of one clinical grade (see Chapter 15). Patients were usually no weaker than they had been before the first series of plasma exchanges, although two patients (not at the MGH) required a ventilator for the first time during a limited relapse. Cerebrospinal fluid (CSF) reexamination showed an increase in protein concentration in 5 of 7 patients with limited relapses, perhaps related only to the duration of illness. A second course of 3 to 5 plasma exchanges in 8 MGH patients resulted in marked improvement over 5 to 10 days. Two patients again relapsed (a triphasic course) and a third course of exchanges resulted in similar improvement (Table 10–1). Patients not treated with further exchanges have also improved, but it has appeared to take longer for them to gain a clinical grade. None of our patients have developed a chronic or recurrently relapsing course typical of CIDP, but others[557a] have. The course of one of our patients with infection-associated relapse and improvement after plasma exchange is shown in Figure 10–2.

This limited relapse phenomenon supports the hypothesis that plasma exchange removes a circulating factor that persists if treatment is stopped early. The existence of several patients with relapses that were worse than the original illness raises the possibility that exchanges also cause a rebound of the underlying immunologic disease.

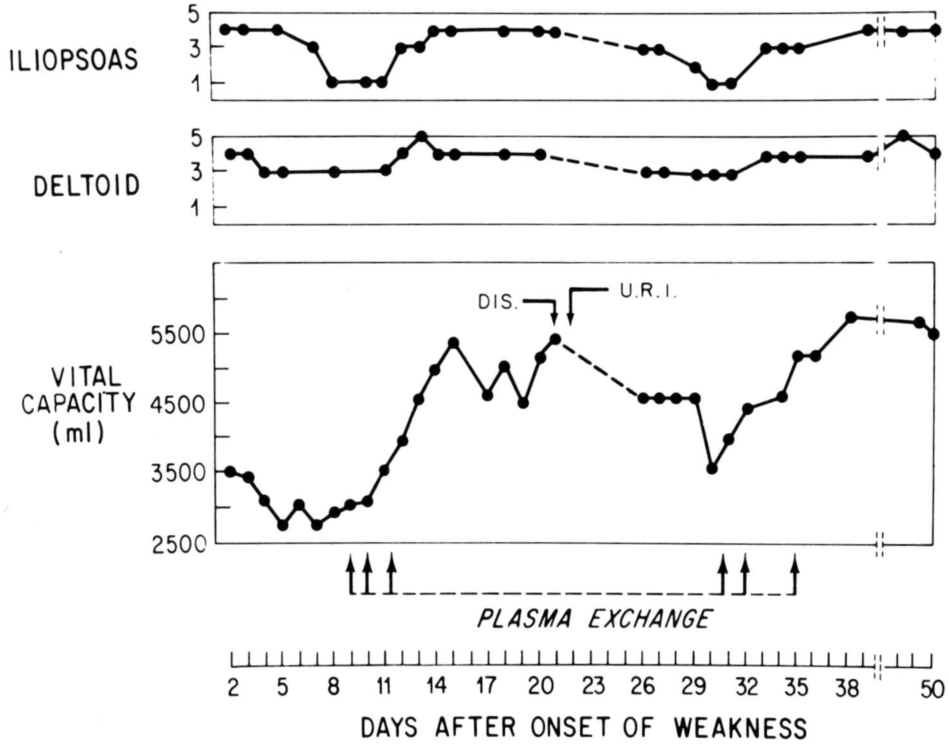

Figure 10–2. Muscle power (MRC scale), vital capacity, and timing of plasma exchanges in a 28-year-old man who had a limited relapse 2 weeks after a first course of plasma exchange. DIS. = discharged; U.R.I. = upper respiratory infection. (Reprinted from Neurological and Neurosurgical Intensive Care by A. Ropper and S. Kennedy [eds.], p. 265, with permission of Aspen Publishers, Inc., 1988.)

One research group[1238] has found preliminary evidence of an antibody rebound after exchange. More often, a severe early relapse indicates an underlying symptomatic GBS, as from Hodgkin's disease or systemic lupus erythematosus.

Most of the major randomized trials of plasma exchange have shown similar incidences of various types of relapses in placebo– and plasma exchange–treated patients. The French Cooperative Study,[380] however, showed more relapses during the first year in the treated group. Early relapses were associated with steroid treatment in acute GBS in one controlled trial.[547] There is insufficient evidence to confirm that steroids increase the risk of acute relapse or the induction of a chronic progressive course. There is, however, clinical worsening when steroids are withdrawn rapidly in some cases of CIDP and of acute GBS.

Biphasic courses of a slightly different nature were described in older series in which no specific therapy for GBS was used. One of Guillain's original patients relapsed after an intercurrent infection.[466] In Haymaker and Kernohan's series,[501] one patient improved, then relapsed 1 month after onset, with quadriparesis, respiratory failure, aspiration, and death, approximately 2 days after the onset of the relapse. Others[124] have described a biphasic course with complete quadriplegia, sensory loss, and muscle pain after influenza B infection. This patient gradually recovered but worsened after a chickenpoxlike eruption, with new oropharyngeal and respiratory weakness, followed again by complete recovery in 2 months. Several similar cases have been reported with acute GBS that improves and then relapses within approximately a month, unassociated with plasma exchange or steroid treatment. In some cases, the region affected has changed between the acute episode and the relapse, as in rare cases of ophthalmoplegia[590] or Fisher's syndrome[582] in which patients relapsed with more generalized weakness.

RELAPSING ACUTE GBS SEPARATED BY LONG ASYMPTOMATIC INTERVALS

In many large series of patients with acute GBS, 1% (to an extreme in one series of 10%) recovered completely and had acute relapses several months to a decade later (Table 10–2). Detailed descriptions are rarely given. A postmortem examination showed perivascular lymphocytic infiltration of spinal roots, cranial nerves, and peripheral nerves in one patient who recovered from initial quadriparesis and cranial nerve involvement but died after a similar acute illness 35 years later.[52] One reported patient relapsed with respiratory failure, bilateral facial weakness, and papilledema, similar to an initial acute episode 6 months previously.[1186] Another had several acute relapses over 31 years—each preceded by an upper respiratory infection or surgical procedure—severe enough to cause quadriplegia with increasing degrees of disability after each episode.[121] One relapse occurred several days after a nerve biopsy under local anesthesia. At least two acute relapsing cases have been described after influenza vaccination[1085] (see Chapter 6), and one after tetanus toxoid.[937] A patient with systemic lupus erythematosus, manifest only as pleural effusions, had three acute GBS episodes in 3 years, perhaps related to steroid withdrawal. Sural nerve biopsy showed no vasculitis.[804] In another, more complex case the patient showed features similar to those of Fisher's syndrome, with several recurrent attacks over 10 years of diplopia, ptosis, and ataxia, lasting 5 to 10 days each.[590] A similar case has been reported with autopsy features.[265]

Acute relapsing GBS with extremely long intervening asymptomatic intervals has also been mentioned in some large series. One of 23 patients in one series[957] had an initial acute episode, recovered, and relapsed gradually with progressive weakness 31 years later. Three patients in the retrospective MGH series had acute relapses 6, 12,

Table 10–2 ACUTE RELAPSES IN MAJOR SERIES OF GBS

Author, Year	*N*	*No. of Relapses (%)*	*Interval*
Peterman et al.,[915] 1959	26	2 (8)	5 mo; 9 mo
Wiederholt et al.,[1278] 1964	97	10 (10)	Not stated
McFarland and Heller,[777] 1966	100	4 (4)	Not stated
Castaigne et al.,[179] 1966	457	14 (4)	6 mo–24 yr
Pleasure et al.,[932] 1968	49	3 (6)	12; 13; 13 yr
Samantray et al.,[1053] 1977	302	6 (2)	2–6 yr
Loffel et al.,[714] 1977	123	4 (3)	4–5 mo; 1, 2, 8 yr
Hughes et al.,[547] 1978	40	3 (8)*	Within 1 yr
Kennedy et al.,[606] 1978	40	1 (2)	4 yr
Andersson and Siden,[31] 1982	60	2 (3)	Between 3 and 5 mo in both
Guillain-Barré Syndrome Study Group,[469] 1985	245	5 (2)†	Within 6 mo
French Cooperative Group,[380] 1987	220	7 (3)‡	Within 1 yr

*All in steroid treatment group.
†Three in plasma exchange group.
‡Six in plasma exchange group.

and 18 years after their initial episode. A fourth had two relapses at 5 and 8 years after the first bout. There have been an additional 5 patients with acute relapses after many intervening years, one of whom is included in the prospective series.[1279] The progression and distribution of weakness were usually similar between the initial and the second acute episodes (Table 10–3). Re-

Table 10–3 CLINICAL CHARACTERISTICS IN PATIENTS WITH ACUTE RELAPSING GUILLAIN-BARRÉ SYNDROME†

Patient No.	*Antecedent Illness*	*Interval*	*Clinical Features*	*Time to Walk*
1	URI		Bifacial weakness, quadriparesis, on ventilator within 24 hr, for 40 days	3 mo
	URI	15 yr	Bifacial weakness, quadriparesis, on ventilator within 24 hr for 16 days	1 mo
2	Diarrhea, fever		Numbness in legs, arms, mouth; leg weakness	8 mo
	Diarrhea, vomiting	10 yr	Numbness in legs; leg weakness, inability to walk	1 mo
	Diarrhea, fever	1½ yr	Numbness in legs; leg weakness, inability to walk	1 mo
3	URI		Quadriparesis, on ventilator for 10 wk	6 mo
	URI	4 yr	Bifacial weakness, ophthalmoplegia, quadriparesis, on ventilator for 5 wk	6 mo
	None	7 mo	Bifacial weakness, ophthalmoplegia, quadriparesis, on ventilator for 10 days	2 mo
	None	1 yr	Bifacial weakness, ptosis, quadriparesis, no respiratory failure	2 mo
4	None		Distal limb weakness and numbness	Several weeks
	URI	36 yr	Facial weakness, quadriparesis, ptosis, pharyngeal weakness, on ventilator for 29 days	4 mo
5	Diarrhea, malaria	23 yr	Virtually pure motor GBS, mild	3 mo
			Pure motor GBS, severe	2 yr

*URI = Upper respiratory infection.
†From Wijdicks and Ropper,[1279] p. 83, with permission.

lapses were triggered by a variety of events including, in one patient, acute malaria.

The pathogenesis of acute relapsing patients is unknown, but a "smoldering" persistent inflammation in the nerves of autopsied GBS that re-emerges during a relapse has been suggested.[52] Similar symptoms and signs with each episode support the theory of persistent inflammatory lesions, but the long symptom-free intervals and virtual or complete recovery in some patients are inconsistent with this explanation. Another possibility is a proclivity for some patients to get relapsing GBS, on the basis of persistent clones of B cells that re-emerge to produce a pathogenic antibody. This may be supported by the provocation of repeated attacks after similar acute infectious illness. One report[4] found an increased frequency of HLA-A1, -B8, -DRw3, and -Dw3 haplotypes in CIDP, whereas no consistent HLA pattern is known to occur in acute GBS (see Chapter 6).

Illustrative Case 10-1 Relapsing Acute GBS

A 42-year-old woman had diarrhea and fever, followed in 2 days by paresthesias in her hands, legs, and mouth and weakness in both legs. She was hospitalized briefly, and was found to have areflexia and elevated CSF protein concentration. She recovered completely in 8 months except for minor paresthesias; the deep tendon reflexes returned. Ten years after the first episode, the patient had a gastrointestinal illness similar to the previous one, followed in 4 days by leg aching, weakness, and paresthesias. She had proximal limb weakness, absent reflexes, a wide-based gait, and inability to stand. The CSF protein level was 156 mg/dL, with 3 mononuclear cells per mm^3. Nerve conduction velocities were slightly slowed (ulnar 32 m/s, median 30 m/s), and median nerve F-wave responses were absent. She recovered completely without any specific therapy after 1 month. A third identical episode occurred 19 months later, again preceded by a gastrointestinal illness. There were no palpable nerves or signs of systemic disease.

CHRONIC INFLAMMATORY DEMYELINATING POLYNEUROPATHY (CIDP)

CIDP Beginning as Acute GBS

In many major series of CIDP 10% to 15% of patients have had an initial rapid onset of weakness indistinguishable from acute GBS;[453,773,936,957] however, in two series of CIDP none of the clinical courses began in this fashion.[240,310] The major differences from acute GBS are continued worsening for more than a month (sometimes for up to 4 months) or minimal recovery before continued worsening. Distinguishing true worsening of CIDP from the effect of steroid withdrawal is often difficult in reported series, as well as in clinical practice. For example, one patient was described as having CIDP with six major relapses associated with steroid withdrawal, each several months apart, and all beginning as acute GBS.[936]

CIDP with Subacute Onset (Typical CIDP)

Numerous reports in the 1960s and 1970s differentiated a chronic as well as a relapsing variant of GBS from the acute monophasic type. Until Dyck and colleagues' paper in 1975,[310] a disarray of descriptive terms existed: recurrent polyneuropathies,[60] relapsing motor polyneuropathy,[55] recurrent and chronic relapsing Guillain-Barré polyneuritis,[1186] relapsing corticosteroid-dependent polyneuritis,[764] steroid-responsive recurrent polyneuropathy,[274] and relapsing hypertrophic neuritis,[279]—all identifying the same illness. Dyck and associates[310] reviewed the clinical features of 53 patients and categorized slowly progressive or relapsing demyelinating polyneuropathy as a distinct clinical entity, despite pathologic and laboratory findings similar to those of acute GBS. Subsequent papers[240] have offered other diagnostic criteria for chronic relapsing-demyelinating poly-

Table 10–4 DISTINGUISHING FEATURES BETWEEN ACUTE GUILLAIN-BARRÉ AND CIDP*

Features	*Typical GBS*	*Typical CIDP*
Antecedent event	70%	20–30%
Onset to maximal deficit	4 wk	6 mo to several years
Fluctuations	Uncommon	Common
Ophthalmoplegia	10–20%	<5%
Respiratory failure requiring ventilation	30%	Seldom
Autonomic dysfunction	50%	Seldom
Normal CSF protein level	10%	90%
Early electromyographic (EMG) findings	Proximal conduction block	Marked slowing of motor nerve conduction
HLA association	None	A1; B8 DRw3

*Adapted from McLeod;[781] Dyck et al.;[310] and McCombe et al.[773]

neuropathy (CRIP or CIDP). Some of the distinctive clinical and laboratory features of CIDP in comparison to acute GBS are summarized in Table 10–4, and the diagnostic criteria we have used are shown in Table 10–5.

CLINICAL FEATURES

CIDP occurs at all ages, with patients ranging from 2 to 70 years.[310,773,957] The literature suggests that men are more frequently affected than women. Well-defined antecedent events are less common in CIDP than in acute GBS, although 19% to 32% have typical preceding acute illnesses (upper respiratory infection, vaccination, and surgery).[310,773] Serologic evidence of preceding CMV infection occurred in a higher proportion of CIDP patients than in a control population in one series.[773] Several authors have suggested that pregnancy produces relapses.[772,863]

Table 10–5 DIAGNOSTIC CRITERIA OF CIDP*

Bilateral relatively symmetric limb weakness
Paresthesias in toes and fingertips
Progression over ≥6 wk, followed by episodes of improvement and worsening of limb weakness for at least 3 mo, or slow progression of limb weakness over 6 wk to several months
Hypoflexia in weak limbs by 1 month; areflexia at ankles
The following laboratory abnormalities confirm the diagnosis:
Elevated CSF protein concentration >100 mg/mL during clinical deterioration
Slowing of motor nerve conduction and prolonged distal latencies in at least 2 limbs (<60% of lower limit of normal), or multifocal conduction block

*After exclusion of associated disorders in Table 10–9.

The most common clinical features of CIDP in large series are summarized in Table 10–6. Relatively symmetric proximal and distal limb weakness tend to equal or eclipse sensory abnormalities early in the illness. A predominantly sensory variant may exist, and up to 85% of patients in one series (higher than in the MGH experience) have eventually had prominent sensory loss.[80] Several authors have highlighted proximal weakness as a characteristic feature. A few exceptional cases with severe quadriplegia have had ventilatory failure, but the illness generally tends to be less severe than typical cases of acute GBS. The reflexes are usually absent in limbs that have been weak for over a month. Patients with very slowly progressive disease that begins in the legs, however, can retain reflexes in the arms, even months after onset. Approximately 10% have areflexia only at the ankles. Various types of pain occur in a quarter of patients. Facial and oropharyngeal weakness or ophthalmoplegia have occurred in less than 15%—far less frequently than in acute GBS. Unusual relapsing variants have been described with ptosis and lateral rectus

Table 10–6 CLINICAL FEATURES IN CIDP/CRIDP IN LARGE SERIES*

Series, Year	*N*	*Time to Peak*	**Deficit† (Predominantly)**		*VII*	*Oropharyngeal Involvement*	*Ophthalmoplegia*	*Papilledema*	*Tremor*	*Ventilator*	*Nerve Enlargement*
			Motor	*Sensory*							
Dyck et al.,[310] 1975	53	—	5 (9)	3 (6)	3 (6)	5 (9)	2 (4)	4 (7)	—	—	6 (11)
Prineas and McLeod,[957] 1976	23	3 wk–16 mo	6 (26)	0 (0)	6 (26)	3 (13)	1 (4)	—	2 (9)	3 (13)	0 (0)
Dalakas and Engel,[240] 1981	25	6–12 mo	0 (0)	0 (0)	2 (8)	0 (0)	2 (8)	0 (0)	6 (24)	—	2 (8)
McCombe et al.,[773] 1987	92	16% <1 mo	20 (22)	6 (6)	14 (15)	6 (7)	4 (4)	1 (1)	3 (3)	Some	—
Barohn et al.,[80] 1989	60	—	—	—	8 (13)	—	2 (3)	2 (3)	—	0 (0)	—

*No. of patients (%).
†Remainder have both motor and sensory involvement.

weakness or a relapsing dysphagia, areflexia, and quadriparesis.[280,590] Dysautonomia is uncommon.[773] One series had a quarter of patients with action and postural tremor at the onset,[240] a feature alluded to by others. This irregular tremor, unrelated to weakness, severe proprioceptive loss, or high doses of corticosteroids, more often appears after the second relapse. Four of twenty MGH patients with CIDP have had severe tremor. Papilledema, though still rare, is more common than with acute GBS, and has been attributed to the greatly elevated CSF protein concentration typical of many cases of CIDP. The pseudotumor-papilledema syndrome in GBS and its relation to CSF protein level are discussed more extensively in Chapter 7.

Pure motor CIDP simulating amyotrophic lateral sclerosis is uncommon and chronic motor neuropathy may suggest circulating antibodies to GM-1 ganglioside or another paraproteinemic neuropathy[675a,913] (see later). A similar possible variant of CIDP, multifocal demyelinating neuropathy with persistent conduction block, has been recognized.[692] The clinical picture simulates mononeuritis multiplex, with wrist or foot drop, primarily large fiber sensory involvement, pain, Tinel's sign, focal nerve tenderness, and areflexia. The arms are generally more severely and frequently affected than the legs. The temporal course is otherwise similar to typical CIDP. Electrophysiologic testing shows multiple focal conduction blocks.[692] Sural nerve biopsy in one patient has shown incomplete lesions in many fascicles, with relative sparing of subperineural fibers, similar to ischemic neuropathy.[865] Uncommon chronic demyelinating-inflammatory sensory or ataxic[239] neuropathies may be variants of CIDP,[239,597] but many of these patients are subsequently found to have a paraproteinemia, some with Sjögren's syndrome.

COURSE AND PROGNOSIS

The duration of progression, number of relapses, and severity of CIDP are unpredictable at the onset, particularly when the course is altered by treatment (Table 10–7). The two major temporal profiles are a chronic progressive and a relapsing-remitting type. The variable courses described in the literature are illustrated schematically in Figure 10–3. In two series, 64%[310] and 53%[80] had a stepwise worsening or monophasic course, in contrast to only 35% in another.[773] The remainder had variants of a relapsing-remitting temporal course. One series suggested an earlier age of onset in patients with a relapsing course. Barohn and colleagues[80] have made the salient point that the longer patients are followed, the more likely relapses are appreciated. Many relapsing cases resolve after a few years[957] and patients with a relapsing course tend to have a more favorable prognosis than

Table 10–7 OUTCOME IN LARGE CIDP SERIES

Author	*No.*	*Follow-up*	*Outcome*	
Dyck et al.,[310] 1975*	53	Mean 7.4 yr	Complete recovery	4%
			Moderately disabled	68%
			Wheelchair-bound	28%
Prineas and McLeod,[957] 1976	23	Mean 3 yr (range 0.5–31 yr)	Complete recovery	26%
			Moderately disabled	74%
McCombe et al.,[773] 1987	76	10 yr (range 1–41 yr)	Complete recovery	30%
			Minimal impairment	43%
			Moderate impairment	18%
			Wheelchair-bound	2%
			Died	7%
Barohn et al.,[80] 1989	60	34 mo (range 6–142 mo)	Responded to treatment	95%
			Died	3%

*Twelve percent died (6 related to CIDP, 3 to other diseases).

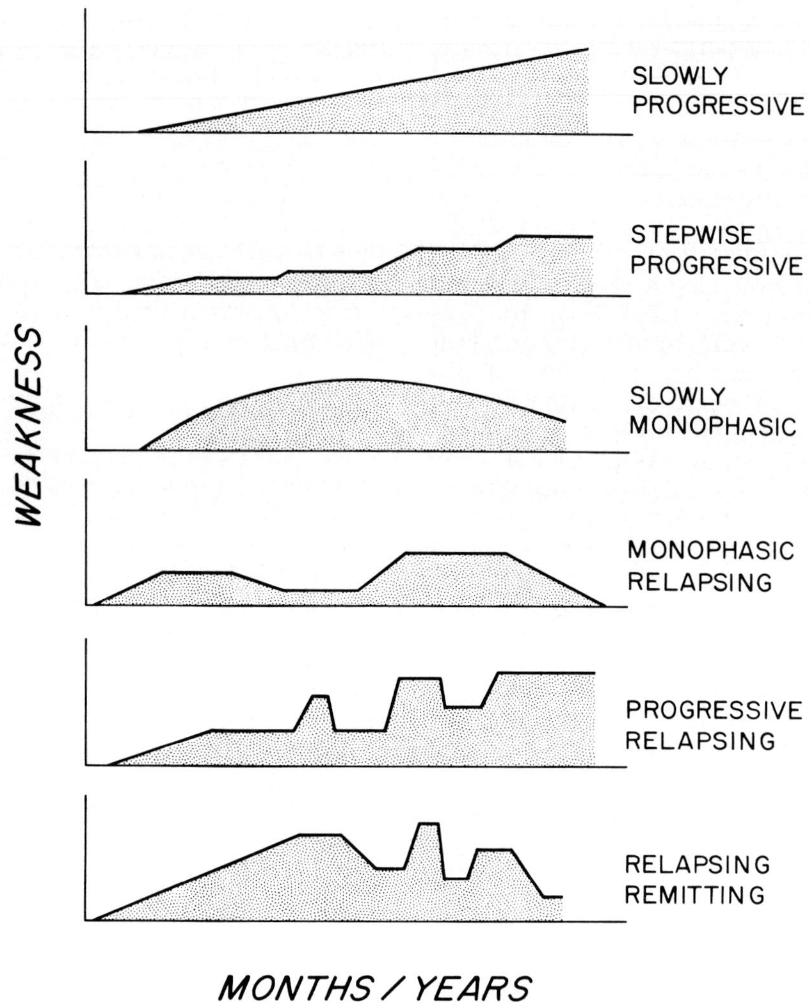

Figure 10–3. Temporal courses of CIDP (see also Fig. 10–1).

those with a chronic progressive course.[773] The clinical course may be influenced by corticosteroid or plasma exchange treatment, but it is clear from reports without treatment that a stepwise or relapsing course occurs naturally in some patients. Two thirds of MGH patients with CIDP have had a relapsing course, though their overall function worsened slowly as the illness progressed.

In many, however, plasma exchange or steroid responsiveness has obscured the natural course of illness. In two large series, up to 30% of patients eventually made a complete recovery with steroid treatment, plasma exchange, or both. In one series,[773] 43% of patients with CIDP were only mildly disabled 10 years after the onset of symptoms. The overall mortality from CIDP has been approximately 5% to 10%, usually attributable to intercurrent infections. The number of relapses probably declines over decades; however, life-threatening relapses requiring ventilatory support have occurred rarely after several stable years.[957]

CIDP in Children

CIDP has been reported in infants; it occurs more often in older children (see

Table 10–8 LABORATORY FINDINGS IN CIDP*

Investigation	***Dyck et al.,[310] 1975***	***Prineas and McLeod,[957] 1976***	***Oh,[872] 1978***	***Dalakas and Engel,[240] 1981***	***McCombe et al.,[773] 1987***	***Krendel et al.,[648] 1989***	***Barohn et al.,[80] 1989***
CSF/N	44	23	10	25	72	14	59
Elevated protein	40 (91)	20 (87)	7 (70)	25 (100)	0.23–5.50 g/L	11 (79)	56 (95)
Pleocytosis	5 (11)	2 (9)	0 (0)	0 (0)	—	0	2 (3)
EMG MNCV†/N	53.0	23.0			25.0		60.0
Ulnar (m/s)	26.2	27.8	28.4	10–28	29.3	—	35.2
Median (m/s)	30.8	30.2	28.8		30.4		35.1
Peroneal (m/s)	27.3	25.6	23.9		29.5		29.7
Sural nerve/N	26	26	10	25	—	14	56
Mononuclear cells	14 (54)	6 (23)	0	0		4 (29)	6 (11)
Demyelination‡	23	23	33	NA§		7 (50)	27 (48)
Onion bulbs	4 (15)	10 (38)	1	NA		5 (36)	—

*No. of patients (%).
†Mean values.
‡Percentage of leased fibers.
§NA = Not available.

Chapter 9).[162,1112] Ten children with CIDP were reported in one large series (aged 2 to 10 years), with minor residual disability in only one child.[773] In a large study of 112 children with a variety of demyelinating neuropathies (collected over 7 years),[1112] 13 had CIDP, 7 with a chronic relapsing and 6 with a slowly progressive course. The natural history in children has been as variable as in adults; self-limiting, progressive, and steroid-dependent courses have been reported.[207] Two sisters, aged 4 and 9, have had CIDP[387] without a family history of neuropathy, both with chronic progressive courses. Sural nerve biopsy demonstrated mononuclear cell infiltrates.

Laboratory Findings

Most patients with CIDP have elevated CSF protein concentrations, often greater than 150 mg/dL, and sometimes up to 1 g/dL; however, CSF protein levels may be normal at various times during the illness (Table 10–8). In a recent series,[80] 95% had elevated CSF protein concentratons at unselected times during the illness. Persistent mild elevation of CSF protein (75 mg/dL) has been described in two patients 7 and 9 years after onset.[518] There is no pleocytosis in most patients, but a few cells are often present (up to 5 cells per mm^3). Monoclonal and oligoclonal bands have been found in a few patients but are not a regular feature of the disease.[241,310]

Slowing of motor nerve conduction velocities and prolonged distal latencies in several nerves, often below 60% of normal, almost always occurs once CIDP is well established, but these signs may not be apparent for up to 6 months. Severe slowing may allow a distinction between CIDP and acute GBS, in which this degree of slowing is uncommon until several weeks of illness (although one quarter of patients with acute GBS have some slowing early in their course; see Chapter 13). Multifocal conduction block, not located at common regions of nerve entrapment, has been emphasized as a typical electrophysiologic phenomenon in CIDP even without the clinical features of multifocal demyelinating neuropathy discussed earlier.[692] Using a definition of the disease that is probably too broad, one series[80] found that only two thirds of patients had at least one nerve with slowing to less than 70% of normal conduction velocity, and only 13% had conduction block. The electrophysiologic uniformity and clinical variability of CIDP therefore remain important questions. Severe slowing may be a function of the long duration of illness, and it is not clear if patients with acute GBS and residual deficits retain their conduction blocks for long after the acute illness.

Pathology

Nerve biopsies in CIDP show demyelination in 20% to 40% and onion bulb formation in 10% to 40%, indicating repeated episodes of remyelination (Fig. 10–4). The material surrounding nerve fibers is predominantly connective tissue. Several series[648] have found mononuclear cell infiltrates in as many as half of nerve biopsies (see Table 10–8), but others[80,241] have not found inflammation. The combination of cellular infiltrates and onion bulb formation in sural nerve biopsies, and the clinical features, have been fairly certain indicators of CIDP.[648] Up to 20% of patients in some series have had purely axonal neuropathies, but the literature is sullied by many cases of axonal neuropathies, clinically indistinguishable from CIDP that are symptomatic of underlying systemic disease. In particular, the paraproteinemic neuropathies are not usually inflammatory. The inclusion of symptomatic noninflammatory neuropathies, and the unreliability of sural nerve biopsies in reflecting the overall nature of disease, makes interpretation of the literature on the pathology of CIDP difficult.

The few postmorten studies of CIDP have shown clusters of endoneural lymphocytes and monocytes and myelin de-

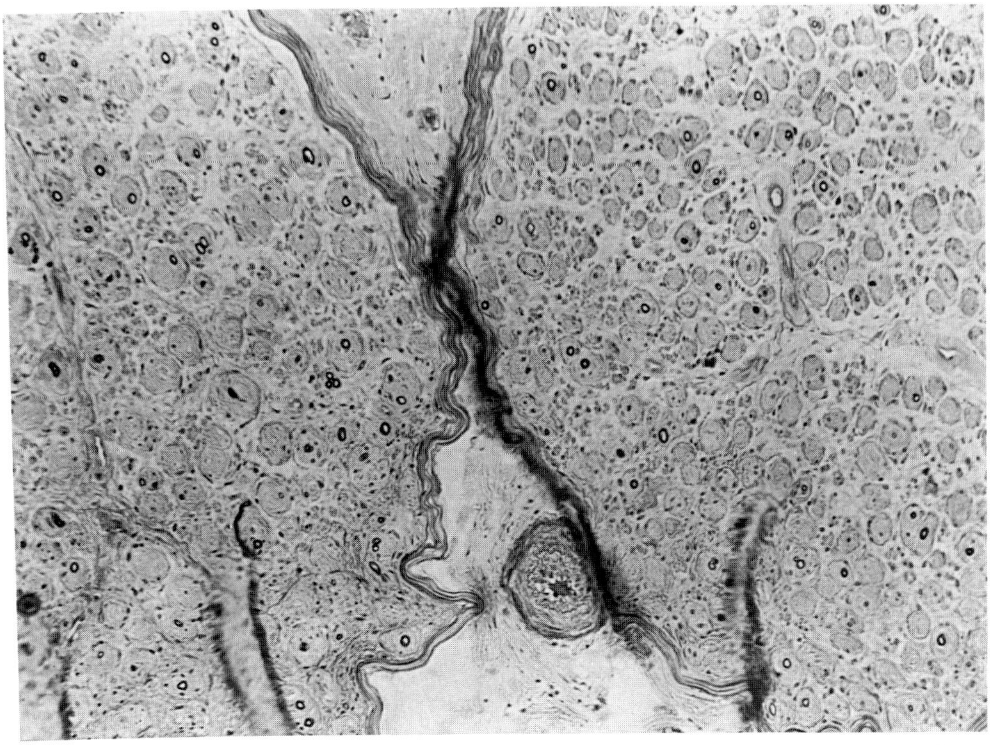

Figure 10–4. Sural nerve biopsy from a patient with relapsing CIDP, showing "onion bulb" formation. The material surrounding the fibers is predominantly connective tissue. This reaction, thought to result from repeated demyelination and remyelination, gives rise to an "onion bulb" appearance on microscopy.

generation in posterior roots and peripheral nerves. There is occasional inflammatory reaction in the meninges. One autopsy, of a patient with CIDP and eye movement abnormalities 1 month before death,[310] revealed scattered lymphocyte collections in the brainstem. Pallor of the posterior columns occurred in another case.[764]

Immunocytochemical staining in CIDP sometimes demonstrates linear IgM, IgG, and C3 deposition.[241] In a case with high titers of anti-GM1 antibody, IgM deposition was found at nodes of Ranvier.[675a] Inflammatory lesions in systemic organs, as in a few cases of acute GBS, have not been reported[310] (see Chapter 4), but several cases,[794,1188] usually of long duration, have shown T-2 signal abnormalities in periventricular white matter on magnetic resonance imaging (MRI) scans, without clinical correlates. Most patients in the MGH series, studied in the first 3 years of illness, have not had cerebral MRI changes on cerebral or spinal cord MRI scans.

Treatment

Several controlled and uncontrolled trials* have claimed a beneficial effect of corticosteroids in CIDP, an impression shared anecdotally by most clinicians. In one study with limited numbers of patients, azathioprine (2 mg/kg) added to prednisone was no more effective than prednisone alone.[312]

After initial reports of successful treatment with plasma exchange, often with rapid effect,† benefit was con-

*See references 60, 80, 240, 311, 773, 872, and 957.

†See references 282, 375, 403, 453, 689, 1084, and 1197.

firmed in a randomized, sham treatment trial[307] of 29 patients with progressive or recurrent CIDP. There were significant differenccs favoring plasma exchange in return of reflexes and improvement in electrodiagnostic studies, although overall improvement in neurological disability, measured on an average disability scale, was comparatively small. Approximatley half of the plasma-exchanged patients did not improve.

Of 21 patients with CIDP seen at the MGH from 1982 to 1988, 13 had mixed motor and sensory signs, 2 had a predominantly sensory neuropathy, and one had a virtually pure sensory polyneuropathy (Table 10–9). Improvement occurred in 7 of 16 patients treated with a series of 3 to 5 plasma exchanges over 1 to 2 weeks. Three patients continue to receive episodic plasma exchanges, supplemented by small doses of steroids, to treat symptomatic deterioration.

Studies of plasma exchange, and probably of other therapies in CIDP, identify two discrete populations: one that responds clearly and another that receives no benefit from plasma exchange. Attempts to demonstrate statistical changes in clinical state obscure these definite differences by combining the groups. Some patients legitimately act as their own control subjects, improving consistently after exchanges at different intervals and levels of neurologic deterioration.

Rapid symptomatic improvement has also been reported after plasma or gamma globulin infusions in uncontrolled and controlled cross-over studies. Improvement occurred repeatedly after reinfusion.[339,1233] Our preliminary experience with gamma globulin infusions in 10 patients suggests that patients who have had CIDP for less than approximately 2 years may benefit from treatment. The degree of improvement has been comparable to (but longer lasting than) that following plasma exchange in four patients and less than that following plasma exchanges in the others. Three patients with polyneuropathy associated with monoclonal or biclonal serum gammopathies have also benefitted from gamma globulin infusion. Other treatments such as cyclophosphamide;[957] nitrogen mustard;[957] and poly ICLC, a synthetic polynucleotide[241] (in a few patients each), have not

Table 10–9 PLASMA EXCHANGE IN CIDP*

	Responders† (N=7)	***Nonresponders (N=9)***
Age		
Mean	47	51
Range	29–73	20–71
Sex		
Male	4	5
Female	3	4
Duration of illness (mo)		
Mean	11	17
Range	(1–42)	(3–48)
MRC limb power <4 in all limbs	6	5
CSF Protein (mg/dL)		
Mean	83	123
Range	34–169	44–300
Electrophysiology (N=14)		
NCV		
<30 m/s in 2 nerves	3	4
>30 m/s	3	4
Active denervation	4	5
Steroids with exchanges	3	5

†At least 1 grade improvement in 3 muscles; or improvement of 1 functional grade; or major improvement.

*MGH (1981–1988); patients not included in prospective or retrospective series.

had a major effect, but these have not been systematically studied.

We currently use gamma globulin infusion 0.4 g/kg per day for 3 or 4 consecutive days before beginning steroids in patients who are worsening with CIDP. If unsuccessful, we follow with plasma exchanges. This approach may be unorthodox, but it is probably preferable to committing patients prematurely to high doses of steroids (care should be taken to exclude IgA deficiency in patients receiving pooled gamma globulin). If exchanges or globulin infusion are associated with adequate symptomatic improvement, we attempt to limit them to 3 or 4 courses per year. Patients who require more frequent treatment are given small doses of prednisone (eg, 20 to 30 mg daily) and plasma exchanges are continued at longer intervals. This may be supplemented with steroids. Alternatively, prednisone 80 to 100 mg daily, or 2 mg/kg body weight in children, may be administered for 3 to 4 weeks, followed by 5-mg decrements every week until clinical symptoms limit the patient. Though reportedly successful, an entirely alternate-day schedule has not been useful in most of our patients. Several patients with intolerable steroid side effects have been treated with azathioprine, 2 mg/kg body weight, and more recently, with cyclosporin, initially 5 to 7 mg/kg. As experience is gained, gamma globulin may become the preferable first treatment.

Three of 16 MGH patients with CIDP who became bed-bound after tapering prednisone failed to improve after increasing the drug dosage, but improved after plasma exchange (Fig. 10–5). Dalakas and Engel[240] have recom-

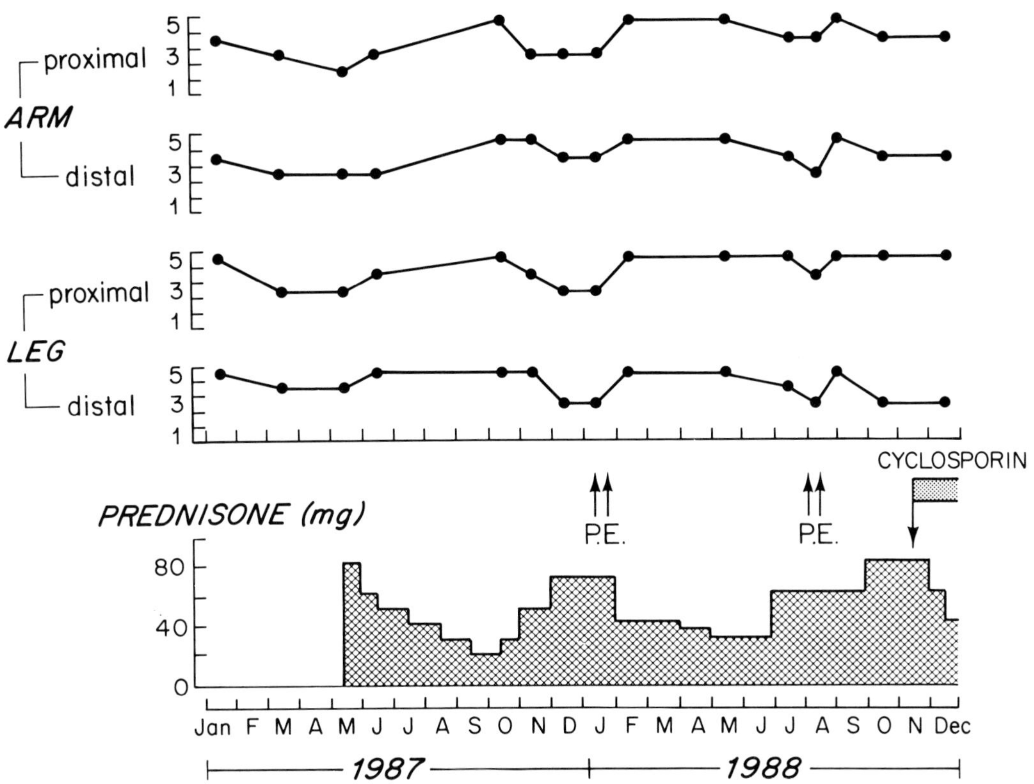

Figure 10–5. Relationship of limb power (MRC scale) and combined plasma exchange and steroid treatment in a 39-year-old man. Increasing steroid doses in late 1987 and mid 1988 did not result in improvement, whereas exchanges apparently did. Cyclosporin allowed a reduction in steroid doses without clinical deterioration.

mended increasing the prednisone dose to starting levels if tapering is associated with deterioration. The course of a representative patient is shown in Figure 10–5.

Differential Diagnosis

Chronic progressive or chronic relapsing polyneuropathy that is clinically indistinguishable from CIDP is occasionally associated with an underlying systemic disorder (guidelines for the evaluation of a CIDP patient are shown in Table 10–10). Dyck and colleagues[313] have emphasized that demyelinating hereditary neuropathy (HMSN-type 1) is the most common unrecognized chronic polyneuropathy, and a subset of familial cases are steroid-responsive.[314,810] Associations have been reported between a CIDP-like illness and HIV,[221] nonsystemic vasculitis,[305] systemic lupus erythematosus,[415,975,1065] lymphoma, particularly Hodgkin's disease and sarcoidosis. An MGH patient with CIDP has had Hodgkin's disease and Castleman's disease (angioimmunoblastic lymphadenopathy), a lymphomalike illness that has been associated with CIDP.[155,281] The relationship of systemic disease to CIDP—and the nomenclature—then becomes problematic. Without a biopsy (and sometimes even with one), the inflammatory component of the illness cannot be documented. For the present, it is advisable to evaluate most new CIDP patients who have had neuropathic symptoms for less than 6 months for an underlying systemic disease and paraproteinemia.

Table 10–10 DIFFERENTIAL DIAGNOSIS OF CHRONIC DEMYELINATING POLYNEUROPATHIES

Hereditary
HMSN-1 neuropathy
Dejerine-Sottas disease
Refsum's disease
Leukodystrophies
Systemic Disorders
HIV
Carcinomas, lymphomas
Systemic lupus erythematosus
Hypothyroidism
Porphyria
Lyme
Plasma Cell Dyscrasias and Paraproteinemias
Benign IgM monoclonal with or without anti-MAG or anti-GM1
Malignant IgM monoclonal
Waldenström
Osteosclerotic myeloma
B-cell leukemia
Lymphomas
Sarcoidosis
Toxic
Diphtheria

Patients with a monoclonal IgM antibody may have a neuropathy that is indistinguishable both clinically and pathologically from CIDP. Several subtypes of this illness have been described including IgM-lambda, IgM-kappa, monoclonal benign gammopathy, cryoglobulinemia, osteosclerotic myeloma, plasmacytoma, and a polyneuropathy associated with multiple myeloma.[15,241,677,1116,1143] The major clinical features of most paraproteinemic cases are a slowly progressive motor-sensory polyneuropathy, usually with spared cranial nerves;[1144] marked muscle weakness; wasting in advanced cases; and ataxia or intention tremor. Approximately 5% of patients have a motor neuropathy that is almost indistinguishable from amyotrophic lateral sclerosis often associated with high titers of anti-GM1 antibody, and a similar number have a multifocal motor conduction block that simulates mononeuritis multiplex. A mild, predominantly sensory neuropathy has also been reported.[476]

Particular IgM monoclonal antibodies that bind to myelin-associated glycoprotein (MAG)[379,602] or GM1[675a,913] may be present in the absence of detectable serum M protein, but most show abnormal serum immunoelectrophereses.[859] Sural nerve biopsies in most paraproteinemic polyneuropathies have shown demyelination with IgM deposits and a paucity of perivascular inflammatory mononuclear cells, in contrast to foci of inflammation at IgM-binding sites in osteosclerotic myeloma and polyneuropathy.[603] The response to cytotoxic agents[858] or plasma exchange[473] has been excellent in some patients, with an occasional concomitant decrease of anti-MAG or specific anti-GM1[675a,913] IgM levels; however, experience with these therapies is limited.[473,602]

Despite similarities, some paraproteinemic chronic neuropathies seem to be primarily demyelinating, while others are large fiber axonopathies,[1143] and the possibility of Schwann's cell destruction has not been excluded. It is therefore still difficult to draw salient conclusions about the pathogenesis of CIDP from paraproteinemic neuropathies, but the possibility should not be overlooked that some cases of typical CIDP may be the result of undetected antimyelin antibodies.

Chapter 11

SYSTEMIC DISORDERS RESULTING FROM GUILLAIN-BARRÉ SYNDROME

Most of the systemic manifestations of GBS are due to immobilization (Chapter 16), respiratory failure (Chapter 17), or dysautonomia (Chapter 7). The many viral infections that precede GBS can cause hepatitis, myocarditis, or secondary glomerular damage, but it appears that there are also primary inflammatory lesions in organs other than the nervous system in GBS. Some lesions may be apparent only indirectly—for example, by serum enzyme elevations, electrocardiographic (ECG) changes, or abnormalities of the urinary sediment. An underlying inflammatory lesion is then inferred because of a few well-documented pathology cases, but there have been no direct clinicopathologic correlations linking clinical or laboratory findings to inflammation in the corresponding organ. Circulating antibodies have also been reported against kidney, liver, and heart antigens in GBS.[1223] This chapter reviews the systemic features of GBS that are not the direct result of the neuropathy or its complications.

CARDIAC INVOLVEMENT

Arrhythmias occur in 10% to 75% of patients with GBS, depending on the population studied (see Table 7–11). Morphologic ECG changes have also been reported in as many as 50% to 80% of GBS patients[137,250,440,697,860] (Table 11–1). These changes occurred but were less frequent in the Massachusetts General Hospital (MGH) series (see farther on). Some of these reported changes were due to hypoxia or pulmonary embolus, but most others were presumably related to dysautonomia.

Morphologic ECG changes were found in 64% of 28 patients with other evidence of autonomic dysfunction in one series that studied dysautonomia in GBS.[697] Flat or inverted T waves in the lateral leads were most common in this series, and in one case the changes disappeared after administering atropine, thus implying a repolarization abnormality from vagal dysfunction. Other patients had ST-segment depression, QT-interval prolongation, increased R-wave voltage in lateral leads, and left axis deviation. Another group[655] noted three common ECG abnormalities in GBS: (1) depressed ST segments, (2) inverted or flat T waves, and (3) preterminal T-wave inversion, which they considered most characteristic of this syndrome. ECG changes correlated with the severity of paralysis but not with tachycardia, mechanical ventilation, cranial nerve deficits, cerebrospinal fluid (CSF) findings, serum electrolytes, or cardiac enzymes. Slight depression of ST segments, anteroseptal inversion of T waves, and flattened T waves in lateral leads that were not present on the admission ECG were

Table 11–1 MORPHOLOGIC ECG CHANGES IN GBS

Series, Year	No. of Patients with ECGs	T-Wave Abnormality (% of Patients)	ST-Segment Abnormality (% of Patients)	AV Block (No. of Patients)		Bundle Branch Block (No. of Patients)
				1st or 2nd Degree	3rd Degree	
Chuttani et al.,[199] 1968	63	0	22	0	0	0
Kunst and Grosser,[655] 1974	58	71	57	5	0	3
Bredin,[137] 1977	24	80	80	0	0	8
Nolte et al.,[860] 1979	30	33	50	10	3	0
Greenland and Griggs,[440] 1980	16	6	50	6	0	6
Ahmad et al.,[10] 1985	25	16	4	0	0	0
de Jager,[259] 1980	43	51	14	—	—	5
Prospective MGH Series	89	8	6	3	2	0

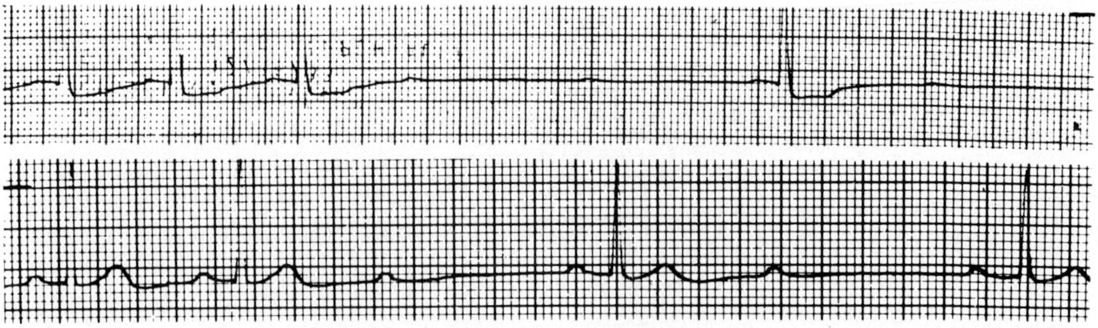

Figure 11–1. Acquired heart block in a 52-year-old hypertensive GBS patient without prior heart disease.

prominent in another study.[812] The following have also been reported, but infrequently: widening of the QRS complex and bundle branch block;[137,440,655] first-degree heart block; [440,860] and second- and third-degree heart block.[655,860,1165] Tall peaked T waves[1108] and prolongation of the QT interval,[697] often described in association with central nervous system (CNS) catastrophies, can occur but are rare in GBS.

In the MGH study, 5% had heart block (see Table 11–1); (Fig. 11–1). None of these patients had more than minor features of other types of dysautonomia. Minor nonspecific ST-T segment changes occurred in 60% of 89 prospectively studied patients (Fig. 11–2), usually those receiving mechanical ventilation, with most abnormalities appearing within the first week of onset.

Myocarditis may be an alternative explanation to dysautonomia for the ECG changes in some cases. Focal collections of perivascular lymphocytes and macrophages in the myocardium have been found at autopsy in a few cases.[322,501,524,761,1038] One well-documented autopsy study of myocarditis was reported in a childhood case of GBS.[524] After an upper respiratory infection, a 12-year-old boy developed symmetrical quadriparesis, facial diplegia, and marked loss of proprioception, followed by tachycardia, hypertension, paralytic ileus, and inappropriate antidiuretic hormone secretion. He died of sudden ventricular tachycardia, but there was no comment about preceding morphologic ECG changes. The major postmorten findings were extensive destruction of dorsal root ganglia and massive infiltration of myocardium by granulocytes, eosinophils, lymphocytes, and plasma cells, with some areas of necrosis.

Most autopsied cases of GBS have not shown myocardial abnormalities, including some in which morphologic ECG changes had been demonstrated,[137] but a systematic study has not been performed. It has been suggested that the "myocarditis" seen by Haymaker and Kernohan (in 7 of 50 autopsied cases) and others may actually have been inflammatory infiltration of small intramyocardial nerves.[354] The hearts in three GBS patients with sudden death had patchy mononuclear infiltrates in subepicardial and intramyocardial nerves, often near the conduction system and cardiac ganglia, but no primary myocardial cell damage.

Creatine phosphokinase (CPK) elevations, seen in approximately one third of patients in the first week of GBS, have not been due to an increase in the myocardial isoenzyme. Although this CPK rise has been associated with the presence of pain, this was not always the case.[1017] Serum CPK concentrations may reach four times normal, whereas other muscle-associated enzymes are usually less elevated. Despite a search for evidence of myocardial infarction in many MGH patients with CPK elevations, we found only two cases, and these were painless, one in a diabetic.

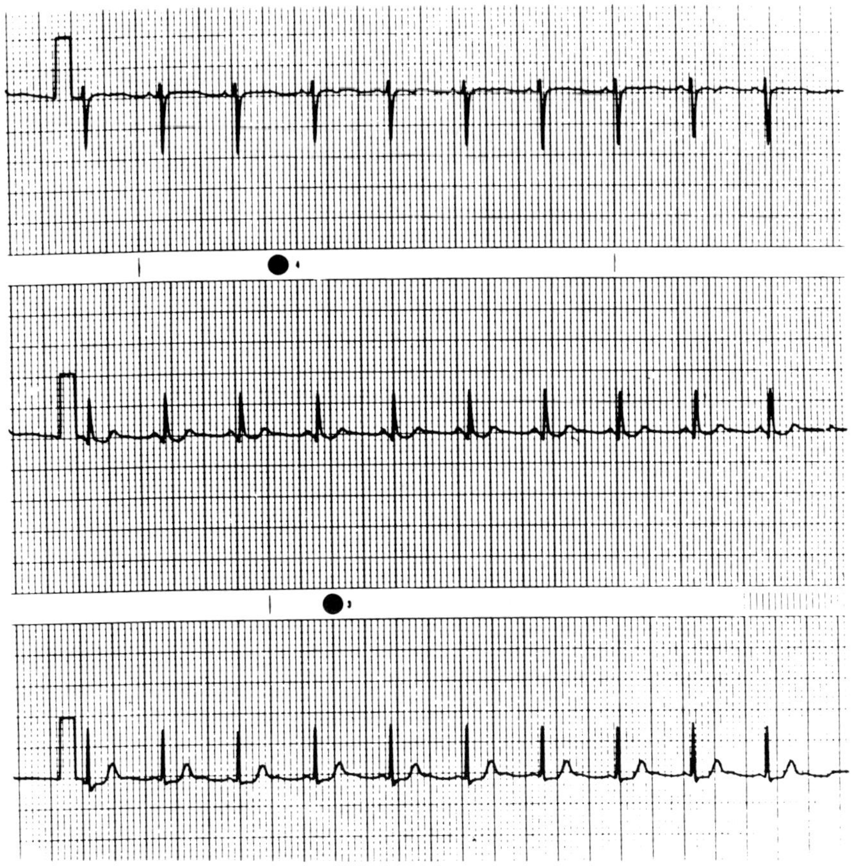

Figure 11–2. Typical, but nonspecific, ST-segment and T-wave changes in a GBS patient. Similar changes occurred in 60 percent of prospectively studied MGH patients.

Pericarditis or valvular lesions have not been reported in GBS, though myocardial inflammation has extended to the pericardium in a few cases. Other aspects of cardiovascular dysfunction related to dysautonomia were discussed in Chapter 7.

RENAL INVOLVEMENT

Mild transient proteinuria is common in GBS (see Chapters 12 and 16). True nephrotic syndrome or active urinary sediments, however, are uncommon. In the MGH prospective series, there was only one patient with urinary casts and none with nephrotic syndrome. In addition to an autopsy report of six GBS patients with glomerulonephritis,[131] several case reports of nephrotic syndrome or acute glomerulonephritis have appeared.[92,101,384,916,998,1178] In one report,[998] 8 of 9 consecutive patients had biopsy evidence of acute glomerulonephritis. There was microscopic hematuria in two and erythrocyte and granular casts in five patients, but serum urea and creatinine measurements were normal in most. One patient with definite histologic changes in the glomeruli had normal blood pressure, creatinine clearance, and urine sediment. This and other pathologic studies have shown membranous and proliferative changes with focal fusion of podocytes, basement membrane thickening, and endothelial cell swelling. Persistent glomerular changes were seen for up to 3 years in some follow-up renal biopsies.[998]

Others[1178] have found membranous glomerulonephritis with IgG, IgM, and C3 deposits along the basement membrane and occasional extensive fusion of epithelial foot processes on electron microscopy. Light microscopy in another case[92] was normal except for slight thickening of mesangial cells and small arterioles that contained hyaline material in their walls. Proteinuria usually subsides during improvement of limb weakness but may persist,[92] or return with a relapse of GBS.[916]

In two reports of patients with renal changes,[92,384] simultaneous lymphocytic and plasma cell infiltration was found in liver biopsy specimens but not in skin, muscle, or sural nerves. IgA has been demonstrated in the renal biopsy of a patient with Henoch-Schönlein–associated GBS, without evidence of vasculitis in a nerve biospy specimen.[819]

GASTROINTESTINAL AND HEPATIC INVOLVEMENT

Ileus and gastric retention, the result of dysautonomia, are the most common gastrointestinal manifestations in GBS and are usually encountered in patients with severe limb weakness and respiratory failure (Chapter 7). Chronic diarrhea, persisting after recovery from limb weakness, has been documented in one report.[768] Diarrhea began one day after the onset of neurologic symptoms, and persisted 2 years, causing marked weight loss and impaired rehabilitation. Stool cultures and diagnostic tests failed to reveal a cause, but it seems unlikely that GBS or bowel inflammation was the cause of the diarrhea (see Chapter 3 for discussion of *Campylobacter* and other enteral infections preceding GBS). GBS has also been associated in a few cases with ulcerative colitis, perhaps due to a proclivity for these autoimmune diseases to occur together, as discussed in Chapter 6.[641,1314]

A number of patients have transient abnormalities of liver function tests, which probably represent preceding cytomegalovirus (CMV), Epstein-Barr virus (EBV), hepatitis A or B, or hepatitis non-A, non-B infection. Interlobar mononuclear infiltration in the liver of a GBS patient and occasional focal necrosis and focal fatty degeneration and infiltration have been found,[1038] but extensive liver cell necrosis leading to hepatic failure has not been reported in GBS (see Chapter 12). In the prospective MGH series, several patients had abnormal liver function test results without clinical or serologic evidence of CMV, EBV, or hepatitis A or B. These cases may have been due to non-A, non-B hepatitis, or alternatively, to hepatic inflammation as a rare systemic manifestation of GBS.[384]

ENDOCRINE DISTURBANCES

At least three cases of diabetes insipidus have been reported in patients with GBS.[912,1053,1228] Postmortem inflammatory changes in the supraoptic and paraventricular nuclei in one patient with a very atypical case of GBS should be interpreted cautiously. The precise cause of diabetes insipidus and the relationship to dysautonomia remain unclear.

GBS occurs in patients with diabetes mellitus;[633,1263] three patients in the prospective series were insulin-requiring diabetics. Hyperglycemia, especially associated with steroid use or formula alimentation, may also appear during the course of GBS.* In addition, glucose intolerance occurred in 16% of 172 GBS patients in one series,[426] presumably acquired as a result of the stress of the illness, and associated with elevated 17-hydroxycorticosteroids. Seven of 25 GBS patients in another series[10] had glucose intolerance, hypertension, and tachycardia, elevated plasma cortisol and norepinephrine levels, and urinary vanillilmandelic acid (VMA) levels. Glycosuria and impaired glucose tolerance occurred at the time of maximal weakness in 5 GBS patients with dysautono-

*See references 10, 112, 250, 426, 860, and 968.

mia.[250] Four had increased urinary excretion of VMA and 17-hydroxycorticosteroids that returned to normal with clinical improvement. Another had elevated plasma cortisol levels with loss of normal diurnal variation. Corticosteroids and catecholamines were thought to have played a role in producing the glucose intolerance. Whether hypoglycemia simply reflects the stress of illness exposing latent diabetes or is an autonomic endocrine dysregulation is not known. Transient glucose intolerance has also been reported in pure pandysautonomia (see Chapter 8).

The autonomic nervous system may influence glucose homeostasis by a number of direct and indirect mechanisms that are disrupted in GBS, including cholinergic and beta-adrenergic innervation, which promotes insulin release, and alpha-adrenergic innervation, which inhibits it. The temporary acquired hyperglycemia of GBS rarely requires treatment unless it is exaggerated by hyperalimentation, sepsis, or high doses of corticosteroids.

Hyperthyroidism has reportedly occured with or shortly after the development of GBS,[145,641,948] and recovery from GBS has occurred after treatment of the thyroid abnormality.[145] Some of these cases have been due to Hashimoto's thyroiditis[948] or Graves' disease,[641] as discussed in Chapter 6. Three cases of GBS with Addison's disease have also been reported,[1,1133] with both disorders apparently responding to administration of steroids. There have been instances of hypercalcemia from immobilization in GBS (discussed in Chapter 16) but not primary parathyroid or calcitonin abnormalities. A numer of electrolyte disturbances that may simulate GBS by causing acute areflexic paralysis are discussed in Chapter 14.

Syndrome of Inappropriate ADH Secretion (SIADH)

Hyponatremia (serum sodium concentration less than 130 mEq/L), usually due to the syndrome of inappropriate ADH secretion (SIADH), has been reported frequently in single cases and large series of GBS* (Table 11–2). Hyponatremia occurred in 7% of patients in the MGH retrospective series and in 26% in the prospective series. It was more common in mechanically ventilated patients (see Table 16–4). SIADH may occur despite relatively mild motor paralysis, absence of respiratory failure, or autonomic dysfunction.[522] Hyponatremia, usually mild and transient, occurs most often at the time of maximal motor impairment. Two patients we have seen not in the MGH series had hyponatremic seizures. Profound hyponatremia has been reported rarely,[250,909,947] with serum sodium concentrations of 105 to 110 mEq/L (in one instance, as low as 91 mEq/L).[952] The lowest recorded serum sodium in MGH patients was 118 mEq/L. Treatment with fluid restriction is usually successful, but hypertonic saline can be used to correct severe hyponatremia. Posner and co-workers[947] postulated that SIADH resulted from afferent abnormalities in nerves from volume receptors and found other evidence of autonomic dysfunction in their patients. Continued urinary sodium excretion and relative urine hyperosmolality despite declining plasma sodium levels and osmolarity have been documented in one patient.[249] During fluid restric-

Table 11–2 INCIDENCE OF HYPONATREMIA IN LARGE GBS SERIES

Series, Year	*No. of Patients*	*Hyponatremia (%)*
Goulon et al.,[426] 1975	172	7.0
Samantray et al.,[1053] 1977	302	0.7
Winer et al.,[1291] 1988	100	12.0
Retrospective MGH Series	169	7.0
Prospective MGH Series	120	26.0

*Na <130 mEq/L

*See references 249, 426, 515, 522, 524, 817, 909, 947, 952, 968, 984, 1053, and 1291.

tion, plasma sodium levels and osmolality rose despite reduction in sodium intake. It has been hypothesized that the osmostatic mechanism may become reset to a lower level due to afferent dysfunction.[909] This is plausible because the shape of the curve describing the relationship between volume and sodium excretion remains normal (ADH secretion is appropriately suppressed after free water challenge), but the system behaves as if it has a new homeostatic setpoint.

Afferent input from cardiovascular receptors inhibits ADH release with the participation of both low-pressure (atrial) receptors and high-pressure (carotid and aortic) baroreceptors.[640,995,1184] Positive pressure ventilation also impairs venous return, thereby stimulating ADH excretion.[1275] Elevated venous renin levels, documented in a few cases of GBS with hypertension, may also play a role in SIADH, but some authors[995] have questioned the importance of the renin-angiotensin system for ADH release. An interesting and unexplained feature was the development of pulmonary edema in 4 of 5 hyponatremic patients in one series.[249]

In a study of 12 consecutive MGH patients with GBS, serum ADH concentrations in 7 ventilated patients were higher than in 5 nonventilated patients.[1280] None, however, developed hyponatremia. Changes in atrial natriuretic factor concentration in GBS are discussed in Chapter 7 in relation to blood pressure lability.

Part IV

LABORATORY INVESTIGATION AND DIFFERENTIAL DIAGNOSIS

Chapter 12

SPINAL FLUID AND OTHER LABORATORY FINDINGS

CSF Protein
Cell Count
Routine Laboratory Findings

Elevated spinal fluid protein concentrations were observed before 1920 in association with spinal cord compression and in Pott's disease. However, Guillain, Barré, and Strohl's seminal description was the first of "hyperalbuminosis of the cerebrospinal fluid (CSF) without cellular reaction," or "albuminocytologic dissociation" in the context of a neuropathy[466] (see Chapter 1). After the original contribution, Guillain re-emphasized, in 1936, his refusal to recognize GBS ("my syndrome") in the presence of an increased CSF cell count. He stated that slight hyperalbuminosis was also inconsistent with the syndrome, or must be regarded as an "abortive form." This restrictive definition initially aided in further delineation and study of GBS, but the absolute inclusion of the typical CSF abnormalities has since been debated and is now recognized as too extreme (see Chapter 2).

CSF PROTEIN

The CSF findings in major series of GBS are summarized in Table 12–1 and exceptions to the typical pattern of albuminocytologic dissociation are shown in Table 12–2. CSF protein is said to be virtually always normal in the first 2 days of illness,[51] even in severe cases, but 18 (16%) Massachusetts General Hospital (MGH) patients had elevated protein values during this time (Fig. 12–1). These patients were otherwise indistinguishable from cases with the expected later protein elevations. According to Haymaker and Kernohan,[501] 4 of their own patients and 8 patients from other reports had early CSF protein elevations. They emphasized 2 patients with protein elevation 2 and 6 days after the onset of paresthesias. One had an initial CSF protein concentration of 40 mg/100 mL, and 6

Table 12–1 CSF FINDINGS IN LARGE SERIES OF GBS

Author, Year	***Protein mg/dl (Range)***	***Cells/mm³ (Range)***
Haymaker and Kernohan,[501] 1949	18–372	0–110
Marshall,[751] 1963	<50–1000	0–50
Wiederholdt et al,[1278] 1963	<50–1800	0–66
McFarland and Heller,[777] 1966	25–133	3–4
Ravn,[973] 1967	<40–796	0–87
Loffel et al.,[714] 1977	48–795	<5 in most cases
Samantray et al.,[1053] 1977	46–>400	1–5 (1 case >10)
Kennedy et al.,[606] 1978	<50–>200	<4 in most cases
Andersson and Siden,[31] 1982	60–780	6–60
Winer et al.,[1291] 1988	10–600	6–103
Retrospective MGH Series	21–645	0–30
Prospective MGH Series	20–692	0–230

Table 12–2 INCIDENCE OF NORMAL CSF PROTEIN VALUES OR INCREASED CELLS IN LARGE GBS SERIES

Author, Year	No. Patients Tested	Normal Protein [No. Patients (%)]	Elevated Cell Counts: No. Patients (%)	Elevated Cell Counts: No. Cells/mm³
Haymaker and Kernohan,[501] 1949	33	11 (33)*	5 (15)	>20
Marshall,[751] 1964	34	7 (21)†	7 (21)	>10
Wiederholdt et al,[1278] 1964	93	17 (18)†	2 (2)	>15
McFarland and Heller,[777] 1966	100	32 (32)†	0 (0)	>10
Ravn,[973] 1967	125	19 (15)‡	34 (26)	>4
Loffel et al.,[714] 1977	117	14 (11)	15 (12)	>15
Samantray et al.,[1053] 1977	302	0 (0)	0 (0)	>5
Kennedy et al.,[606] 1978	36	5 (14)	4 (11)	>4
Andersson and Siden,[31] 1982	60	3 (5)	16 (27)	>6
Winer et al.,[1291] 1988	92	18 (20)	11 (12)	>5
Retrospective MGH Series	164	14 (9)	38 (22)	>4
Prospective MGH Series	111	30 (27)	14 (13)	>4

*Four normal after repeat sampling.
†All protein values were elevated after repeated sampling.
‡Six normal after repeat sampling.

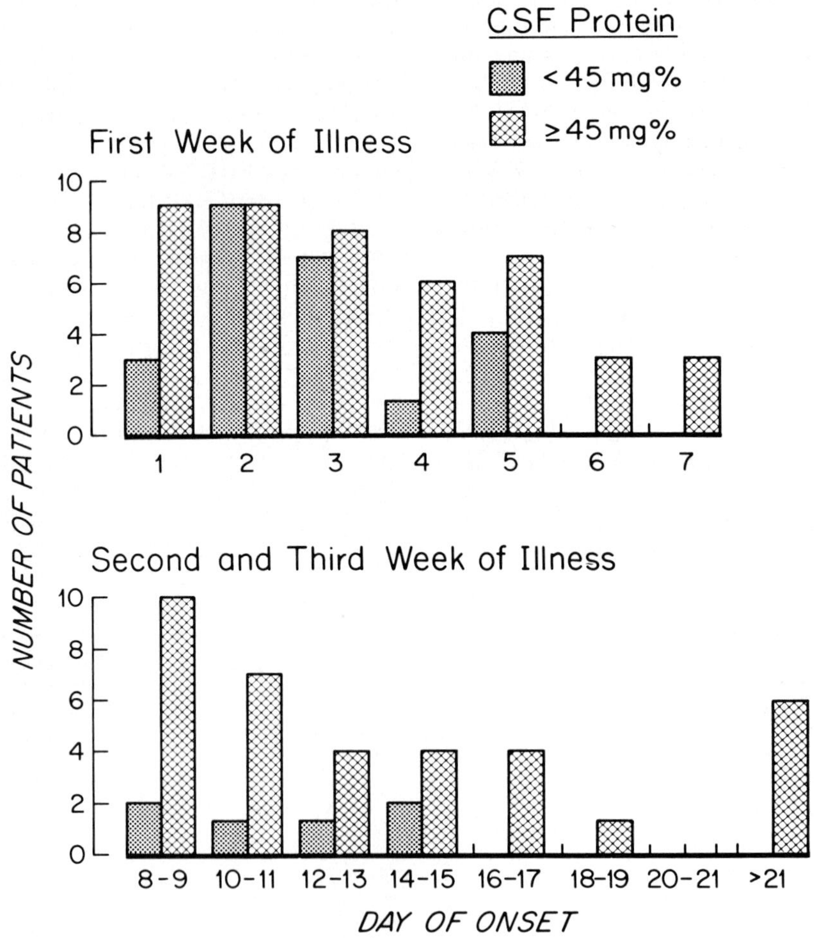

Figure 12–1. CSF protein concentration by day from onset in first week of illness *(top)* and in second and third weeks of illness *(bottom)* in MGH prospective series.

days later of 280 mg/100 mL. The CSF protein can rise rapidly in the first week. In another series,[751] the CSF protein level in one patient rose from 330 to 1000 mg/100 mL between the second and seventh days. The highest protein concentrations (up to 1000 mg/100 mL) were found between the 4th and 18th days, and in another series,[31] between the 10th and 19th days. Seventeen of 32 patients with serial examinations in two series from the same authors[1277,1278] had elevated CSF protein concentrations 1 to 25 days after the onset of the plateau phase; these levels remained elevated for approximately another 20 days. Only 4 had declining CSF protein values during the period when clinical signs were improving or stable. The majority of patients in another large series[777] had normal protein concentrations in the first week, that rose to a peak between 2 weeks and 2 months and gradually declined thereafter, although in some patients values remained high when sampled years later. Normal protein concentrations were found in 11% of 117 patients in a series;[714] 9 still had normal values 3 weeks or more after the onset of illness.

The protein values in the MGH retrospective and prospective series are summarized in Tables 12–3, 12–4, and Figure 12–1. Considering only CSF results measured in the MGH, 30 (27%) of 111 prospective patients had normal CSF protein concentrations on the first sample, all in the first 3 weeks of illness. The incidence of normal protein values (below 45 mg/dL) in the initial CSF sample generally declined from 34% in the first week to 18% in the second week. There was a weak correlation in the prospective series between CSF protein values and the duration of illness ($r = .50$ for CSF protein versus day of illness for the first 3 weeks). In 6 of 9 patients with initially normal CSF protein values who had a second lumbar puncture, protein concentrations were found to have increased; in the other 3 patients, however, the values remained normal after 5, 8, and 35 days of illness. The outcome in patients with persistently normal test results was no different from that in patients who had normal CSF protein levels in the first 2 days.

Table 12–3 MAXIMUM CSF PROTEIN

	No. of Patients (%)	
Max Protein (mg/dl)	***MGH Retrospective Series (N=164)***	***MGH Prospective Series (N=111)***
0–45	14 (9)	30 (27)
46–100	53 (32)	51 (46)
101–200	59 (36)	19 (17)
201–300	20 (12)	5 (5)
301–400	9 (6)	2 (2)
401–500	7 (4)	2 (1)
>500	2 (1)	2 (2)

CSF protein concentrations in patients with Fisher's syndrome and with pharyngeal-cervical-brachial variants (see Chapter 8), however, were generally lower, and more often normal, than those in patients with typical GBS who had CSF examinations at similar times (Table 12–4; $P < .01$).

Extremely high protein values, up to 1800 mg/dL, have been described in GBS patients, usually after 2 weeks of illness.[1278] There may be an association between greatly elevated CSF protein concentration and the pseudotumor-papilledema syndrome, as discussed in Chapter 7. In the prospective MGH series, the highest protein value (692 mg/dL) was found in a patient with papilledema, but pseudotumor did not occur with sustained values of 500 to 600 mg/dL in two other patients, indicating that these concentrations alone are inadequate to cause pseudotumor.

Protein concentration has not been associated with specific electrophysiologic abnormalities. In the prospective series, CSF protein level was generally highest in patients with diffuse slowing of motor conduction velocity, but the differences from other groups were not significant (Table 12–5). We were also unable to find an association between CSF findings and outcome (Table 12–6).

Table 12–4 PROTEIN VALUES IN GBS VARIANTS*

Variants	*No. of Patients*	*Day LP from Onset*	*Protein (mg/dl)*
Fisher's syndrome	7	2–9 (mean, 3)	21–55 (mean, 40)
Pharyngeal-cervical-bracheal	4	2–10 (mean, 4)	20–39 (mean, 28)
Paraparetic	2	4, 5	42, 133
Pure motor†	3	2, 5, 10	22, 40, 49
Pure sensory	1	2	57
Typical GBS with CSF sampled in 1st wk	86	0–10 (mean, 3)	20–320 (mean, 80)‡

*In prospective MGH series.
†Protein value unavailable in one patient.
‡$p<0.01$ typical GBS vs. variants.

Table 12–5 RELATION OF CSF PROTEIN TO ELECTROMYOGRAPHIC FINDINGS*

		Lumbar Puncture (LP)	
	No. of Patients	*Day LP from Onset (Mean ± SD)*	*Protein (mg/dl) (Mean ± SD)*
Diffuse slowing of motor nerve conduction velocity†	29	16 ± 15.0	157 ± 176
Proximal conduction block only	29	10 ± 11	94 ± 98
Distal demyelination	6	10 ± 10	132 ± 144

*In prospective MGH series; SD = standard deviation. (See Chapter 13 for electrophysiologic definitions.)
†Protein values unavailable in two patients.

Increased CSF protein concentration has been explained as the result of breakdown of the blood-CSF barrier. Abnormalities of the CSF amino acid profile have been most marked in patients with a raised CSF protein concentration,[224] suggesting a breakdown in the barrier. In the presence of normal CSF protein levels, however, amino acid composition was also abnormal in some patients, making interpretation of these results difficult.

Table 12–6 RELATIONSHIP OF INITIAL PROTEIN VALUES AND CELL COUNTS TO OUTCOME*

	Initial Protein		Initial Cell Count	
Outcome	*≥45*	*<45*	*>3/mm³*	*≤3/mm³*
Good recovery	64	20	18	66
Poor outcome	10	5	2	13
Death	2	3	0	5

*In 104 GBS patients in prospective MGH series with follow-up period of more than 6 mo.

Increased CSF, IgG, IgM, and IgA concentrations have been demonstrated in some patients with GBS.[704,1120] Serum IgG, IgM, and IgA were normal in these studies, suggesting intrathecal synthesis of immunoglobulin. The highest concentrations of immunoglobulins were found in patients with high CSF protein concentrations and in samples obtained early in the disease. Oligoclonal banding in CSF has also been described in 10% to 30% of patients with GBS.[26,651,1081] Study of serum and CSF samples in one GBS patient confirmed high relative CSF concentrations of IgG, IgA, and IgM at the end of the second week, at a time when total protein concentration was highest.[705] Oligoclonal IgG bands, found in the CSF during the first 2 weeks, disappeared by 4 weeks and reappeared 2½ months later.[705] In one study,[1081] the presence of oligoclonal bands was correlated with the severity of the disease. Myelin basic protein has been present in approximately half of GBS patients and 70% of patients with chronic inflammatory demyelinating polyneuropathy (CIDP) possibly representing peripheral nerve P1 protein.[220]

CSF CELL COUNT

The absence of cells in the CSF was considered to be the second hallmark of acute GBS in the original report by Guillain, Barré, and Strohl.[466,467] When Guillain later described 10 new cases seen over 20 years, he implicitly accepted, without further comment, a case with 7 mononuclear cells per mm^3.[459] Nevertheless, he adopted a position that is no longer widely accepted—that CSF pleocytosis precludes the diagnosis of GBS. Haymaker and Kernohan's 1949 review[501] included patients with up to 340 cells per mm^3, even 4 months after the onset of illness. Others[31,751] have found elevated cell counts within the first 2 weeks of illness but not thereafter. The incidence of increased CSF cells in the major published series is summarized in Table 12–2; however, definitions of normal have varied between series. The cell counts in the MGH retrospective and prospective series are given in Table 12–7. In the prospective series, 14 patients had more than 4 cells per mm^3 in the first 2 weeks (4 had more than 10 cells per mm^3). One patient had 230 cells per mm^3 but no cells 6 days later. In all the major series, cells in the CSF have been predominantly lymphocytes. A systematic cytologic study of CSF has not been made in GBS.

No correlation has been found in the literature, or in the MGH experience, between the number of cells in the CSF and clinical grade, pain, distribution of weakness, meningeal signs, or outcome (see Table 12–6). Several unusual infections, however, have been associated with an increased CSF cell count or peculiar cellular morphology. GBS in human immunodeficiency virus (HIV)–positive patients is often associated with a pleocytosis.[221] The relatively high incidence of cytomegalovirus (CMV) infection, sometimes with meningitis in HIV-positive patients, may be a confounding factor that also causes a meningitis (see Chapter 6). An increased cell count also makes the distinction from Lyme disease difficult, particularly in the very rare case that cannot be distinguished clinically from GBS[203] (see Chapter 14). Elevated Lyme disease titers, persistent pleocytosis (often with hundreds of cells), a lymphocytic pleocytosis, and particularly immunoblasts and plasma cells, suggest Lyme disease.[974,1296]

Table 12–7 MAXIMUM CSF CELL COUNT

	No. of Patients (%)	
Maximum Cells	***MGH Retrospective Series (N=161)***	***MGH Prospective Series (N=111)***
0–4/mm^3	123 (76)	97 (87)
5–10/mm^3	24 (15)	10 (9)
11–20/mm^3	9 (6)	2 (2)
21–30/mm^3	4 (2)	0 (0)
>30/mm^3	1 (1)	2 (2)

The diagnostic sensitivity and specificity of the classic CSF formula in GBS therefore has limitations and must be regarded only as supportive evidence for the diagnosis. Failure to find the expected albuminocytologic dissociation, even after repeated CSF sampling, does not preclude the diagnosis in an otherwise typical case. Conversely, in perplexing cases with clinical and electrophysiologic evidence suggesting GBS, the classic CSF criterion may be helpful in correctly classifying the illness. We have routinely performed HIV and Lyme disease serologic testing if there are more than approximately 10 cells per mm^3 in the CSF of a GBS patient.

ROUTINE LABORATORY FINDINGS

A small number of GBS patients have elevations of erythrocyte sedimentation rate (ESR) and white blood cell (WBC) counts that cannot readily be explained by coexisting illness. In an older series,[501] 7 of 10 patients had an ESR greater than 20 mm/h, with further elevations as GBS progressed. Approximately 10% to 20% of patients also had a leukocytosis, often with a pronounced lymphocytosis, independent of an upper respiratory infection. In large series of 302 cases,[1053] however, in which both ESR and WBC counts were determined consistently, the incidences of elevation were much lower, 2% and 1%, respectively. One group[1290] has reported that peripheral WBC counts and ESR are often elevated in patients with a poor outcome at 3 months. They did not take into account preexisting or coexisting infections. In the retrospective MGH series, ESR was greater than 50 mm/h in 16% of patients, and WBC counts greater than 20,000 per mm^3 were only encountered in patients with concomitant infections (Table 12–8). A persistent ESR over 100 mg/h resulted from temporal arteritis and Hodgkin's disease in one patient each.

Table 12–8 HEMATOLOGY FINDINGS IN MGH RETROSPECTIVE SERIES (N = 162)

WBC >10,000	36%
WBC <4000	1%
Abnormal differential	34%
Lymphocytosis (10%)	
Atypical lymphocytosis (15%)	
Monocytosis (4%)	
Left shift (3%)	
Eosinophilia (2%)	
Anemia	5%
Elevated ESR	16%

Many patients with severe pain have mild elevations of serum creatine phosphokinase (CPK) levels, possibly reflecting some degree of myonecrosis.[1017] In a previous report of MGH cases, the serum CPK concentration was elevated in 77% of 13 patients with, and in 13% of patients without, pain. Elevations up to seven times the upper limit of normal occurred without obvious explanation.

Another relatively frequent observation has been mild proteinuria without impaired renal function during the first week. Increased urine protein concentration was reported in 6% of 50 fatal cases.[501] Acute glomerulonephritis and nephrotic syndrome with subepithelial immunoglobulin deposits have been described (see Chapter 11).[92,998] One-quarter of patients in the MGH retrospective and prospective series had minimal proteinuria.

Approximatley 10% of patients have abnormal liver function tests as a result of preceding or coexistent hepatitis, most often from CMV or Epstein-Barr virus (EBV). The existence of a primary hepatitis as a manifestation of generalized inflammatory process in GBS is doubtful (see Chapter 11).

Chapter 13

ELECTROPHYSIOLOGIC STUDIES*

Nerve conduction studies and needle electromyography (EMG) have become invaluable for the diagnosis and understanding of GBS. These tests are probably more sensitive than raised cerebrospinal fluid (CSF) protein concentration in confirming the clinical diagnosis, particularly early in the disease. Segmental demyelination and other features of inflammatory neuropathy are reflected by several characteristic abnormalities. In the presence of demyelination, conduction block in individual fibers produces heterogeneous slowing of electrical impulses, resulting in temporal dispersion, desynchronization, slowing of nerve conduction velocity (NCV) in the largest fibers, and, when extreme, complete failure of conduction. Perhaps the most typical electrophysiologic evidence of conduction block, reflecting the current use of the term, is a progressive decline in compound muscle action potential (CMAP) amplitude with nerve stimulation at successively more proximal sites. The expected electrophysiologic finding with severe demyelination, and slowing of conduction velocity, also occurs but is less common early in the illness.

The type and extent of electrophysiologic findings in GBS depend on the stage of the disease, the number of nerves studied, and the types of investigation—particularly evaluation of late responses. Patients tested early often will have predominantly proximal nerve demyelination, which is not detected with conventional studies of distal nerve segments. This explains the high incidence of normal electrophysiologic tests in studies that do not investigate late responses or fail to systematically seek evidence of conduction block (Table 13–1). Thorough testing of several nerves, including the use of late responses, will show abnormalities in essentially all patients with acute GBS (Table 13–2). With this type of extensive testing protocol, a recent study[14] found a completely normal electrophysiologic pattern in only 1 of 70 GBS patients.

A comprehensive electrodiagnostic study for GBS includes:

- Stimulation of two or more motor nerves each in the arms and legs, with recording of CMAP distal latency, duration, and amplitude, as well as calculation of NCVs
- Examination of two or more sensory nerves with recording of amplitude, duration, and NCV
- Proximal and distal motor stimulation to assess conduction block
- Recording of F responses from several nerves with attention to minimal and maximal latencies, and to persistence during 10 consecutive supramaximal stimuli
- Recording of the H reflex
- Needle examination for fibrillation potentials and recruitment in at least one proximal and distal muscle, with confirmation of any abnormality in at

*With the assistance of Dr. Bhagwan Shahani, Clinical Electrophysiology Service, Massachusetts General Hospital.

Table 13–1 CONVENTIONAL ELECTRODIAGNOSTIC STUDIES IN GBS

Author/Year	*No. Patients*	*Age (Yr) (Range)*	*Time from Onset*	**Abnormal Conduction Velocity (%)**		*Patients with Fibrillation Potentials (%)*	*Patients with Normal Conventional Studies (%)*
				Motor	*Sensory*		
Lambert and Mulder,[662] 1964	49	NA	<3 wk	61	—	—	14
McQuillen,[785] 1971	20	1.5–73	2–107 d	55	—	—	45
Eisen and Humphreys,[324] 1974	19	16–69	<3 wk	74	53	26	26
Raman and Taori,[963] 1976	47	3–70	<4 wk	87	66	34	13
McLeod,[781] 1981	114	3–78	1–128 d	30	76	—	9
Takeuchi et al.,[1177] 1984	39	8–55	<3 wk	26	—	—	2
Walsh et al.,[1248] 1984	17	16–81	2–45 d	88	59	—	2
Albers et al.,[14] 1985	70	3–82	<5 wk	87	82	3	1
Cornblath et al.,[222] 1988	210	NA	<4 wk	24	—	—	—
Winer et al.,[1291] 1988	94	2–79	<44 d	68	Many	15	10

Table 13–2 ABNORMAL F-WAVE LATENCIES IN GBS PATIENTS WITH NORMAL MOTOR NCVs

Author, Year	*Time of Study from Onset*	*No. Patients*	*Abnormal F Waves (%)*
Kimura and Butzer,[615] 1975	<4 wk	9	23
Lachman et al.,[660] 1980	<2 wk	11	18
Walsh et al.,[1248] 1984	2–45 days (mean 16 days)	17	12
Mills and Murray,[807] 1985	<3 wk	21	24

least one contralateral muscle (in many cases, however, where confirmatory evidence only is required, a truncated protocol is appropriate)

PATTERNS OF ELECTROPHYSIOLOGIC ABNORMALITIES

The demyelination pathoanatomy of GBS probably causes pathophysiologic changes in single nerve fibers, but clinical electrophysiologic tests examine many fibers simultaneously. The important abstracted patterns of electrophysiologic abnormalities derived from these examinations are:

- One of the various forms of conduction block
- Slowed motor NCVs
- A pattern of axonal damage
- The relative degree of involvement of sensory and motor fibers

Additional information from somatosensory evoked potentials, blink reflexes, RR interval variation, and sympathetic skin responses is valuable but not as useful for routine diagnosis.[911,1012,1086]

Motor Nerve Conduction Block

Conduction block was first described by Erb,[333] and later by McDonald,[774] who showed that focal demyelination produced by diphtheria toxin caused local conduction block. Others[1047,1163] have subsequently demonstrated a similar block in regions of segmental demyelination induced by intraneural injection of GBS or experimental autoimmune neuritis sera. Proximal stimulation of injected nerves results in a progressive decline in CMAP without appreciable slowing in NCV, suggesting early vulnerability of intermediate-sized fibers (Fig. 13–1). The degree of conduction block, however, does not clearly correlate with pathologic change in nerve, and subtle demyelination is at times associated with complete conduction block.[1163]

Two leading groups in this field[153,1163] have concluded that motor conduction block causes the acute weakness of GBS (see Chapter 7). Their definition of conduction block, generally accepted in practice, is a decline in CMAP amplitude of more than 20% between the proximal and distal sites of stimulation, without a parallel increase in duration or dispersion of the CMAP, thus excluding phase cancellation from heterogeneous conduction velocities in different fibers as the cause of the amplitude reduction.[153] Conduction block can be further delineated into three types, based on the segment of nerve most affected—proximal, intermediate, and distal—any of which may coexist. The expansion of conduction block to these implicitly anatomic types is a useful shorthand for clinical study, but differences between them are not always clear, and, with the exception of intermediate block, they have not yet been shown definitely to correspond to lesions in a certain portion of nerve, or to clinical phenomena.

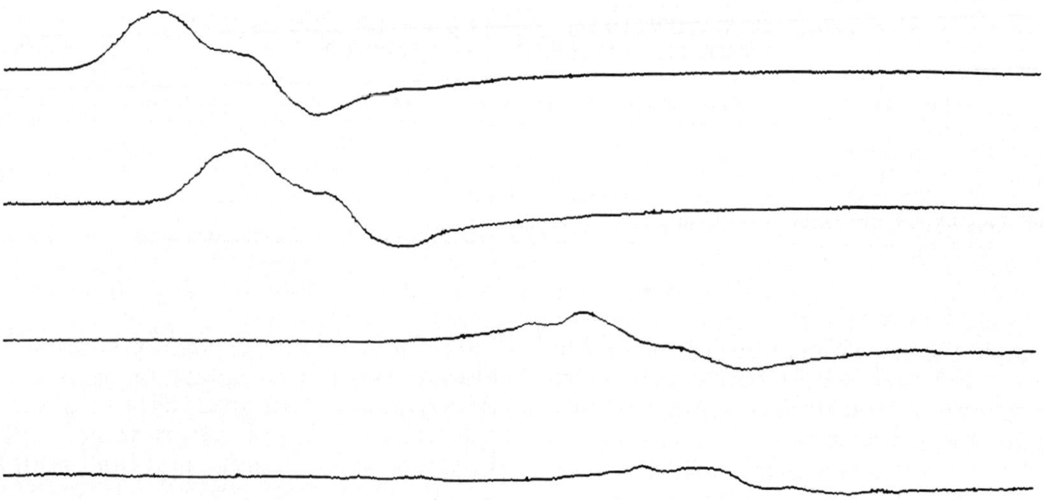

Figure 13–1. Progressive decline in CMAP recorded from ADM with ulnar nerve stimulation at the wrist *(top line)*, above the elbow *(second line)*, axilla *(third line)*, and Erb point *(bottom line)*. This shows the archetypal conduction of GBS.

PROXIMAL CONDUCTION BLOCK

Demonstration of a proximal nerve lesion in roots or plexus depends primarily on the recording of late responses. The H reflex and F wave reflect nerve conduction along the entire nerve. The H reflex is the electrical representation of the reflex, usually tested from the gastrocnemius-soleus. The F wave is an electrical volley that follows the CMAP after supramaximal nerve stimulation and results from centrifugal discharge of anterior horn cells.[767] F-wave latency interpretation must be normalized for height (paralleling nerve length).[660] By comparing late response latencies with the conduction time for directly measured intermediate and distal segments, conduction in proximal segments can be deduced. The precise anatomic dividing line between proximal and intermediate block is vague, but most workers have considered the nerve roots and perhaps the plexus as proximal.

Proximal conduction block is demonstrated by prolonged, dispersed, or absent F waves, in the presence of normal distal conduction. Minimal and maximal F-wave latencies or impersistence of F waves with repetitive stimuli may be abnormal in demyelinating disease.[1087] In order to evaluate proximal conduction, a ratio of motor nerve conduction from the spinal cord to the stimulus site compared with conduction in the distal nerve segment can be calculated as follows:[614]

$$\text{F ratio} = \frac{\text{(F latency} - \text{M latency)} - 1\text{ (millisecond)}}{\text{M latency} \times 2\text{ (milliseconds)}}$$

A delay of 1 millisecond in the numerator is estimated for the recurrent discharge of motor neurons and the refractory period of motor axons. A normal F ratio, indicating that the nerves are affected similarly proximally and distally, occurs in half of GBS patients.[614] Approximately equal numbers of the others have predominantly proximal or distal slowing.[614] Proximal conduction block can also be demonstrated by stimulation in the axilla, Erb's point, or cervical roots. One study[153] found proximal delay in 6 of 16 nerves stimulated at Erb's point. Others[807] have demonstrated conduction block restricted to the segment between the cord and the axilla as the sole finding in some GBS patients after percutaneous cervical root stimulation. Proximal conduction block has also been demonstrated more directly by needle stimulation of the cervical motor roots at C7.[95] Rapid motor recovery after plasma exchange was associated with reversal of proximal block[95] (Fig. 13–2). Newly devised magnetic motor evoked potential techniques may be useful in demonstrating proximal block by stimulation of central structures or by transcutaneous stimulation of proximal nerve segment or roots.

In several relatively small series of GBS patients, abnormalities of F-wave latencies have been described in 12% to 24% of patients with normal motor NCVs, depending on the timing of the study (Table 13–2). In Albers' extensive study,[14] absent F waves were common early in GBS but the incidence of prolonged F-wave latencies was highest 3 to 5 weeks after onset. F waves were absent (or latencies increased more than 120% of the upper limit of normal) in 46% of 210 electrodiagnostic studies from different centers participating in the Guillain-Barré Syndrome Study Group.[222] The F wave abnormalities in these series were not clearly separated from abnormalities of motor NCV.

Proximal conduction block occurred in 68% of patients in the MGH prospective series tested early after onset, making it the most common electrophysiologic abnormality, but it occurred in isolation in only 27%.[1021] In 10 (9%) patients with otherwise typical early GBS, CSF protein concentration was normal and F-wave abnormalities were the only abnormal findings on electrodiagnostic testing (see later).

INTERMEDIATE CONDUCTION BLOCK

Intermediate block probably corresponds best to the original use of the term *conduction block* and is characterized by a decline in the CMAP amplitude at progressively more proximal stimulation sites, without a concomitant increase in the duration or a decrease in NCV. In normal motor nerves, distal CMAP amplitude may be 20% to 40% less than proximal CMAP amplitude.[153,222,800] Intermediate block (CMAP decrease of more than 20%) occurred in 13 of 19 patients within 2 weeks of on-

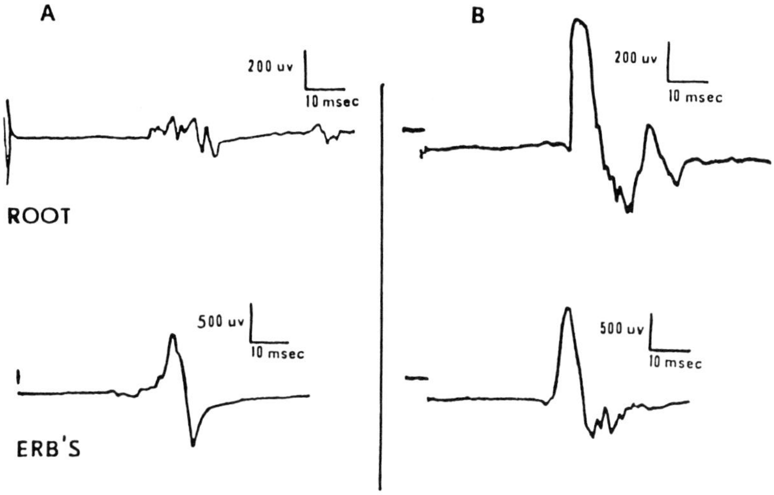

Figure 13–2. Proximal conduction block before and after plasma exchange in a GBS patient, with stimulation of cervical roots. (From Berger et al.,[95] p. 1041, with permission.)

set of illness in one study,[153] and in 30% of 210 patients reported in the Guillain-Barré Syndrome Study Group.[222] Phase cancellation may have contributed to an apparent intermediate block in the GBS Study Group's report because approximately 20% of the patients had slow motor conduction velocity or markedly decreased distal CMAP amplitude.

Six percent of the patients in the Massachusetts General Hospital (MGH) prospective study had intermediate conduction block in some nerves, usually associated with distal or proximal conduction block in other nerves. Isolated intermediate block occurred rarely, in only 1 of 113 consecutive patients.[1021] Others[1222] have made the interesting observation that intermediate or proximal conduction blocks were associated with normal conventional electrophysiologic sensory testing in most patients with typical GBS. The MGH results, discussed farther on, do not entirely confirm this. (Sensory conduction block may occur more frequently than appreciated because it is not measured by conventional tests.)

DISTAL CONDUCTION BLOCK

This is the least common type of block, though it may be difficult to detect in isolation. A very low amplitude or absent CMAP with distal stimulation implies axonal degeneration. Without extensive fibrillations, however, it is difficult to distinguish from distal conduction block. Block in distal motor nerve segments is reflected by increasing CMAP amplitude with stimulation at very distal sites (for example, distal to the flexor retinaculum of the median nerve).[153] There was no response in the median motor nerve in 2 and in the peroneal nerve in 6 of 50 patients in one series;[783] in 2 of 22 patients in another series;[785] and in only 1 patient in Albers' study.[14] In the prospective MGH series, 9% had distal block in combination with proximal conduction block at other sites (see later).[1021]

Slowed Nerve Conduction Velocity

Between the first and fourth week of illness, half of GBS patients have slowing of motor conduction or prolonged distal motor latency.[781] Slowing may be found as early as 3 days after onset;[963] it is usually widespread and varies in degree from one nerve to another. Approximately a quarter of patients tested within 3 weeks of illness in the prospective study had severe slowing in several or all nerves. Slowing is usually most marked distally or across sites of typical nerve compression.[662] Marked distal slowing (below 70% of normal, or less than 40 meters/sec in the arms and less than 30 meters/sec in the legs, or median nerve distal latency more than 7 milliseconds) has been attributed to segmental demyelination.[781,783] In the MGH prospective series, approximately one quarter of patients tested early had diffuse slowing (motor NCV below 80% of lower limit of normal in at least two nerves).[1021]

Slowing of sensory NCV, probably almost as common as slowing in motor nerves, may not be evident for several weeks.[14,833] In the first 4 weeks, more than three quarters of typical GBS patients in Albers' study[14] had normal sural sensory, and approximately one quarter, normal median sensory conduction studies. Sensory studies seem to be abnormal very frequently in Fisher's syndrome (see farther on and Chapter 8).

EMG and Patterns of Axonal Damage

Electromyographic (EMG) fibrillations and positive sharp waves almost certainly indicate axonal damage in GBS. Some sharp waves and fibrillations, however, may be detected during early GBS without necessarily implying a poor outcome. Denervation potentials appear as early as the second to fourth week of illness but are most frequent 11 to 15 weeks after onset. They usually occur simultaneously in distal and proximal muscles.[14] Varying degrees of fibrillation potentials have been reported in 20% to 64% of patients in the first month.[14,153,324,963] One particularly careful study[153] found fibrillation potentials in one or more of the thenar, hypothenar, and extensor digitorium brevis muscles in two thirds of patients as early as 9 days following the onset of weakness, more common distally and in the legs. There was an association between reduced distal motor amplitudes and denervation. When CMAP was less than 50% of normal, fibrillation potentials occurred in virtually all muscles tested.

Myokymic discharges, occurring early in GBS in facial or limb muscles, consist of spontaneous 30 to 60 Hz bursts of potentials that individually resemble motor unit action potentials, usually recurring almost regularly at intervals of a few seconds.[14]

ACUTE AXONAL GBS

An infrequent acute axonal form of GBS has been described,[348] with poor recovery, probably from widespread axonal damage. Motor nerves are inexcitable or CMAP amplitudes are extremely low with widespread denervation within days of onset of the illness.[153,803,1007] As noted earlier, distinction from distal block is difficult. Sensory responses are usually abnormal but may be present. These patients often become severely and rapidly paralyzed (the eye movements may be spared), ventilator dependent, and eventually have profound atrophy and a prolonged recovery. A relationship to typical GBS is presumed from the initial course, areflexia, raised CSF protein concentration in some patients, preliminary pathologic evidence, and the absence of alternative diagnoses. The presence of widespread and severe denervation makes distal conduction block an unlikely alternative explanation to extensive axonal damage. A careful study of such a case[586] found scant inflammation considering the degree of demyelination. There was also more small myelinated than large fiber damage and frequent vesicular demyelination (see Chapter 4). If this case is representative of other cases with similar clinical and electrophysiologic features, it must be considered another type of GBS, perhaps predominantly humorally mediated.

In the MGH prospective series, 2 patients (2.5%) had inexcitability in all nerves and, later, extensive denervation.[1021] Absent CMAP and extensive denervation were demonstrated only on repeated testing 2 and 16 days after onset. Initial studies showed normal NCV and proximal and distal conduction block.

CHANGES IN ELECTROPHYSIOLOGIC FINDINGS OVER TIME

Changes in electrophysiologic findings over time are unpredictable and generally do not parallel the clinical course.[499,783,785,963] F waves may spontaneously reappear without simultaneous clinical improvement.[615] In contrast, several MGH patients have had rapidly improving weakness that paralleled a reduction in the severity of distal block after plasma exchange. Reversal of proximal conduction block has been demonstrated,[95] coinciding with improvement of strength, but without changes in distal or intermediate conduction.

Albers and colleagues[14] grouped 180 electrodiagnostic studies as a function of time and found similar incidences of abnormal nerve conduction studies from the 2nd to the 20th week. Increasing slowing of motor nerve conduction occurred in some patients despite recovery of motor function. In the first 4 weeks of illness, abnormal sensory conduction study results occurred less frequently than abnormal motor conduction study results. Others[963,1222] have demonstrated consistently normal sensory studies during the course of some cases, despite progressive motor involvement.

Abnormal NCVs can persist for years after recovery. In one study,[757] completely normal nerve conduction was found in only 1 of 10 patients more than 2 years after complete recovery. In contrast, others[783] have found that most patients had normal motor conduction studies 6 months to 5½ years (mean 3 years) after onset.

ANCILLARY ELECTROPHYSIOLOGIC STUDIES

Blink Reflexes

Blink reflex first-component (R1) latencies were mildly prolonged in 2 of 10 GBS patients, with normal second-component (R2) latencies in one study,[385] suggesting slowing of facial nerve conduction. Almost half the patients in the MGH prospective study had blink reflex abnormalities[1021] (see farther on). Virtually all patients with prolonged R1 latencies had facial weakness, making these tests largely confirmatory (similar to others' findings[613]), rather than detecting occult areas of conduction block. Central abnormalities of evoked responses or blink reflexes, usually reported without clinical correlates, have been rare. (See Chapter 8 for a discussion of putative central nervous system lesions in GBS.)

Brainstem Evoked Potentials

Short-latency brainstem auditory evoked potentials (BAEP) have occasionally been abnormal in GBS. Three of twenty one MGH patients had abnormal study results: one with bilateral I-III interwave latency prolongation, one with unilateral I-III interwave latency prolongation, and another with unilateral III-V latency prolongation.[1012] Others,[1066] however, have found prolonged I-III interwave latencies in 5 of 6 patients and have attributed this to focal demyelination in the extramedullary portion of the auditory nerve. Two patients with abnormal peripheral BAEP conduction had acquired deafness, which is rare in GBS.[842] BAEPs are usually normal in patients with Fisher's syndrome[385,1012] (see Chapter 8).

Visual Evoked Potentials

Pattern shift visual evoked potentials (VEPs) have not been systematically studied in large GBS series, but normal VEPs occurred in three patients with Fisher's syndrome.[561] Ten patients with typical GBS in the MGH series had normal VEPs, another had abnormal VEPs bilaterally as a result of papilledema.[1012]

Somatosensory Evoked Potentials

Somatosensory evoked potentials (SEPs) can detect proximal sensory conduction block in the presence of normal distal conduction. The most common finding suggesting proximal sensory nerve demyelination is an increase in the EP-P/N13 (Erb's point to cervicomedullary) conduction time (Fig. 13–3).[1248] Prolonged EP-P/N13 conduction time or reduction in P/N13 amplitude, and dispersion, occurred in 12 of 17 GBS patients; 6 had normal F-wave latencies and 3 had normal median nerve conduction.[1248] Conversely, two patients had abnormal F-wave latencies and normal SEPs. Others[154] have found abnormal SEPs in 10 of 11 GBS patients, usually using normal conventional studies.

As previously reported, approximately half of a limited series of MGH patients with GBS had peripheral abnormalities of median nerve SEPs, and approximately three quarters had peripheral abnormalities of lower extremity SEPs.[1012] In a minor difference from previous studies,[1248] all 10 MGH patients with abnormal median nerve SEPs had absent, dispersed, or prolonged F-wave latencies from median

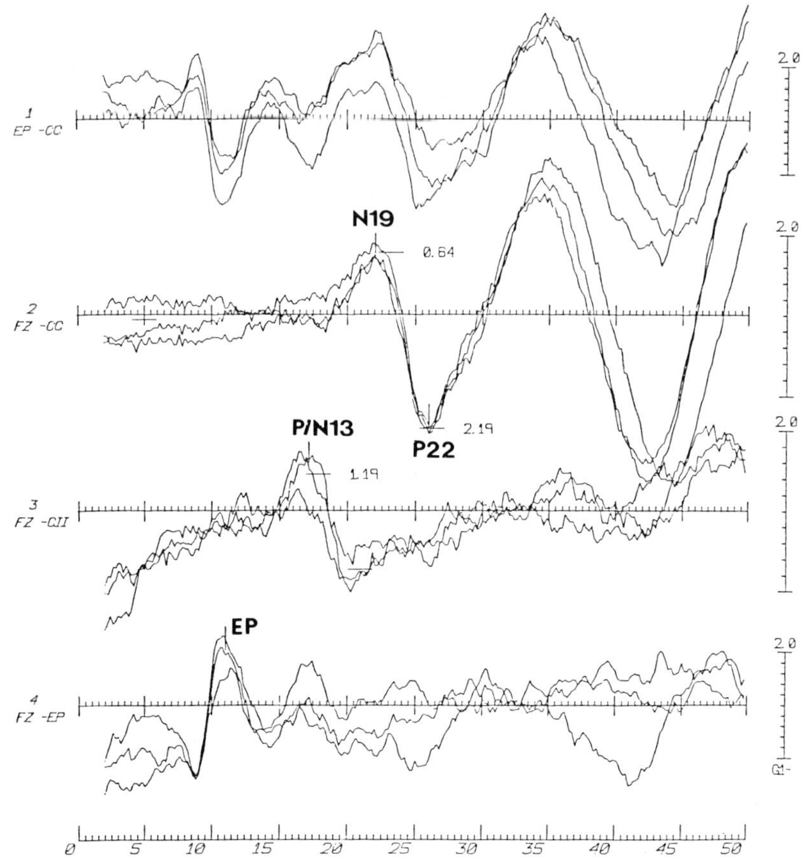

Figure 13–3. Median nerve somatosensory evoked potentials, following stimulation at the wrist, showing an increased EP-P/N13 interwave latency (6.2 milliseconds; upper normal 5.2 milliseconds) brachial plexus to cervicomedullary junction, with normal P/N13-N19 latency. This corresponds to a proximal conduction block in sensory nerves. There was normal sensory nerve conduction by conventional studies, but prolonged median F waves. (From Ropper and Chiappa,[1012] p. 589, with permission.)

nerve stimulation, whereas 6 of 8 patients with abnormal F waves had normal somatosensory responses.[1012] The frequency of proximal sensory and motor abnormalities has therefore been similar as gauged by the two types of studies but there is little point in comparing the sensitivity of the two techniques since they study different systems.

Sympathetic (Galvanic) Skin Response and RR ECG Interval

These tests are valuable adjuncts in detecting and quantifying autonomic failure in GBS. Small fiber sympathetic function in cutaneous blood vessels and sweat glands can be tested by measuring the sympathetic skin response (SSR) from surface electrodes on the palm, dorsal hand, and sole in response to deep inspiration and to cutaneous electrical stimuli.[1086] Normal variability in the test makes a completely absent response the only definite abnormality.[1086,1125]

The expected variation in RR interval is often absent in GBS, probably representing vagal afferent dysfunction[727] (see Chapter 7). The interval between successive QRS complexes is measured by triggering an oscilloscope sweep with alternate R waves and measuring RR variation in response to deep breathing and the Valsalva maneuver.[831,911] The responses at rest and to deep breathing are inversely and linearly related to age in controls.[727]

Thirteen of 17 patients had abnormal SSR and 10 of 15 had abnormal RR testing in a limited series of MGH patients.[1085a]

Recently developed techniques for sweat testing [quantitative sudomotor axon reflex test (Q-SART)] remain to be explored in GBS patients, but such test results have been normal in those with other primarily demyelinating neuropathies.[724]

Phrenic Nerve Conduction

Prolonged phrenic nerve conduction time has been demonstrated[848] in GBS patients with quadriplegia and cranial nerve involvement. Motor NCV in the limbs was related to phrenic nerve conduction time. In another small series,[429] most patients with prolonged latency of the diaphragmatic muscle action potential—some with initially normal vital capacities—developed respiratory failure, whereas none of the patients with normal phrenic nerve latencies did so. The predictive value of phrenic nerve conduction abnormalities for respiratory failure has not been systematically studied but these observations may be valuable in the future for intensive care unit practice.

PROGNOSTIC ELECTROPHYSIOLOGIC FEATURES

Fibrillation potentials have been associated with poor recovery in a few studies.[324,963] One careful evaluation[153] correlated low-amplitude distal CMAP and fibrillations with residual motor disabilities, results confirmed in two recent retrospective studies.[222,800] A greatly reduced CMAP (below 10% of the lower limit of normal) predicted a poor outcome.[800] Multivariate analysis of the Guillain-Barré Syndrome Study Group's data[222] also found a poor outcome in patients with greatly reduced (below 20%) mean amplitude of compound muscle on distal stimulation early in the disease. Few patients were tested for concomitant fibrillation. Prognostication of the outcome of GBS from electrophysiologic features in children is discussed in Chapter 9.

ELECTROPHYSIOLOGIC STUDIES IN EARLY GBS: THE MGH PROSPECTIVE STUDY

In order to analyze completely the patterns of electrophysiologic abnormalities in GBS, 113 of the 120 consecutive GBS patients in the MGH prospective study were studied with a uniform electrophysiologic protocol. The methods and more complete findings are described in another publication.[1021] Of the 120 MGH prospectively studied patients, 103 (90%) had electrodiagnostic studies within 3 weeks of the onset of illness. (An excellent similar but retrospective study by Albers and associates[14] contains useful similar data and should also be consulted by interested readers.) In brief, the MGH uniform electrodiagnostic protocol included motor and sensory nerve conduction studies in ulnar, median, and peroneal nerves; late responses from several nerves (H reflex and F wave); sensory action potentials in at least two nerves; and EMG of at least four muscles. Tests of blink reflexes,[1089] RR interval, and sympathetic skin responses were performed in selected patients. Values above 3 standard deviations (SD) from the laboratory mean were considered abnormal. F waves were elicited 10 times for each test by supramaximal stimulation and were considered abnormal if they were delayed for the patient's height; were dispersed, with a maximum to minimum latency more than 3 milliseconds in the arms or 5 milliseconds in the legs; or were impersistent, with less than 5 responses to 10 stimuli.

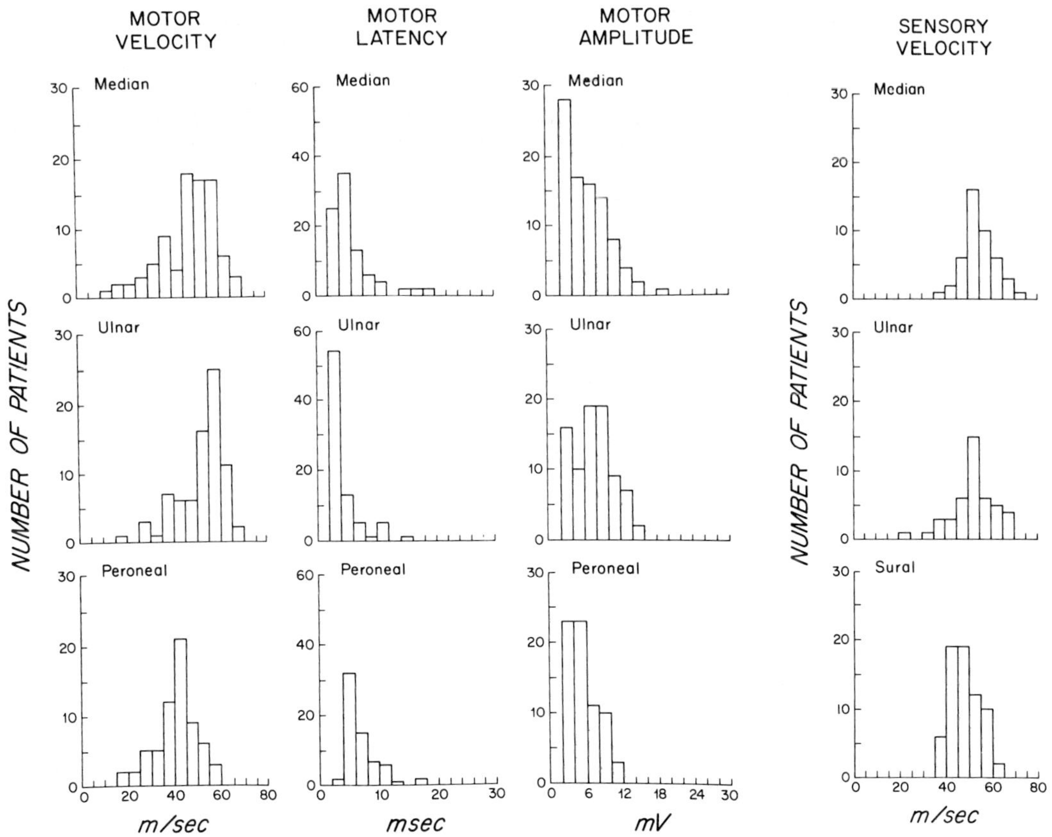

Figure 13–4. *A*, Distribution of motor nerve conduction velocity, latency, and amplitude in median, ulnar, and peroneal nerves in MGH prospective series. Only patients with a measurable motor response are shown. *B*, Sensory nerve conduction velocities in median, ulnar, and sural nerves in patients with a measurable response. (From Ropper et al.,[1021] with permission.)

Table 13–3 ELECTROPHYSIOLOGY IN EARLY GBS*†

Nerve	*No. Absent*	*No. Present*	*Mean Conduction Velocity (ms)*	*Mean Distal Latency (ms)*
Median motor	2	88	47±12	6.1±3.6
Ulnar motor	4	81	51±10	4.1±2.3
Peroneal motor	4	65	40±9	7.2±3.9
Median sensory	33	45	54±7	3.3±2.2
Ulnar sensory	27	45	52±10	2.9±1.7
Sural sensory	30	69	47±6	2.8±1.6

*MGH experience in 113 consecutive patients. Only worst shown; often both sides tested.
†From Ropper et al.,[1021] with permission.

Table 13–4 ELECTROPHYSIOLOGIC MOTOR NERVE FINDINGS RELATED TO CLINICAL FEATURES AND IN VARIANTS*

Clinical Features or Variants	*No. Patients*	*Motor Abnormalities (No. Patients)*		*No. Patients with Sensory Abnormalities*
Fisher's syndrome only	3	PCB + DL	(1)	3
		PCB	(2)	
Pharyngeal-cervical-brachial	3	Normal†	(1)	3
		DL + PCB	(1)	
		PCB	(1)	
Pharyngeal-cervical-brachial and ophthalmoplegia	1	DL + PCB	(1)	1
Paraparetic	2	Slowing	(2)	2
Ataxia only (initial)	1	PCB + ICB	(1)	1
Pure motor	4	Slowing	(2)	0
		PCB	(1)	
		DCB + PCB	(1)	

*From Ropper et al.,[1021] with permission.
†Increased F-wave latencies in several nerves in repeated EMG 3 days after onset. DL = distal lesion, PCB = proximal conduction block, DCB = distal conduction block, ICB = intermediate conduction block.

The mean motor and sensory nerve conduction velocities, amplitudes, and distal motor latencies are summarized in Figure 13–4 and Table 13–3. The combined electrophysiologic findings are shown in Tables 13–4 and 13–5.

Motor Nerve Abnormalities

The main findings on early initial testing were proximal conduction block as an isolated finding in 27%, proximal conduction block combined with a distal lesion in 27%, and generalized slowing in 22%. These three categories together, therefore, accounted for three quarters of electrophysiologic abnormalities. Two patients had inexcitable motor nerves in all nerves tested. One patient (with an oropharyngeal-brachial GBS variant) had a completely normal study result on the first day of illness; however, prolonged F-wave latencies were noted in several nerves 2 days later.

Approximately one third of patients had electrodiagnostic abnormalities in only one nerve segment. After combining the electrodiagnostic abnormalities, another 47 (42%) of 113 patients had electrophysiologic evidence of demyelination in two or more nerve segments. In the first week of illness, multiple ab-

Table 13–5 OUTCOME AND ELECTRODIAGNOSTIC FINDINGS*

Electrodiagnostic Findings	*No. Patients*	*Good Recovery†*	*Poor Outcome‡*
Diffuse slowing	20	13	7
Multifocal demyelination	33	23	10
Median motor amplitude ≤1000 μV	17	11	5
Ulnar motor amplitude ≤1000 μV (N = 10)	10	8	2
Peroneal motor amplitude ≤700 μV (N = 11)	11	6	5
Proximal conduction block only	24	22	2
Absent response	2	2	0
Distal demyelination only	5	4	1

*In 86 consecutive patients tested within 2 wk of illness. (Adapted from Ropper et al.[1021])
†Good recovery includes minor weakness or paresthesias.
‡Poor outcome includes need for braces, splints, or crutches; wheelchair-bound patients; or death.

normalities (16 of 41) and proximal conduction block (15 of 41) were the most frequent patterns. Diffuse slowing occurred less often (5 of 41). Of the 30 patients with normal CSF protein concentration in the first 3 weeks, 5 had prolonged F-wave latencies or impersistent F waves, 5 had absent F waves, and 20 had a variety of other abnormalities.

Sensory Nerve Abnormalities

Forty (37%) of 107 patients had normal sensory latency, amplitude, and velocity in at least two nerves in the first 2 weeks (mean 8 days). A pure motor variant of GBS, characterized by the absence of sensory signs or paresthesias, was present in 4 patients (see later and Chapter 8). Normal sensory nerve conduction occurred in combination with several types of motor abnormalities in other patients, but 22 of 25 patients with diffuse slowing had abnormal sensory nerve studies, compared with only 9 of 27 with proximal conduction block.

EMG

Upon EMG, 2 of 105 patients had sporadic (1+) denervation potentials; 10 had more extensive (2+, 3+, and 4+) early denervation in at least two muscles in the arm and legs. Of these patients 4 became severely quadriparetic (grade 4) and 6 developed respiratory failure (grade 5).

Relation of Electrophysiologic Features to Clinical Variants

A synopsis of motor electrophysiologic findings in relation to GBS variants appears in Table 13–4. All six patients who had Fisher's syndrome at onset (three progressed to generalized weakness) had a proximal conduction block and abnormal sensory tests. (One patient with Fisher's syndrome had only blink reflexes tested, and is not included in this series.) Normal sensory NCVs persisted in patients with the pure motor variant of GBS despite severe slowing of motor conduction (see Chapter 8). Two patients with a paraplegic GBS variant had normal motor conduction in the arms.

Follow-Up Studies

Twenty MGH patients (18%) had studies repeated during their hospital stay. Four of five with progressing weakness had further slowing of motor nerve conduction; in the other patient, proximal conduction block remained unchanged several weeks later. Eight of 15 patients with second studies after the acute progressive phase of illness had progressive conduction block or increased nerve conduction slowing.

Ancillary Studies (Blink Reflex, SSR, RR Interval)

Fifty-six of the 113 patients had blink reflex testing; of these, 26 (46%) had abnormal results. All but one of these had facial weakness—20 symmetric and 5 asymmetric. Abnormal blink reflexes were not associated with any consistent pattern of conduction block or diffuse slowing in other nerves, but the latency of the blink R1 response correlated closely with median motor nerve distal latencies.

Twenty-six patients underwent SSR and RR interval studies; 12 (46%) had abnormal study results. Ten of 15 patients with quadriplegia had abnormal autonomic study results, as did 7 or 8 patients with diffuse motor nerve conduction slowing; Other electrodiagnostic features were approximately equally distributed between groups with and without SSR and RR abnormalities.

Outcome Related to Electrophysiologic Studies

Chapter 18 provides a more extensive discussion of features pertaining to outcome. For the purposes of electrophysiologic analysis, good recovery was considered to be the ability to walk without impediment and to perform independent self-care, albeit with possible minor weakness or paresthesias. Poor outcome included those requiring orthoses or appliances. Patients with diffuse slowing and multifocal abnormalities generally had poorer outcomes than those with conduction block in one segment (Table 13–5). Poor outcomes in our patients with very low CMAP amplitude in median motor, ulnar motor, and peroneal motor nerves partly confirmed earlier published observations that patients with low CMAP had poorer outcomes. However, many did make some improvement. Only a few patients composed each category of conduction block, which made outcome comparisons difficult, but 22 of 24 with early proximal block had good outcomes. Two of 3 patients with inexcitable nerves and extensive fibrillations (1 on initial testing and 2 after follow-up studies several days later) remained wheelchair bound. Of the 10 patients with early extensive fibrillations, including 1 with absent responses, 6 made good recoveries after 3, 6, 7, 7, 11, and 12 months, respectively. Outcomes were similar in patients with initially normal sensory study results and those with absent or slowed sensory nerve conduction.

Extensive electrophysiologic testing is virtually always abnormal in GBS, even very early in the illness. The major patterns of motor abnormalities tend to be isolated proximal conduction block (reflected in aberrant late responses), proximal conduction block with prolongation of distal conduction, or widespread slowing of NCV. The temporal course of electrophysiologic changes is unpredictable and has only a limited relationship to clinical outcome.

Chapter 14

DIFFERENTIAL DIAGNOSIS

GBS is readily recognized in its typical form, but atypical manifestations extend the differential diagnosis to many neuropathies, myopathies, and neuromuscular diseases. Atypical GBS, however, is more common than most of the relatively rare diseases that simulate GBS.

This chapter is divided into two sections. The first section deals with individual clinical or laboratory features or clinical settings that should make the physician consider alternative diagnoses to GBS. The second section includes brief descriptions of the diseases in the differential diagnosis, many but not all of which are neuropathies. The tables, organized according to approximate order of frequency or importance of each sign, enable the clinican to use atypical features of apparent GBS to focus on a more limited differential diagnosis, and then to consult the second portion of the chapter concerning alternative diagnoses. We have focused on features that help differentiate GBS from diseases that resemble it. Some material is unavoidably repeated in the two sections of the chapter in order to facilitate rapid reference.

DIFFERENTIAL DIAGNOSIS BASED ON CLINICAL SIGNS

Asymmetric Limb Weakness

Weakness in GBS is relatively symmetric. Subtle asymmetries (a "neurologist's asymmetry") are common, and occasionally more marked asymmetries occur due to superimposed compressive neuropathies. Substantial asymmetry, however, suggests an alternate diagnosis (Table 14–1), particularly transverse myelitis or another acute myelopathy. Acute spinal shock is necessary to produce areflexia, so this sign remains a relatively dependable sign of GBS. Polio, rabies, and cutaneous diphtheria resemble GBS but may cause markedly asymmetric weakness.

The vasculitic neuropathies may progress so rapidly that the clinical picture is dominated by a relatively symmetric polyneuropathy, but focal weakness or some asymmetry is usually present. Paralysis in Lyme disease and carcinomatous meningitis may also be asymmetric.

Asymmetric Sensory Loss

Sensory symptoms and signs in GBS are invariably symmetrical (see Chapter 7). Asymmetries suggest the diseases listed in Table 14–2, including myelitis or other acute myelopathies. In rabies, the initial symptom is often pain or paresthesias near the site of the bite. Uni-

Table 14–1 ASYMMETRIC LIMB WEAKNESS

Transverse myelitis
Other acute myelopathies
Polio
Rabies
Vasculitic neuropathies
Mononeuritis multiplex
Diphtheria
Carcinomatous meningitis
Tick paralysis (rare)
Periodic paralyses (rare)
Lyme disease

Table 14–2 ASYMMETRIC SENSORY LOSS

Transverse myelitis
Other acute myelopathies
Rabies
Vasculitic neuropathies
Lyme disease
Carcinomatous meningitis

lateral or asymmetric sensory loss is common in the distribution of a single peripheral nerve in vasculitic neuropathy and Lyme disease, or conforming to multiple spinal roots in carcinomatous meningitis.

Asymmetric Cranial Nerve Weakness

Facial paralysis in GBS may be asymmetric but other cranial nerve palsies are typically symmetric. Persistent asymmetry of cranial nerve signs suggests other diagnoses (Table 14–3). Unilateral or asymmetric palatal paralysis is a hallmark of diphtheria and may occur in Lyme disease and sarcoidosis. Rabies may begin with asymmetric cranial nerve involvement when the bite is on the face or when the disease is transmitted by corneal transplantation. Acute mass lesions near the foramen magnum may also produce asymmetric paralysis of lower cranial nerves and limb weakness. Cranial nerve involvement in Lyme disease and carcinomatous meningitis may be asymmetric, and the latter may involve the acoustic nerve, rare in GBS. Basilar artery occlusive disease, most relevant in the differential diagnosis of Fisher's syndrome (see later), typically produces asymmetric cranial nerve palsies.

Table 14–3 ASYMMETRIC CRANIAL NERVE WEAKNESS

Diphtheria
Rabies
Foramen magnum mass lesions
Lyme disease
Carcinomatous meningitis

Table 14–4 FACIAL SENSORY ABNORMALITIES

Acute sensory neuronopathy syndrome
Rabies
Vasculitic neuropathies
Ciguatera, paralytic shellfish poisoning
Hypophosphatemia
Thallium intoxication
Arsenic intoxication (rare)
Tick paralysis
Barium toxicity
Hyperkalemic periodic paralysis
Perhexiline neuropathy
Carcinomatous meningitis

Facial Sensory Abnormalities

While facial paralysis is common in GBS, paresthesias or loss of sensation on the face is uncommon. Occasional patients have paresthesias on the tip of the tongue, the nose, or in the skin over the vertex (see Chapter 7). Loss of facial sensation or widely distributed facial sensory symptoms are hallmarks of the acute sensory neuronopathy syndrome. Trigeminal neuropathy has been described in the connective tissue diseases but usually occurs independently of the other signs of neuropathy. Early symptoms of ciguatera and paralytic shellfish poisoning include a tingling or burning of the lips, tongue, gums, mouth, or face, or a loose feeling in the teeth. In hypophosphatemia, paresthesias may affect the limbs, perioral, and periorbital areas. Abnormal facial sensations have rarely been reported in the other entities listed in Table 14–4.

Prominent Sensory Abnormalities

The diseases listed in Table 14–5 resemble GBS but have more prominent sensory symptoms and signs than in typical GBS. Disproportionate sensory symptoms, like facial paresthesias, may be an important clue that the underlying process is not GBS.

Table 14–5 PROMINENT SENSORY ABNORMALITIES

Acute sensory neuronopathy syndrome
Rabies
Vasculitic neuropathies
Ciguatera poisoning
Paralytic shellfish poisoning
Hypophosphatemia
Thallium intoxication
Arsenic intoxication
Vacor neuropathy
Perhexiline neuropathy

Table 14–7 PURE OR PREDOMINANTLY MOTOR SYMPTOMS AND SIGNS

Lead poisoning
Poliomyelitis
Polymyositis
Other acute myopathies
Myasthenia gravis
Botulism
Hypermagnesemia
Tick paralysis
Periodic paralyses
Organophosphate poisoning

Prominent Ataxia

Fisher's variant of GBS is characterized by limb and, to a lesser extent, gait ataxia. Gait ataxia may also be seen in almost any neuropathy with significant impairment of sensation but has been most prominent in some of the diseases listed in Table 14–6.

Pure or Predominantly Motor Symptoms and Signs

Motor symptoms and signs predominate over sensory ones in typical GBS and in the pure motor GBS variant (discussed in Chapter 8). Acute pure motor neuropathy may be caused by other diseases, particularly polio, lead poisoning, and muscle diseases (Table 14–7), all less common than GBS.

Prominent Pain

Aching pain in the axial muscles occurs in more than two thirds of patients with GBS. Table 14–8 lists other acute diseases in which various types of pain are common or very prominent. Deep aching pain in limb and axial muscles, often associated with tenderness, suggests polymyositis or other myopathies associated with acute rhabdomyolysis, or poliomyelitis. Radicular pain may occur in patients with transverse myelitis and carcinomatous meningitis (as well as sciatica that occurs in GBS). Focal pain along the course of a nerve occurs in mononeuritis multiplex and vasculitic neuropathies. Painful paresthesias are also characteristic of some of the neuropathies listed in Table 14–8.

Table 14–6 ATAXIA

Hypophosphatemia
Tick paralysis
Thallium intoxication
Vacor neuropathy
Acute sensory neuronopathy syndrome

CSF Pleocytosis

CSF pleocytosis occurs in 10% to 20% of GBS patients (see Chapter 12). Transverse myelitis is the process that most commonly resembles GBS and produces a CSF pleocytosis. Rabies and polio are major considerations for quadriparesis and pleocytosis in nonindustrialized countries. Lyme disease

Table 14–8 PROMINENT PAIN

Painful Paresthesias	*Focal or Multifocal Pain*
Acute porphyrias	Mononeuritis multiplex
Thallium intoxication	Rabies
Arsenic intoxication	Snake and other envenomations
Perhexilene neuropathy	Vasculitic neuropathies
Muscle Pain	*Radicular Pain*
Polymyositis	Transverse myelitis
Rhabdomyolysis	Carcinomatous meningitis
Hypokalemic myopathy	Polio
Polio	

Table 14–9 CSF PLEOCYTOSIS

Polio
Rabies
Transverse myelitis
Trichinosis
Lyme disease
Carcinomatous meningitis

and acquired immunodeficiency syndrome (AIDS) may cause a neuropathy that, at times, is indistinguishable from GBS (see later, and Chapter 6) except that both typically have an associated aseptic meningitis. Table 14–9 summarizes diseases that typically have cerebrospinal fluid (CSF) pleocytosis and simulate GBS.

Increased CSF Protein Level

Elevated CSF protein concentration is a hallmark of GBS but is also very nonspecific, as many other neuropathies can have albuminocytologic dissociation. Table 14–10 lists diseases with elevated CSF protein concentrations that are likely to be considered in the differential diagnosis of GBS.

Differential Diagnosis of Fisher's Syndrome

The primary entities in the differential diagnosis of Fisher's syndrome, discussed further in Chapter 8, are disorders of neuromuscular transmission

Table 14–10 INCREASED CSF PROTEIN LEVEL

Acute porphyrias
Thallium intoxication
Arsenic intoxication
Gold neuropathy
Lead poisoning
Vacor neuropathy
Perhexiline neuropathy
Vincristine neuropathy
Acute sensory neuronopathy syndrome
Carcinomatous meningitis

(botulism, myasthenia gravis, hypermagnesemia, antibiotic-induced weakness, snake envenomations), and other peripheral nerve diseases with external ophthalmoplegia as a prominent feature (diphtheria, hypophosphatemia, thallium intoxication, and tick paralysis). Only the disorders of neuromuscular transmission are likely to produce the severe, often complete external ophthalmoplegia seen in Fisher's syndrome. Hyporeflexia or areflexia, however, may occur in severe cases of any of these disorders, and all but myasthenia and the snake envenomations have occasionally been reported with ataxia. Prominent or isolated ataxia can occur with a number of diseases, including neuropathies, discussed earlier.

Three disorders of the central nervous system—Wernicke's encephalopathy, brainstem encephalitis, and basilar artery occlusion, in limited circumstances—may also simulate Fisher's syndrome. Ophthalmoplegia and ataxia are characteristics of Wernicke's encephalopathy, and occasional patients may also have global areflexia. Nystagmus, however, is rare in Fisher's syndrome. The ataxia of Wernicke's encephalopathy affects primarily gait and the trunk, whereas ataxia in Fisher's syndrome usually involves the limbs. The abnormal laboratory studies of GBS, CSF albuminocytologic dissociation and sensory nerve electrophysiologic changes, common in Fisher's syndrome, are not seen in uncomplicated Wernicke's encephalopathy, basilar artery ischemia, or brainstem encephalitis.

Ophthalmoplegia, ataxia, and areflexia may occur in patients with large bilateral lesions in the mid-brain and pons, such as infarction or brainstem encephalitis. Other signs, however, give clinical evidence of brainstem localization. Almost all central nervous system (CNS) parenchymal lesions producing total external ophthalmoplegia also produce alteration in wakefulness and when global areflexia occurs (rarely) there is almost always limb weakness. The controversy over the site of the lesion in Fisher's syndrome and its relation to brainstem encephalitis is discussed extensively in Chapter 8. In our opinion, the triad of ophthalmoplegia, ataxia, and areflexia should not be considered Fisher's syndrome if coma, obtundation, nystagmus, internuclear ophthalmoplegia, quadriplegia, or bilateral Babinski's signs also exist.

Internal Ophthalmoplegia

Pupillary dysfunction is uncommon in typical GBS. It may occur with complete ophthalmoplegia, quadriplegia, and respiratory failure, or in patients with Fisher's syndrome. Early or isolated internal ophthalmoplegia also occurs in the diseases in Table 14–11. Classic diphtheria and some forms of botulism are associated with accommodation paralysis, evident most commonly as blurred vision or near visual tasks such as reading. Pupillary reactions to light and convergence may, however, be normal in patients with botulism.

External Ophthalmoplegia

Partial external ophthalmoplegia occurs in 10% to 15% of GBS patients. Complete external ophthalmoplegia, however, is less common in typical GBS, occurring in cases with severe quadriplegia and respiratory failure or in those with Fisher's syndrome. Early or disproportionate external ophthalmoplegia suggests a disorder of neuromuscular transmission (Table 14–12.)

Table 14–11 INTERNAL OPHTHALMOPLEGIA

Diphtheritic neuropathy
Botulism
Anticholinergic toxicity
Barium toxicity
Antibiotic-induced paralysis
Snake envenomations
Lambert-Eaton syndrome

Table 14–12 EXTERNAL OPHTHALMOPLEGIA

Botulism
Myasthenia gravis
Hypermagnesemia
Antibiotic-induced weakness
Diphtheria
Hypophosphatemia
Thallium intoxication
Tick paralysis
Snake envenomations
Organophosphate poisoning

Ptosis

Ptosis is relatively uncommon in typical GBS without complete ophthalmoplegia but has probably been underreported. Perhaps less than complete ophthalmoplegia, ptosis suggests a disorder of neuromuscular transmission or one of the diseases in Table 14–13.

Respiratory Failure Disproportionate to Limb Weakness

Respiratory failure in GBS is associated with severe limb paralysis. When respiratory failure occurs with little limb weakness, alternative diagnoses include disorders of neuromuscular transmission such as myasthenia gravis, botulism, hypermagnesemia, and antibiotic-induced weakness (Table 14–14). Rabies may either cause paralysis of the respiratory musculature, with severely paretic limbs, or directly involve the medullary respiratory centers, with

Table 14–13 PTOSIS

Botulism
Myasthenia gravis
Hypermagnesemia
Antibiotic-induced weakness
Hypophosphatemia
Thallium intoxication
Tick paralysis
Barium toxicity
Snake envenomations
Lambert-Eaton syndrome

Table 14–14 RESPIRATORY FAILURE DISPROPORTIONATE TO LIMB WEAKNESS

Myasthenia gravis	Rabies
Botulism	Acid maltase deficiency
Antibiotic-induced weakness	ALS
Hypermagnesemia	High cervical intramedullary lesions
Hypophosphatemia	Barium intoxication
Critical illness polyneuropathy	Snake envenomations

minimal associated limb weakness. Patients having adult acid maltase deficiency may present with pure respiratory paralysis. Amyotrophic Lateral Sclerosis (ALS) or intermedullary spinal processes such as syringomyelia or tumor confined to the C2–4 region of the cervical spinal cord rarely produce bilateral diaphragmatic paralysis without substantial limb weakness.

Prominent Oropharyngeal Paralysis

Weakness of the pharyngeal muscles is common in GBS, but its severity usually parallels limb weakness. Oropharyngeal weakness disproportionate to limb weakness is a feature of several other diseases that simulate GBS (Table 14–15). Disorders of neuromuscular transmission, diphtheria, or rabies are the major considerations when bulbar paralysis is prominent. Nasal speech and a diminished gag response have also been noted in hypophosphatemia and polymyositis. In the acute porphyrias, pharyngeal weakness seldom appears before significant limb paralysis. There are rare cases of localized tetanus or hyperthyroidism with prominent pharyngeal dysfunction. Some cases of sarcoid have laryngeal paresis and hoarseness as prominent features of a generalized polyneuropathy.

Constipation and Ileus

Both constipation and ileus are common in GBS patients, usually with severe motor deficits. Acute intermittent porphyria and botulism are alternative diagnoses in patients with suspected GBS and prominent or persistent constipation or ileus (Table 14–16).

Nausea, Vomiting, and Abdominal Pain

Nausea, vomiting, and abdominal pain are uncommon in GBS. The gastrointestinal (GI) prodrome has usually resolved several days prior to onset of GBS. *Campylobacter* enteritis has been recognized as a common preceding pathogen in GBS. Ingestion of biologic and inorganic toxins commonly causes GI symptoms hours or days after ingestion, and before neurological symptoms (Table 14–17).

Dry Mouth or Eyes

Impaired salivation or lacrimation, uncommon in GBS, raises the possibil-

Table 14–15 PROMINENT OROPHARYNGEAL PARALYSIS

Botulism	Tetanus
Diphtheria	Hyperthyroidism
Myasthenia gravis	Thallium intoxication
Hypermagnesemia	Tick paralysis
Antibiotic-induced weakness	Barium toxicity
Rabies	Snake envenomations
Hypophosphatemia	Lambert-Eaton syndrome
Polymyositis	Carcinomatous meningitis
Acute porphyrias	

Table 14–16 CONSTIPATION AND ILEUS

Acute intermittent porphyria
Botulism
Transverse myelitis
Other acute myelopathies
Thallium intoxication
Lead poisoning
Polio
Vincristine neuropathy
Lambert-Eaton syndrome
Carcinomatous meningitis

Table 14–17 NAUSEA, VOMITING, AND ABDOMINAL PAIN (GI PRODROME)

Acute intermittent porphyria
Botulism
Thallium intoxication
Arsenic intoxication
Lead poisoning
Barium toxicity
Polio
Fish poisoning

Table 14–19 ABNORMAL MENTAL STATUS

Acute intermittent porphyria	Thallium intoxication
Rabies	Arsenic intoxication
Anticholinergic toxicity	Gold neuropathy
Hypophosphatemia	Lead poisoning
Hypermagnesemia	Vacor intoxication
"Overlap" syndromes	Lyme disease
Vasculitides	Carcinomatous meningitis

ity of the neuromuscular disorders that also affect cholinergic transmission at autonomic synapses (Table 14–18). Sjögren's syndrome may also be associated with a subacute or chronic sensory neuropathy, more similar to chronic inflammatory demyelinating polyneuropathy (CIDP) than to GBS.

Abnormal Mental Status

Confusion in patients with GBS is usually the result of secondary medical complications such as hypoxia, hypercapnia, or hyponatremia. When confusion or stupor are prominent features of an illness and their cause cannot be found, the alternative diagnoses in Table 14–19 should be considered. Acute intermittent porphyria with neuropathy that is severe enough to mimic GBS, and rabies, are almost always associated with agitation or an abnormal mental state. Mental status abnormalities are also typical of intoxication with heavy metals. Confusion has been reported inconsistently with botulism, hypermagnesemia, hypophosphatemia, and antibiotic-induced weakness, probably secondary to retention of carbon dioxide rather than to the underlying process. Rarely confusion occurs in a few cases of "overlap" syndromes that produce both peripheral and CNS demyelination or inflammation.

Seizures

Seizures are not a feature of GBS unless due to complications such as hypoxemia, hyponatremia, or hypertensive encephalopathy. Acute intermittent porphyria or toxins are the primary alternative diagnoses (Table 14–20). In the AIDS patient with GBS, a variety of other processes affecting the CNS may cause seizures (eg, toxoplasmosis, Progressive Multifocal Leukoencephalopathy [PML], opportunistic meningitis). Of the vasculitic processes that cause an acute polyneuropathy mimicking GBS, systemic lupus erythematosus (SLE) is most likely to cause seizures. Other autoimmune diseases may cause seizures indirectly after renal involvement has led to hypertension

Table 14–18 DRY MOUTH OR EYES

Botulism
Hypermagnesemia
Antibiotic-induced weakness
Anticholinergic toxicity
Sjögren's syndrome with vasculitis/cryoglobulinemia
Thallium intoxication
Arsenic intoxication
Barium toxicity
Lambert-Eaton syndrome

Table 14–20 SEIZURES

Acute intermittent porphyria
Anticholinergic toxicity
"Overlap" syndromes
AIDS
Vasculitides
Hypophosphatemia
Thallium intoxication
Arsenic intoxication
Carcinomatous meningitis

and uremia. Seizures have been reported in patients with hypophosphatemia, but concomitant electrolyte and acid-base disturbances may play a role.

Fever

Fever has generally been considered an exclusionary criterion for the diagnosis of GBS. An antecedent febrile illness or complications such as pneumonia, atelectasis, pulmonary embolism, or urinary tract infection may, however, cause fever at the onset of GBS. Otherwise, the diseases in Table 14–21 should be considered if fever is greatly elevated or protracted. Polio characteristically includes fever in both the prodromal and paralytic phases. Patients with diphtheria may be febrile with palatal or accommodation paralysis but are afebrile once the neuritis evolves. Fulminant thyrotoxicosis, the type likely to cause either Basedow's paraplegia or acute bulbar paralysis, may also be associated with fever. Vasculitis associated with mononeuritis multiplex or fulminant polyneuropathy may cause a low-grade fever.

Mucocutaneous Abnormalities

Abnormalities of the skin and mucous membranes are uncommon in GBS. Facial flushing occurs occasionally in GBS with dysautonomia but is more common in anticholinergic toxicity or hypermagnesemia (Table 14–22). Purpura and petechiae are characteristic of mixed cryoglobulinemia and a variety of cutaneous manifestations may be seen with other vasculitic neuropathies. Dermatomyositis classically causes a heliotrope orbital rash, Gottron's sign, or other rashes. An erythematous scaly rash of the face and scrotum has been described in thallium intoxication. Morbilliform or maculopapular rashes on the trunk or proximal legs are common in arsenic poisoning; a classic manifestation is desquamation and hyperkeratosis of the palms and soles. Palmar dyshydrotic keratosis has also been seen in hexacarbon (glue sniffer's) neuropathy. Rashes or urticaria may be seen with the neurologic marine toxins, often due to concomitant intoxication with other marine toxins (scombroid). Local tissue reactions are common at the site of injury in rabies, snake bites, other envenomations, and Lyme disease. Stomatitis often occurs in patients with thallium intoxication, and perioral herpetiform lesions may be seen in those with arsenic poisoning. Mees' lines (transverse white nail bands) are seen in those with arsenic and thallium poisoning and hexacarbon neuropathy. Alopecia is a classic, albeit delayed, feature of thallium intoxication (Table 14–22).

Table 14–21 FEVER

Polio
Diphtheria
Rabies
Anticholinergic toxicity
Vasculitides
Hyperthyroidism
Acute porphyrias
Trichinosis

Table 14–22 MUCOCUTANEOUS ABNORMALITIES

Fish poisonings
Cryoglobulinemia
Other vasculitic neuropathies
Hypermagnesemia
Anticholinergic toxicity
Thallium intoxication
Arsenic intoxication
Lead poisoning
Polio (during prodrome)
Hexacarbon (glue sniffer's) neuropathy
Dermatomyositis
Trichinosis

Postoperative or In-Hospital Onset

Approximately 5% or less of GBS cases occur postsurgically. However, a variety of other diseases resembling

GBS develop in patients hospitalized for other reasons (Table 14–23). Previously undiagnosed myasthenia gravis may be evident for the first time with difficulty weaning from an artificial respirator after a surgical procedure, especially if neuromuscular blocking drugs have been used. Weakness due to the neuromuscular blockade induced by aminoglycoside antibiotics may occur in patients with or without preexisting disorders of neuromuscular transmission. Hypermagnesemic weakness occurs in patients with impaired renal function who receive magnesium-containing antacids or cathartics. Treatment of toxemia with parenteral magnesium may also lead to hypermagnesemic paralysis. Several cases of acute areflexic paralysis with cranial nerve dysfunction and respiratory paralysis associated with hypophosphatemia have occurred during parenteral hyperalimentation. Wound botulism may appear in patients with compound fractures or crush injuries. The incubation period is 4 to 14 days, longer than for food-borne botulism. An unclassified form of botulism, probably due to bowel colonization by *Clostridium botulinum*, with endogenous production of toxin, has followed gastrointestinal surgical procedures. There are cases of botulism in which constipation at onset was so prominent that bowel obstruction was suspected and patients underwent exploratory laparotomy before other neurologic features had developed. Attacks of acute intermittent porphyria often appear in hospitalized patients after the use of drugs known to precipitate attacks.

An axonal neuropathy occurs in intensive care unit (ICU) patients who have had recurrent septic episodes (see Chapters 8 and 13).[118,119,1315] The illness becomes evident when patients have difficulty weaning from the ventilator. There is generalized weakness and depressed reflexes, but usually no cranial nerve abnormalities.

Travel and Geographic Considerations

A history of recent travel in a patient with suspected GBS suggests that one of the diseases listed in Table 14–24 may be responsible. For example, paresthesias beginning shortly after a trip to the Carribean or Pacific Islands raises the possibility of ciguatera or other marine intoxication. Travel to underdeveloped nations exposes patients to rabies, polio (in unvaccinated patients), and diphtheria. Botulism might be considered in a patient returning from a trip to a high-altitude region (where temperatures required for boiling may be insufficient to kill *C. botulinum* spores) or to an area where local dietary, canning, and cooking practices do not eliminate botulism. A history of a recent camping trip or outing in a wooded area (or other area known to have ticks) suggests tick paralysis or Lyme disease in endemic areas. Snake envenomation obviously requires exposure to snakes but occurs primarily in certain areas such as the tropical regions of Asia.

Table 14–23 POSTOPERATIVE OR IN-HOSPITAL ONSET

Neuropathy of critical illness polyneuropathy
Hypermagnesemia
Hypophosphatemia
Myasthenia gravis
Acute intermittent porphyria
Antibiotic-induced weakness
Botulism

Table 14–24 TRAVEL AND GEOGRAPHIC CONSIDERATIONS

Fish poisonings
Polio
Diphtheria
Botulism
Tick paralysis
Rabies
Snake envenomations
Trichinosis
Lyme disease

Underlying Cancer

The differential diagnosis of GBS in patients with known cancer (Table 14–25) includes not only paraproteinemic and paraneoplastic neuropathies but also other complications such as acute epidural spinal cord compression or complications of cancer therapy such as vincristine neuropathy. Carcinomatous meningitis is most likely to occur in patients with undifferentiated lymphoma, oat cell carcinoma, breast cancer, malignant melanoma, or a variety of adenocarcinomas. Other associated diseases such as polymyositis/dermatomyositis and Lambert-Eaton syndrome occur in patients with known or occult neoplasms.

Vincristine or suramin, antineoplastic agents discussed later, can produce neuropathies that simulate GBS. Suramin infusions are associated in a few patients with progressive quadriparesis over 1 or 2 months, raised CSF protein levels, and electrophysiologic changes similar to those of GBS. Cisplatin may produce an axonal sensory neuropathy with paresthesias that initially raise the possibility of GBS. The syndrome does not otherwise conform to GBS or its variants.

Hypokalemia

Hypokalemia (Table 14–26) suggests, in addition to periodic paralysis or hypokalemic myopathy, the possibility of intoxication with either barium salts or thallium.

Table 14–25 UNDERLYING CANCER

Paraproteinemic neuropathies
Paraneoplastic neuropathy
Vincristine neuropathy
Suramin neuropathy
Spinal cord compression
Carcinomatous meningitis
Polymyositis/dermatomyositis
Myasthenia gravis
Lambert-Eaton syndrome

Table 14–26 HYPOKALEMIA

Barium intoxication
Thallium intoxication
Familial periodic paralysis
Thyrotoxic periodic paralysis
Other acute hypokalemic states

MAJOR DISEASES SIMULATING GBS

(Table 14–27).

Table 14–27 MAJOR DISEASES SIMULATING GBS

Spinal Cord Disorders
Transverse Myelitis
Other Acute Myelopathies
Disorders of Neuromuscular Transmission
Myasthenia Gravis
Antibiotic-Induced Paralysis
Lambert-Eaton Myasthenic Syndrome
Botulism
Hypermagnesemia
Snake Envenomations
Myopathic Disorders
Polymyositis
Other Acute Myopathies
Vasculitic Neuropathies
Acute Intermittent Porphyria
Carcinomatous and Lymphomatous Meningitis
Acute Sensory Neuropathy (Neuronopathy) Syndrome
Infections and Biological Toxins
Diphtheritic Polyneuritis
Lyme Disease
Tick Paralysis
Poliomyelitis
Cytoplasmic and Nuclear Neuronopathy
Botulism
Rabies
Tetanus
Other Animal and Plant Toxins
Marine Toxins
Buckthorn Neuropathy
Snake Envenomations
Hymenoptera Stings
Miscellaneous Animal Toxins
Environmental Toxins and Drugs
Organophosphate Poisoning
Vincristine Neuropathy
Suramin Neuropathy
Hexacarbon (Glue-Sniffer's) Neuropathy
Perhexilene Neuropathy
Disulfiram Neuropathy
Vacor Neuropathy
Lithium Neuropathy
Nonorganophosphate Insecticides
Heavy Metal Toxic Neuropathies

(continued)

Table 14–27—*Continued*

Thallium Neuropathy
Arsenic Neuropathy
Gold Neuropathy
Lead Neuropathy
Barium salt intoxication
Metabolic Abnormalities
Periodic Paralyses
Hypokalemic Myopathy
Hyperthyroidism
Hypermagnesemia
Hypophosphatemia
Critical Illness Polyneuropathy
Hysteria

Spinal Cord Disorders

Transverse Myelitis

Acutely evolving spinal cord disorders initially may mimic GBS. Once the classic features of a myelopathy—hyperreflexia, Babinski's signs, and a sensory level—are evident, the correct diagnosis becomes apparent. Transverse myelitis (TM) is the spinal cord disorder most likely to be confused with GBS, as attested to by the inclusion of myelopathies in the category of "Landry's ascending paralysis" in many older papers. GBS may occasionally have fleeting features suggesting a myelopathy, but the remainder of the illness indicates an acute peripheral neuropathy. One potentially confusing feature is the tendency in TM for numbness or paresthesias to begin in the feet and progress proximally. Myelopathies with an abrupt onset may be associated with spinal shock, a flaccid areflexic paralysis below the level of the lesion. Five of 11 patients with TM of catastrophic onset had spinal shock in a series from the Massachusetts General Hospital (MGH),[1015] but these cases were easily distinguishable from GBS by the acute paraplegia or quadriplegia and clear sensory level without facial weakness.

Several features beyond the classical features of spinal cord disease are useful in differentiating TM from GBS (Table 14–28). Early urinary retention that persists for several days may be seen in patients with TM when limb paralysis is minimal, whereas in those with GBS, transient retention usually occurs with substantial limb paralysis. Urinary incontinence is far more common in TM than in GBS. In the MGH retrospective series, urinary incontinence and uninhibited contractions on cystometrogram were the first features to suggest a myelopathy in several excluded cases. Patients referred with such symptoms as "numbness from the waist down" are often incorrectly diagnosed as having GBS. This symptom reflects a lumbar or low thoracic sensory level of myelitis. Since most cases of TM are in the thoracic cord, only the legs are weak. GBS is often thought of as an ascending paralysis with the legs often more involved, but there is usually simultaneous arm weakness. An exception is the uncommon paraparetic form of GBS in which weakness and areflexia are con-

Table 14–28 DIFFERENTIATING GBS FROM TRANSVERSE MYELITIS

	GBS	*TM*
Muscles affected	All limbs	Below level of lesion; not facial or oropharyngeal
Reflexes	Often absent	Absent only with spinal shock, increased later
Sensory symptoms and signs	Distal	Segmental, long level on trunk
Bladder	Urinary retention, transient, occurs at time of peak weakness	Incontinence, common, persistent, often occurs early
Respiratory failure	Common with quadriplegia	Rare
Pain	Proximal muscles and trunk	Segmental radicular

fined to the legs (see Chapter 8). The weakness in TM follows a corticospinal distribution, but this is not particularly helpful in distinguishing it from early GBS. Asymmetry, however, suggests a myelopathy. Respiratory failure, common in the GBS patient with quadriplegia, is rare in TM. Back pain may occur in GBS but is usually vaguely localized and associated with similar pain in the proximal limb muscles. A few exceptional cases have severe acute mid-line back pain that simulates the pain in a few cases of TM.[1017] A CSF pleocytosis may suggest TM. Eighteen of 52 TM patients had a CSF pleocytosis, generally lymphocytic, 6 having more than 200 white blood cells (WBC) per cm^3. Eight cases had elevated CSF protein levels without cells—the same pattern seen in GBS—but a pleocytosis is more often present in TM.[1015]

Other Acute Myelopathies

Other spinal cord disorders seldom cause confusion with GBS, though early acute upper cervical cord compression may be superficially similar. One patient referred to MGH as having GBS, had quadriplegia that evolved over several days and was associated with a high CSF protein level but no cells. Unilateral weakness of the tongue and an asymmetric sensory loss led to a myelogram that showed cord compression near the foramen magnum due to a hemangiopericytoma. In order to avoid this potentially egregious error, we always suggest that the diagnosis of GBS should be reconsidered if there is moderate or severe weakness of all limbs but no facial weakness.

DISORDERS OF NEUROMUSCULAR TRANSMISSION

Myasthenia Gravis

Myasthenia gravis, frequently considered in the differential diagnosis of GBS, is an immune-mediated disorder of the neuromuscular junction characterized by presence of acetylcholine receptor antibodies. The slow onset of weakness and typical regional pattern in myasthenia gravis usually allows a distinction between the two diseases (Table 14–29). Certain muscle groups are preferentially involved in myasthenia gravis: extraocular, levator, pharyngeal, jaw, neck, and respiratory muscles. Fatigue is a characteristic feature, and symptoms and signs may vary considerably throughout the day. Ptosis is one of the most common manifestations, and myasthenic fatigue of eyelid elevation can often be demonstrated even in the absence of resting ptosis. Ptosis occurs in some patients with GBS but does not fatigue, though it may be ameliorated briefly with edrophonium (see Chapter 7). Weakness of facial muscles is often confined to the orbicularis oculi and has a different

Table 14–29 DIFFERENTIATING GBS FROM MYASTHENIA GRAVIS

	GBS	*Myasthenia Gravis*
Respiratory failure	When limbs weak	Often before weakness onset
Reflexes	Absent	Preserved
Ptosis	Rare, no fatigue	Common, fatiguing
Neck weakness	Only when severe	Common early
External ophthalmoplegia	Uncommon	Common
Objective sensory loss	Common	No
Bladder involvement	Common	No
CSF protein concentration	High	Normal
NCV	Slow, may be normal early	Normal
Repetitive nerve stimulation	Normal	Decremental

appearance than the more generalized facial weakness of GBS. Pharyngeal weakness is manifested by a nasal hypophonic voice, often worsening with prolonged talking, and dysphagia. In myasthenia gravis neck weakness may be profound and disproportionate to limb weakness, whereas in GBS neck weakness occurs only with severe limb weakness. Respiratory failure appears insidiously, sometimes in the absence of severe limb weakness. Limb weakness in myasthenia, worse proximally, usually occurs after it appears in the other typical regions just mentioned. Preservation of reflexes, and the absence of sensory features, bladder dysfunction, or dysautonomia are most helpful in distinguishing myasthenia from GBS. The CSF albuminocytologic dissociation seen in patients with GBS is not a feature of myasthenia gravis.

Electrophysiologic studies clearly differentiate the two disorders. Studies of nerve conduction in myasthenia are typically normal. The classic decremental response to repetitive nerve stimulation is usually present and single-fiber electromyogram (EMG) may show abnormal "jitter" and "blocking" in myasthenia.

At the bedside, Tensilon (edrophonium) or neostigmine tests may be useful. However, quantifiable signs must be chosen for monitoring. Appropriate cautions are justified in performing Tensilon or neostigmine tests in a patient with suspected GBS, since anticholinesterases increase saliva production and may cause aspiration in a GBS patient with pharyngeal paresis. Patients with dysautonomia also may have adverse reactions to anticholinesterases but we encountered this only once in our patients (see under dysautonomia in Chapter 7).

Antibiotic-Induced Paralysis

Several drugs, notably aminoglycoside or polymyxin antibiotics, can partially block neuromuscular transmission and cause generalized weakness.[38] Respiratory failure 1 hour to 1 day after administration of the antibiotic is the clinical hallmark in most cases. However, two thirds of antibiotic-associated cases have additional, underlying neuromuscular abnormalities.[702] Limb weakness, often flaccid,[786,929] may be associated with normal or absent deep tendon reflexes. External ophthalmoplegia, ptosis, or ataxia have been reported,[702] and pharyngeal dysfunction may cause dysphagia or dysarthria. Blurred vision[702,929] and fixed dilated pupils[786] may occur in extreme cases. Paresthesias, though uncommon, may involve the face as well as the limbs.[702] Most cases become evident, however, through difficulty being weaned from the mechanical ventilator.

Mild improvement may occur after anticholinesterase administration, but more typically lack of improvement is the clue that the paralysis is not simply due to the persisting effect of the neuromuscular blocking agent that had been used during anesthesia. Intravenous calcium often produces both clinical and electrophysiologic improvement.

Electrophysiologic studies show a defect in neuromuscular transmission.[786,1173,1253] The polymyxins tend to show features of postsynaptic blockade with low-amplitude muscle action potentials and decremental responses to low and high rates of repetitive stimulation. Aminoglycosides produce a presynaptic block in the release of acetylcholine similar to that seen in hypermagnesemia (see farther on).

The majority of reported cases of antibiotic paralysis occur in severely ill patients who have undergone surgery and have respiratory weakness. Other important factors are impaired renal function, hypocalcemia, use of neuromuscular blocking agents with anesthesia, and preexisting disorders of neuromuscular transmission (particularly myasthenia gravis). The antibiotics most often implicated are neomycin, kanamycin, gentamicin, streptomycin, colistin, and polymyxin B. In vitro neuromuscular blocking properties have also been shown for amikacin, netilmicin,

Table 14–30 DIFFERENTIATING GBS FROM ANTIBIOTIC-INDUCED PARALYSIS

	GBS	*Antibiotic Induced Paralysis*
Time postoperatively	About 10 days	Hours to days
Respiratory failure	When limbs weak	Often before weakness onset
Ptosis	Rare	Common
Neck weakness	Only when severe	Common
Internal ophthalmoplegia	Rare	May occur
Objective sensory loss	Common	Rare
CSF protein	High	Usually normal
Tensilon test	Negative	May be positive
NCV	Slow, may be normal early	Normal
CMAP	Normal*	Low
Repetitive nerve stimulation	Normal	Decrement or increment

*May be reduced if conduction block or temporal dispersion present.

and lincomycin. Conflicting results have been found for tobramycin.[172,269]

Several features help differentiate antibiotic-induced weakness from that of GBS (Table 14–30). Although GBS does occur after surgery in approximately 5% or less of cases, there is typically a latent period of several days to 2 weeks before the first neurologic symptoms occur. Antibiotic-induced paralysis, on the other hand, is usually evident in the immediate postoperative period. The pattern of weakness in antibiotic-induced disorders suggests a defect in neuromuscular transmission, affecting the respiratory, neck, pharyngeal, and extraocular muscles. Ptosis is common. In antibiotic paralysis, respiratory failure occurs early and may be the predominant clinical problem, whereas in GBS it occurs when limb weakness is severe. Preservation of reflexes in the presence of respiratory failure also suggests the disorder is not GBS. The CSF protein level in antibiotic paralysis is presumably normal, but there have been isolated reports of its elevation.[786] Electrophysiologic studies differentiate GBS from neuromuscular blockade.

Lambert-Eaton Myasthenic Syndrome

The Lambert-Eaton myasthenic syndrome (LEMS) is a disorder of neuromuscular transmission characterized by a defect of the presynaptic release of acetylcholine.[849] Though it is often associated with a neoplasm—particularly oat cell carcinoma—it may also appear independently or with autoimmune disorders. Several of its clinical features may resemble GBS, but the evolution of LEMS is usually much slower (Table 14–31). The hallmark is limb weakness, usually most pronounced proximally and in the legs and neck. Ptosis and pharyngeal dysfunction may occur, but respiratory failure is uncommon. The reflexes are typically reduced or absent. However, they show the unique phenomenon of potentiation after exercise or contraction. As in GBS, bladder dysfunction and other autonomic features[610,741,1032] may occur. However, the most consistent autonomic symptom in LEMS, dry mouth, does not occur in GBS. The lack of objective sensory loss in LEMS (unless a paraneoplastic neuropathy is also present) is an important feature distinguishing this syndrome from GBS, though paresthesias may occur and sensory loss has been noted rarely. The CSF is usually normal in LEMS.

As with myasthenia gravis, electrophysiologic studies readily distinguish LEMS from GBS. The hallmark of LEMS is a low-amplitude compound muscle action potential (CMAP) after a single supramaximal nerve stimulus, with an increase in CMAP amplitude af-

Table 14–31 DIFFERENTIATING GBS FROM LAMBERT-EATON MYASTHENIC SYNDROME

	GBS	LEMS
Respiratory failure	Common	Rare
Reflexes	Absent	Reduced but potentiated by contraction
Neck weakness	In severe cases	May occur
Objective sensory loss	Common	No
Dry mouth	Rare	Common
CSF protein	High	Normal
NCV	Slow, may be normal early	Normal
CMAP amplitude	Normal*	Reduced
Repetitive nerve stimulation	Normal	Incremental response

*May be reduced if conduction block or temporal dispersion present.

ter voluntary contraction or repetitive stimulation at high frequencies. Single-fiber EMG may be normal in both diseases.

Botulism

(See p. 277).

Hypermagnesemia

(See p. 303).

Snake Envenomations

(See p. 286).

Myopathic Disorders

Polymyositis

The combination of symmetric proximal weakness and pain, common in early GBS, often suggests polymyositis (Table 14–32). It usually begins with gradual symmetric proximal muscle weakness, though acute forms that evolve over 4 weeks or less are known.[538,1229] Pain and muscle tenderness may be severe, usually in the shoulders and upper arms, described as soreness, aching, or cramping.[538] In our experience, neurologists often see cases of polymyositis without pain, whereas painful cases are usually first seen by rheumatologists. Flexor neck muscle weakness is common and may be disproportionate to limb weakness, whereas neck weakness in GBS usually occurs only with quadriparesis. Weakness of cranial musculature is much less common in polymyositis. Though dysphagia occurs in 28%,[273] it often reflects esophageal dysmotility, and true pharyngeal weakness occurs in only 6%. Ptosis and weakness of the orbicularis oculi muscles, a pattern suggesting neuromuscular junction or primary muscle disease, occurs in only 4%. Severe respiratory muscle paresis occurs infrequently, generally occurring only with severe limb paresis. Sensory symptoms and signs, common in GBS, are not seen in pure polymyositis, but cases associated with collagen vascular disease or malignancy may rarely have a concomitant peripheral neuropathy. Raynaud's phenomenon and skin changes of dermatomyositis, including the classic heliotrope lesion and eyelid edema, may be present. Although not characteristic of GBS, these features occur particularly in polymyositis associated with other collagen vascular diseases.

Elevation of the erythrocyte sedimentation rate (ESR) is common in polymyositis, but it is not of much differential utility. In one series, 45% of patients had normal ESRs, and only 19% had ESRs greater than 50 mm/h.[273] In our retrospective GBS series, 16% had

Table 14–32 DIFFERENTIATING GBS FROM POLYMYOSITIS

	GBS	*Polymyositis*
Neck and trunk weakness	Only when severe	Common
Objective sensory loss	Common	No
Reflexes	Absent	Usually normal, may be reduced
Muscle tenderness	Uncommon	May occur
Autonomic dysfunction	Common	Rare
Cranial nerve involvement	Common	Uncommon
Raynaud's phenomenon	Rare	Common
Skin changes	No	Heliotrope, rashes
Systemic features	Rare	Common
CSF protein	High	Normal
NCV	Slow, may be normal early	Normal
EMG	Normal or neuropathic	Myopathic, positive sharp waves, fibrillations

ESRs greater than 40 mm/h and 6%, greater than 50 mm/h (see Chapter 12). Serum concentrations of muscle enzymes are usually elevated in polymyositis but may be elevated in up to one third of GBS patients (see Chapter 3). The level of creatine phosphokinase (CPK) elevations tends to be less in GBS than in polymyositis.

Electrodiagnostic studies may differentiate polymyositis from GBS. Nerve conduction velocities (NCVs), distal latencies, and late responses are normal in polymyositis, but EMG shows myopathic changes (small amplitude, short duration polyphasic units) and often fibrillations, positive sharp waves, and bizarre high-frequency discharges.

Muscle biopsy ultimately confirms the diagnosis of polymyositis, with muscle fiber destruction and regeneration, with perivascular and interstitial inflammatory infiltrates of lymphocytes and plasma cells. The inflammatory component is typically minimal in the severe acute form that most resembles GBS.[1229]

Other Acute Myopathies

Most other myopathic disorders are gradually progressive and do not resemble GBS. A few may simulate neuropathy when they are acute.

Acute myopathies with pain and tender muscles, weakness, and elevated serum muscle enzymes have been reported with clofibrate[671,925] or lovastatin administration for the reduction of serum cholesterol, sometimes leading to inability to rise from a chair. Postinfluenza myositis has caused quadriparesis evolving over several days.[213] However, normal reflexes and sensory function and serum CPK elevation demonstrate the myopathic nature of the illness. Acute rhabdomyolysis with diffuse muscle pain, severe weakness, markedly elevated serum muscle enzymes, and myoglobinuria have been reported rarely after infection with other viruses and *Mycoplasma pneumoniae.*[760] Acute rhabdomyolysis has been reported with muscle pain, weakness, and myoglobinuria after heavy alcohol consumption, certain snake envenomations (particularly the sea snake and Russell's viper), or without obvious etiology.[1180] Muscle biopsy shows severe muscle necrosis without inflammation. (Acute hypokalemic myopathy and barium intoxication are discussed elsewhere in this chapter.)

Trichinosis may rarely simulate GBS, producing a rapidly evolving myositis,[760] and may involve cranial nerves, particularly the sixth and seventh, with facial diplegia.[721] The usual gastrointestinal prodrome may be absent but clues to the diagnosis include leukocytosis, eosinophilia, periorbital edema, chemosis, subconjunctival hemorrhages, facial erythema, and macular rash.[760] Preserved reflexes distinguish such cases from GBS. The CSF in trichinosis may show a mild lymphocytic pleocytosis.

Vasculitic Neuropathies

Rapid and widespread vascular disease in nerves may resemble a symmetric generalized polyneuropathy more than typical mononeuritis multiplex.[621] Polyarteritis nodosa, rheumatoid arthritis, SLE, and Wegener's granulomatosis are the diseases most likely to be associated with vasculitic polyneuropathy. Neuropathy occurs less frequently with Sjögren's syndrome (often a sensory syndrome), scleroderma, giant cell arteritis, or Churg-Strauss angiitis.[214,621]

Some patients seen in the MGH Neurology Service and initially thought to have GBS, have had instead Wegener's granulomatosis, cryoglobulinemia, or polyarteritis nodosa with sequential involvement of peripheral nerves resulting in a pattern that simulated a diffuse symmetric sensorimotor polyneuropathy within 24 hours. Careful examination also demonstrated focal neuropathies such as asymmetric wrist or foot drops, manifestations of vasculitic ischemia of large nerve trunks. Peripheral neuropathy occurred in 52% of 25 patients with polyarteritis nodosa in one large series.[818] Four clinical patterns were identified: (1) mononeuritis multiplex; (2) a more extensive form of mononeuritis multiplex; (3) patchy areas of altered sensation in the distribution of cutaneous nerves; and (4) a subacute or chronic distal sensorimotor polyneuropathy. The second category most resembled GBS. One patient had limb pain and a sensorimotor neuropathy that ascended over 2½ weeks, resulting in a severe flaccid quadriparesis with sensory loss. The CSF was normal. Two other patients had subacute flaccid weakness and sensory loss from the elbows and knees downward. Patients often had mid-arm or mid-thigh pain before onset of the other symptoms, roughly corresponding to the watershed areas in nerves where ischemia occurs. Sensory levels often occurred at mid-thigh and mid-arm. Other researchers[356] have reported similar cases as a source of diagnostic error in GBS.

Mononeuritis multiplex may occur in rheumatoid arthritis, but a distal symmetric sensory or sensorimotor neuropathy is more common.[87,214,417] Both patterns occur in patients with severe disease; arthritis, often with rheumatoid nodules; high titers of rheumatoid factor; and other evidence of vasculitis such as digital arteritis.

Neuropathy in primary and secondary cryoglobulinemia usually evolves slowly with a distal sensorimotor pattern.[229,391,715] Initial symptoms are usually distal pain and paresthesias, more prominent in the legs, followed in weeks or months by distal weakness. All sensory modalities may be impaired in a glove-stocking distribution, sometimes paralleling the level of cutaneous purpura.[715] Weakness is usually confined to the wrist and ankle extensors and intrinsic hand and foot muscles. The reflexes are lost, first at the ankles. Cranial nerve, bladder, and autonomic dysfunction do not occur.[391] A more rapidly evolving mononeuritis multiplex may also occur with acute asymmetric weakness involving proximal or distal muscles. The neuropathy may fluctuate, worsening in cold weather, but is generally progressive.

CSF is usually normal, but mild elevations of protein may occur. Nerve conduction studies may show absent or reduced amplitude sensory responses. Motor NCVs, where recordable, are usually normal but prolonged distal latencies and reduced-amplitude CMAP in the legs may occur. Cases with mononeuritis multiplex show changes in a pattern conforming to nerves involved. Nerve biopsies often show loss of myelinated fibers with disruption of myelin and myelin ovoids and debris but regular internodal lengths and no evidence of segmental demyelination. Perivascular inflammatory infiltrates and thickening may be seen in the epineurium and perineurium.[391]

A case of cryoglobulinemia has been reported because it closely resembled (or may simply have been) GBS.[535] The patient had hereditary angioedema with SLE-like nephritis and cryoglobulinemia. Four months after treatment with prednisone and Danazol he developed asymmetric weakness, progressing to areflexic quadriplegia, facial diplegia, and respiratory failure over 10 days. The CSF protein concentration was normal on two examinations in the first 10 days. Nerve biopsy showed segmental demyelination with a mononuclear round cell infiltrate essentially indistinguishable from that of GBS. Typical cryoglobulinemic neuropathy is, however, easily distinguishable from GBS by its slower evolution; distal sensorimotor distribution; lack of cranial nerve, bladder, or autonomic dysfunction; and electrophysiologic features. The mononeuritis multiplex causes asymmetric involvement of individual peripheral nerves alluded to earlier. Ultimately, the systemic nature of cryoglobulinemia is the most important differential feature. Characteristic cutaneous lesions consist of petechiae and purpuric lesions of varying age, more common in the lower extremities. Raynaud's phenomenon, arthralgias, abdominal pain, bleeding from mucous membrane bleeding, cutaneous ulcers (especially submalleolar), or ischemic lesions of the digits, nails, and nose are common. Glomerulonephritis with microscopic hematuria and proteinuria, as well as renal failure, is characteristic. Aside from obvious detection of cryoglobulins in the serum, other laboratory abnormalities include anemia, elevated ESR, and presence of high titers of rheumatoid factor.

Neuropathies occur in about 10% of patients with SLE.[355,572] They may produce chronic or subacute distal symmetric sensorimotor, or predominantly sensory neuropathies or mononeuritis multiplex. Acute and chronic demyelinating polyneuropathy have also been reported in patients with SLE. A number of cases have had acute generalized, areflexic, predominantly motor neuropathies with acellular CSF and raised CSF protein levels. A sensorimotor neuropathy closely resembling GBS was associated with areflexia and CSF albuminocytologic dissociation in a patient with pathologic features of SLE.[514] Another two patients had a monophasic demyelinating neuropathy as the initial presentation of SLE.[975] These cases, like others, all progressed over 5 weeks to 5 months with weakness and sensory loss more pronounced distally, areflexia, and CSF albuminocytologic dissociation. One patient had a facial diplegia. Electrophysiologic tests were consistent with GBS. Patients with discrete bouts of GBS over years have also been reported.[415,804] The demyelinating neuropathies of SLE, however, usually resemble CIDP more than acute GBS.[1065] The distinction of these acute and chronic demyelinating neuropathies associated with SLE from acute GBS and CIDP, respectively, may be semantic, since they can be similar in all respects, including showing an inflammatory demyelinating process at autopsy.[415] The underlying systemic process, like a preceding infection, may simply serve as the immunologic trigger for inflammatory demyelination. The association of SLE with GBS and CIDP may occur frequently enough to make an antinuclear antibody test part of the evaluation of any atypical cases.

DIFFERENTIATION OF VASCULITIC NEUROPATHIES FROM GBS

Though some of the cases just mentioned resemble GBS, most cases have features of vasculitic neuropathy that distinguish the two entities (Table 14–33). Asymmetry, seldom seen in GBS, is common in vasculitic neuropathies. Even when symmetric, the distribution of sensory and motor signs tend to occur below the watershed regions for ischemia,[306] causing weakness and multimodality sensory loss distal to the

Table 14–33 DIFFERENTIATING GBS FROM VASCULITIC NEUROPATHIES

	GBS	*Vasculitic Neuropathy*
Systemic signs	Rare	Usually present
Fever	Rare	Common
Sensory symptoms and signs	Distally symmetric	May be asymmetric often to knee, thigh
Weakness	Symmetric	Often asymmetric, often distal
Bladder involvement	Common	Rare
Reflexes	Often absent even before weakness	Reduced proportionate to weakness
Cranial nerves	Often involved	Rare, asymmetric
Respiratory failure	Common	Rare
Pain	Proximal muscles and trunk	Occurs in distribution of nerves involved
CSF protein	Usually elevated	Usually normal
Denervation on EMG	In severe cases, late	Usually present

elbow, knee, or mid-thigh. In GBS, the proximal muscles are weakest and sensory loss seldom extends to the elbow, mid-arm, knee, or mid-thigh. Cranial nerve involvement, usually symmetric, is common in GBS but uncommon in the vasculitic neuropathies. Respiratory paralysis or sphincter dysfunction are uncommon in the vasculitic neuropathies compared with GBS.

The CSF analysis may be useful since the albuminocytologic dissociation typical of GBS is unusual in the vasculitic neuropathies, with the exception of SLE with demyelinating neuropathy. Electrophysiologic study results may provide ambiguous information. Evidence of denervation is more likely to be seen in the vasculitic neuropathies, in which axons are affected, but may occur in severe cases of GBS. Nerve conduction studies and late responses are often abnormal in both conditions.

Ultimately, recognition of multisystem involvement or vasculitis on biopsy material leads to correct diagnosis of vasculitic neuropathy. Whole sural nerve biopsy is preferable to fascicular biopsy when investigating arteritis, as the latter may contain too few blood vessels.[214]

Acute Intermittent Porphyria

The acute porphyrias are autosomal dominantly inherited disorders with acute neurologic manifestations. Acute intermittent porphyria (AIP) is the prototype but similar features may occur in variegate porphyria, hereditary coproporphyria, and acute porphyria due to severe deficiency of delta-aminolevulinic acid (ALA) dehydrase.[120] Clinical disease occurs more frequently in women. Attacks occur most often during the third and fourth decades but may appear any time after menarche in women. A precipitating factor such as any of a variety of drugs, intercurrent infections, or fasting is identifiable in 67% to 75% of acute attacks.[989,1145] Some women have a tendency for attacks to occur premenstrually.

The first symptoms of an attack are almost always gastrointestinal or mental,[414,747,989,1145] rather than those of somatic neuropathy (Table 14–34). The hallmarks are abdominal pain (90%), often associated with nausea or vomiting (50% to 70%), and constipation (50% to 90%). Diarrhea is less common. Though there is often a disparity between the severity of the abdominal pain and the findings on physical examination, symptoms are often severe enough to lead to surgical procedures.[747] Pain may occur in other areas, including the back, flank, chest, and extremities. Sinus tachycardia and hypertension are common. The exact incidence of motor neuropathy in porphyria has varied due to selection

Table 14–34 DIFFERENTIATING GBS FROM ACUTE INTERMITTENT PORPHYRIA

	GBS	*AIP*
Evolution	1–3 wk	Longer
Pattern of weakness	Usually ascending	Often begins in arms
Reflexes	Usually absent	Occasionally preserved AJ
Sensory loss	Distal	Often proximal
Abdominal pain	Uncommon	Almost always present
Constipation	At maximal deficit	Early, prominent
Abnormal mental status	No	Very common
Seizures	Rare	May occur
Recovery	Weeks to months	May be rapid
CSF protein	Elevated	Normal or <100 mg/dL in most
Urine pigmented	No	Most
NCV	Abnormal	Normal or slight slowing
CMAP amplitude	Normal*	Reduced

*May be reduced if conduction block or temporal dispersion present.

criteria, from 15%[16] to 100%[989] with most series reporting 50% to 70%.[120,414,1128,1145]

Compared with GBS, the weakness in porphyric neuropathy more commonly begins in the upper arms; all the limbs are eventually affected (Table 14–33). Acute quadriparesis characterized the neuropathy in 11 of 20 patients in one series.[16] Weakness is generally symmetric, with a greater distribution proximally than distally at onset, thus simulating GBS. A distribution greater distally than proximally may occur later in the course, with wrist and ankle dorsiflexors disproportionately involved. Muscle tone is reduced and hyporeflexia or areflexia are characteristic. In contrast to GBS, however, ankle reflexes are often preserved longer than other deep tendon reflexes.[120,990] Other researchers[747] have commented on a day-to-day variability in reflexes. Severe quadriparesis with preservation of at least some reflexes has been reported. Oropharyngeal weakness or other cranial nerve dysfunction is relatively uncommon and seldom appears before limb paralysis.[120] The face and pharynx may, however, be weak, and rare cases have had extraocular paresis. A high-pitched voice, uncommon in GBS, may be secondary to vocal cord paresis,[747] though a hoarse whispering voice may also be seen.[1182] In severe cases, the axial musculature may be involved, with respiratory failure in 10% to 25%.[414,990,1145] Ventilatory failure is the most common cause of death during an acute attack. Limb pain, a common feature of some patient's attacks, is intermittent and has a sharper, and more focal quality than the pain associated with GBS. It also tends to be worse in the distal muscles than in the proximal fleshy muscles.

Some of the sensory symptoms of AIP are similar to those of GBS—typically numbness, paresthesias, or dysesthesias. Objective sensory loss occurs in 25% to 65%. Although a glove-stocking distribution may occur, proximal sensory loss is common and unusual distributions such as "bathing trunk," "long johns," or "arm band" patterns are characteristic.[989] The head and neck may be involved.[414,989] (See Chapter 7 for further contrasts with GBS in the patterns of sensory loss.)

Bladder dysfunction has been reported in 10% to 15% of patients in most series,[120,414,1145] but it occurs in up to half of patients experiencing neuropathic crises.[989] As in GBS, urinary retention rather than incontinence occurs.

Depending on the study, tachycardia occurs in from 51%[747] to nearly 100% of patients with porphyric neuropathy.[990,991] As in GBS, tachycardia in porphyria often precedes clinical weakness.[990,991] Hypertension is noted in approximately 50% of attacks;[747,990] postural hypotension occurs in about 20% of cases.[120,1145]

Psychiatric syndromes or confusion occur in 40% to 86% of cases,[120,414,990,1145] and some authors have emphasized that psychosis rarely occurs in patients without paralysis. Features that help to distinguish AIP from GBS include confusion, hallucinations and delusions, delirium, sleep disturbances, anxiety, and depression. The level of arousal is sometimes decreased, and coma may occur rarely. Seizures occur in 10% to 20% of cases, owing either to the porphyria or to hyponatremia or hypomagnesemia.

The most characteristic electrophysiologic feature is reduction of the CMAP.[16,1295] Motor NCVs and distal latencies are generally normal, unlike those in patients with GBS, although temporal dispersion and occasional mild slowing of conduction or prolonged latencies may be seen. F waves are usually normal in patients with porphyrias, in contrast to their early absence or prolongation in those with GBS (see Chapter 13). Sensory nerve latencies are usually normal, though amplitudes may be low. The EMG shows fibrillations (especially in proximal muscles), reduced recruitment, and later polyphasic units. The presence of high-amplitude, long-duration polyphasic units early in an acute attack of AIP has been attributed to prior attacks of porphyric neuropathy. The CSF is usually normal in the acute porphyric neuropathies; however, mild elevations of protein concentration occur, sometimes over 200 mg/dL.[1182]

During attacks of AIP there is increased urinary excretion of both ALA and porphobilinogen (PBG). Screening tests such as the Watson-Schwartz and Hoesch reactions are simple methods for rapid diagnosis of increased urinary PBG levels. These tests should be supplemented by quantitative determination of urinary PBG excretion. Urinary excretion of both ALA and PBG may be normal between attacks or even during recovery. In these circumstances, the diagnosis of AIP rests upon documenting a low level of erythrocyte uroporphyrinogen-I-synthetase.

Carcinomatous and Lymphomatous Meningitis

Diffuse leptomeningeal spread of carcinoma, poorly differentiated lymphoma, or leukemia, and rarely, primary CNS neoplasms may produce a combination of cranial and spinal nerve involvement superficially resembling GBS.[443,710,877] The syndrome usually evolves over several weeks or months, less rapidly than GBS. Any cranial nerve may be involved in carcinomatous meningitis; however, they are most often affected asymmetrically, compared with the relatively symmetric involvement in GBS. The motor and sensory findings in carcinomatous meningitis are also often asymmetric and may conform to dermatomal or radicular distributions. Compared with the global areflexia of GBS, reflex loss in carcinomatous meningitis is patchy. Pain in carcinomatous meningitis may be radicular, whereas in GBS a more diffuse, deep, aching limb and axial pain is seen. Headache, signs of meningeal irritation, seizures, and mental status abnormalities are present in many patients with carcinomatous meningitis. A CSF pleocytosis with elevated protein concentration, reduced glucose concentration, and positive cytology are characteristic of neoplastic involvement. Only one of these abnormalities may be present, particularly early in the course. Repetitive CSF examinations, using proper cytopathologic specimen collection and identification techniques, are necessary to confirm the diagnosis. Non-Hodgkin's lymphomas generally do not invade the meninges unless they are highly undifferentiated. Inflammatory cells may appear in the CSF in paralymphomatous neuropathy and in lymphomatous meningitis.

Acute Sensory Neuropathy (Neuronopathy) Syndrome

This syndrome, reported by Sterman and co-workers,[1149] has several features in common with GBS and is often indistinguishable from a sensory variant of GBS (see Chapter 8). It is characterized by rapid evolution of sensory symptoms and signs (often following an infectious process) and areflexia, autonomic dysfunction, and CSF albuminocytologic dissociation. Numbness or paresthesias—often beginning in the face, mouth, or tongue—spread to the limbs over several days. Position and vibratory sense are usually affected disproportionately to other sensory modalities; sensory ataxia and pseudoathetosis occur in some cases. Patients may be areflexic, without weakness or EMG evidence of motor involvement. Motor NCVs are unremarkable, but sensory conduction shows absent or reduced amplitude responses. The CSF has shown elevated protein levels in most cases. Autonomic dysfunction (acute urinary retention, orthostatic hypotension, tachycardia without fever) was seen in some of the originally described cases. As discussed in Chapter 8, there is cross-over between acute sensory neuropathy and pandysautonomia. For example, some cases[208,524] had rapid evolution of parasympathetic and sympathetic dysfunction in association with diffuse sensory loss, areflexia, and weakness. The disorder described in this category was probably a neuronopathy, affecting nerve cell bodies in the dorsal roots with abnormalities of sensory conduction. Sterman's patients received penicillin or semisynthetic penicillin derivatives for 3 to 8 days before neurological symptoms began.[1149] Similar subsequent cases have occurred without antibiotics. Neoplasms, especially lymphomas, have been associated with a similar syndrome.

The neuronopathies are distinguishable from GBS by the striking predominance of sensory signs, particularly on the face and trunk. Early dysautonomia may also be a useful differential feature. The CSF may be acellular with raised protein concentration, or there may be mild pleocytosis, but motor nerve conduction study results are usually normal.

Infections and Biological Toxins

DIPHTHERITIC POLYNEURITIS

Diphtheritic polyneuritis is a toxin-mediated sensorimotor neuropathy that occurs after tonsillar, pharyngeal, or cutaneous diphtheria. Despite its rarity, the syndrome of areflexic limb weakness, raised CSF protein level, and electrophysiologic evidence of a demyelinating polyneuropathy closely simulates GBS. Typical diphtheria begins with a sore throat, fever, and systemic symptoms such as headache and nausea. Cervical lymphadenopathy may be prominent, causing a characteristic "bull neck" appearance. There is usually, but not always, a membranous exudate on the tonsils and pharynx that eventually becomes the adherent grayish, greenish, or black membrane characteristic of diphtheria. Local airway obstruction can be fatal, but most deaths have been related to myocarditis and polyneuritis. The risk of polyneuritis in adults varies with the severity of the original pharyngeal involvement and may be as high as 80% in severe cases.[1000,1064]

Palatal paralysis, almost always the initial sign of neuritis, may appear within the first 14 days[1064] (Table 14–35). Though many patients with diphtheria have difficulty swallowing, initially owing to the inflammation and membranes, palatal and pharyngeal paralysis is characterized by nasal regurgitation of liquids and a hypophonic voice with a nasal quality. These features are similar to GBS that descends from oropharyngeal weakness. Of all patients with palatal paralysis, 44.4% subsequently develop polyneuritis, compared to only 4.8% of those without

Table 14–35 DIFFERENTIATING GBS FROM DIPHTHERIA

	GBS	*Diphtheria*
Rapidity of evolution	1–3 wk	Longer
Respiratory failure	Common	Uncommon
Palatal paralysis	Symmetric	Early, asymmetric
Accommodation paralysis	Rare	Very common
Congestive heart failure	Rare	May occur
ECG changes	Occasional	Conduction disturbances more common

it.[894] While the palatal paralysis may be bilateral, it is often asymmetric, with more weakness ipsilateral to the more prominent pharyngeal membrane. These signs are due to the local action of diphtheria toxin.

Paralysis of accommodation usually appears a few days later, between the second and third week of illness in half of cases[152,366] (Table 14–35), but may be the initial symptom in cases related to wound or cutaneous diphtheria, where palatal paralysis is absent.[1249] Patients report blurred vision with reading or near tasks such as threading a needle.[1000] Pupillary responses to light and convergence are often normal on examination. Walshe[1249] commented that vision may become blurred with accommodation fatigue after about 2 minutes of reading.

Extraocular and facial muscle weakness occur less frequently. Of 53 patients with diphtheritic polyneuritis, however, paralysis of muscles innervated by the trigeminal nerve occurred in 12 and oculomotor nerve paralysis in 8; 11 had facial paralysis, and a few had involvement of the 9th, 11th, and 12th nerves.[152] Weakness of the neck flexors and extensors or weakness and tenderness of the sternocleidomastoids also occurs.

Limb paralysis usually appears between the fifth and seventh weeks after pharyngitis.[1064] Weakness is usually symmetric but rarely may begin in one limb in cases of wound diphtheria.[1249] Similar to GBS, proximal muscles are affected earlier than distal, but distal weakness eventually predominates. In milder cases only the legs are involved. The respiratory muscles may be involved in severe cases. Maximum weakness usually occurs as late as the 12th week,[1064] though the peak of respiratory failure may occur earlier. The absence of muscle atrophy has been emphasized,[366] but it may occur.

The deep tendon reflexes are ultimately diminished or absent but may be normal when weakness is mild.[1064] Early disappearance of reflexes has been emphasized by others.[152,775] In 10 cases in which examination was possible prior to onset of weakness, loss of reflexes preceded severe weakness by 4 to 12 days.[152]

As in early GBS, mild paresthesias are common,[1064] though objective sensory loss occurs infrequently. Abnormalities of position and vibration sense tend to be more prominent than loss of cutaneous sensibility,[366] and a sensory ataxia (diphtheritic pseudotabes) has been reported.[775] Sphincter dysfunction is rare,[366] but temporary loss of bladder or bowel control has been reported.[1000,1064] Sinus tachycardia, with heart rates of 85 to 100 beats per minute, occurred in most of Walshe's patients,[1249] and the electrocardiogram (ECG) is said to be abnormal in the majority of cases.[366]

The CSF in diphtheritic neuropathy may be normal but usually shows albuminocytologic dissociation similar to that of GBS,[152,366,1064] with maximum CSF protein concentration approximately 75 to 300 mg/dL.

Much of the understanding of demyelinating neuropathies has been gleaned from experimental models using diphtheria toxin, but there is little clinical electrophysiologic information from patients. Most studies[656,775] have shown typical changes of a demyelinating polyneuropathy with prolonged terminal latencies and later slowing of motor NCVs. Late responses and sensory action potentials may be absent. Like the CSF abnormalities, these findings are almost indistinguishable from those of GBS.

Myocarditis, a dangerous complication of diphtheria, may coexist with neuropathy. The myocarditis usually appears earlier, about a week after onset of pharyngeal symptoms, in 20% of cases. It may be evident by ECG changes, arrhythmias, or congestive heart failure. T-wave changes are the most common ECG abnormality, but bundle branch blocks and any degree of atrioventricular block have also occurred.[835]

Differentiation of diphtheritic neuropathy from GBS may be nearly impossible if the original faucial involvement is not appreciated (Table 14–34). The features of the paralysis, CSF, and electrophysiologic tests are very similar, but the rarity of diphtheria in developed countries makes it a far less likely cause than GBS of generalized areflexic paralysis or of pharyngeal weakness. The evolution of the paralysis in diphtheria is generally slower than in GBS and unilateral or bilateral asymmetric palatal paralysis, accommodation paralysis, or myocarditis are important clues to the diagnosis of diphtheritic neuropathy.

Lyme Disease

If *Borrelia burgdorferi* produces a neuropathy like GBS, it must be rare. A case of Lyme disease with an acute demyelinating polyneuropathy resembled GBS, except for a CSF pleocytosis.[1148] Two months after the appearance of a rash, systemic symptoms, symmetric progressive leg weakness, and meningitis occurred over 2 weeks. Sensory and motor NCVs were slow, with prolonged distal latencies, prolonged F waves, and absent sural sensory conduction. The CSF had more than 100 WBC per mL and the patient recovered. This case perhaps comes closest of the many reported Lyme neuropathies to the clinical features of GBS.

The meningoradiculopathies and other peripheral neuropathies of Lyme disease superficially resembling GBS[363, 482,892] are discussed in more detail in Chapter 6. The neuropathic complications of Lyme disease are generally progressive, asymmetric, or focal, unlike those of GBS. Lyme disease, however, may be a diagnostic consideration in cases of GBS presenting initially with cranial nerve dysfunction, especially asymmetric facial palsy, or with a mild to moderate sensorimotor neuropathy with CSF pleocytosis. The latter is particularly suggestive of Lyme neuropathy (and of HIV-associated neuropathies).

Tick Paralysis

Tick paralysis, a rare neurologic disorder caused by a toxin secreted by the gravid female tick, may closely resemble GBS. It occurs most commonly in the northwestern United States and western Canada but has also been reported in the southeastern United States, Australia, South Africa, Crete, France, Yugoslavia, and other European countries.[2] The wood tick *(Dermacentor andersoni)* is most often implicated in Canada and the northwestern United States, the dog tick *(D. variabilis)* in the southeastern United States, and *Ixodes holocyclus* in Australia; less frequently implicated are the Lone Star tick, the Gulf Coast tick, and the black-legged deer tick. Most cases of tick paralysis occur in April, May, and June, when nymphs and mature wood ticks are most prevalent. Most cases have been in children between the ages of 2 and 5 years. A reported overall mortality of 10%, mainly in children, reflected cases in the prerespirator era.

Tick paralysis is usually a rapidly progressive ascending paralysis after the tick has been attached for 5 to 7 days.[2,904,1140] A biphasic course is common, with ataxia and areflexia occur-

Table 14–36 DIFFERENTIATING GBS FROM TICK PARALYSIS

	GBS	*Tick Paralysis*
Rapidity of evolution	1–3 wk	Often 1–2 days
Sensory loss	Common	Rare
Ptosis	Uncommon	Common
Neck weakness	Uncommon early	Common
Speed of recovery	Generally weeks to months	Hours to "days" (once tick removed)
Facial paresthesias	Rare	May occur
Abnormal movements	Do not occur	Muscle twitches, chorea, myoclonus
Nystagmus	Rare	Common
CSF protein	Elevated	Normal or minimally elevated
CMAP amplitude	Normal*	Reduced
Repetitive nerve stimulation	Normal	May show increment or decrement

*May be reduced if conduction block or temporal dispersion present.

ring a day or two before weakness. The first symptom is difficulty walking, owing either to ataxia or to leg weakness. An ascending, symmetric, flaccid, areflexic paralysis, similar to GBS but evolving more rapidly (over 1 to 2 days), may involve the bulbar, extraocular, facial, and respiratory muscles. As in GBS, paralysis may be worse proximally than distally (Table 14–36). Ptosis and weakness of the neck muscles are often more prominent than in GBS, suggesting a disorder of neuromuscular transmission. Severe gait, truncal, and appendicular ataxia occurs in a few cases. Early paresthesias are common but objective sensory loss is not. Paresthesias may affect the face and perioral region, a phenomenon rarely found in GBS. Sphincter disturbances and sinus tachycardia may occur rarely.[1174] Cerebrospinal fluid is usually normal, though occasional mild pleocytosis or slight protein elevation (50 to 60 mg/dL) have been encountered.[1140]

Electrodiagnostic studies have shown a prominent reduction in the amplitude of muscle action potentials.[191,1174] Although usually no change occurs in the CMAP on repetitive nerve stimulation, a slight decrement or increment at high rates of stimulation has been noted in some cases. Mild to moderate slowing of motor (and occasionally sensory) nerve conduction velocities are seen in most cases, with prolongation of terminal latencies.[191,1174] The overall electrophysiologic appearance of tick paralysis is therefore similar to that of GBS.

Differentiating GBS from tick paralysis purely on the basis of the neurologic examination may be nearly impossible. Very rapid progression, prominent ptosis, neck weakness, low-amplitude muscle action potentials, or incremental responses to repetitive nerve stimulation particularly suggest tick paralysis. A high index of suspicion and meticulous physical examination are required to exclude ticks, not only in endemic areas, since 5 to 7 days elapse between the time of tick attachment and the onset of clinical symptoms. A careful search for ticks, particularly in areas of the scalp, neck, pubis, and other hair-covered areas, is essential. The cure for this disease, removing the tick, is both simple and nearly miraculous.

Poliomyelitis

Paralytic poliomyelitis now most often results from oral polio vaccine[857] rather than from "wild" poliovirus, although the latter remains a problem in underdeveloped nations. A similar clinical illness may be caused by other RNA viruses such as coxsackie virus, echovirus, and enterovirus. The median interval between the oral vaccine and the onset of paralysis is 20 days for vaccine recipients and 35 days (range 11 to 58 days) for contacts. A history of absent or inadequate immunization against polio is common in contacts who develop polio.

The disease begins with fever, headache, nausea, and coryza or sore throat, sometimes with diarrhea, constipation, or rash; then anxiety, photophobia, sonophobia, muscle or body pain, muscle twitching or tremor, and nuchal rigidity.[59,242,728,1285] This prodromal phase usually lasts 3 to 4 days before progressing to the paralytic phase. Up to 25% of cases have a "dromedary" or bimodal course with remission of fever and other symptoms, then recurrence.[59]

Flaccid paralysis is often preceded by hyporeflexia or twitching of the affected limbs. In contrast to GBS, paralysis in polio is almost always asymmetric, and the legs are twice as often involved as arms (Table 14–37). All limbs are affected in only 10%. Differential involvement of muscle groups within a limb is also common. Total paralysis of a limb is unusual. Paralysis may involve the abdominal, respiratory, paraspinal, and neck muscles. Deep tendon reflexes may briefly be accentuated but rapidly become diminished, eventually leading to areflexia of the weak limbs. Involvement of brainstem motor nuclei causes facial, palatal, pharyngeal, or laryngeal paralysis. Muscles of mastication or extraocular muscles are occasionally weak. Pain, indistinguishable from that of GBS, is common as paralysis evolves (Table 14–36). Muscle atrophy develops within 2 to 3 weeks, and often as early as 1 week.[1285] As in GBS, urinary retention is common but incontinence rare. Autonomic dysfunction, less common than in GBS, includes transient hypertension, hyperhidrosis and hypohidrosis, vasomotor instability, and localized thermoinstability. Although polio is primarily a motor disorder, sensory symptoms may occur without objective sensory loss.

The CSF in polio characteristically shows a mild to moderate pleocytosis, usually less than 200 WBC per cm^3.[1285] Polymorphonuclear cells may predominate early but lymphocytes are more frequent after 3 days, when paralysis appears. The cells gradually diminish and usually disappear within 3 weeks. CSF protein concentration is slightly increased at the onset and rises over 2 to 3 weeks to levels as high as 200 mg/dL; glucose level is usually normal. A peripheral leukocytosis is common but other routine hematologic and chemistry determinations are generally unremarkable.

Nerve conduction studies in polio may show no muscle response in a severely affected limb. When a response can be elicited, the motor NCV is usually normal.[570] EMG shows a reduced interference pattern and reduced recruitment, but abnormal spontaneous activity is absent early in the illness. Fibrillations generally begin after 2 to 4 weeks. Late in the course, motor unit

Table 14–37 DIFFERENTIATING GBS FROM POLIOMYELITIS

	GBS	***Polio***
Prodromal illness	1–2 wk prior	1–3 days prior
Evolution	1–3 wk	3–4 days
Symmetry of weakness	Symmetric	Asymmetric
DTRs	Often absent even before weakness	May be normal in nonparetic limbs
Muscle atrophy	Uncommon, late	Common, early
Fever	Uncommon	Common
Sensory symptoms and signs	Common	Rare
CSF pleocytosis	No	Yes
NCVs	Slow, especially late	Normal

action potentials become polyphasic and increased in duration and amplitude, eventually giving rise to the giant motor units characteristic of anterior horn cell disease. Occasionally, a decremental response of the CMAP amplitude to repetitive nerve stimulation may be seen.

Polio, formerly a purely clinical diagnosis, is now confirmed serologically or by isolation of the virus.[879] The virus is seldom isolated from CSF (unlike the other enteroviruses that may produce a polio-like syndrome). Isolation from the gastrointestinal (GI) tract should be attempted early in the course of the disease. A rise in serum antibody titers is usually required for diagnosis. Later in the illness, documentation of serum IgM antibodies against polioviruses supports the diagnosis.

Several clinical features help differentiate polio from GBS, the foremost being asymmetry of the paralysis (Table 14–37). Paresthesias are common in GBS but rare in polio. Reflexes may be present in the nonparetic limbs in polio, compared with the more common uniform areflexia seen in GBS. Muscle atrophy occurs early in polio but late, if at all, in GBS. Fever is characteristic of polio as it enters the paralytic phase, whereas GBS patients are afebrile unless an infectious complication has occurred (or the antecedent illness is one such as infectious mononucleosis). The prodromal illness in GBS has usually resolved more than a week prior to onset of paralysis, whereas in polio the prodromal symptoms have begun only 1 to 3 days prior to onset of paralysis. In polio, the paralysis seldom progresses beyond 3 to 4 days, whereas in GBS the typical period of progression is 10 to 12 days. The CSF is of greatest differential diagnostic value, as the characteristic pleocytosis of polio occurs infrequently in GBS (see Chapter 12). However, after 5 to 6 days the CSF formula in polio may be similar to that of GBS, with a slightly elevated protein level.[570] Nerve conduction velocities are generally normal in polio but are slowed in GBS, particularly later in the course.

CYTOPLASMIC AND NUCLEAR NEURONOPATHY

A poliomyelitis surveillance autopsy series in children in Mexico found 25 cases of "acute paralytic illness" lacking inflammatory changes in the CNS.[966] Ten cases had pathology compatible with GBS, 8 others had extensive chromatolysis of lower motor neurons (called "cytoplasmic neuronopathy"), and 7 others had little chromatolysis but a peculiar argyrophilic degeneration of the nuclei of lower motor neurons (called "nuclear neuronopathy"). Clinically, these three groups were indistinguishable. All presented with weakness, usually beginning in the legs and ascending to produce quadriplegia and respiratory failure. Involvement of the pharyngeal and facial muscles also was seen. Muscle pain and tenderness were common. Though an elevated CSF protein concentration was sometimes seen in all three groups, the elevation occurred earlier in the GBS group. Death occurred sooner in the cytoplasmic and nuclear neuronopathy groups. Virologic studies were unrevealing and the etiology of these neuronopathies remains unknown.

Botulism

Botulism results from a neurotoxin elaborated by *Clostridium botulinum* types A, B, and E (rarely types F and G). For a detailed analysis of the actions of botulinum toxin, we refer the reader to Simpson's review.[1105] There are four clinical forms: (1) food-borne botulism, (2) wound botulism, (3) infant botulism, and (4) a rare type that may be the adult equivalent of infant botulism. The neurologic syndrome results from the toxin's combined action on neuromuscular junctions and the autonomic system. Botulism initially simulates the oropharyngeal and ocular types of regional GBS, but later causes generalized weakness.

The illness usually begins 12 to 72 hours after ingestion of contaminated food (range 6 hours to 8 days). The earliest symptoms are nausea, vomiting, and, occasionally, diarrhea. Constipation and neurologic symptoms follow. Blurred vision is usually an early symptom, followed by dry mouth, ptosis, dysphagia, and dysphonia. Dilated pupils, with poor response to light and accommodation, are a hallmark of botulism but may be absent or appear late. Diplopia and weakness of the extraocular, facial, and neck muscles and proximal limb muscles then appear in a pattern that is compatible with regional GBS or myasthenia gravis. The lateral rectus is the most commonly affected eye muscle but the triad of ptosis, medial rectus weakness, and dilated or poorly reactive pupils has been reported to be valuable in predicting respiratory failure.[1183] The paralysis usually descends from the cranial muscles to the limbs, reaching a peak over several days. Weakness tends to be more pronounced in the proximal arms. Respiratory muscle weakness is often disproportionate to limb weakness, and the reflexes are preserved even in the presence of significant weakness (but may become diminished in severe cases). Constipation often remains prominent and patients may have urinary hesitancy or retention.[636,1183] Impairment of lacrimation and salivation, orthostatic hypotension, sore throat, and erythema of the tongue and pharynx may be present.[635] Atypical features of botulism have included paresthesias (15%), nystagmus, ataxia, and Babinski's signs.[542] Ptosis and limb weakness may be asymmetric.

The CSF is generally normal in botulism, though slight CSF protein level elevations have been reported, particularly in type A[542] and type E.[636] Electrodiagnostic studies reveal increased numbers of myopathic units (low amplitude, short duration, polyphasic). There are often low-amplitude CMAPs, with a decremental response at low rates of repetitive stimulation and facilitation after exercise or repetitive nerve stimulation at higher rates (a pattern also seen in Lambert-Eaton syndrome). The typical electrophysiologic features may be found only in some muscles and are absent in patients without limb weakness. Single-fiber EMG may reveal increased jitter and blocking.[756,1218] Fibrillations may appear during the recovery stages. Nerve conduction velocities and terminal latencies are usually normal. F waves may be absent in cases with very low CMAP. H reflexes are usually normal but low-amplitude H reflex with prolonged latency or prominent H reflexes have been reported.[1207] The presence of brief small abundant motor-unit potentials (BSAPs) have been particularly emphasized in infant botulism. Edrophonium may cause brief clinical and electrophysiologic improvement.[542]

The diagnosis of botulism is readily considered in multiple-case outbreaks. It may be overlooked when the incubation period is prolonged, severity of the illness variable, or victims geographically disseminated, as exemplified by outbreaks in which cases were not readily recognized before publicity in the media.[636]

Electrophysiologic studies just outlined distinguish botulism from GBS, but there are clear clinical clues as well. Botulism produces a descending paralysis, beginning in the cranial nerve–innervated musculature, then in the arms, and then the legs—such a pattern is seen in only approximately 15% of GBS cases. The relatively higher frequency of GBS compared to botulism nonetheless makes GBS a more likely cause of this pattern of weakness (Table 14–37). Respiratory failure in botulism may occur when limb weakness is mild or moderate, whereas in GBS, limb weakness is severe when respiratory failure occurs. Tendon reflexes are reduced or absent in one quarter to one half of patients with botulism, but may be preserved even with significant limb or respiratory weakness. Ptosis, present in most, if not all, cases of botulism, is less common in GBS (see Chapter 7). (Ptosis or disproportionate neck muscle weakness compared to limb strength raise suspicion of a disorder of the neuromuscular junction.) The pupils are characteristically dilated and poorly reactive, but this sign may be absent or appear late.[189,542] A distinguishing feature may be the consistent association of pupillary findings with ophthalmoplegia in GBS, compared with their occurrence without ophthalmoplegia in one third to one half of botulism cases (Table 14–38). Dryness of the tongue and pharynx occurs in most botulism cases[542] but is rare in GBS. GBS may follow a nonspecific gastroenteritis (or a specific enteritis such as *Campylobacter*), but the GI symptoms have usually resolved by the time the neurologic syndrome evolves. In botulism, however, the GI symptoms are rapidly followed by the neurologic symptoms. Paresthesias occur in less than 15% of patients with botulism, and objective sensory loss virtually excludes botulism. The CSF is usually normal. Laboratory confirmation of botulism requires detection of botulinum toxin in the stool or serum, detection of the toxin in contaminated food, or culture of *C. botulinum* from the stool. Toxin is more likely to be detected early. In one study,[683] there was a 52% rate of detection of botulinum toxin in the serum initially but none during or after the third week.

Wound botulism produces all the classic signs of botulism except constipation (the latter usually reflecting local toxin action on the GI tract).[797] In the United States there were only 19 reported cases of wound botulism from 1976 to 1986, and 15 from 1943 to 1976. Two thirds of cases were associated with compound fractures or crush injuries.[1169] The incubation period for wound botulism is 4 to 14 days, longer than for food-borne botulism. Electrophysiologic features are most useful in making the correct diagnosis. Botulism in chronic drug abusers may be a form of wound botulism.[736,969]

Infant botulism begins at a mean age of 15 weeks (range 3 weeks to 6 months) and occurs almost exclusively in white breast-fed infants.[44,717,718] Constipation is typically the first symptom and may occur up to 3 weeks prior to onset of the neurologic symptoms. Weak sucking reflex, difficulty swallowing, pooling of secretions, and a feeble cry are the usual early neurologic symptoms, followed by generalized weakness. Examination reveals decreased spontaneous movement, hypotonia, ptosis, extraocular weakness, facial weakness, absent gag and suck reflexes, and generalized weakness. Weakness of the neck flexors is often striking. Deep tendon reflexes are diminished or absent in more than half the patients. Pupil-

Table 14–38 DIFFERENTIATING GBS FROM BOTULISM

	GBS	*Botulism*
Other community cases	No	Sometimes
Pattern	Ascending	Descending
Respiratory failure	When limbs weak	Often early
Reflexes	Absent	May be preserved
Ptosis	Uncommon	Common
Neck weakness	Only when severe	Common, early
Internal ophthalmoplegia	Rare	Common
Dry mouth	Rare	Common
Constipation	May occur late	Common, early
Objective sensory loss	Common	Rare
CSF	Raised protein	Normal
NCV slowing	May be normal early	Normal
Distal latencies	Prolonged	Normal
EMG	Normal early	BSAPs (see text)
CMAP	Normal*	Reduced amplitude
Repetitive nerve stimulation	Normal	Decrement at low rates and incremental at high rates

*May be reduced if conduction block or temporal dispersion present.

lary reaction to light may or may not be impaired and impaired salivation and lacrimation, vasolability, and labile blood pressure and pulse may be seen. Respiratory failure is common. Full recovery is the rule if complications do not supervene. Botulinal toxin is not found commonly in the serum in infant botulism but is consistently found in the stool, along with growth of *C. botulinum*, often for many weeks or months after clinical recovery has occurred. Electrophysiologic studies may reveal the classical features of botulism seen in the adult. BSAPs are particularly common.[44]

Infant botulism differs from adult food-borne botulism in that it is due to colonization of the gut with *C. botulinum* prior to toxin production. *C. botulinum* is not a part of the normal intestinal flora, and the prevailing theory is that the changes in intestinal flora that occur at the time of weaning allow for a period in which *C. botulinum* (the spores of which are ubiquitous) can colonize the GI tract.

The unclassified form of botulism (where neither a wound nor ingestion of preformed toxin can be identified) may be the adult equivalent of infant botulism (ie, associated with colonization of the gut by *C. botulinum* with endogenous production of toxin).[192] Several cases have followed gastrointestinal surgical procedures (often with postoperative antibiotic therapy) such as vagotomy/antrectomy/Billroth I anastomosis, jejunoileal bypass, resection of gangrenous bowel, and surgical blind loops, when it may simulate postsurgical GBS; other cases occurred following regional enteritis.[1127] Toxin and organism remain in the stool for prolonged periods. Clinical features are the same as in other forms of botulism, though persistent constipation is typical.

Rabies

Domestic canine rabies vaccination programs in the United States have led to a decline in human rabies, from an average of 22 cases per year from 1946 to 1950, to less than 5 cases per year since 1960. Because of its relative rarity, 4 of 87 cases from 1930 to 1979 were misdiagnosed as GBS, and more than 25% of cases in the United States since 1960 were not diagnosed in life.[29,301]

An incubation period of 1 to 2 months (range 9 days to several years) follows the animal bite. The typical illness may begin with a prodromal phase characterized by fever, malaise, myalgias, headache, photophobia, nausea, or sore throat. Pain or paresthesias at the site of the bite occur in 35% to 80% of cases,[1254] often with local hypesthesia or hyperpathia and abnormal muscle movements, variably described as tics, twitches, spasms, or fasciculations, in the bitten limb. An excitement phase classically ensues in several days, characterized by agitation, insomnia, apprehension, aggressive behavior, disorientation, and hallucinations, interspersed with periods of relative calm and lucidity. Paralytic (or "dumb") rabies, lacking a typical excitement stage, is common in animal rabies but accounts for less than 20% of human rabies cases.[1254] Signs of brainstem polioencephalitis follow: dysphagia, dysarthria, drooling, and excessive salivation, hoarseness and a voice with a "barking" quality from pharyngeal, palatal, and laryngeal paralysis.[1254] The unique phenomenon of hydrophobia occurs in less than 50% of the cases. Inspiratory spasms due to contractions of the diaphragm and accessory respiratory muscles[1255] are often precipitated by drinking water, the sight of water, a draught of cold air, pharyngeal stimulation, splashing water on the face, tracheal stimulation, speaking, or swallowing, or they may occur spontaneously. Breathing rhythm abnormalities are common, with apneustic, periodic, or cluster breathing, or a pattern resembling respiratory myoclonus.[1254] Nystagmus, ophthalmoplegias, ptosis, and gaze paresis may occur, reflecting brainstem dysfunction in other areas. A number of prominent dysautonomic signs, a few similar to GBS, occur in most patients.

The paralytic stage follows brainstem abnormalities in 1 to 5 days if death does not occur. Increased muscle tone and reflexes occur, with Babinski's signs, followed by flaccid areflexic paralysis, often as the patient becomes obtunded or comatose. It is only at this stage that the illness resembles GBS, but abortive prodromal and excitement stages and the inconsistency of all the classic signs, have led to the incorrect diagnosis. Paralysis of the legs is complete by the end of the first week, and of the arms by the end of the second week.[412] Respiratory failure often has been the cause of death. CSF protein level elevation has occurred in one-quarter of patients during the first week, and in the majority later. CSF cell counts greater than 5 per cm^3 have occurred early in more than half of cases, and in almost all cases after the first week.

Paralytic (or "dumb") rabies, lacking a typical excitement stage, has been well described in humans,[551,632,722] but cases had myelopathic features that clearly distinguished them from GBS.

Several cases resulting from corneal transplantation have been misdiagnosed as GBS because the typical index event, an animal bite, was absent. These patients had facial, oropharyngeal, and areflexic limb paralysis with raised CSF protein.[64,536] Other features would have been atypical for GBS such as retro-orbital pain, masticatory weakness, facial sensory changes, asymmetric ataxia, delirium, and coma.

Verma and colleagues[1232] described a case with areflexic weakness in both legs, extending to arms, face, and oropharyngeal muscles over 6 days. The legs were weak disproportionately to the arms. The CSF contained two lymphocytes per cm^3 and CSF protein was 32 mg/dL. Respiratory failure and death soon followed. Banerjee and Chopra[70] described two cases of rabies resembling GBS in India, where the two diseases are comparably frequent. Both patients had fever, areflexic quadriparesis, and respiratory failure, one with oropharyngeal dysfunction; neither had hydrophobia. Mild CSF pleocytosis (20 to 80 WBC per cm^3) was seen in each, and one had a moderately elevated CSF protein level (113 to 257 mg/dL).

In a pathology study of the peripheral and central nervous systems from 11 cases of paralytic rabies, 8 had motor weakness beginning in the affected limb, but 3 had simultaneous onset in all four limbs.[195] The CNS pathology was typical of rabies. However, a surprising feature in peripheral nerve was loss of axons and myelinated fibers, segmental demyelination and remyelination, and infiltration with inflammatory cells. Though some nerves showed wallerian degeneration in addition to segmental demyelination, none showed wallerian degeneration only.

Several clinical points, in addition to the relative rarity of rabies in most countries, help differentiate it from GBS (Table 14–39). GBS patients have usually recovered completely from their antecedent illness when their neurologic symptoms appear, whereas prodromal symptoms are still present when the neurologic symptoms of rabies appear. Fever, uncommon in uncomplicated GBS, is almost always present and persistent in rabies. Pharyngeal paralysis is common in both diseases, but GBS patients do not have pain on swallowing or the characteristic spasms seen in rabies. Oropharyngeal paresis is symmetric in GBS but often asymmetric in rabies (as in diphtheria). Initial sensory symptoms or pain in rabies is usually confined to one limb, compared with the bilateral distal symmetric paresthesias in GBS. Sensory and motor signs in rabies are also likely to be asymmetric. Discrete sensory levels, especially on the trunk, occur very infrequently in GBS but indicate the ability of rabies to produce a myelopathy. Bowel and bladder dysfunction occur early in rabies compared with GBS, where they are seldom seen in the nonquadriparetic patient. Severe leg paralysis in GBS is virtually always associated with at least moderate arm weakness.

Table 14–39 DIFFERENTIATING GBS FROM RABIES

	GBS	*Rabies*
Prodrome	1–2 wk prior	1–4 days prior
Fever	Rare	Common
Sensory symptoms and signs	Distally symmetric	Unilateral early
Sensory levels	No	Common
Muscles affected	All limbs symmetric	Legs weakest early, asymmetric
Bladder involvement	Usually urinary retention, transient, occurs at time of peak weakness	Incontinence common, often occurs early
Reflexes	Often absent before weakness	Arm reflexes normal with paraplegia
Bulbar paresis	Flaccid, symmetric	Spasms, hydrophobia, asymmetric
Facial pain	No	May occur
Respiratory failure	Only when arms and shoulders weak	Early
Respiratory patterns	Hypoventilation due to respiratory paralysis	Periodic, irregular breathing
Mental status abnormal	No	Common
Pain	Proximal muscles	Asymmetric
CSF pleocytosis	No	Common

In rabies, there is often a disparity between arm and leg strength. The reflexes are usually absent globally in GBS by the time severe leg weakness has developed, whereas in rabies, upper extremity reflexes may be preserved even with flaccid areflexic paraplegia. Respiratory failure may occur in rabies when arm strength is normal, whereas such patients with GBS have profound shoulder and arm weakness. Facial pain, sometimes encountered in rabies, is not a feature of GBS. The unusual breathing patterns and the mental status changes seen in rabies (either the excitement or depression of arousal) are not features of GBS.

Early in either illness, the CSF may be normal and in both, relative albuminocytologic dissociation occurs. In rabies, however, pleocytosis eventually occurs in almost all patients. Completely normal electrophysiologic studies, unusual in GBS at any stage of the illness, are expected in rabies.

Antemortem laboratory confirmation of rabies may be difficult, particularly early in the course.[549] Attempts should be made to isolate the virus from saliva, throat swab, urine, CSF, and conjunctival and nasal secretions. Brain biopsy is seldom helpful but it has on occasion demonstrated rabies by the fluorescent rabies antibody (FRA) test. Vital antigen may also be demonstrated by the FRA test in biopsies of facial or nuchal skin or on corneal impressions,[158,634] but false-positive results do occur.

Virus isolation from tissues or body fluids, through mouse inoculation, generally takes more than a week. Nevertheless, 4 of 7 patients with rabies had virus isolated in the first 4 days (earliest on day 2) and 6 of 19 by 8 days in one report.[29] Isolation of virus after the second week was rare. Serum antirabies antibody titers may not be detected before the eighth day of illness, and interpretation is difficult in patients who received preexposure or postexposure vaccination or rabies immunoglobulin. Nevertheless, detection of serum antirabies antibody was the most successful method of laboratory confirmation of cases in the United States.[29] In unvaccinated patients, the earliest the antibody was found was the sixth day, and all cases were positive by the end of the second week.

Tetanus

Tetanus, except in limited forms, seldom enters the differential diagnosis of GBS, as full-blown tetanus has characteristic features. A patient has been described, however, with localized tetanus presenting with progressive difficulty swallowing and a soft hoarse voice that simulated early GBS.[1071] The typical limb and axial muscle spasms and stiffness characteristic of tetanus were absent. However, trismus and visible contraction of the platysma were clues to the correct diagnosis. The EMG showed continuous muscle activity, even on attempted relaxation, lack of inhibition when antagonistic muscles were activated, and absence of a silent period in the masseter following a jaw jerk.

Other Animal and Plant Toxins

Neurotoxic Fish Poisoning

(CIGUATERA, NEUROTOXIC SHELLFISH POISONING, PARALYTIC SHELLFISH POISONING, AND PUFFER FISH POISONING)

These related illnesses, resulting from ingestion of marine toxins that have direct effects on nerve and muscle sodium channels, may be the most common poisoning in the world. Several excellent reviews have appeared on the subject.[543,805,1049,1130] All of these illnesses occur minutes to hours after ingestion of toxic fish. The illness occurs after eating reef fish that have ingested toxic dinoflaggelates. Several cases have been reported from imported fish, but travel in the Carribean or South Pacific are index features for American and European patients. Several patients have been referred to the MGH, usually recently returned from vacations, because of paresthesias that have raised the possibility of GBS. Despite apparent clinical differences and specific toxins associated with each fish poisoning, the illnesses are neurologically similar. Many of the symptoms thought to be characteristic of each syndrome are also seen with the others, the main differences being epidemiologic and the relative severity of gastrointestinal and neurologic features. A recent review made this point and proposed a unifying term of *pelagic paralysis* (perhaps a misnomer, as "pelagic" refers to the open seas).[805]

All four illnesses are typified by paresthesias, often beginning perioral1y, or in the mouth, tongue, gums, and throat, and almost always involving the distal limbs (the hands as much as, or more than, the feet). In some cases, an unusual but characteristic reversal of hot and cold sensation occurs (cool objects feel hot, and vice versa, or local temperature changes cause intense paresthesias). An electric or other paresthetic feeling may be elicited by running water over the hands. In MGH patients' experience, the paresthesias have been described as "large" pins and needles, or a prickly, or tight burning sensation, unlike most patients with GBS, who report finer, numbness symptoms (see Chapter 7). Muscle aches such as a charley horse have been described, particularly in ciguatera,[196] similar to the pains of GBS and polio (see Chapter 7). Shooting pains in the limbs have also been mentioned.

Weakness is prominent in pufferfish poisoning and in severe cases of ciguatera; paralysis has not been reported in humans with neurotoxic shellfish poisoning, which causes a predominantly paresthetic syndrome. Respiratory failure is rare but occurs in occasional cases with severe paralysis. Ataxia, apparently on a peripheral basis, has been reported in patients with ciguatera.[574] In general, there are few CNS features in these patients, but severe cases of paralytic and neurotoxic shellfish poisoning and ciguatera have included vertigo, cerebellar tremor, and nystagmus. Transient blurred vision, blindness, and headaches have occurred in a few patients. A few cases of unexplained respiratory failure without weakness have been attributed to central depression of breathing. The illnesses are usually transient but severe cases may persist for weeks or longer.

The weakness, paresthesias, and

muscle aches probably have a peripheral origin, but it is not clear if reflex changes are to be expected. Several case reports with adequate neurologic detail have indicated that deep tendon reflexes have been active, though others have shown them to be depressed. We have seen a case with transient depression of tendon reflexes and persistent depression of knee reflexes. Gastrointestinal symptoms, particularly diarrhea, vomiting, and abdominal cramping—approximately in that order of frequency—are invariable accompaniments, usually preceding the paresthesias; the GI symptoms may be mild. Common cholinergic and adrenergic symptoms include mydriasis, tachycardia, bradycardia, and dry mouth (and perhaps the GI symptoms).

Tetrodotoxin (pufferfish), ciguatoxin (ciguatera), saxitoxin (paralytic shellfish poisoning), and brevitoxin (neurotoxic shellfish poisoning) lower the conductance of sodium current and have become important neurologic research tools for identifying sodium channels. The early and prominent perioral distribution of paresthesias, abrupt onset, associated enteritic symptoms while in endemic coastal areas, and generally normal electrophysiologic study results[169] all allow distinction from GBS. As a static phenomenon, however, neurotoxic fish poisoning may simulate early GBS.

Buckthorn Neuropathy

A rapidly progressive and sometimes fatal polyneuropathy follows ingestion of the fruit of the buckthorn shrub, a plant found in central and northern Mexico, Texas, and New Mexico.[164,502] The disorder begins with weakness in the lower extremities that rapidly ascends to produce a symmetric flaccid, areflexic quadriplegia incuding pharyngeal, masticatory, facial, neck, paravertebral, and respiratory muscles. Distal sensory loss is overshadowed by the motor signs. The CSF is typically normal. Early reports suggested segmental demyelination as the primary pathophysiologic mechanism,[164] although subsequent reports have suggested a primary effect of the toxin on the axon. The disorder clinically resembles GBS, and distinction rests on recognition of ingestion of the fruit in endemic areas and on the normal CSF protein concentration.

Snake Envenomations

Bites of certain poisonous snakes have neurotoxic features. The neurotoxins interfere with either presynaptic or postsynaptic transmission at the neuromuscular junction.[924,1260] The clinical manifestations therefore resemble myasthenia gravis and other disorders of neuromuscular transmission more than a neuropathy. Ptosis is the most common and usually the earliest manifestation.[1256,1260] External ophthalmoplegia may be complete or may produce more weakness of upward than of downward gaze.[1256] Pharyngeal, tongue, neck, paravertebral, and respiratory weakness is common. Limb weakness is usually worse proximally but flaccid complete quadriplegia may occur. The reflexes may be relatively preserved, diminished proportionate to weakness, or absent despite normal limb power.[978] Though patients may complain of numbness, there is no objective sensory loss. The pupils may be fixed and dilated. A classic myasthenic decremental response to repetitive nerve stimulation occurs.[1260] Clinical and electrophysiologic improvement occurs with the administration of anticholinesterases when the toxin acts postsynaptically but seldom when the activity is presynaptic.

Depending on the species of snake, muscle tenderness, rhabdomyolysis, myoglobinuria, oliguria, hemolysis, defibrination, and excessive bleeding may be present. Local reactions at the bite location and cardiac toxicity also vary depending on the species.

Hymenoptera Stings

A variety of neurologic syndromes have been reported following stings by *Hymenoptera* species (bees, wasps, fire ants). Apparently typical cases of GBS have very rarely followed such stings by 1 to 2 weeks[63,699,1043] (see Chapter 6). Fisher's syndrome also has been reported, although the latent period has been as short as 1 day.[699] Inflammatory and demyelinating changes of both the peripheral and central nervous systems have occurred after yellow-jacket stings.[788]

Though both axonal and myelin changes have been induced experimentally by local application of bee venom, there is no convincing evidence that GBS-like illnesses result from a toxin in the venom. In view of the latent period between the sting and the onset of neurologic symptoms, this may be a delayed hypersensitivity response. Bee venom contains a phospholipase A[1043] different from the phospholipase A found in snake venom that causes a presynaptic blockade of neuromuscular transmission.[537]

Miscellaneous Animal Toxins

Envenomation from bites of the Gila monster and Mexican beaded lizard cause local pain, inflammation, paresthesias, and hyperesthesia.[1138,1245] The systemic effects of neurotoxin may produce profound weakness, dysphonia, dyspnea, and blurred vision, among other symptoms. Certain salamanders (newts) contain tetrodotoxin, and poisoning by ingestion has been reported,[133,144] similar to puffer poisoning discussed earlier.

Other Toxins and Drugs

Organophosphate Poisoning

Organophosphate esters, used mainly in insecticides, have two main neurotoxic manifestations: (1) an easily identifiable acute syndrome due to inhibition of acetylcholinesterase, and (2) a delayed distal axonal neuropathy.[837,1063] An intermediate syndrome most closely resembling GBS, appearing shortly after the cholinergic phase, also has been described.[1083,1241]

Signs of acute organophosphate toxicity include miosis, fasciculations, salivation, diaphoresis, altered consciousness, seizures, and pulmonary edema. Paralysis was reported in 52 of 200 cases of organophosphate poisoning, present in 16 cases on admission and later (9 to 85 hours) in 36 (5 cases had initial paralysis, resolution, then recurrent paralysis).[1241]

In delayed or intermediate cases (most of whom received atropine for the cholinergic phase), weakness was greater proximally than distally, and greater in the legs than in the arms—the same pattern seen in most GBS cases. The reflexes were reduced and global areflexia occurred in half of these patients. Cranial nerves were commonly involved, including oropharyngeal, facial, and extraocular muscles. Ophthalmoplegia, usually bilateral sixth nerve palsies, occurred more commonly than in GBS (50% of cases) (Table 14–40). Paralysis of neck and trunk muscles was very common. Respiratory insufficiency occurred early in some series.[1083] NCVs and EMG were generally normal. Repetitive nerve stimulation, however, showed decremental responses at high rates of stimulation, none at low rates, and no evidence of post-tetanic facilitation.

Two cases have been reported of areflexic quadriparesis with normal sensation and CSF albuminocytologic dissociation after organophosphate exposure.[7,367] In one case, no acute cholinergic phase occurred. Both cases clearly resembled GBS rather than the typical distal delayed axonal neuropathy that may follow organophosphate exposure and were called "GBS" by the authors. Motor nerve conduction velocities were slowed in one patient.

In another case of acute areflexic quadriplegia with respiratory failure,

Table 14–40 DIFFERENTIATING GBS FROM ORGANOPHOSPHATE POISONING (INTERMEDIATE SYNDROME)

	GBS	*Organophosphate Poisoning*
Miosis	No	Common
Fasciculations	Rare	Common
Objective sensory loss	Common	No
Respiratory failure	When limbs weak	Often before limbs weak
Ophthalmoplegia	Unusual	Common
Neck weakness	Only when severe	Common early
NCV slowing	May be normal early	Normal
Distal latencies	Prolonged	Normal
Repetitive nerve stimulation	Normal*	Decremental in many

*May be reduced if conduction block or temporal dispersion present.

botulism was at first suspected.[758] However, a decremental response to repetitive nerve stimulation at higher rates and worse after edrophonium suggested organophosphate poisoning. Erythrocyte cholinesterase levels were reduced and methylparathion was identified in a spray used mistakenly on the patient's hair.

In the absence of known organophosphate exposure, the typical clinical symptoms and signs of poisoning may lead to the mistaken diagnosis of GBS (Table 14–39). Indeed, several titles in the literature have misnamed cases of organophosphate poisoning. Prodromal symptoms and signs such as fasciculations, miosis, salivation, and diaphoresis exclude GBS and suggest the correct diagnosis. Other features suggesting organophosphate poisoning are neck and respiratory muscle weakness disproportionate to limb weakness, lack of sensory symptoms and signs, and rapid progression of paralysis. A decremental response to repetitive nerve stimulation may assist in the differential diagnosis.

Vincristine and Suramin Neuropathy

Vincristine, widely used as a cancer chemotherapeutic agent, usually produces a slowly progressive axonal neuropathy that does not resemble GBS,[177] though it often is considered in the differential diagnosis in cancer patients with neuropathy. Paresthesias generally begin in the fingers, ankle jerks are lost early, and weakness develops later. There is a predilection for distal extensor weakness. Constipation, ileus, urinary retention, orthostatic hypotension, and syndrome of inappropriate secretion of antidiuretic hormone (SIADH) may occur. Motor conduction velocities may be normal or mildly slowed and sensory nerve amplitudes are typically reduced, even when latencies are normal. Nevertheless, weakness may rarely become severe enough in some to resemble GBS. Six of the patients described by Casey and coworkers[177] had significant proximal leg weakness, and two were unable to stand. Weakness may progress rapidly over 2 weeks. Rapidly progressive weakness, often with quadriparesis, as well as respiratory and cranial nerve involvement in patients treated with vincristine have been reported;[827] several also had elevated CSF protein levels. The more typical axonal neuropathy occurs in patients receiving chronic vincristine therapy and may be dose related; the rapidly progressive quadriparetic cases have often followed one or two doses. Whether these truly represent vincristine neuropathy or are simply cases of GBS in immunosuppressed cancer patients, as some have been designated, remains uncertain.[861] Obviously, however, vincristine should be discontinued in such cases.

Suramin, an experimental cancer

and AIDS chemotherapy drug derived from an antihelminthic drug, can produce a spectrum of neuropathies, from paresthesias (including on the face) to quadriplegia and respiratory failure. The CSF protein level often is elevated and electrophysiologic testing may reveal conduction block indistinguishable from that of GBS. The risk of neuropathy may be related to peak drug serum levels rather than to the total drug dose. The few nerve biopsies that have been performed have shown noninflammatory demyelination. The main difference from GBS has been a long progression of weakness, usually 1 to 2 months in severe cases.

Glue Sniffer's Neuropathy

The hexacarbons *n*-hexane and methyl-butyl-ketone cause an axonal neuropathy in industrial workers and in glue sniffers.[22,1136] The neuropathies are characterized by distal symmetric sensory loss, loss of ankle jerks, and distal weakness. Weakness is occasionally more prominent in those cases due to glue sniffing, and then may superficially resemble GBS. A remarkable series of glue sniffer's neuropathy appeared in 18 patients in Germany in 1975 after glue thinner containing *n*-hexane was altered by the addition of methyl-ethyl-ketone.[25] Symptoms began with paresthesias in the feet and foot weakness. However, weakness progressed in an ascending fashion with progressive areflexic quadriparesis over 6 weeks. Muscle atrophy, striking in most cases, began early. The cranial nerves and bladder were unaffected. Two quadriplegic patients had reduced vital capacities, but respiratory assistance was not required. CSF protein level was normal in all but one case. NCVs and distal latencies were slowed proportionate to the weakness, and EMG showed prominent denervation. Nerve biopsy showed axonal loss. Four similar cases were reported previously.[423]

Points distinguishing this severe toxic neuropathy from GBS are the striking early atrophy, predilection for distal extensor muscles, lack of cranial nerve or respiratory involvement despite quadriplegia, normal CSF protein concentration, and the more prolonged period of progression.

Perhexilene Neuropathy

A demyelinating neuropathy has been associated with perhexiline maleate, a drug used to treat angina pectoris.[126] Paresthesias and pain begin in the legs. Global areflexia or loss of ankle jerks may occur. Facial diplegia, sphincter disturbances,[1042] and orthostatic hypotension[378] have been reported. Paresthesias and sensory loss on the face and trunk, uncommon in GBS, have also been noted.[1042] Papilledema occurs in 20%.[126] The CSF protein level is commonly elevated. Motor NCVs are typically slowed, often severely. Nerve biopsies show segmental demyelination and wallerian degeneration. This neuropathy shares some clinical features with GBS but generally evolves more slowly and produces less severe maximum motor deficits. Weakness often only appears several weeks after paresthesias, compared with its early onset in GBS.

Disulfiram Neuropathy

Disulfiram is another drug that may be associated with a mild sensorimotor neuropathy. At least one case of a fulminant neuropathy resembling GBS has been reported.[1029] The patient had been receiving disulfiram for 4 months when she overdosed on alcohol, disulfiram, and amitriptyline. She recovered from the acute toxic encephalopathy but 2 weeks later developed tongue numbness, dysarthria, and dysphagia. Over 3 days, limb paresthesias and progressive weakness with areflexia developed and by day 20 she could no longer walk. CSF on day 21 showed no white blood cells (WBC) and a protein level of 104 mg/dL; on day 37, there were 8 WBC per mL and a protein level of 990 mg/dL. NCVs were normal both early and later, but sensory and motor amplitudes were reduced and later EMG showed evidence of denervation. Sural nerve biopsy showed extensive degeneration but no segmental demyelination.

Vacor Neuropathy

A rapidly progressive neuropathy following ingestion of the rat poison PNU (Vacor) causes nausea, vomiting, and abdominal pain within hours of ingestion.[694] Weakness, paresthesias, and prominent autonomic dysfunction develop in one to several days. Generalized areflexic weakness often lasts for weeks. However, sensory changes are usually more prominent. An autopsy in one case showed myelin ovoids in the dorsal roots with normal ventral roots. Elevated CSF protein concentration has been noted in some cases. Several patients have developed cerebellar ataxia, tremor, nystagmus, or altered mental status, including two patients with a delayed encephalopathy.

The hallmark of Vacor toxicity, however, is diabetes and ketoacidosis, developing in all patients within hours or days after ingestion. Although glucose intolerance can occur in patients with GBS, it is usually mild and unassociated with ketoacidosis. The predominance of sensory and autonomic manifestations early in the course would be unusual in someone with GBS.

Lithium Neuropathy

Two reported cases of rapidly progressive lithium-related neuropathy have resembled GBS. One occurred in a patient who developed acute symptoms of lithium intoxication.[157] Limb, face, tongue, and pharyngeal weakness and distal sensory loss developed over several days, followed by areflexic quadriplegia with respiratory failure. CSF protein level was 166 mg/dL. Motor NCVs, distal latencies, sensory nerve latencies, and amplitudes were all normal. EMG showed insertional irritability, fibrillations, positive waves, and pseudomyotonic discharges. Serum lithium levels were within the accepted therapeutic range. Another case of a rapidly evolving severe polyneuropathy followed an acute encephalopathy due to very high serum lithium levels.[898] At the peak of illness, there was oropharyngeal weakness, severe distal arm weakness, flaccid paraplegia, and distal sensory loss. Reflexes were absent distally and reduced proximally. The CSF was acellular with a protein concentration of 70 mg/dL. CMAP and sensory amplitudes were reduced, and nerve biopsy showed acute axonal degeneration.

NONORGANOPHOSPHATE INSECTICIDES

A case strongly resembling GBS, with rapidly progressive quadriplegia, facial diplegia, respiratory failure, and CSF albuminocytologic dissociation, occurred after exposure to the insecticides DDD (a halogenated hydrocarbon) and Aldrin (a cyclodiene).[566] The patient had been working in fields sprayed with Aldrin and dusting tobacco with DDD in the preceding 1 to 2 months. Myoclonic jerks for 3 to 4 weeks prior to onset of paralysis and a mild recurrence of symptoms on re-exposure a year later suggested a causal relationship to the Aldrin. A second patient, exposed to DDT and Endrin, presented with predominantly distal limb weakness, minimal sensory loss, and CSF albuminocytologic dissociation but preserved reflexes except for ankle jerks.[566]

HEAVY METAL TOXIC NEUROPATHIES

The majority of toxic neuropathies related to drugs or toxins produce distal "dying-back" axonal neuropathies that do not resemble GBS other than that some may be associated with elevated CSF protein concentrations. We will limit our discussion to those agents producing a neuropathy that may, in a limited number of cases, more closely resemble GBS. Most of these are rare, and the correct diagnosis becomes evident by other circumstantial evidence.

Thallium Neuropathy. Thallium intoxication causes an axonal neuropathy, but its rapid evolution and clinical features may lead to a misdiagnosis of GBS.[181] Thallium poisoning has become rare since the agent has been removed from commercially available depilatory preparations and rat or insect poisons in the United States, but two cases of American students returning from abroad have been recently referred to the MGH. The clinical manifestations depend upon the dosage and chronicity of exposure, but most cases resembling GBS occur after a large single intoxication with thallium. Alopecia, the characteristic sign of thallitoxicosis, may not appear until after neurologic features have evolved.

Gastrointestinal symptoms typically begin within hours or days of ingestion. Nausea, vomiting, anorexia, abdominal pain, and diarrhea are common. There may be diffuse abdominal tenderness without rebound tenderness.[72] In contrast, GI symptoms in GBS appear late, as autonomic complications, or as part of the antecedent illness, in which case they precede the neurologic symptoms by 1 to 2 weeks (Table 14–41).

Painful paresthesias usually herald the neuropathy, beginning several days after the exposure; they may occur within hours after massive exposure. They tend to affect the hands and feet, particularly the soles, although cases confined to the hands have been noted. Pain and muscle tenderness may also occur in other areas such as the back, abdomen, chest, proximal limbs, and joints.[72] Sensory symptoms and signs predominate early and in mild cases. Proximal and axial muscle pain is common in GBS but the painful distal dysesthesias characteristic of thallium poisoning are uncommon in early GBS. Fatigue and malaise are often present before weakness.

A motor neuropathy subsequently evolves. There is early, distally predominant weakness, compared with the proximal weakness early in GBS. In most cases, the legs are weaker than the arms.[181] Overwhelming cases may evolve rapidly and produce severe quadriplegia. Respiratory failure occurs rarely as the neuropathy progresses.[181,605] In contrast to GBS, there is a relative preservation of deep tendon reflexes in thallium neuropathy. Ankle reflexes are suppressed earliest;[72,181] other reflexes may subsequently become depressed or absent, but they may be normal[823] or even hyperactive in the presence of significant weakness.

Sensory loss affecting all modalities tends to have a glove-stocking distribution, usually more pronounced in the legs.[72] Superficial sensation may be more affected than deep sensibility in some patients.[181] A few patients have

Table 14–41 DIFFERENTIATING GBS FROM THALLIUM NEUROPATHY

	GBS	*Thallium Neuropathy*
Rapidity of evolution	1–3 wk	Days or weeks
Pattern of weakness	Often proximal > distal	Distal > proximal
DTRs	Usually absent	Often preserved
Painful paresthesias	Uncommon	Typical
Nausea/vomiting/abdominal pain	Uncommon	Common early
Abnormal mental status	Rare unless complication	Common
Seizures	Rare	May occur
CSF protein	Elevated	Normal or <100 in most
Skin abnormalities	No	Rash common
Alopecia, stomatitis, Mees' lines, gingival line, dry mouth	No	Common

been reported with more prominent sensory abnormalities than motor.[181]

Facial diplegia and oropharyngeal paresis are common and trigeminal-innervated muscles may be weak. External ophthalmoplegia and ptosis have been reported frequently.[181,828] As in GBS, internal ophthalmoplegia is uncommon in thallium neuropathy; pupillary dilatation has been noted, however.[828] Impaired corneal and facial sensation, uncommon in GBS, may occur in thallium poisoning.[252,605] Optic nerve dysfunction, not a feature of GBS, is common in thallium poisoning.[72] The following have been reported sporadically: impaired visual acuity, centrocecal scotomata, loss of color vision, hyperemic discs, and optic atrophy. Ophthalmoscopy may show any of a number of retinal changes. As in GBS, sinus tachycardia and hypertension are common. Orthostatic hypotension, xerostomia, priapism, and hyperhidrosis have also been reported. Urinary retention has not been a feature.

Mental status abnormalities are often characteristic. Irritability, enhanced startle responses,[72] confusion, agitation, insomnia, hallucinations, delusions, lethargy, obtundation, or coma[72,828,976] have all been reported. Seizures have occurred in 20% of children in Reed's series.

Alopecia, a unique clinical sign that often leads to consideration of thallium poisoning, unfortunately does not usually appear early, and some cases may occur without alopecia.[181] Though scalp hair seems the most vulnerable, hair in other areas can be easily and painlessly plucked out. Mucocutaneous manifestations of thallium poisoning include fissures at the corners of the mouth, stomatitis, xerostomia, and an erythematous (and often scaling) rash of the face and scrotum. Mees' lines (transverse white nail bands) occur, as seen in arsenic poisoning, but often only after 3 to 4 weeks of illness recovery. A bluish or purplish line along the gingiva may appear at the same time as Mees' lines.[976]

Hypokalemia has been attributed to displacement of K^+ by thallium ions but might also reflect GI losses of K^+.[181,823] However, the presence of a low K^+ or ECG changes suggestive of hypokalemia may be clues to the diagnosis of thallium poisoning.[252,823]

The CSF is usually acellular with a normal protein concentration, but cases with modest elevations of protein (50 to 130 mg/dL) have been recorded.[181,823] Urinary excretion of delta aminolevulinic acid (ALA) and porphobilinogen (PBG) may be mildly increased,[72] causing confusion with the acute porphyrias. The neuropathy of thallium poisoning also clinically resembles acute porphyric neuropathy in many respects—including the autonomic features and abdominal signs and symptoms—and worsening has been reported following use of barbiturates.[72] Nerve conduction is slightly slowed.[72,181] In cases with severe weakness, there may be no response to nerve stimulation.[181] Autopsy studies have suggested a primary axonal neuropathy with secondary myelin breakdown.[181,605] Sural nerve biopsy in one case[72] showed prominent changes in the myelin sheaths with relative sparing of axons, but others[252] have reported extensive axonal pathology with large vacuoles and distended mitochondria, consistent with a "dying-back" axonal neuropathy.

The diagnosis is made by determination of urinary excretion of thallium. Since thallium is cleared slowly from the body, persistent urinary excretion is usually detectable for weeks after the neurologic manifestations.

Arsenic Neuropathy. Exposure to arsenic generally produces an axonal neuropathy and characteristic systemic manifestations.[200,516] Acute exposure causes a polyneuropathy that evolves rapidly and may be misinterpreted as GBS.[283] Clinical or subclinical neuropathy may follow chronic exposure.[357] In one series, 9 patients had a rapid evolution of neurologic symptoms, peaking within 24 hours, and 22, within 10 days.[200] Nine had quadriparesis and sensory symptoms within 10 days, resembling GBS. Many similar acute cases have been reported, including several with quadriplegia and respiratory failure simulating severe acute GBS.[438,516]

The initial symptoms of arsenic intoxication are usually gastrointestinal with nausea, vomiting, diarrhea, and, in some, abdominal pain within minutes or hours after exposure. There may be a metallic taste and garlic-like odor to the breath. Severe cases show vascular collapse and periorbital edema. These prodromal symptoms may resolve spontaneously after a few days and the neurologic symptoms may not appear for 7 to 14 days, similar to the course of GBS following a gastrointestinal or respiratory illness.

The initial neuropathic symptoms are usually paresthesias or dysesthesias, occasionally painful or burning. They may appear within hours of the GI symptoms or be delayed for more than a week. Numbness and tingling typically involve the hands and feet initially. Distal aching or burning pain is common.[200,1286] All sensations may be diminished, most commonly producing a glove-stocking distribution. The sensory manifestations tend to be more prominent in arsenic neuropathy than in GBS. Weakness usually begins distally,[283] compared with that of GBS, in which an early proximal pattern is more common. However, the weakness may spread to involve the proximal musculature and can cause a flaccid quadriplegia with respiratory failure. Early in the course, only the ankle jerks may be lost, a situation not uncommon in early GBS.

One clinical feature distinguishing GBS from arsenic intoxication is the relative rarity of cranial nerve involvement. Most GBS patients with quadriplegia and respiratory failure have facial diplegia and oropharyngeal paresis, in contrast to those having arsenic intoxication[283,438,516,1286] (Table 14–42). The mental status abnormalities common in arsenic poisoning are another distinguishing feature. Autonomic dysfunction seen in GBS such as sinus tachycardia, hypertension, and orthostatic hypotension has not been mentioned in reports on arsenic neuropathy. Heyman and colleagues[516] found urinary retention in 4 of 41 cases, but it has been otherwise rare. The period of progression of the neuropathy in arsenic intoxication is generally more prolonged than in GBS, in some cases continuing for 4 to 6 weeks, longer than acute GBS.

Early electrodiagnostic studies may

Table 14–42 DIFFERENTIATING GBS FROM ARSENIC NEUROPATHY

	GBS	***Arsenic Neuropathy***
Neuropathy evolution	1–3 wk	Up to 6 wk
Pattern of weakness	Proximal > distal	Distal > proximal
Reflexes	Absent	Only AJ lost early
Painful paresthesias	Uncommon	Typical early
Sensory loss	Late	Distal and early
Cranial nerves	Commonly involved	Involvement uncommon
Gastrointestinal symptoms	Uncommon	Prominent
Abnormal mental status	Rare unless complication	Common, though mild
CSF protein	Elevated	May be elevated
Skin abnormalities	No	Rash, desquamation
Mees' lines, dry mouth	No	Common
Anemia	No	Common
Basophilic stippling	No	May occur
Limb edema	No	Common
Prolonged QT interval	Rare	Common
CMAP amplitude	Normal*	Low

*May be reduced if conduction block or temporal dispersion present.

show absent or reduced sensory nerve potentials, partial motor conduction block, and prolonged F-wave latencies.[283] Later, absence of sensory potentials, slowed motor NCVs, prolonged distal latencies, and reduced CMAP amplitudes may be found. Serial electrodiagnostic studies[283] have suggested that the neuropathy of arsenic intoxication has demyelinating features early, and later becomes the more typical distal axonal sensorimotor neuropathy.

The CSF may be normal in arsenic neuropathy,[283,438,516] or may show a moderately elevated protein concentration (up to 270 mg/dL) without pleocytosis,[200,283,516,566] and is therefore not helpful in distinguishing arsenic neuropathy from GBS.

As in thallium neuropathy, the major clinical clues to arsenic intoxication (Table 14–41) are the preceding involvement of other body systems. Mucocutaneous abnormalities are common, including a morbilliform or maculopapular rash on the trunk or proximal legs. A classic manifestation is desquamation and hyperkeratosis of the palms and soles. Pitting edema of the feet and legs is common.[283,516] Burning of the mouth and tongue and herpetiform lesions around the mouth may occur.[516] Mees' lines (transverse white nail bands) are characteristic but not pathognomonic. However, these typically do not occur until 30 to 40 days after exposure to arsenic.[516]

Hematologic abnormalities are present in most cases and include anemia, leukopenia, and occasionally thrombocytopenia.[1073] The anemia is usually normochromic and normocytic but may be megaloblastic or sideroblastic with basophilic stippling of red cells[283] or eosinophilia.[516]

Gold Neuropathy. A polyneuropathy has been rarely associated with gold salt treatment for rheumatoid arthritis. It is usually characterized by distal sensory loss, predominantly distal weakness, autonomic involvement, and elevated CSF protein concentration, all closely simulating acute GBS.[595,1247,1286] Several cases have been cited as GBS. One patient had symmetric ascending weakness, respiratory failure, areflexia, distal sensory loss, and CSF albuminocytologic dissociation.[1234] Two patients with similar cases, one with generalized areflexic weakness, had distal sensory loss.[1067] However, fasciculations were prominent, NCVs were normal, denervation was seen on EMG, and nerve biopsy showed abnormalities of both myelinated and unmyelinated fibers. The other case had rapidly progressive limb weakness, distal sensory loss, and a unilateral facial paresis. CSF albuminocytologic dissociation was present in both. An unusual patient had rapidly progressive neuropathy characterized by distal paresthesias, distal upper extremity weakness but proximal lower extremity weakness, generalized areflexia, and oropharyngeal involvement.[276] CSF albuminocytologic dissociation was present, and there was mild slowing of motor NCVs. Another case apparently had typical Fisher's syndrome after gold therapy.[1022]

Other than the recognition of administration of gold salts, distinction from GBS may be difficult. Though myokymic fasciculations may occur in GBS, they have been reported more frequently in cases of gold neuropathy. Mental status abnormalities are not seen in uncomplicated GBS but may occur in patients with gold neurotoxicity. There is a poor correlation between gold neuropathy and duration or total dose of gold therapy. Vernay and associates[1234] suggested that there may have been a chance combination of GBS and rheumatoid arthritis treated with gold salts (likely for the Fisher's syndrome case cited earlier), but one patient had a previous reaction to gold, suggesting a more specific relationship.

Lead Neuropathy. Classic lead neuropathy only superficially resembles GBS.[1286] It is a predominantly motor neuropathy with striking distal weakness and a predilection for the extensors of the wrists, fingers, and feet. Nevertheless, rare atypical cases may cause

Table 14–43 DIFFERENTIATING GBS FROM LEAD NEUROPATHY

	GBS	*Lead Neuropathy*
Sensory symptoms and signs	Common	Rare
Cranial nerves	Commonly involved	Involvement uncommon
Gastrointestinal prodrome	1–2 wk prior	Days prior
Nausea/vomiting	Uncommon	Common early
Abdominal pain	Uncommon	?Common
Constipation	May occur late	Early, prominent
Abnormal mental status	No	May occur
CSF protein	Elevated	May be elevated
Anemia, basophilic stippling, hepatic dysfunction, renal involvement	No	May occur

confusion with GBS.[84,701] A patient has been described who had injected lead and opium parenterally. Systemic signs improved but flaccid generalized paralysis appeared after 2 weeks, progressing to respiratory failure within 2 days.[84] Other patients have had nausea, vomiting, abdominal pain, mild azotemia, hematemesis, and anemia followed by proximal greater than distal progressive areflexic paralysis.[356,701] The CSF in those cases was acellular, with a protein level of 120 mg/dL. Toxicology studies confirmed lead toxicity, subsequently traced to an old embedded bullet. Strength gradually improved after chelation therapy.

The absence of cranial nerve involvement in the setting of near-complete quadriplegia with respiratory paralysis and the purely motor nature of this illness distinguish lead neuropathy from GBS (Table 14–43). Signs of autonomic dysfunction, common in GBS, are uncommon in lead toxicity. In GBS, the antecedent illness typically occurs 10 to 14 days prior to onset of neurologic symptoms, whereas in lead toxicity, neurologic symptoms appear within days of the GI symptoms. Hypochromic microcytic anemia, basophilic stippling, and transient hepatic dysfunction are typical. A blue line along the gums is often present, though not pathognomonic of lead toxicity.

BARIUM TOXICITY

Barium salt intoxication produces an acute areflexic quadriplegia possibly related to an associated hypokalemia.[920] Aside from its hyperacute evolution, it may simulate GBS (Table 14–44). It occurs from massive ingestion or inadvertent aspiration during radiographic use.[1091] Nausea, vomiting, abdominal

Table 14–44 DIFFERENTIATING GBS FROM BARIUM TOXICITY

	GBS	*Barium Toxicity*
Evolution	1–3 wk	Hours
Early neck weakness	Uncommon	Common
Reflexes	Absent when quadriplegic	May be relatively preserved
Internal ophthalmoplegia	Uncommon	Common
Sphincter involvement	Common	Rare
Circumoral paresthesias	Rare	Common
Dry mouth	Rare	Common
Testicular pain	No	May occur
Muscle twitching	Uncommon	Common
Gastrointestinal prodrome	1–2 wk prior	Hours prior
Nausea/vomiting/abdominal pain	Uncommon	Common early
Serum potassium	Normal	Extremely low
ECG changes	Variable	Prominent

pain, diarrhea, and dry mouth are early symptoms, appearing within hours of exposure. Flaccid areflexic quadriplegia with or without respiratory and bulbar involvement, evolves over several hours. Neck and respiratory muscle weakness are often prominent early.[425] Paresthesias are common and circumoral paresthesias[690] or a stiff feeling around the mouth[255] may occur. Mental status and sensory examination are usually normal. Cranial nerve weakness most often involves oropharyngeal muscles, but all motor cranial nerves may be involved.[425,920] Miscellaneous signs include salivation and diaphoresis[1091] and testicular pain and tenderness.[690] Transient oliguric renal failure[920] and azotemia with hematuria and casts in the urinary sediment[1091] may occur (Table 14–43).

Profound hypokalemia due to the passive movement of potassium into cells is present in most cases. This may be reflected on the ECG with prominent U waves, flat or biphasic T waves, or ventricular irritability. Paralysis is reversible if potassium is replaced, usually within days, suggesting that it is due to the hypokalemia. However, depolarizing blockade of muscle or the neuromuscular junction by the combined effects of barium and hypokalemia have been suggested as alternative mechanisms.[920]

A very low serum potassium level may be the initial clue to barium intoxication. In barium toxicity, the prodromal GI symptoms are present only hours before the weakness develops (compared with the delay in weakness of GBS) and the paralysis evolves much more rapidly than in GBS. Though areflexia is characteristic of both conditions, relative preservation of deep tendon reflexes despite severe quadriplegia may occur in barium intoxication. Objective sensory loss is absent in barium intoxication, but it may also be absent early in the course of GBS. Muscle twitching, circumoral paresthesias, and dry mouth are unusual in GBS and common in barium toxicity; testicular pain and tenderness are unique to barium intoxication. The ECG may be useful when it shows changes of hypokalemia.

Metabolic Abnormalities

PERIODIC PARALYSES

The periodic paralyses are classified as (1) hypokalemic, (2) hyperkalemic, (3) normokalemic, and (4) thyrotoxic.[161] A possible hypermagnesemic periodic paralysis has been reported in a patient who also had the hyperkalemic form.[329]

Most attacks of hypokalemic periodic paralysis begin nocturnally with the patient awakening paralyzed.[161,905] A symmetric flaccid quadriplegia with depressed or absent reflexes may be present. Despite sometimes total paralysis of limbs and trunk, respiratory or cranial nerve involvement is rare. The mental status, sensory examination, and sphincters are normal during attacks. The duration of attacks varies from several hours to 8 days, but seldom exceeds 72 hours.[161] Common precipitating factors are resting after exertion and eating carbohydrate-rich meals. The disorder is inherited as an autosomal dominant trait with males more severely affected. Sporadic cases may exist.[161]

In hyperkalemic periodic paralysis, attacks are shorter and seldom cause as complete a paralysis as in the hypokalemic form. Most attacks occur during the daytime, but noctural episodes are more severe and prolonged. Weakness tends to be more pronounced in the legs. The reflexes are commonly reduced in the legs but global areflexia is uncommon. Facial and pharyngeal muscles may be affected, but respiratory failure is uncommon. Percussion myotonia may be present, and transient diplopia or blurred vision has been ascribed to myotonic phenomena in the internal and external ocular muscles. The paralysis persists for minutes to hours. As in the hypokalemic variety, rest after exertion is a common precipitating factor. The disease is autosomally dominant, with equal involvement of males and females; sporadic cases are rare.

Attacks of normokalemic periodic paralysis are similar clinically to the hypokalemic type, although this type of paralysis can last for a week before gradually improving over 1 to 2 weeks, thereby simulating GBS.[946] The disease is autosomally dominant, with equal penetrance in both sexes. Weakness usually begins in the legs, then spreading to the arms and trunk muscles. Facial, masticatory, and neck muscles can be affected, but oropharyngeal weakness and respiratory failure do not occur. Muscle stiffness is sometimes present at the onset, giving way to flaccid weakness with reduced reflexes. Myotonia does not occur. One patient developed sensory deficits in a glove-stocking distribution with attacks. Carbohydrate intake has played neither a precipitating nor a preventive role. The most common precipitating factors have been resting after exercise, sleeping late in the morning, ingesting alcohol, sitting or standing for prolonged periods, going out in cold damp weather, and enduring severe emotional stress.

The first attacks of the hyperkalemic and normokalemic periodic paralyses usually occur during the first decade but are commonly delayed to the second or later decades in the hypokalemic variety.[905] Some patients show a characteristic change in serum potassium level during most attacks, yet have no change or a paradoxical alteration in other attacks.[905] Thyrotoxic periodic paralysis is essentially indistinguishable from hypokalemic periodic paralysis, including a marked decline in serum potassium during attacks.[361,776] The risks of cardiac arrhythmias may be higher than in other types.[558,776] This disease has a predilection for males, especially Orientals.

The EMG in all periodic paralyses shows low-amplitude myopathic potentials with some polyphasic activity.[445,946] In the normokalemic variety, a few larger, long-duration polyphasic units have been seen, but the spontaneous discharges and mechanical irritability seen in the hyperkalemic type have not occurred. There are several discussions in the literature[706,1199] on interictal electrophysiologic abnormalities in the periodic paralyses.

Several features allow distinction of the periodic paralyses from GBS (Table 14–45); a past history (or family history) of similar recurrent attacks is the most persuasive. The paralysis evolves more rapidly than in typical GBS, with weakness usually maximal within hours. Even the rare "ultra-rapid" form of GBS is generally not this fulminant. The deficits resolve far more rapidly than in GBS, with improvement several hours or days after onset. Although patients with the periodic paralyses may have near-total limb paralysis, cranial

Table 14–45 DIFFERENTIATING GBS FROM PERIODIC PARALYSES

	GBS	*Periodic Paralyses*
Evolution	Days to weeks	Hours
Duration of paralysis	Weeks to months	Hours to days
Sensory loss	Common	No
Facial paresthesias type	Rare	May occur in hyperkalemic
Respiratory failure	Common	Rare
Cranial nerve involvement	Common	Rare
Masticatory weakness	Rare	May occur
Myotonia	No	Present in hyperkalemic form
Serum potassium	Normal	Usually abnormal
CSF protein	Elevated	Normal
EMG	Normal early	Myopathic features
NCV	Abnormal	Normal

nerves and respiratory muscles are usually not affected. While the reflexes are commonly depressed or absent in periodic paralyses, they may be preserved despite significant weakness. Asymmetric weakness may occur rarely in periodic paralyses,[776,946] often affecting muscles most that had been more vigorously exercised. Paresthesias and objective sensory loss—common in GBS—do not occur in periodic paralyses. Determination of serum potassium level during paralysis is usually helpful, but not always conclusive unless a baseline serum potassium value before paralysis is known. The CSF is presumably normal in the periodic paralyses. If the diagnosis is not already evident on clinical grounds, the EMG in the periodic paralyses shows myopathic features with normal nerve conduction, both unlike those of GBS.

Hypokalemic Myopathy

Profound hypokalemia (serum potassium concentration below 2 mEq/L) may produce quadriparesis, evolving over days or weeks, severe enough to mimic GBS.[108,270,449,815,1226] Hypokalemia of this degree most often occurs with diuretic therapy but may occur with use of other drugs, as well as through malabsorption, villous adenoma, hyperaldosteronism, renal tubular defects, and chronic laxative abuse.[629] The few cases brought to our attention at the MGH have occurred in young women who dieted excessively and abused diuretics. The initial diagnosis was GBS until the serum electrolyte values were known. Licorice abuse is a rare cause.[108,449] Barium salt poisoning, thallium neuropathy, and periodic paralysis (discussed in other sections of this chapter) are all associated with hypokalemia (though barium intoxication is unique in that there is no intracellular deficiency of potassium). For a discussion of the physiologic and cellular effects of hypokalemia on the neuromuscular apparatus, we refer the reader to Knochel's review.[629]

Vague, aching pains in the back and limb muscles often precede an episode of hypokalemic paralysis.[815] Weakness is generally symmetric and affects primarily axial and proximal muscles. Profound weakness of neck flexion is frequent and patients often cannot sit up from the supine position.[449,1226] Muscle tenderness may be present.[815,1226]

Several features help distinguish hypokalemic myopathy from GBS (Table 14–46). The reflexes may be normal or hypoactive but are seldom completely absent. Preservation of ankle jerks with loss of other reflexes, a pattern almost never seen in GBS, has been noted in hypokalemic myopathy.[449] Cranial nerve involvement is uncommon, al-

Table 14–46 DIFFERENTIATING GBS FROM HYPOKALEMIC MYOPATHY

	GBS	*Hypokalemic Myopathy*
Neck and trunk weakness	Only when severe	Common
Sensory loss	Common	Rare
Cranial nerve involvement	Common	Rare
Polyuria	No	Common
Reflexes	Absent	Reduced but present
Muscle tenderness	Uncommon	May occur
Bladder dysfunction	Common	Uncommon
CSF protein	High	Normal
EMG pattern	Normal or neuropathic	Myopathic
CPK	Occasional slight rise	May be elevated
ECG	Variable	Hypokalemic changes
Myoglobinuria	No	May occur
Renal abnormalities	Rare	Common
Muscle biopsy	Normal or denervation	Myopathy-vacuolar

though weakness of facial and masticatory muscles has been reported.[449] Paresthesias are rare, but objective sensory loss is not. Unlike in GBS, bladder dysfunction is rare, but bowel and bladder distension have been noted.[449] Though the CSF should be normal, an elevated protein level was found in a case referred to MGH.

Polyuria with dilute urine,[1226] secondary renal effects of hypokalemia, may occur. The ECG usually shows changes typical of hypokalemia, including prominent U waves, prolonged QT interval, prolonged QU interval, flat T waves, and ST segment depressions. Ventricular irritability may be found.

Aside from the obvious determination of greatly reduced serum potassium concentration, other laboratory features useful in making the differentiation from GBS include a usually normal CSF;[449,1226] marked elevations of serum CPK or myoglobinuria;[270,449,815] and normal NCVs, terminal latencies, and late responses. The EMG may show the low-amplitude potentials characteristic of myopathy, and muscle biopsy may show areas of muscle necrosis and vacuolar myopathy.[270,449,815,1226]

An acute ascending paralysis resembling GBS has been reported with hyperkalemia in a patient with acute renal failure.[712] However, pertinent information about other electrolytes, particularly magnesium and calcium, were not included in this report.

Hyperthyroidism

Hyperthyroidism may enter into the differential diagnosis of GBS in several ways. It may be associated with myasthenia gravis or periodic paralysis, discussed earlier. In addition, acute weakness of oropharyngeal muscles or acute limb weakness, predominantly of the legs (Basedow's paraplegia), may occur with thyrotoxicosis and can superficially simulate regional or typical GBS.

Four patients in whom myasthenia gravis was excluded[585] had dysphagia, dysphonia, and dysarthria related to hyperthyroidism. Weakness of the trapezii and sternocleidomastoids existed in most patients, as well as variable weakness of the face, jaw, and tongue. Two patients had proximal muscle weakness and one had reduced reflexes. Oropharyngeal dysfunction improved following treatment with propranolol and ultimately resolved with control of the hyperthyroidism. Other investigators reported severe, flaccid, areflexic paraparesis in a patient with thyroid storm; this report includes a review of the literature on Basedow's paraplegia.[353] Electrophysiologic tests and muscle biopsy showed evidence of a neuropathy.

Hypermagnesemia

Magnesium intoxication, by its effects at the neuromuscular junction, may produce a flaccid, areflexic paralysis resembling GBS. For detailed descriptions of the numerous other neurophysiologic actions of magnesium, we refer the reader to reviews by Chutkow[198] and Fishman.[368] Hypermagnesemia occurs most commonly with the use of magnesium-containing antacids or cathartics in patients with impaired renal function,[180] in the treatment of patients with toxemia of pregnancy with parenteral magnesium, and rarely, in otherwise normal individuals exposed to large amounts of magnesium in either antacids or cathartics. Coexisting conditions in chronic renal failure such as hyperkalemia, hypocalcemia, acidosis, hyperphosphatemia, or concomitant drug administration may allow symptoms and signs of magnesium intoxication to occur at relatively lower serum magnesium concentrations.[967]

One of the earliest symptoms is a sensation of increased warmth, often associated with visible flushing of the skin[1126,1151] (Table 14–47). Dizziness or lightheadedness, probably due to cutaneous vasodilatation and hypotension, dry mouth and thirst, and difficulty initiating micturition or defecation are

Table 14–47 DIFFERENTIATING GBS FROM HYPERMAGNESEMIA

	GBS	*Hypermagnesemia*
Respiratory failure	When limbs very weak	Before severe weakness
Ptosis	Rare	Common
Neck weakness	When severe	?Common
Internal ophthalmoplegia	Rare	Common
Dry mouth	Rare	Common
Facial flushing	Rare	Common
Hypotension	At peak of dysautonomia	Early
Objective sensory loss	Common	No
CSF protein	Raised	Normal
Tensilon test	Negative	Often positive
NCV	Abnormal	Normal
Repetitive nerve stimulation	Normal	Increment at high frequency

other early features.[967,1151] Nausea and vomiting have been reported at serum magnesium levels higher than 10 mEq/L[967] but at lower levels by others.[1126]

The earliest signs may include systolic and diastolic hypotension, orthostatic hypotension, or loss of the normal sinus arrhythmia. Flaccid, areflexic weakness appears at serum magnesium levels above 10 mEq/L, but has been reported in unusual circumstances with levels as low as 4 mEq/L. Limb weakness, initially more pronounced proximally, may become complete and affect oropharyngeal, facial, extraocular, and respiratory muscles.[1172] Early ptosis and pupillary dilatation with sluggish light responses have also been reported.[21,1126] Speech becomes dysarthric or hypophonic and respiratory failure may develop insidiously. Drowsiness, possibly due to hypotension and respiratory failure rather than to direct effects of magnesium, may begin at serum levels of 7 to 14 mEq/L, and coma occurs at higher levels. Numerous ECG abnormalities occur in magnesium intoxication.

Electrophysiologic studies in magnesium intoxication show a presynaptic disorder of neuromuscular transmission with reduced CMAP and decremental response at low rates of repetitive stimulation, and facilitation after exercise or repetitive stimulation at higher frequencies.[965,1172]

In contrast to patients with GBS, magnesium intoxication does not cause sensory symptoms or signs, aside from the aforementioned frequent flushing or warm sensation (Table 14–46). Dry mouth, facial flushing, ptosis, pupillary abnormalities, early hypotension, and ECG changes should suggest hypermagnesemia. Improvement in strength following edrophonium injection is also consistent with intoxication, as the defect appears to be at the neuromuscular junction. EMG with repetitive nerve stimulation therefore may confirm the diagnosis. CSF and nerve conduction studies are normal unless they are affected by coexisting disease (eg, uremia).

Hypophosphatemia

Severe hypophosphatemia may produce acute flaccid, areflexic paralysis with respiratory and cranial nerve paralysis—a syndrome that mimicks GBS[386,526,847,1265] (Table 14–48). The mechanism of weakness is probably reduction of high-energy phosphate stores. (For a review of the cellular pathophysiologic mechanisms of hypophosphatemia, see Knochel's review.[628]) Neurologic manifestations occur with serum inorganic phosphate levels below 1 mg/dL (usually 0.2 to 0.5 mg/dL). The most common clinical situations resulting in hypophosphatemia are paren-

Table 14–48 DIFFERENTIATING GBS FROM HYPOPHOSPHATEMIA

	GBS	*Hypophosphatemia*
Rapidity of evolution	1–3 wk	Days
Respiratory failure	With severe limb weakness	Early
Ptosis	Rare	?Common
Neck weakness	When severe	?Common
Facial paresthesias	Rare	Common
Nystagmus	Rare	May occur
Gaze paresis	Rare	May occur
CSF protein	Raised	Usually normal
NCV	Abnormal	Usually normal
Clinical setting	Varied	Highly selected: hyperalimentation, refeeding, alcohol, ketoacidosis, postburn diuresis, respiratory alkalosis, antacid use

teral hyperalimentation, large glucose loads after starvation, and acute alcohol intake. Other potential factors include use of phosphate-binding antacids, postburn diuresis, diabetic ketoacidosis, and prolonged severe respiratory alkalosis.

Paresthesias, usually the first symptom of acute hypophosphatemia, typically involve the hands and feet but also may be perioral[386,526] or periorbital.[1103] There may be prominent objective sensory loss.[386,1103] Areflexic limb weakness, often more pronounced proximally, evolves rapidly over 24 to 48 hours or less. Ptosis and weakness of the oropharynx and neck muscles are often prominent.[386] Respiratory failure may appear precipitiously, often with only moderate limb weakness.[847]

Additional features, noted less frequently, have included ataxia and tremor, gaze paresis, nystagmus, and bilateral abducens paresis,[1103] sometimes suggesting Wernicke's encephalopathy (Table 14–48). Seizures and coma have been reported but concomitant electrolyte and acid-base disturbances may play a role. Phosphate repletion produces improvement in limb power and other symptoms within hours,[847] days,[526] or, rarely, weeks.[386,1265]

The CSF is usually normal, but mildly elevated protein levels (perhaps unrelated) have been reported.[386,1265] Nerve conduction studies may be normal,[386] but at least one patient had reduced motor NCVs that improved during recovery.[847] The EMG shows few if any abnormalities. One study found minor neurogenic changes in a muscle biopsy.[386]

Differentiation from GBS is not difficult if the physician recognizes the clinical setting and measures the serum organic phosphate concentration. Rapid evolution, facial paresthesias, ptosis, nystagmus, gaze paresis, and early respiratory failure suggest hypophosphatemia rather than GBS.

Critical Illness Polyneuropathy (CIP)

An axonal polyneuropathy of yet-unknown etiology may complicate critical illness, most often in patients who are intubated and having sepsis and multiple organ failure.[118,119,1315] It is often first recognized by failure of ventilatory weaning. Muscle weakness and wasting with reduced or absent tendon reflexes are found in most patients. Mild facial weakness may occur but muscles innervated by other cranial nerves are typically spared. Glove-stocking distribution loss of all sensory modalities may occur, but autonomic dysfunction has not been evident.

Electrophysiologic studies consistently reveal attenuated compound muscle and sensory nerve action potential amplitudes and widespread denervation on needle EMG. Motor and sensory NCVs, distal latencies, and F-wave latencies are usually normal or nearly normal. Conduction block and temporal dispersion are not seen. Repetitive stimulation reveals no evidence of a defect in neuromuscular transmission. Diaphragmatic responses to phrenic nerve stimulation may be absent. Needle EMG shows fibrillations and positive waves, and often myotonic or other complex repetitive discharges. With recovery over several months there is an increase in the amplitudes of the compound muscle and nerve action potentials. EMG shows the appearance of numerous polyphasic motor unit potentials, consistent with reinnervation.

Autopsy studies show widespread primary axonal degeneration of motor and sensory fibers, with extensive denervation atrophy of limb and respiratory muscles. Neither inflammatory changes nor segmental demyelination are seen.

Differentiation from GBS may be difficult, particularly in those with global areflexia (Table 14–49). Bacterial sepsis is most often associated with CIP, whereas GBS is more often preceded by a viral syndrome, surgery, or vaccination. The CSF protein level is usually normal or only minimally elevated in CIP, compared with the more striking elevations seen in GBS. Whereas most patients with GBS have slowing of motor NCVs, prolongation of distal latencies, prolonged-latency or absent F waves, and temporal dispersion, such parameters are usually normal or nearly normal in CIP. The hallmark of CIP, a reduction in the amplitudes of the CMAP and sensory nerve action potential (SNAP), may be seen also in GBS patients. In CIP, widespread denervation is evident on needle EMG, with fibrillations, positive waves, and complex repetitive discharges—features rarely seen in early GBS. Conduction block, commonly found in GBS, is not seen in CIP.

Hysteria

Early GBS is commonly misdiagnosed as anxiety or hysteria. In assembling the MGH retrospective series we encountered a number of patients who had been discharged from emergency rooms before the correct diagnosis was made. In many, the clinical impression was hysteria, anxiety, hyperventilation syndrome, or other functional illness. One scenario is a young person who comes to the emergency room complaining of weakness and paresthesias in the limbs. When sensory examination is found to be normal and no objec-

Table 14–49 DIFFERENTIATING GBS FROM CRITICAL ILLNESS POLYNEUROPATHY

	GBS	*CIP*
Antecedent illness	Viral syndrome, surgery, vaccination, etc.	Bacterial sepsis, ICU, intubation, multiple organ failure
Cranial nerve dysfunction	Common	Rare (face may be weak)
DTRs	Absent	Variably reduced or absent
CSF	High protein	Normal or slightly elevated
NCV	Slow, may be normal early	Near normal
Distal latencies	Prolonged	Near normal
F-wave latency	Prolonged or absent	Near normal
CMAP amplitude	Normal*	Consistently reduced
SNAP amplitude	May be reduced	Consistently reduced
Temporal dispersion	Often	Not seen
Conduction block	Often	Not seen
Denervation on EMG	Late if at all	Common, early
Spontaneous EMG activity	Uncommon	Myotonic or complex repetitive discharges

*May be reduced if conduction block or temporal dispersion present.

tive weakness can be demonstrated, the patient is often asked if there has been a recent spat with a spouse, boyfriend, or girlfriend (to which many answer "yes"), and is then sent home with a diagnosis of a functional disorder—only to return later with generalized weakness. Even experienced clinicians may mistake true weakness for the "give-way" weakness usually seen in functional disorders. Hoover's sign may be useful in diagnosing patients with functional hemiparesis, but not patients with bilateral leg weakness. Although weakness and objective sensory loss truly may be undetectable in the first days of GBS, hyporeflexia, areflexia, or a sinus tachycardia are clues to the early diagnosis of GBS. The tendon reflexes initially may feel, to the examiner, as if they are slightly delayed. It is rare for GBS patients to progress from normal strength to quadriplegia and respiratory failure over 24 hours; however, it is sometimes advisable to admit patients with suggestive symptoms but no objective signs for observation, or alternatively to arrange for follow-up the next day by phone.

Part V

TREATMENT AND REHABILITATION

Chapter 15

SPECIFIC TREATMENTS

Plasma Exchange
Corticosteroids
Other Immunomodulating Treatments

PLASMA EXCHANGE

Brettle and coworkers[141] have been credited with the first report of an apparently beneficial effect of plasma exchange in acute GBS. Many anecdotal reports followed, both in adults* and in children.[607,1108,1155a,1308] A patient with renal failure and apparent improvement in GBS after hemodialysis has also been reported.[1236] Several large randomized trials have demonstrated a shortened length of illness, and other improvements as measured by a number of criteria, but at least one smaller study has shown no benefit.[442] The Guillain-Barré Study Group, organized by Dr. Guy McKhann at Johns Hopkins University, conducted an open, nonsham, randomized trial in 245 patients from 13 North American centers, including the Massachusetts General Hospital (MGH), between 1980 and 1984.[469] A six-point functional grading scale devised by Hughes and associates[547] was adopted for the study (Table 15–1), using strict clinical criteria for entry to the trial. Plasma exchange volumes totaled 200 to 250 mL/kg, in 3 to 5 treatments, over 7 to 14 days, beginning within 30 days from the onset of illness. The number of patients who had improved at 1 month was greater in the treated group (59%) than in the control group (39%), and the time for patients to improve one grade was reduced (19 versus 40 days, median) (Table 15–2). The treated subgroup on ventilators did similarly better (50% versus 35% one grade improvement at 1 month; 24 versus 48 days median to improve one grade). The median time to reach grade 2 (the point at which patients were able to walk unassisted) was most dramatically reduced by treatment from 85 to 53 days. Deaths, serious complications, and relapses were similar among groups, and the patient groups had similar overall outcomes at 6 months.

In a smaller Swedish study of 38 patients,[886] muscular weakness, measured by the sum of power (0 to 5 scale) in seven muscles, improved more rapidly, and to a greater extent at 1 month. This trial used 6 kilograms of plasma exchanged in five or more sessions, with an intermittent flow system.

A similar third trial, performed by a French Cooperative Group,[380] in 220 patients treated within 17 days of onset with four exchanges of 2 plasma volumes each, showed an improvement in

*See references 6, 216, 261, 302, 304, 364, 451, 604, 883, 1018, 1035, 1074, 1214, and 1215.

Table 15–1 DISABILITY SCALE USED IN MAJOR TREATMENT TRIALS*†

0	No symptoms
1	Minor signs or symptoms
2	Able to walk 15 ft (5 m) without support but incapable of manual work
3	Able to walk 15 ft (5 m) only with a cane, appliance, or support
4	Bed- or chair-bound
5	Requiring assisted ventilation
6	Dead

*A variant of this scale devised by Hughes et al.,[547] has been used in the Guillain-Barré Syndrome Study Group Plasma Exchange Trial and other clinical trials.[469]

†Adapted from Hughes et al.,[547] p. 751.

Table 15–2 PLASMA EXCHANGE TRIALS IN GBS

NORTH AMERICAN STUDY[469]	*Plasma Exchange (N=122)*	*Conventional (N=123)*
Days to reach grade 2 (median)*	53	85
Days to improve one grade (median)*	19	40
Percentage of patients improved at least 1 grade		
At 1 mo*	59%	39%
At 6 mo*	97%	87%
Percentage of patients walking independently, 6 mo*	82%	71%
Mortality (no. of patients)	3	4
SWEDISH STUDY[886]	***N=20***	***N=18***
Days to improvement in limb weakness* (mean)	8.5	17.1
No. of patients improved 2 grades or more, 1 mo*	12	4
No. of patients improved 3 grades or more, 2 mo*	12	5
Mortality (no. of patients)	1	1
FRENCH STUDY[380]	***N=111***	***N=109***
Days to onset motor recovery (median)*	6	13
Days to weaning (median)*	18	31
Days to recover walking without assistance (median)*	70	111
Mortality (no. of patients)	7	7
BRITISH STUDY[442]	***N=14***	***N=15***
No. of patients, improved 1 grade or more, 1 mo	7	6
Full recovery, 1 yr	4	4
Walking independently	7	5
Mortality (no. of patients)	2	4

*Statistically significant difference from conventional therapy.

the treated group, particularly in the onset of recovery, the time to unassisted walking, and the duration of mechanical ventilation (see Table 15–2). This trial focused on the differences between replacement fluids, comparing fresh frozen plasma (FFP) to albumin with saline. Of the 52 patients in the group treated with FFP, 5 got hepatitis and more untoward incidents occurred during exchanges, but neurological outcome was not better than in the group treated with albumin and saline.

None of the large cooperative trials of plasma exchange have been blinded or used sham exchanges. This fact, among other potential flaws in these studies, has been extensively editorialized.[308] The authors of the North American trial recognized some of these potential shortcomings and had data collected by an individual not involved with patient care. In addition, post hoc analysis showed that vital capacities were similar at the time of initiation and cessation of mechanical ventilation between the two groups, suggesting that investigator bias had little effect. (At the final data meeting of that trial, before the results were known, a straw poll indicated that only 2 of 30 investigators thought from their anecdotal experience that the treatment had worked.)

Two British trials that failed to demonstrate benefit from plasma exchange[442,832] may have simply been too small to detect an effect (see Table 15–2). One trial[832] is of interest despite negative results because it used "intensive" exchanges, 10 treatments over 15 days in 7 patients, without complications. In another trial, the addition of steroids to plasma exchange showed no effect compared with no-treatment within 4 weeks of onset of illness.[793] Prednisone 100 mg/d for 1 week was followed by the same dose on alternate days for 2 weeks, and subsequent reduction over 3 weeks. Only 12 patients were treated and compared with 13 control subjects, a number probably too small to support firmly the conclusion offered that steroids were ineffective or negated the beneficial effect of plasma exchange.

The temporal course of recovery in patients who respond to plasma exchange is variable, as reviewed in Chapter 10. Rare patients have a marked but transient improvement in power within hours of each exchange. A larger number, though not the majority, improve and continue gaining strength over several days, too quickly to be due to remyelination. In others, the improvement is apparent only by comparison to control groups, and the remaining patients probably do not respond to treatment at all. There is no evidence that plasma exchange results in chronic or chronic-relapsing polyneuropathy. An unusual short-term relapsing course occurs in approximately 10% of treated patients,[884,885,1011] perhaps related to a rebound in antibody concentration[1238] (see Chapter 10 and Fig. 10–2). In exceptional cases the relapse is worse than the initial illness and requires the institution of mechanical ventilation; the majority of relapses are milder. Most patients with limited relapses benefit from another course of exchanges.[1011]

The precise regimen of plasma exchange that is most effective has not been established, but most investigators have used approximately 150 to 250 mL/kg of total plasma removed over 7 to 10 days (larger volumes than typically used to treat myasthenia gravis and other illnesses). Exchanges of less than 3 to 3.5 L each have been less effective. Gammaglobulin supplementation (ostensibly to prevent infection) has generally not been used since the North American and Swedish trials showed similar benefit of plasma exchange without it (see farther on). FFP, initially believed to give superior results to albumin-saline as a replacement fluid,[1097] has not been shown to be useful and has greater risks for transmitting viral infection.[127,380,550] The albumin-saline replacement fluid is therefore currently preferred because of its simplicity and cost.

There is evidence that patients who begin treatment too late have worse outcomes; instituting therapy in a group of patients more than 2 weeks after the onset of illness has had limited effect.[469] The use of continuous flow machines has been associated (tentatively) with better results than use of intermittent flow machines.[780] The most powerful predictor of poor outcome in the North American trial was the presence of compound muscle action potentials (CMAPs) less than 20% of normal with distal stimulation,[222,780] but plasma exchange was still beneficial in this poor-prognosis group (see Chapters 13 and 18).

The large trials included only patients who were unable to walk unaided within a predetermined time, 2 to 4 weeks from the onset of illness. This, coupled with evidence that beginning exchanges earlier is beneficial, creates a dilemma about the proper timing of exchanges in patients who are still able to walk but are deteriorating toward the end of the second week of illness. Similarly, patients who are unable to walk because of ataxia or who have Fisher's syndrome have not yet been shown, as a group, to benefit from plasma exchange, although anecdotes suggest they do.[401,452,557] Our practice has been to institute exchanges if it appears that the patient is worsening and will be unable to return home within 2 weeks, approximately the time it would take to complete a course of exchanges. Therefore, only patients with the mildest cases and with a brief period of progression would not receive plasma exchanges. At the time of this writing, plasma exchange is considered the initial therapy of choice in those with acute GBS, if it can be performed safely and consistently.

Comparisons between groups in the several large trials and series favored treatment largely because the complication rates were low. There tend to be more frequent episodes of hypotension in treated patients, not always coincident with the exchange. These usually respond to fluid infusion. The risks of exchanging patients with severe cardiovascular dysautonomia are excessive. Theoretical risks of exchange in other patients include an increased infection rate because of hypoglobulinemia, bleeding (urinary, nasal, gastrointestinal) from hypoprothrombinemia,[601] cardiac arrhythmias or myocardial infarction from the stress of the procedure. None of these has occurred more frequently in treated patients in large series, but individual cases of hematuria, epistaxis, or disseminated herpes zoster have been reported or are anecdotal. Hepatitis, and perhaps acquired immunodeficiency syndrome (AIDS) are risks only if plasma is used as a replacement fluid.[127] Otherwise, patients can be told with confidence that plasma exchange does not expose them to these viruses. Mortality has been similar in both arms of the major plasma exchange studies (see Table 15–2) (approximately 3% to 7% overall in most series), but more than 40 deaths directly associated with plasma exchange in other disorders have been reported.[539] Plasma exchange has been performed safely in children[607,1308] (see Chapter 9) and without complications in several pregnant patients,[334] but safety is probably predicated on the availability of an experienced team. Patients with poor venous access require temporary femoral vein catheters, or more sustained subclavian catheters. The risk is reduced if only experienced physicians insert and care for these lines.

Relative contraindications to plasma exchange include hepatic failure (where citrate toxicity is a risk), severe electrolyte abnormalities that have been associated with arrhythmias, the use of drugs that require constant serum concentrations (antibiotic therapy is not usually a contraindication), or active bleeding.[1099] Hypotension that cannot be quickly remedied by fluid replacement, recent myocardial infarction (within 6 months) or suspicion of myocardial infarction, or severe hepatic or renal failure are serious contraindications to treatment. Alternative treatment or no active therapy may be more prudent in these cases.

The rationale for plasma exchange in GBS patients has been the presence of pathogenetically important circulating agents—probably antibodies; alternatively, the immune reaction in nerves may be modified in some other way that ultimately reduces peripheral nerve damage (see Chapter 5 for a discussion of immunologic features of GBS pertinent to plasma exchange). Plasma exchange has also improved the clinical deficit and pathologic lesions in experimental allergic neuritis (EAN) in a controlled trial[450] and in uncontrolled experiments.[32]

CORTICOSTEROIDS

Various corticosteroids have been used to treat GBS on the premise that the inflammatory response in GBS would subside. Stillman and Ganong's first report[1154] of the apparently successful use of adreno corticotropic hormone (ACTH) and cortisone to treat GBS was followed by numerous anecdotal reports and reviews. Early influential reviews[507,560] (of almost 200 patients) suggested that outcome was improved with treatment. In a subsequent retrospective, uncontrolled series of 687 patients,[179] steroids were thought to be beneficial in those with acute GBS. All of these analyses were based on clinically heterogeneous cases and various regimens of steroid administration.[116,435,844] In contrast, many others either failed to find benefit in small series or expressed an opinion that they were of no value.* One study, a harbinger of more recent trials,[418] suggested steroids were detrimental and prolonged the illness in 37 patients. The authors of most recent, retrospective, large, personally collected series have tentatively concluded that

*See references 322, 934, 1053, 1055, and 1100.

†See references 418, 714, 973, 1053, and 1278.

steroids or ACTH were of no value in shortening the course of the illness or reducing residual neurologic deficits.†

In a prospective, randomized trial to settle this issue, Hughes and colleagues[547] treated 21 patients with 60 mg of prednisolone daily for 1 week, 40 milligrams for 4 days, and 30 milligrams for 3 days, compared with 19 untreated control patients (Table 15–3). They failed to demonstrate a benefit of treatment using a six-point clinical scale (see Table 15–1). Three months after entry, the treated group was slightly worse off, particularly patients who had been randomized within a week of onset. In addition, 17 of 19 patients in the untreated group were virtually asymptomatic at one year, compared with 15 of 21 who were treated. Three patients among those treated with prednisolone had relapses during the first year, whereas no relapses occurred in the control group. This study has been criticized because of its small size, which did not preclude a type II error; slightly different entry times into the study between the groups; and the generally mild disease among the subjects, among other points. The trial has added to the controversy over steroids by suggesting, as had some previous studies,[418] that they may be deleterious. Nevertheless, this study remains the best trial of corticosteroids to date, and the functional grading system devised for it was an important contribution to subsequent trials.

Table 15–3 MAJOR ENDPOINTS IN STEROID TRIAL*

	Prednisolone (N=21)	***Control (N=19)***
Days to onset improvement (median)	8	10
No. of patients grade 2 or worse, 1 yr	7	1
No. of patients with relapses, 1 yr (no significant difference between groups)	3	0

*Adapted from Hughes et al.,[547] p. 752.

A smaller, blinded, randomized trial of corticotropin (ACTH), 100 U intramuscularly for 10 days, in 9 patients, compared with 7 control subjects,[1171] showed a reduction in mean time to recovery from 9.0 to 4.4 months but no difference in the duration of hospitalization. Patients with respiratory failure were excluded from the trial. An analysis of patients treated with steroids (of varying type) outside the trial, but during the same period, produced the same results. The interval between the onset of illness and initiation of steroids had no effect on the duration of illness. There were three deaths, all in corticotropin- or steroid-treated patients.

The generally discouraging or uncertain results of recent trials using conventional anti-inflammatory doses of steroids is balanced by a provocative anecdotal observation[285] of marked and rapid improvement (within 4 days) in 3 of 5 patients treated with high doses of steroids (125 mg intravenously of methylprednisolone every 6 hours for 24 to 48 hours followed by slowly reduced doses of orally administered prednisone). Improvement with these high doses is consistent with the observations of some other clinicians. Treatment with 500 to 1000 milligrams of methylprednisolone daily within 14 days of the onset of illness was associated with marked improvement in 8 of 11 patients (without the benefit of a control group).[472] Premature reductions in steroid dose led to clinical deterioration, which, like the limited relapses seen after premature cessation of plasma exchange, suggests some biologic effect. On occasion, a remarkable and prompt improvement has been seen in deteriorating patients within 12 or 24 hours of the institution of high-dose steroid therapy.

On the other hand, numerous patients have developed GBS while receiving steroids for other illnesses, particularly asthma; while receiving other immunosuppressive drugs;[167,433,626] or while suffering from Cushing's syndrome.[140] Six patients in the MGH experience were receiving steroids in varying doses at the onset of GBS, including one patient receiving high-dose steroids for asthma. This finding, of course, does not discount the possibility that steroids are beneficial, but it demonstrates that they do not prevent GBS by pretreatment.

A trial to determine if steroids (100 mg oral prednisone for 10 days) are useful as a supplement to plasma exchanges demonstrated no difference between 12 patients treated with both modalities and 13 untreated patients.[793] The authors suggested that a deleterious effect of steroids may have obscured the anticipated beneficial effects of plasma exchange, but the trial may have been too small to demonstrate a difference between groups (even from plasma exchange alone). In contrast, a Japanese trial[821] claimed a significant benefit of high-dose methylprednisolone (500 to 1000 milligrams for 3 days) with plasma exchange over high-dose steroids alone.

At this time, there is no evidence that conventional doses of corticosteroids (in the range of 60 mg of prednisone daily) are effective in shortening the course of, or reducing residual deficits in, acute GBS. Neither can it be definitively stated that steroids or corticotropin are ineffective. This uncertainty is particularly evident in comparing the small sizes of the major randomized trials of steroids. (Approximately as many patients were entered into Hughes' trial of plasma exchange that also found no effect, as participated in the United Kingdom steroid trial.) The magnitude of the steroid effect may therefore require a large trial, or large doses, to be detected. Also, any beneficial effect of corticosteroids, particularly high-dose treatment, must be considered in the context of potential complications. Serious infection and bowel perforation (particularly dangerous risks) may have a higher incidence in debilitated bedbound and respirator-dependent patients. Nevertheless, the ease of administration of corticosteroids and their lesser cost compared with plasma exchange still make them an attractive alternative treatment, should they prove beneficial in appropriate trials. Categoric statements that corticosteroids are contraindicated in GBS[1062] may be too severe, but the absence of convincing benefit from conventional doses makes their routine use in acute GBS unappealing. High-dose steroids are perhaps currently best used in patients who cannot tolerate plasma exchange—for example, because of severe cardiovascular dysautonomia—or when this treatment is unavailable. Hughes and colleagues are conducting a British trial of high-dose steroids, with or without plasma exchange. The initial experience with methylprednisolone 500 milligrams daily for 5 days has been encouraging and without side effects, but results of the completed trial will be necessary before this aggressive therapy can be recommended for routine use.

OTHER IMMUNOMODULATING TREATMENTS

In keeping with the current concept of an immune mechanism in acute GBS, several investigators have examined immunomodulating treatments other than steroids and plasma exchange. All of these are currently investigational, and the results of treatment remain largely anecdotal. Most of the therapies discussed farther on are used successfully in chronic-relapsing polyneuropathy (see Chapter 10), but the sections that follow pertain to acute GBS.

Azathioprine (Imuran)

Two reports[182,1311] have appeared of the beneficial effects of azathioprine in acute GBS that was refractory to corticosteroid treatment. Five patients with severe quadriparesis improved within 2 weeks of beginning azathioprine, and all had good recoveries despite widespread denervation and slowed nerve conduction velocities (NCVs).[1311] One patient had a relapse after a reduction in the daily azathioprine dosage to 50 milligrams, and again improved after the original dosage of 200 milligrams daily was reinstituted. In the other patients, azathioprine treatment was stopped without subsequent deterioration. One patient had reversible thrombocytopenia and another, dyspepsia, but none had serious or long-lasting side effects of the drug. Azathioprine can be administered orally in a 3 mg/kg single or divided daily dosage. The dosage is usually titrated to cause a reduction in white blood cell (WBC) count (not lower than 1500 to 2000 mm^3). It usually takes 10 to 30 days to cause leukopenia, and 1 to 12 weeks for clinical improvement to occur. Frequent complete blood counts (CBCs) and liver function tests are recommended. Other potential hazards include an increased rate of future lymphoma and an increased susceptibility to infection.

Cyclophosphamide (Cytoxan)

Cyclophosphamide reversed clinical signs and improved the histopathologic appearance of peripheral nerves 1 to 5 days after the onset of paralysis in rats with EAN.[900] This prompted investigations of the effect of intravenous cyclophosphamide 40 mg/kg in 3 or 4 doses, at daily intervals, in severe GBS.[1024] In 15 patients, 22 courses of treatment resulted in stabilization in 13 patients an average of 4 days after beginning treatment. The overall outcome (3 dead, 6 complete recoveries, and 6 severely disabled), however, was no better than expected in conventionally treated patients. Therefore, it did not appear from this preliminary series that a controlled trial was warranted. Side effects—including transient leukopenia, hematuria, and alopecia—occurred in half of patients.

β-Mercaptopurine

A patient with acute GBS treated with β-mercaptopurine had an apparently striking benefit,[896] but enthusiasm was tempered after two subsequent reports[210,388] did not reproduce these results. In both of the latter patients therapy with steroid had failed, and mercaptopurine treatment was begun approximately 1 month after onset. They remained clinically unchanged for 2 months and 6 weeks, respectively. Leukopenia may have caused premature discontinuation of treatment.

Polyunsaturated Fatty Acid Diet

Polyunsaturated fatty acids (PUFAs) inhibit in vitro lymphocyte function (phytohemagglutinin-stimulated transformation and lymphocyte-antigen interaction). Moreover, a PUFA-deficient diet makes animals susceptible to experimental allergic encephalomyelitis, and dietary supplementation appears to be protective. A provocative report[129] claimed virtually complete recovery in two children who were severely disabled after typical GBS for 6 and 12 months. Improvement began after 1 week in both patients, despite EMGs showing considerable slowing of motor NCV and axonal degeneration in one patient. No relapse occurred in one patient after the diet was stopped for 1 year. The timing of treatment makes it unlikely that PUFA had a beneficial effect on the inflammatory demyelination of the acute disease.

Immunoglobulin Treatment

Immunoglobulin therapy with large quantities of human IgG has been used for many years to treat a variety of diseases such as autoimmune thrombocytopenia.[845] The availability of safe intravenous immunoglobulin preparations (IVIG) in the past several years has led to several encouraging reports of IVIG treatment of chronic inflammatory demyelinating polyneuropathy (CIDP). In CIDP, 100 milliliters of FFP per kilogram for 5 to 7 days, or 0.4 g/kg of gammaglobulin infusion daily, for several consecutive days has been recommended[13,339,734,765a,1090a,1233] (details are described in Chapter 10). A preliminary uncontrolled trial of IVIG treatment in 8 patients with severe acute GBS (4 who had plasma infusion) claimed improvement from the treatments.[624] Two patients who deteriorated after an initial improvement from plasma exchange improved again after IVIG or plasma infusion.

Most previous attention concerning immunoglobulin therapy in acute GBS has been directed at differences between replacement fluids for plasma exchange. Preliminary results suggested that FFP might be more effective than albumin as a replacement fluid in the treatment of GBS,[1097] but in a small, randomized trial of 21 patients it was concluded that replacement during exchange was not a critical factor.[550] As discussed earlier, a larger comparative trial[380] found no significant difference in outcome between the group that received albumin and the group that received FFP. Fresh frozen plasma also had important disadvantages, causing nonicteric hepatitis in 10% of patients, and bradycardia, sometimes severe enough to require a temporary pacemaker. Because both groups received gammaglobulin to prevent infection, however, no definite conclusion about the effects of immunoglobulin administration could be made.

The potential advantages of IVIG over plasmapheresis in GBS are its simplicity of administration and its slightly lesser cost. Reactions (hypotension, facial flushing, headache, muscle cramps, fever, and nausea) tend to be mild, occur early, and are generally related to the rate of infusion. Slowing or stopping the infusion for approximately 30 minutes usually allows IVIG administration to resume at a higher rate. Anaphylaxis seldom occurs but is a risk in rare patients who are deficient in IgA. Because IVIG is prepared by pooling plasma from several thousand donors, transmission of viral infections, including AIDS, is an important concern. All commercial plasma collected for IVIG preparation is routinely tested for the human immunodeficiency virus (HIV) antibody in most countries and no transmission has yet been reported during administration for hematologic disorders. Outbreaks of hepatitis B and non-A, non-B hepatitis have been traced to immunoglobulin administration, resulting in severe postnecrotic cirrhosis and chronic active hepatitis in a few patients.[1262] In one study,[1233] 2 of 17 patients with chronic-relapsing GBS developed a benign hepatitis. These risks make this encouraging form of therapy appealing only in controlled trials, with safe, intensely screened donor pools. At this time, IVIG infusion in acute GBS is being compared with plasmapheresis in a Dutch multicenter trial.

Plasma exchange has become the first resort in the treatment of acute GBS because of several large randomized trials validating its consistent effectiveness. The exchanges are cumbersome, expensive, and not applicable to patients with dysautonomia. High-dose steroids, gammaglobulin, or other immunomodulating treatments are promising alternatives under investigation.

Chapter 16

GENERAL CARE

The management of GBS requires special expertise in medical and intensive care, and the patience to be sensitive to the small daily needs of these patients and their families. The neurologist who plans to deal comprehensively with these patients must be familiar with therapy for infections, nutrition, fluid management, and selected aspects of pulmonary medicine. These skills contribute as much, or more, to the overall outcome of an individual patient's condition as do specific anti-inflammatory therapies discussed in Chapter 15. Nursing and psychologic features also constitute a considerable portion of the care required when these patients become seriously ill. In this chapter we discuss the overall management of GBS and provide guidelines for the physician. An overall plan for surveillance and treatment is shown in Table 16–1; more specific criteria for admission to the intensive care unit (ICU) and the details of ICU care is shown in Tables 16–2 and 16–3.

GENERAL MEDICAL MANAGEMENT

Infection Surveillance and Nosocomial Infections

Immobilized patients, especially in an ICU setting, are at high risk of acquiring nosocomial infections. Cross-infection and cross-colonization are often unavoidable but can be minimized by careful surveillance and selective treat-

Table 16–1 SUMMARY OF SURVEILLANCE AND APPROACH TO TREATMENT IN THE ACUTE STAGES OF GBS

Severity of Illness	***Surveillance***	***Treatment***
Mild • Able to walk • VC >25 mL/kg • No cardiovascular dysautonomia	• VC and MIF daily • Weekly infection surveillance: CBC, CXR, U/A • Baseline arterial blood gas	• Observe; treat with plasma exchange if still worsening toward end of second week of symptoms • Active physical therapy exercises as tolerated
Moderate • Unable to walk, but lifts limbs from bed or chair • VC 15–25 mL/kg • Mild or no dysautonomia • Oropharyngeal weakness but swallows safely	• VC every 6–12 h (allow sleep) • Biweekly infection surveillance and blood gas • Move to ICU if deteriorating (see Table 16–2)	• Begin plasma exchange (? or high-dose steroids) • Incentive spirometry • Passive physical therapy
Severe • Unable to lift limbs • VC <15 mL/kg or on ventilator • Aspiration risk • Blood pressure fluctuations	• ICU care (see Table 16–3) • VC q 3–6 h if not intubated • Alternate day infection surveillance and blood gas, or as determined by acuity	• Plasma exchange if hemodynamically stable (? or high-dose steroids) • Passive physical therapy and splinting (see Table 16–3)

Table 16–2 CRITERIA FOR ADMITTING GBS PATIENTS TO ICU*

Deteriorating VC <18–20 mL/kg; signs of diaphragmatic fatigue (see Chapter 17)
Poor cough, accumulating secretions, aspiration pneumonia
Progressive weakness associated with difficulty swallowing
Major dysautonomic features (wide blood pressure and pulse fluctuations; arrhythmias, heart block, pulmonary edema, profound ileus with risk of visceral rupture)
Hypotension precipitated by plasma exchange, or plasma exchange planned in a ventilated or unstable patient
Secondary sepsis
Chest pain

*Neurology—Neurosurgery ICU, Massachusetts General Hospital.

Table 16–4 MEDICAL COMPLICATIONS IN MGH SERIES

	No. of Patients (%)	
	Retrospective Series, N=169	***Prospective Series, N=120***
Pneumonia*	46 (27)	24 (22)
Urinary tract infection†	38 (22)	15 (14)
Hyponatremia‡	12 (7)	29 (26)
Gastrointestinal bleeding	13 (8)	2 (2)
Pulmonary embolism	6 (4)	2 (2)
Sepsis	1 (0)	2 (2)
Tracheal stenosis	5 (3)	1 (1)
Hypercalcemia	0	2 (2)
Pneumothorax	2 (1)	6 (1)
(Miscellaneous, one each: tracheo-esophageal fistula; bowel and urethral obstruction)		

*2–16 days of occurrence of complication, from first day of illness (mean, 8.3 days).
†5–75 days (mean, 24.3 days).
‡0–31 days (mean, 13.5 days).

ment. The most common infections in the MGH series included respiratory infections (pneumonia and tracheobronchitis), urinary tract infections, and, less commonly, sepsis (Table 16–4).

Table 16–3 GUIDELINES IN THE GENERAL INTENSIVE CARE TREATMENT OF GBS

Measure vital capacity as indicated by rapidity of deterioration:
  VC 12–15 mL/kg: intubate
  VC 15–18 mL/kg: intubate if bulbar paralysis (see Chapter 17)
Incentive spirometry to prevent atelectasis
Bronchial clearing and assisted coughing
Chest x-ray examination weekly, or more often
Biweekly serum albumin, sodium, BUN, calcium measurements
Urinalysis weekly
Pulmonary embolism prophylaxis: 5000 U heparin every 12 hours subcutaneously
Peristalsis checked
GI bleeding prophylaxis: magnesium-containing antacid 30–120 mL or sucralfate
Decubitus prophylaxis: frequent position changes; air-floating bed or water mattress and skin care
No antibiotic prophylaxis; urine and pulmonary infections treated with antibiotics after bacterial sensitivities available, unless septic
Tube feeding when swallowing is impaired (start with continously administered fiber-enriched mixtures)
Inquiries daily concerning pain, sleep, and hallucinosis; administration of adequate pain treatment
Limitation of antecubital phlebotomy if plasma exchange anticipated

Urinary infections tended to occur later, on average, than pulmonary infections. More than half of nosocomial infections are caused by organisms that can be cultured from the patient at the time of admission to the ICU.[567] The most important measures that reduce the frequency of these infections are conscientious and frequent handwashing,[17] proper management of urinary catheterization,[931,1139,1257] and disinfection and sterilization of ventilatory equipment, especially nebulizers.[1104]

Respiratory Tract Infections

Nosocomial respiratory tract infections are common in GBS, resulting from organisms of mixed oral flora and anaerobic aspirations.[82,868,1013,1051] Sputum should be collected weekly or more often for culture and Gram's stain in intubated patients, but the results must be interpreted with caution, since most patients have colonized their oropharynx with gram-negative bacteria or staphylococcus aureus after 3 to 5 days in the ICU. Prophylactic antibiotics probably do not prevent pneumonia and only increase the emergence of resistant organisms.[1139]

Aspiration pneumonia that follows intubation may be treated with the combination of a cephalosporin and aminoglycoside, for 5 to 7 days. There is no evidence that the potential neuromuscular blockade caused by aminoglycosides has a clinically detrimental effect in GBS. Other nosocomial pneumonias may be treated with a similar regimen or, if recent surveillance cultures demonstrate an organism that is insensitive to these antibiotics, more specific therapy should be chosen.

Soft polyvinylchloride endotracheal tubes with low-pressure, high volume cuffs obviate the need for early tracheostomy. The optimal timing of intubation, tracheostomy, and their complications in GBS will be discussed in Chapter 17. Patients with endotracheal tubes or tracheostomies are at particularly high risk for colonization and subsequent pneumonia.[504,505,1142] Bacteria adhere to polyvinylchloride, and therefore the sputum of intubated GBS patients is rarely sterile. In a recent study, 57% of intubated intensive care patients had tracheobronchial airway colonization with gram-negative bacilli, mostly *Pseudomonas aeruginosa* and *Serratia marcescens*.[1051] Inappropriate institution or prophylaxis with antibiotics for tracheobronchial colonization may predispose to superinfection with resistent microorganisms and raise overall management morbidity.[351,622,625] The distinction between colonization and nosocomial pneumonia or tracheobronchitis is often difficult. The clinician must be guided by the appearance of an infiltrate on chest radiographs, purulent secretions, fever, leukocytosis, and the presence of intracellular organisms on Gram's stain in tracheal aspirates.[1051] Antibiotic treatment is clearly indicated in tracheitis when fever is accompanied by purulent sputum in the presence of a normal chest roentgenogram. Chest physiotherapy and intermittent positive pressure breathing have little effect on the resolution of pneumonia in intubated patients[432] but may make the patient more comfortable.

Nasally intubated patients are at increased risk of sinusitis, as these cavities may not drain freely.[171] Three MGH patients had severe purulent sinusitis. Paranasal sinusitis can rarely be a source of sepsis.[272] In a series of 27 nasally intubated patients with sinusitis, *Staphylococcus epidermidis* and *Pseudomonas aeruginosa* were frequent causes. Antibiotic treatment and movement of the tube to the oral route, with or without the administration of decongestants, resulted in cure in all patients in one study.[272] Some intensivists advocate suctioning of the respiratory tract only when needed to reduce substantial secretions, rather than routinely, in order to minimize damage to the tracheal mucosa. The differences among various nurses' techniques for endotracheal suctioning are magnified in ICU patients' experience.[130] A sensitive, well-timed and rapid technique with preliminary ventilation keeps the patient comfortable and confident.

Elective tracheostomies in GBS should be performed under aseptic conditions in an operating room. A tracheostomy is a major risk factor for serious *Pseudomonas* and enteric gram-negative pneumonias and requires strict adherence to sterile techniques in subsequent tracheostomy care.[505] In a prospective series of 150 critically ill patients,[1142] the most common problems with tracheostomy were stomal infection (36%), stomal bleeding (36%), excessive cuff pressure requirements (23%), subcutaneous emphysema or pneumomediastinum, and tracheal stenosis (19%), all of which have been seen in GBS patients at MGH.

Urinary Tract Care

Thirty percent of all hospital-acquired infections are urinary tract infections.[930,931] Despite the use of aseptic closed methods for urinary drainage, urinary tract infections are common in GBS patients, primarily because of the use of Foley catheters in persistently bed-bound patients. In the MGH series, 14% to 22% of patients had urinary tract infections at some time during hospitalization, most often during the third week (see Table 16–4). After 10 days of catheterization the incidence of bacteriuria may exceed 50%.[393,1059] Meatal colonization is a major risk for catheter-associated bacteriuria, but use of antibacterial lubricants and cleansing of the meatus have not lowered infection rates and therefore are not routinely recommended. Antibiotic irrigation with a neomycin-polymyxin irrigant similarly has not affected the infection rate in a randomized controlled trial[1257] and may ultimately increase the incidence of *Pseudomonas* infections.

Intermittent urinary catheterization offers some advantages over indwelling catheters, particularly a lower infection rate, but the procedure is time consuming and may eventually irritate the urethral mucosa sufficiently to produce strictures that allow entry of microorganisms. Suprapubic catheters have the advantage of leaving the urethra intact, but are unnecessarily invasive and probably do not obviate the effects of a foreign body on the bladder or prevent infection. Although no controlled trial has been carried out, recent experience suggests that intermittent catheterization, even if done in a nonsterile fashion, may be an improvement over a chronic indwelling catheter.[654,1059] The most important preventive measure is strict maintenance of a closed system and handwashing by personnel handling the system.

Bacteriuria without pyuria usually should not be treated, as removal of the catheter often suffices. Antibiotic treatment of urinary tract infections with the catheter in place is laregly unsuccessful and only results in the emergence of resistant organisms.[1257] Pyuria, fever, flank pain, or other clinical manifestations of pyelonephritis develop in less than 1% of patients with catheter-associated bacteriuria.[1139] A reasonable recommendation in bed-bound GBS patients is to treat urine infections, based on antibiotic sensitivities, if there are more than 15 to 20 white blood cells (WBC) per high-power field. Enterococcal urinary tract infections may be an exception, perhaps justifying therapy at lower urinary bacterial and WBC concentrations.

Intravenous Catheter Sepsis

Treatment of severe autonomic dysfunction with unstable blood pressures or bowel dysfunction often requires the insertion of central venous catheters. The infection rate of these catheters is 2% to 5% when they are left in place longer than 72 hours.[740,1109] Catheters used for parenteral nutrition become infected far more frequently than those used for fluid or drug infusion. A presumptive diagnosis of catheter sepsis is made when 15 or more colonies of bacteria grow from a culture produced by rolling the catheter tip on the medium plate, or when identical organisms are grown from blood obtained from a distant site.[740] If gram-positive bacteremia has been proved or is strongly suspected, vancomycin and an aminoglycoside are usually given for 10 to 14 days. Guidelines for central venous catheter removal have been established, but it is prudent to change all lines, including arterial, when staphylococcal bacteremia has been documented. Changing potentially infected lines over guide wires invites continued infection and bacteremia.

Catheters left in place for up to 48 hours for plasma exchange treatment do not become infected often, but a femoral insertion site and longer periods increase the risks.

Gastrointestinal Complications

Stress ulcers and acute erosive gastritis are potential complications in the immobilized GBS patient. Gastrointestinal (GI) bleeding, usually minor, occurred in 8% of patients in the MGH retrospective series and in 2% of the MGH prospective series. The presence of a nasogastric tube attached to suction (rarely necessary in the GBS patient) has the potential for inducing superficial mucosal lesions of the gastric fundus or duodenum, but an increased risk of major gastric hemorrhage has not been demonstrated convincingly. Prophylaxis for gastric bleeding in patients who are not being fed regularly may be achieved with 30 to 100 milliliters of a magnesium-containing antacid hourly, to maintain the luminal gastric pH above 3.5.[954] Potential complications of this regimen are diarrhea, hypermagnesemia, and possibly aspiration from regurgitation.[424] Intravenous cimetidine apparently does not protect ICU patients as well as antacids from acute GI bleeding.[954] Preliminary work, however, has suggested that the deacidification of the stomach is associated with an increased rate of nosocomial pneumonia in ventilated ICU patients by a presumed mechanism of microaspiration of bacteria that have colonized the unprotected gastric mucosa. Sucralfate, an agent that preserves the natural gastric acid barrier, has been shown to be an alternative to antacids and H-2 blockers in the prevention of bleeding, does not significantly lower gastric pH, and is associated with fewer serious aspiration pneumonias, though sucralfate aspiration can be disastrous.[139,170,294,1202] Sucralfate has few associated side effects but it often clogs feeding tubes. The MGH Neurology-Neurosurgery ICU has generally used sucralfate in preference to antacids in GBS patients. Ranitidine is used in obese or tube-fed unintubated GBS patients who may be at high risk of aspiration, but not otherwise.

Because prolonged immobility, narcotic analgesics, and antacids predispose patients to constipation and ileus, the abdomen should be checked regularly for distention. Although ileus is rare in GBS (2% in the MGH retrospective series) it can be dramatic and has led to bowel perforation (Fig. 16–1). Fecal impaction should be avoided because, in addition to the mechanical risks, a distended cecum and sigmoid

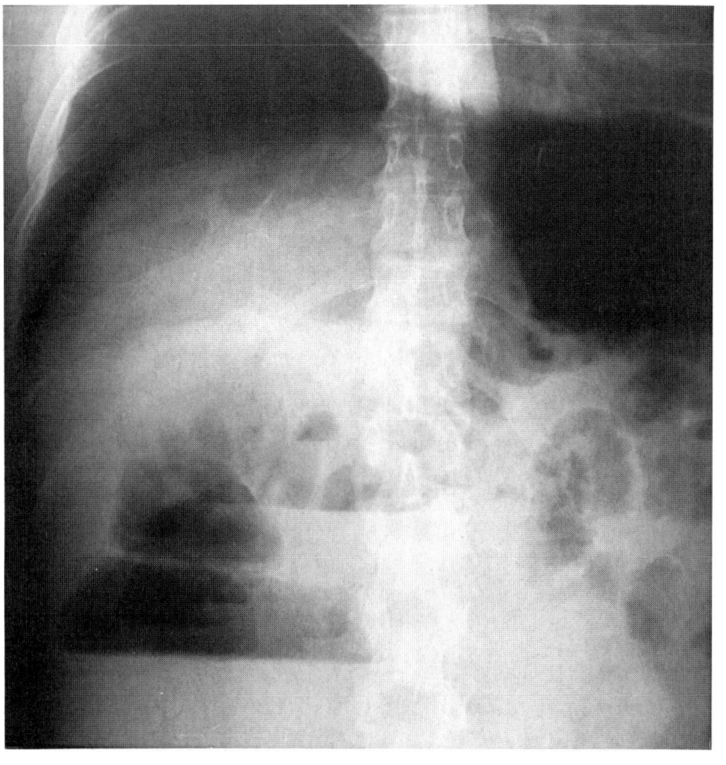

Figure 16–1. Rupture of cecum with free air under the diaphragm of a patient with GBS. The patient had had an ileus for the previous week but no other major dysautonomic features.

may precipitate a vagal response. Recently, GI perforation was recognized as a frequent complication in patients receiving steroid therapy for other neurologic diseases,[338] and constipation was found to be a major risk factor. Stool softeners on a regular basis are probably sufficient prophylaxis for impaction. They are unnecessary if a low-residue feeding formula is used.

Prophylaxis of Venous Thrombosis and Pulmonary Embolism

Pulmonary embolus has occurred as a complication of immobilization in up to 5% of bed-bound patients with GBS.[431,871] In the GBS Study Group trial, 2 of the 7 deaths were from embolism. Reports that up to one third of GBS patients have embolism were based on clinical criteria alone and were probably excessive.[964] Two patients (2%) had angiographically documented pulmonary embolus in the MGH prospective series, 6 (4%) in the retrospective series. Most immobilized patients in the prospective, but not the retrospective, series received prophylactic subcutaneous heparin. Pulmonary embolus should be suspected in a patient who has been bed-bound for more than 2 weeks and has a sudden deterioration in Pa_{O_2} or pleuritic chest pain with dyspnea. The differential diagnosis of hypoxia includes more common instances of bronchial plugging, excessive pulmonary secretions, pneumonia, pneumothorax on positive pressure ventilation, or endotracheal cuff leak. Radionuclide ventilation and perfusion scans have usually been performed before angiography in all but the most convincing cases. Patients with clinically typical cases of pulmonary embolism who had appropriate blood gas, roentgenographic, and ECG features, or those with widespread lung consolidation, have had pulmonary angiography initially. One MGH patient who had a ventilation-perfusion scan that suggested a low probability of embolism subsequently underwent an angiogram that demonstrated a large embolism (Fig. 16–2). Treatment is usually with a transvenously inserted caval interruption device, though there are more invasive surgical alternatives for caval interruption. Most often there is no associated calf phlebitis, but impedance plethysmography testing of the legs may provide circumstantial evidence of more proximal deep venous thrombosis.

Prophylaxis with subcutaneous heparin has been effective in preventing pulmonary embolus in postoperative patients.[212] The risk of bleeding complications is low and independent of the frequency of treatment; 5000 U every 12 hours appears to be effective in preventing deep venous thrombosis and is more convenient than an 8-hour regimen. Thrombocytopenia develops in a few patients and, if severe, may require discontinuation of heparin. After several weeks the heparin dose may need to be increased because of tachyphylaxis. There is as yet little evidence that oral anticoagulants are more effective than subcutaneous heparin. In those few patients who will be bed-bound for many months, however, subcutaneous injections become painful and impractical and warfarin has been used (in 6 MGH patients), attempting to keep the prothrombin time 1.5 times control. One death in the Mayo Clinic series was attributed to the combination of heparin and aspirin.[431] Other methods of prophylaxis for venous thrombosis (eg, the combination of subcutaneous heparin and dihydroergotamine) have not been studied in neurologic diseases associated with long-term immobilization.

Intermittent calf pneumatic compression (air boots) are a potential alternative to subcutaneous heparin in an attempt to reduce the incidence of venous thrombosis, but many patients find these devices uncomfortable, often enough to deprive them of sleep. The anecdotal impression in the MGH Neurology-Neuro-surgery ICU has been that the early use of air boots has left many patients with residual peroneal nerve palsies (Fig. 16–3).

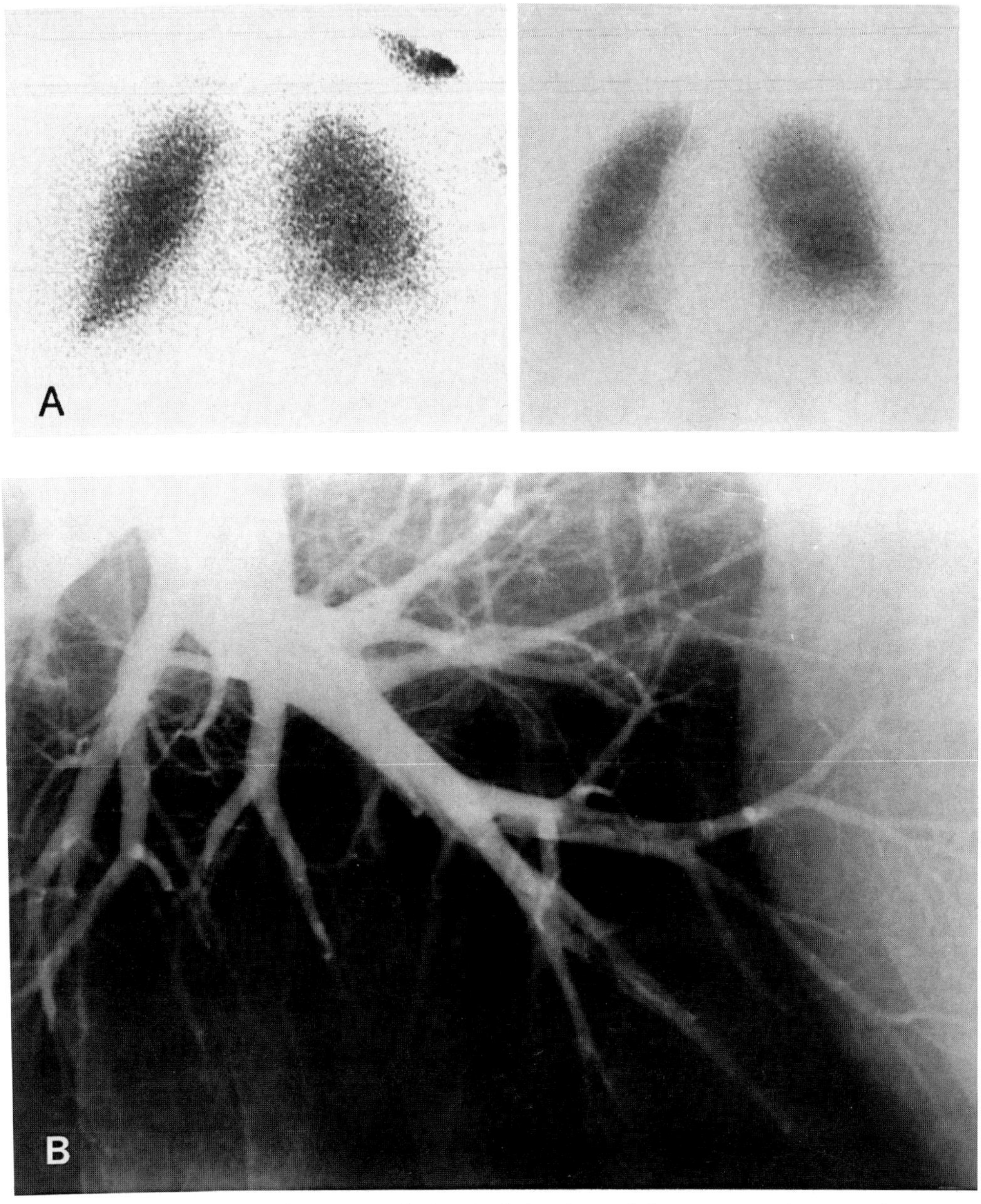

Figure 16–2. (A) Perfusion (left) and ventilation (right) radionuclide scans in a 56-year-old GBS patient with right pleuritic chest pain and an arterial Po_2 of 87 mm Hg breathing room air. The scan was interpreted as having a low probability of pulmonary embolus because of matched perfusion and ventilation defects, but angiography (B) demonstrated clots in pulmonary vessels. The patient was receiving heparin subcutaneously for 3 weeks before the embolus.

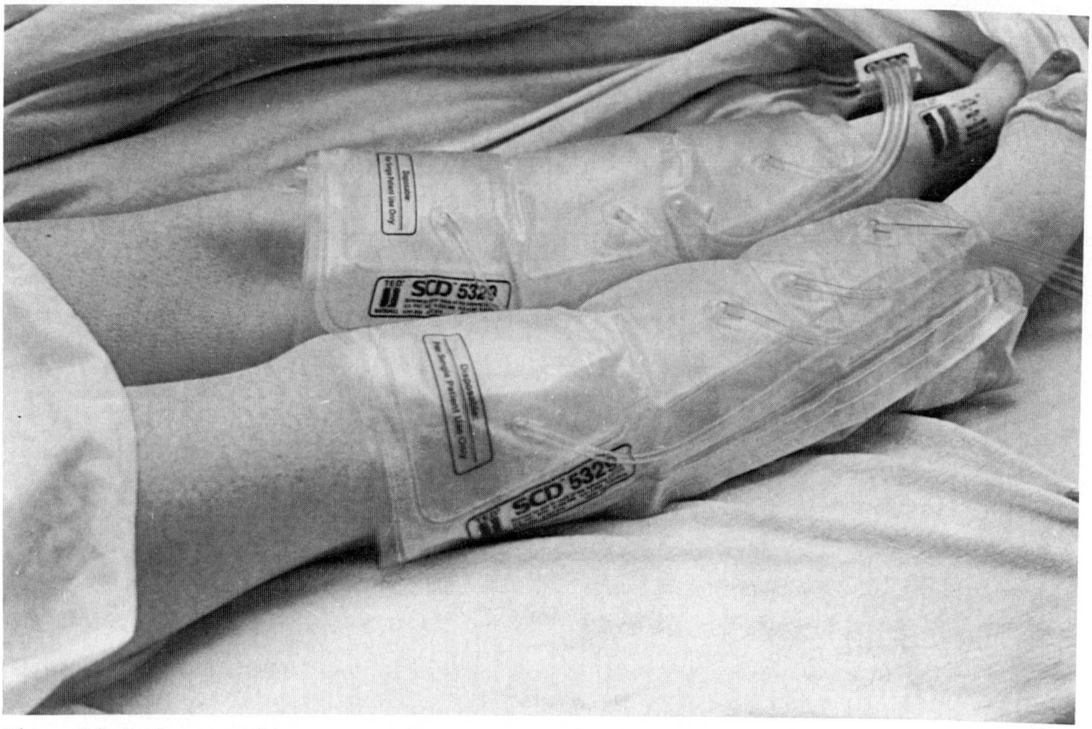

Figure 16–3. Sequential-type pneumatic compression boots, used for the prophylaxis of venous thrombosis, may compress the peroneal nerve at the fibular head and (anecdotally) cause residual foot drop.

Other Aspects of General Medical Care

Dysautonomia is discussed in Chapter 7. As a general rule, avoiding excessive treatment of cardiovascular dysautonomia is safer than attempting to keep all physiologic measurements normal. Intravenous suxamethonium should be avoided (eg, during tracheostomy and other procedures) because in patients with severe weakness it may lead to the release of large amounts of potassium, causing serious ventricular arrhythmias.[357a,360]

Phlebotomy for blood drawing must be minimized, as all severely ill patients sooner or later become anemic and antecubital veins should be spared if the patient is to receive plasma exchange. Anemia virtually never results from plasma exchange. Immobilization hypercalcemia has been mentioned in several well-documented case reports[541,798] and occurred in two patients in the MGH prospective series. This complication may become evident approximately 4 months after the onset of paralysis, as in other states of immobilization that favor resorption of calcium.[1152] Anorexia, nausea, and vomiting were the sole clinical features, but it may be asymptomatic. Subcutaneous calcitonin combined with oral etidronate disodium has been found to be useful if sodium infusions fail.[798]

Hyponatremia (less than 132 mEq/L) attributable to inappropriate antidiuretic hormone is often seen in patients on a ventilator. Seldom severe, it responds to fluid restriction. In the MGH prospective series, hyponatremia was significantly associated with treatment with a ventilator (Table 16–5). The mean sodium concentrations were similar (129 mEq/L) in ventilated and nonventilated hyponatremic patients. Hyponatremia appeared an average of 10 days after intubation.

Table 16–5 RELATION OF HYPONATREMIA (<132 mEq/L) TO VENTILATOR STATUS*†

	Ventilated Patients	Nonventilated Patients	Total
Hyponatremia‡	16	16	32
Normal serum sodium concentration	22	66	88
Total	38	82	120

*MGH Prospective Series.
†$P<.01$.
‡1–23 days (mean, 9.5 days) after intubation.

NURSING CARE AND PATIENT COMFORT

Positioning and Skin Care

The extremities of patients with GBS must be handled carefully because manipulation often produces pain. Further discussion on movement and positioning appears in Chapter 18. The patient should be asked which areas are painful to avoid lifting or turning those areas. Most quadriparetic patients prefer to be supine, but the upper body must not be elevated 30 degrees or more for a prolonged period because the weight at pressure points becomes unacceptably high.[719] Unintubated patients should generally be turned every 2 hours when they are awake; some prefer less frequent movement. Special turning beds (eg, the Stryker frame or the Foster frame) are expensive but have been useful in GBS. The Clinitron bed is based on the principle of air-fluidization of silicon-coated beads and is said to prevent the development of decubitus ulcers (as discussed in Chapter 18), but the MGH unit staff generally prefers the simplicity of water mattresses. Besides these measures, the skin must be kept free from moisture or dryness. Excessive sweating and urine or fecal contamination may lead to skin tissue breakdown. The skin should be washed with mild soap and patted dry without vigorous friction. Talc-based dusting powder and lanolin cream should be applied. Hypoalbuminemia, starvation, and fecal incontinence are particularly important risk factors for the development of pressure sores.[23,719]

Eye and Mouth Care

Bifacial palsy predisposes the patient to corneal abrasions and ulcerations. Lubricating methylcellulose eye drops in the daytime and ointment at night should be applied. At night, and during sleep, the lids may be gently taped closed. Some patients with total ptosis prefer to have their eyes taped open for brief periods in the daytime. However, ointment and artificial tears to prevent ulceration are then needed frequently, unfortunately resulting in blurred vision.

Mouth care consists of regular tooth brushing and flossing to prevent gingivitis and oral ulcers. Simple oral candidiasis responds to oral clotrimazole troches 10 milligrams taken 5 times daily.

Pain Management

Pain was mentioned in up to 50% of patients in many early reports on GBS.[501,751,777] Rice's poignant description of his own illness,[983] from a physician's point of view, is helpful in understanding the devastating effect of pain. GBS pain usually simulates the sensation that occurs hours or a day after strenuous exercise.[1017] Common locations are the low back, large fleshy muscles, anterior or posterior aspects of the thighs, buttocks, and, less often, calves. Low back pain has sometimes been accompanied by sciatica. Pain usually occurs in the most profoundly weak proximal muscles, but there has not been any relationship to severity of limb weakness or sensory changes. Another pain syndrome results from intense distal paresthesias accompanied by severe loss of vibration and joint position sense.

Pain is usually the worst between 10 PM and 4 AM, preventing sleep, and is reported most accurately by hospital night-shift nurses. It is often alleviated when the knees and hips are slightly flexed. Some patients have benefited from cold or warm packs or gentle massage. Pain response to medication is variable; acetaminophen and aspirin may provide temporary, incomplete relief. Antidepressants or anticonvulsants have generally not been effective for dysesthetic distal pain at MGH. Quinine, despite a favorable response in one reported patient,[856] has not been effective in most. Sustained relief for a few days may occur with a single injection of 40 to 60 milligrams intramuscularly of methylprednisolone. Epidural morphine sulfate proved to be successful in a patient who had no response to other pain medication.[1025] Narcotics (oxycodone with acetaminophen orally, meperidine HCl intramuscularly) have been the most effective treatment, and they should be administered liberally at night if necessary. If patients are so marginally compensated that narcotics for pain will cause respiratory failure, then they should be intubated; sleep would probably be disastrous in these patients. Administration of narcotics, however, may contribute to ileus. Limited experience with transcutaneous electrical stimulation[769] suggests that it may be helpful for some patients with back and buttock muscular pain or painful dysesthesias. A number of our patients have had no relief.

NUTRITION

Because most GBS patients have previously been well nourished, early nutrition is easily managed and there is no rush to begin feedings. Severely paralyzed patients with oropharyngeal weakness, however, may rapidly become undernourished, leading to hypoalbuminemia, increased risk of pressure sores, and impairment of respiratory muscle strength. Diaphragmatic mass and power have been shown to parallel peripheral muscle bulk in ICU patients.[47]

Enteric tube feeding should be started after several days in patients with normally functioning GI tracts who have difficulty swallowing. Enteral nutrition is efficient and safer than parenteral nutrition, which has potential complications such as pneumothorax, catheter sepsis, catheter embolus, and metabolic intolerance.[111] Small-caliber, highly flexible plastic tubes with metallic weighted tips allow relatively easy placement with minimal patient discomfort. Insertion should be performed by carefully trained personnel since these tubes have a high risk for misplacement, resulting in complications that include pneumothorax, hydrothorax, empyema mediastinitis, pneumonia, and esophageal perforation[787] (Fig. 16–4). Passage of the tube into the lungs occurs particularly frequently in patients with pharyngeal weakness. Radiographic confirmation of the tube's position should be accomplished immediately after tube placement and before beginning alimentation. The presence of a cuffed endotracheal tube does not preclude bronchial passage or obviate radiographic verification. In a recent study,[787] half the nasogastric tube misplacements were discovered in patients with endotracheal tubes. Misplacement in the lung, particularly if the tube is coiled in the thoracic cavity, should be assumed to have caused a pneumothorax. Ideally, the tip of the tube should be in the duodenum or jejunum because tubes may cause lower esophageal sphincter incompetence, thus increasing the risk of reflux and aspiration. Antral placement is more common and usually safe.

Continuous pump infusions of feeding formulas are well tolerated by pa-

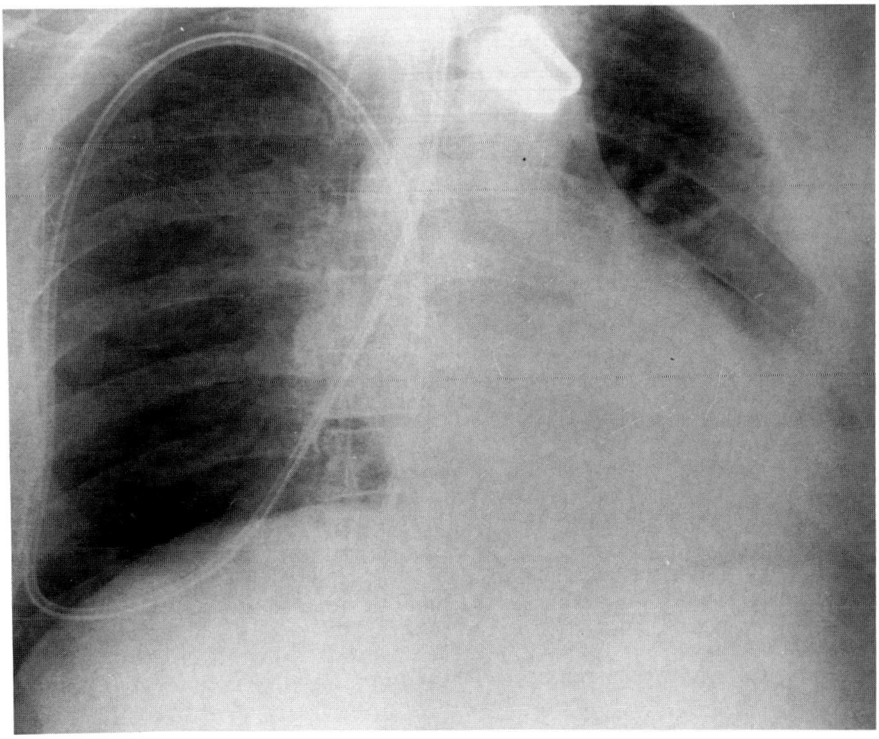

Figure 16–4. Malpositioned small-caliber feeding tube in a GBS patient. The tube has transbronchially punctured the pleura and caused a left pneumothorax. Patients with poor oropharyngeal movement (and those with diminished levels of consciousness) are prone to this type of complication.

tients and easy for nursing staff to manage. Bolus administration often results in abdominal bloating, cramping, a feeling of fullness, and, in some patients, diarrhea.[1181] Regardless of tube location, the patient should not be fed when supine, and if the feeding must be stopped, the tube should be cleared with a small volume of water or ginger ale. Maintaining tube patency may become a problem if sucralfate is used as prophylaxis for gastric bleeding or if medications are not ground finely. A clinical dietitian should be consulted to help choose the optimal diet, meeting complete nutritional requirements. Low-residue, high-calorie, commercial fiber-enriched mixtures (Ensure Plus, Enrich) are delivered continuously by means of a volumetric feeding pump. Hyponatremic patients who require fluid restriction can be fed concentrated formulas such as Two Cal.

Diarrhea, a frequent complication of tube feeding, may lead to fluid-electrolyte imbalances. In a recent prospective study in tube-fed burn patients,[424] diarrhea was associated with antibiotic use and with caloric intake from fat greater than 20 grams. Other causes of diarrhea in GBS patients are *Clostridia difficile* bowel infection and lactose intolerance. Lactinex and similar preparations sometimes help to repopulate the colon with normal organisms and diminish diarrhea. Codeine phosphate is also useful in stopping diarrhea. Several young patients have complained of pharyngeal pain from the pressure of the tube as it curves against the posterior mucosa. Erosions or severe discomfort require replacement through the opposite nostril. If enteral tube feeding is correctly managed, the elastic tubes will be well tolerated for weeks. Gastrostomy is not indicated in GBS patients unless long-term immobilization and mechanical ventilation (more than 2 months) are anticipated.[374,674,1002] Even then, gastrostomy has not been shown to be superior to a nasogastric tube, but the recent inception of endoscopic tube placement has minimal risks and may be suitable for patients who will require feeding for several weeks.

Full nutritional supplementation through a central venous catheter is indicated when ileus, sepsis, or bowel perforation is evident. Total parenteral nutrition (TPN) is safe in the hands of the experienced clinician. Occasionally serous complications such as TPN-associated sepsis are unavoidable, even with the best care. Profound hypophosphatemia is a recognized complication of intravenous hyperalimentation and enhances weakness and respiratory failure.[386,526] Alimentation catheters should not be used for other purposes such as plasma exchange.

PSYCHOLOGIC SUPPORT AND COMMUNICATION

Several physicians' accounts of their own illnesses, especially those by Bowes[130] and Rice,[983] are most helpful in understanding the experience of GBS. As noted in the introduction to this text, they emphasize that small nursing care details and some degree of involvement in or control over decisions about their own care were crucial to psychologic well-being. Rice's description of nighttime GBS pain[983] is poignant and sensitizes physicians and nurses to the travail. These descriptions, and those of others,[1093] if given judiciously to patients and their families, can be used to show them that their fears and concerns are appropriate and typical for the illness, as well as reinforcing the likelihood of recovery. The novel *Bed Number Ten*[66] is perhaps better read by the patient after recovery, but it may be helpful to families of GBS patients during the illness.

Care of the GBS patient involves painstaking psychologic support. During the progressive phase, severe anxiety, fear, and even panic can be encountered, often reinforced by the patient's lack of knowledge about the disease.[325] A particularly strong fear has been that of being unable to obtain another breath should the ventilator become temporarily disconnected. Establishing early and continuing communication with nursing staff builds trust and is helpful. The MGH Neurology-Neurosurgery ICU employs a primary nursing approach, making one team member very familiar with the personal and physical needs of the patient and family.[446,1209] Patients often complain that the staff does not take enough time to interpret their messages or understand their needs.

Communication with a virtually "locked-in" patient is often difficult, but preservation of slight jaw movement, even in the most severely paralyzed patients, can be used to push a button for signaling (Fig. 16–5). A code system for communication must be started as soon as possible and posted above the patient's bed. A physician with GBS, Dr. Kopel Burk, has devised 3 groups of color coded cards that patients chose by nodding or blinking. Two very useful devices at the MGH have been a clear plastic spelling and signaling board, which is used as described in Figure 16–6, and a computer screen with a cursor that can be moved by the jaw or finger to spell out messages. Similar commercial and "homebrew" systems that use personal computers have been described.[846] Fried-Oken (in a personal communication, 1989) and others[102] have assessed various assistive communication devices for use with GBS patients, including an ocularly guided computer that types messages. One such sophisticated device uses electrodes surrounding the orbit to move the cursor among the letter fields (Fig. 16–7). A simpler electrooculographic "Twinkle Switch" has only two states but is correspondingly easier to calibrate and use (Adaptive Communications systems, Pittsburgh, PA).

In the plateau phase, patients often become depressed. Depersonalization may develop, possibly progressing to visual hallucinations. These sometimes

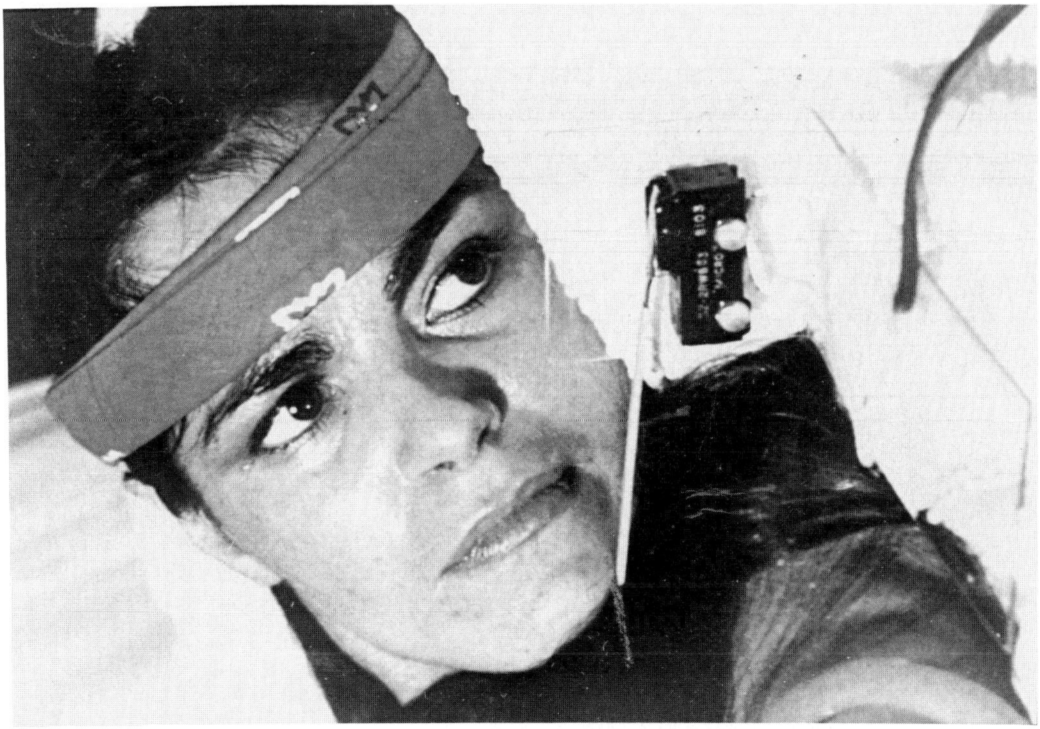

Figure 16–5. Signal switch manipulated by the chin or jaw in a virtually quadriplegic GBS patient.

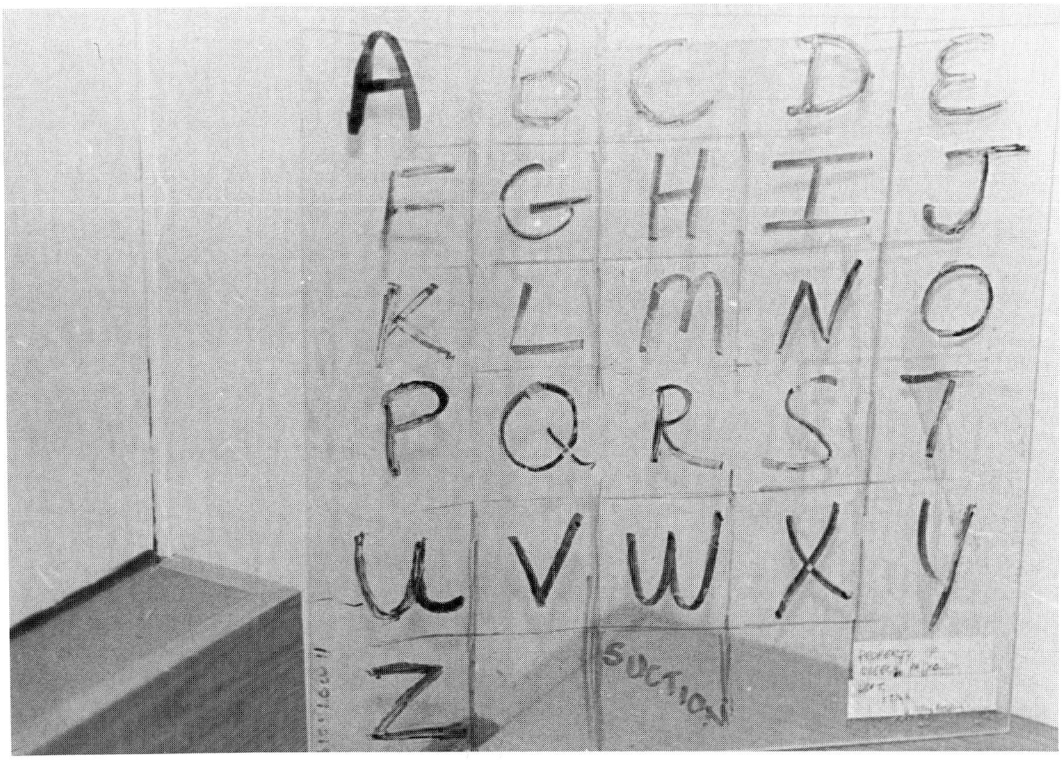

Figure 16–6. A transparent spelling-signal board used in the MGH Neuro-ICU. The nurse stands behind the board while the patient fixes gaze on letters or messages. It is helpful to have messages such as "turn me," "pain," "can't breath" in cells for rapid communication.

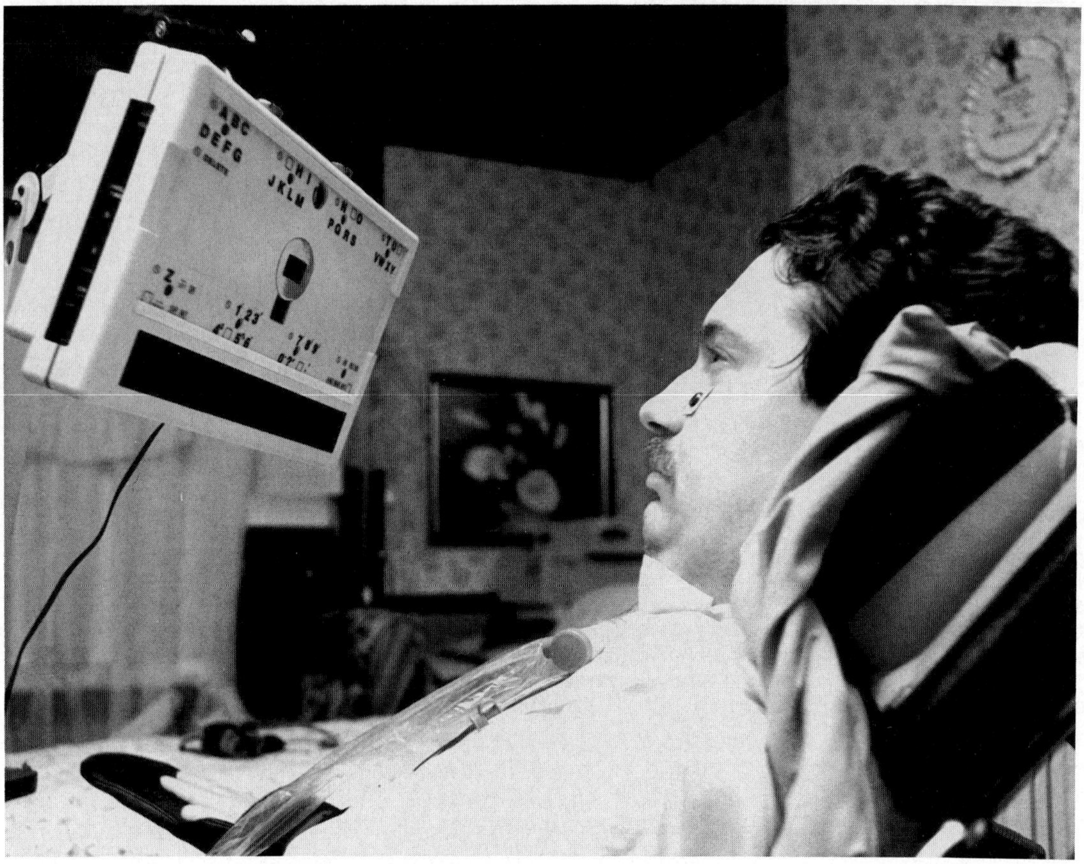

Figure 16–7. An Eye Typer visually guided computerized typing device for augmenting communications in quadriplegic patients. (Courtesy of Sentient Systems Technology Inc., Pittsburgh, PA.)

extremely frightening hallucinations may go unnoticed by the staff. Sleep deprivation and medication are important contributing causes. It is therefore imperative to ask daily about such experiences, which may be helped by treatment with haloperidol 1 to 5 milligrams or lorazepam 1 to 2 mg orally every few hours if the symptoms are extreme. Another major concern during the plateau phase is exacerbation of pain, which may affect the psychologic state of the patients and eventually wear on the nursing staff. Reassurance and support from family members, social workers, and chaplains may contribute to the care during this stressful phase.

The recovery phase is often marked by a dysphoric depression caused by the expectation of a long recovery. In patients who are weaned from the ventilator too early, extubation followed by rapid reintubation can be extremely frustrating. Visits by former GBS patients to offer encouragement has been a very helpful technique at MGH, during both the acute phase and recovery. Some patients can be very demanding and emotionally draining; therefore, continuously emphasizing an optimistic outlook while setting realistic limits is important for patients and staff.[130,1093]

The GBS Foundation (PO Box 262, Wynnewood, PA 19096), an organization founded and run by patients, has a newsletter, other literature, and videotapes for families and patients. Knowing that others have survived and thrived after the ordeal is comforting to patients and families.

PHYSICIAN AND NURSE STRESS

The lengthy ICU admissions, the dysphoric mood of patients from immobilization and pain, and the slow progress of recovery take a toll on physicians and nurses caring for patients with severe GBS. Nurses often switch assignments to prevent "burn-out" from an individual patient with GBS who has been in the ICU for weeks, especially if the patient can manipulate a call button at night to take a disproportionate amount of nursing time. Families are also likely to ask the same questions repeatedly and to leave messages regularly at the physician's office when there is nothing new for the doctor to report. These stresses wear on the physician and nurse and contribute to interstaff conflicts. A study[1213] has demonstrated that physicians involved in direct patient care are more likely than other professionals to have serious personal and social problems. Physician responses to difficult patients with GBS have included apathy, with short or irregular patient visits; passive-aggressive behavior, in delaying responses to call buttons or verbal requests to be turned to another position or for pain medication; and a tendency to be abrupt with nurses or therapists who have legitimate questions about the patient's recovery. An excellent remedy for these stresses is to establish a special team relationship among the physicians, nurses, and therapists caring for the patient. The initial effort to make a weekly plan concerning pain medications, weaning, availability for families, timing of plasma exchanges, and so on, distributes the burden of caring for these patients, while further investing others in the patient's problems. In addition, a regular routine for collecting urine and sputum samples, blood testing, and chest roentgenograms partly absolves the physician from the worry of trying to remember to be constantly vigilant for medical complications. Finally, it is helpful to treat these patients as special cases to be pampered purposely with a bit of extra time and solicitousness during daily visits, because the long, sometimes pastoral relationship that develops during this difficult watershed period of the patient's life can produce rewarding support and confidence in the future.

MANAGEMENT IN PREGNANCY

The management of GBS in the first two trimesters of pregnancy is essentially no different from its management in other patients, with most women delivering healthy, full-term babies (see Chapter 6). Concern arises in the third trimester. During gestation, tidal volume and minute ventilation increase while functional residual capacity decreases. Furthermore, increased respiratory demands during labor, delivery, and recumbency may be anticipated. Induction of labor to improve respiratory difficulty during the third trimester of pregnancy is highly controversial and should be avoided when the disease is still active. There is no strong indication for cesarean section, which has previously been associated with a small number of maternal deaths. We are aware of several instances of precipitous labor in pregnant GBS patients in the third trimester, but most carry the fetus to term without complications. Some obstetricians have advocated forceps delivery to assist during the second stage of labor. Plasma exchange has been used without major incident to treat GBS in all trimesters of pregnancy.[334]

Emphasis on these mundane aspects of daily care has contributed more than have major immunologic therapies to patient well-being and good outcome. Consistency in the management and anticipation of general medical problems reduces morbidity and mortality. Although it may be beneficial to collect patients with the most severe cases of GBS in tertiary centers, where staff has extensive experience and habitual methods are used to treat the major complications of the disease, most patients can be treated well in community hospitals with interested and committed personnel who are willing to manage—directly or by delegation—every detail of general medical care in this multifocal illness.

Chapter 17

RESPIRATORY FAILURE

The most common serious complication of GBS is mechanical respiratory failure that requires positive pressure ventilation. Oropharyngeal weakness, sometimes contributing to aspiration pneumonia, may occur independently or with respiratory weakness. In one series,[444] aspiration was the cause of respiratory failure in 4 of 30 patients with GBS. The recognition and skillful management of these complications are major determinants of overall morbidity and mortality in acute GBS. Familiarity with several basic techniques of respiratory care and with ventilators and their potential complications is necessary to care for these patients successfully. Intensive care units (ICUs) are derived from polio units, which were established largely to provide efficient mechanical ventilation[939,940] (see Chapter 1). The respiratory techniques used currently, including modern ventilators and chest physiotherapy, were a response to the practical needs of patients with neurologic disease in the early 1950s.

OROPHARYNGEAL WEAKNESS, INTUBATION, AND TRACHEOSTOMY

Approximately one quarter of patients with GBS develop difficulty swallowing secretions, continuous minor aspiration of saliva, atelectasis, small bronchopneumonias, or frank aspiration of food with major pneumonias. Oropharyngeal weakness occurs most often with severe generalized limb weakness, but may also be associated with regional variants of the illness, such as pharyngeal-cervical-brachial weakness,[1008] Fisher's syndrome that progresses, or the descending form of GBS (see Chapter 8). Unlike myasthenia gravis, pharyngeal weakness in GBS is usually not associated with the severe tongue and jaw weakness that causes a characteristic velopalatine dysphonia and lingual dysarthria.[1004] Isolated nasal regurgitation is rare. The relationship between oropharyngeal and facial weakness is somewhat inconsistent, but the two usually progress in parallel. There is usually some associated respiratory weakness, but it may not be severe. The patient's palate usually elevates voluntarily and reflexly, but when swallowing, there is a pause in the oral phase as fluid reaches the oropharynx, followed by a slow, incomplete elevation of the thyroid cartilage. Coughing immediately after swallowing may reveal the sounds of fluid collected in the hypopharynx. Hoarseness or airway obstruction from laryngeal paresis is rare in GBS, if it occurs at all.

Endotracheal Intubation

Endotracheal intubation is performed most often for positive pressure ventilation, but some patients have isolated, early, or disproportionate oropharyngeal weakness requiring airway protection alone. Prevention of pulmonary complications probably has more to do with the timing and care of endotracheal intubation than it does with the initiation of mechanical ventilation. Because endotracheal intubation has substantial risks, each instance should be anticipated and the decision made deliberately. Early elective intubation is preferable to a temporizing approach because in GBS, unlike in myasthenia gravis, there is little chance that oropharyngeal weakness will improve rapidly.

General guidelines for endotracheal intubation are (1) requirement for mechanical ventilation; (2) frequent coughing from pooled secretions; (3) inability to swallow comfortably, as reported by the patient or as observed; (4) documented pneumonia acquired after admission to the hospital in a patient with oropharyngeal weakness; and (5) other evidence of inability to clear pulmonary secretions, requiring frequent "blind" endotracheal or pharyngeal suctioning (these patients usually have a diminished vital capacity). Elective nasal intubation is preferred to oral, unless there is a bleeding diathesis or severe nasal-septal obstruction.

Prior to the use of plasma exchange to treat GBS, several ICUs recommended immediate or early tracheostomy.[770,817,852,871] In the plasma exchange era, however, one third to one half of patients with ventilatory failure have been weaned from the ventilator in less than 2 to 3 weeks, thus obviating tracheostomy.[850,1013] In the Massachusetts General Hospital (MGH) prospective series, only half of the patients who were intubated required tracheostomy. Soft, large-diameter, low-pressure cuffed endotracheal tubes infrequently cause complications in GBS because these patients are relatively immobile and do not have abrasion of tracheal tissue. The major risk of endotracheal intubation, cuff overinflation, can be avoided if cuff inflation pressures are kept as low as possible to maintain a seal (less than 20 to 25 centimeters H_20) and are checked regularly to prevent cartilaginous distention. Access to the trachea for suctioning is not as easy as with a tracheostomy but remains adequate for most patients.

Complications of intubation in acute GBS have included minor aspiration pneumonia or atelectasis, evident soon after intubation in up to 50% of patients, and complications of longer-term intubations such as granulomas of the trachea, tracheal stenosis, or tracheomalacia, similar in incidence to that in patients with other respiratory illnesses in the modern era.[503,1142,1191]

Tracheostomy

Tracheostomy may be performed during the third week of intubation or earlier if it is clear that the patient will require mechanical ventilation for a longer period. The complications of tracheostomy are uncommon and have been much the same as in other ICU patients.[503,1142,1191] Tracheo-esophageal or tracheocutaneous fistulas, tracheal stenosis, local hemorrhage,[817] and innominate artery erosion[431] have all been reported in GBS patients. Cuff inflation pressures for tracheostomies must be monitored regularly, as with endotracheal tubes, in order to prevent erosion or tracheomalacia.[1283] In the MGH prospective series, of 19 tracheostomies performed an average of 14 days after intubation, there was one instance of tracheal stenosis from granulation requiring late surgical reconstruction. Four other patients had local revision of the tracheostomy scar for cosmetic purposes.

The tracheostomy is removed when the need for mechanical ventilation or frequent tracheal suctioning has passed. Patients with persistent oropharyngeal weakness risking aspiration or those requiring only intermittent or low-rate ventilation (for example, at night) can benefit from a "talking" tracheostomy[933] (Fig. 17–1) that allows the patient to speak, albeit dysphonically, by blowing air or oxygen through the larynx from a port just above the cuff. This device is useful with ventilator rates below approximately 5 per minute. Another type of fenestrated tracheostomy has an inner trocar that may be removed to allow normal air flow through the larynx when the outer hole is plugged (Fig. 17–2). Speech is then

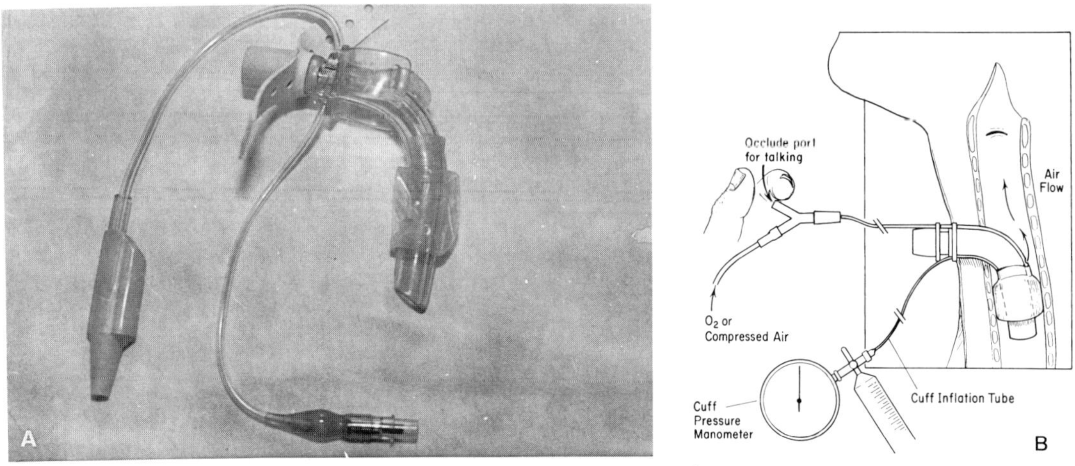

Figure 17–1. *A*, "Talking" tracheostomy with ports above the cuff to allow compressed air or oxygen to traverse the larynx. Speech is dysphonic and monotonous but usually understandable. *B*, Schematic diagram of this type of tracheostomy.

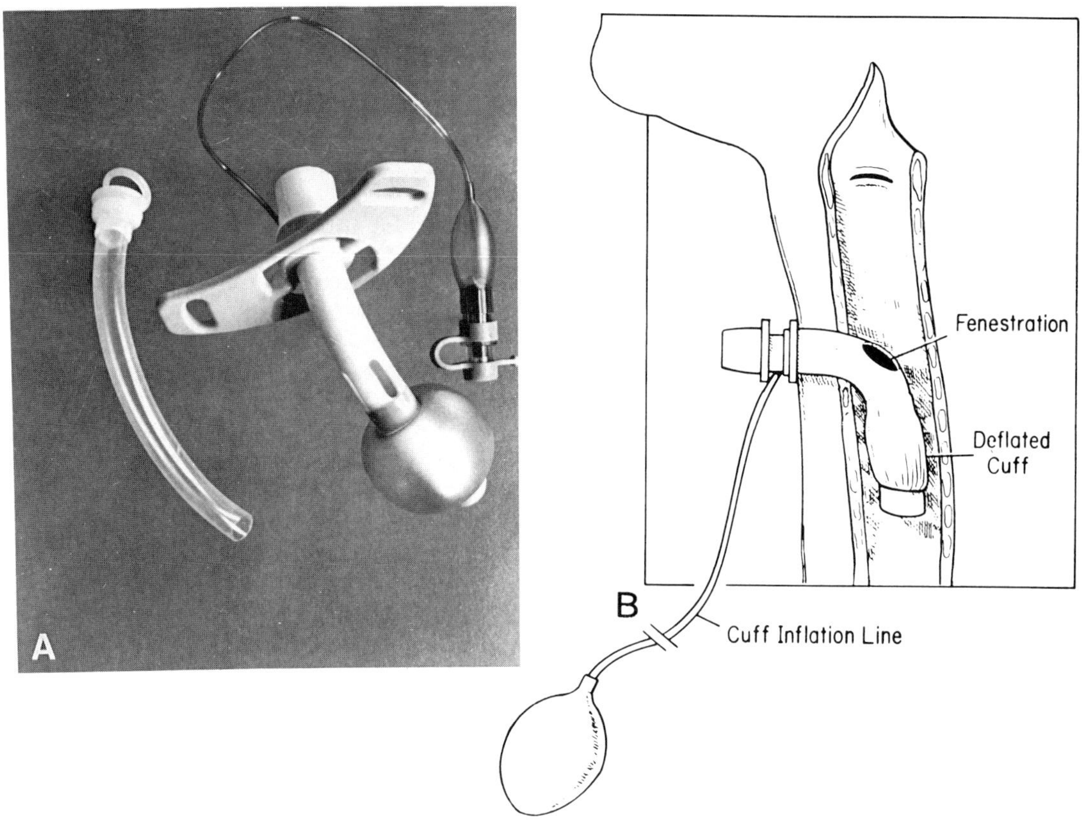

Figure 17–2. Fenestrated trocar tracheostomy that allows normal speech. The inner trocar is removed and the outer hole plugged. The cuff may be left inflated or deflated. Device is shown in *A* and schematic in *B*. (From Wilson,[1283] p. 84, with permission.)

normally modulated, but the patient must be off the ventilator.

By staining small amounts of food with methylene blue dye and allowing patients to swallow with the tracheostomy cuff deflated, it is possible to determine whether or not aspiration is occurring and whether it would be advisable to remove the tube. A modified barium swallow under fluoroscopy is an alternative but more cumbersome technique rarely used in GBS patients. Small-caliber nasogastric feeding tubes do not seem to interfere with this test nor to enhance aspiration in unintubated patients. It is probably best to leave a tracheostomy in place until swallowing is secure and powerful coughing is possible. Access to the trachea for suctioning can be maintained for a week or two after removal of the tube by plugging the stoma with a plastic "button" device. These are often coughed out of place unless secured by cloth tapes.

MECHANICAL RESPIRATORY FAILURE

Clinical Features

Respiratory failure, due mainly to diaphragmatic weakness, is the most common serious complication of acute GBS. It is severe enough to require mechanical ventilation in approximately one third of patients in most large series but occurs to a lesser degree in virtually all patients with generalized limb weakness. Of 120 consecutive patients in the MGH prospective series, 38 (32%)—and 34% in the retrospective series—required intubation and mechanical ventilation; the courses of the first 19 prospective patients are detailed in previous publications.[1013] These patients had more profound limb weakness, longer hospitalization, longer recovery, higher mortality, and more frequent serious residual deficits than patients who do not require ventilation. There was no definite predictive feature for severe respiratory decompensation, except perhaps severe and rapidly progressive limb weakness. Bifacial paresis, suggested in one report[373] as a prognostic feature for respiratory failure, has not been consistently helpful (approximately one third of MGH patients with early facial weakness had ventilatory failure, compared with one fifth of those without facial weakness). As in polio, diaphragmatic weakness usually parallels shoulder weakness early in the illness. If a patient has avoided mechanical ventilation for 2 weeks after the onset of paresthesias, then it is unlikely to be necessary unless another major problem supervenes. The average time to instituting mechanical ventilation in the prospective study was 7 days (SD 5 days; range, 1 to 16 days).

Time on Ventilator

Several reports have highlighted the modern respiratory intensive care aspects of acute GBS* (Table 17–1). The mortality in these patients, which had been over 10% to 30% during the early epoch of respiratory intensive care,[515] is now approximately 3% in large units. These rates are currently considerably lower than ICU mortality for patients with primary pulmonary disease.[918] In the GBS Study Group,[469] 104 (42%) of 245 patients required a ventilator for an average of 26 days. Ventilated patients took substantially longer than patients who did not require mechanical ventilation to be able to walk independently. In other series, the average time on a ventilator has been 37 to 54 days.[431,770,817] Prospectively studied MGH patients were ventilated for a similar average of 49 days.

Virtually all patients are eventually weaned from the ventilator if they survive the medical complications of prolonged ventilation and immobilization. One elderly patient, anecdotally, has required a ventilator for more than 2

*See references 260, 431, 444, 515, 770, 817, 871, and 1013.

Table 17–1 MAJOR ICU—VENTILATION SERIES OF GBS

Series (Yr of Study)	*Total No. Patients*	*No. Ventilated/ Total ICU*	*Mean Days on Ventilator (Range)*	*No. with Tracheostomy*	*Major Complications/ Deaths (%) among Ventilated Patients*
McCleave et al.,[770] 1969–1974	69	13/15	20	NA	NA/2 (15%)
O'Donohue et al.,[871] 1967–1974	32	22/32	NA*	22	9/2 (9%)
Moore and James,[817] 1970–1980	33	9/14	63 (21–210)	8	4/1 (11%)
Gracey et al.,[431] 1974–1979	79	13/21	37 (6–93)	13	3/3 (23%)
Newton-John,[852] 1972–1983	91	67/67	NA	53	NA/16 (30%)
Sunderrajan and Davenport,[1165] 1977–1984	40	18/40	68 (3–396)	11	5/5 (28%)
de Jager[260] 1955–1983	63	63/63	55	60	8/5 (8%)
GBS Study Group,[469] 1980–1984	245	104/160	26	NA	NA/4 (4%)
Prospective MGH Series, 1981–1988	120	38/85	49 (3–247)	19	5/3 (8%)

*NA = Not available.

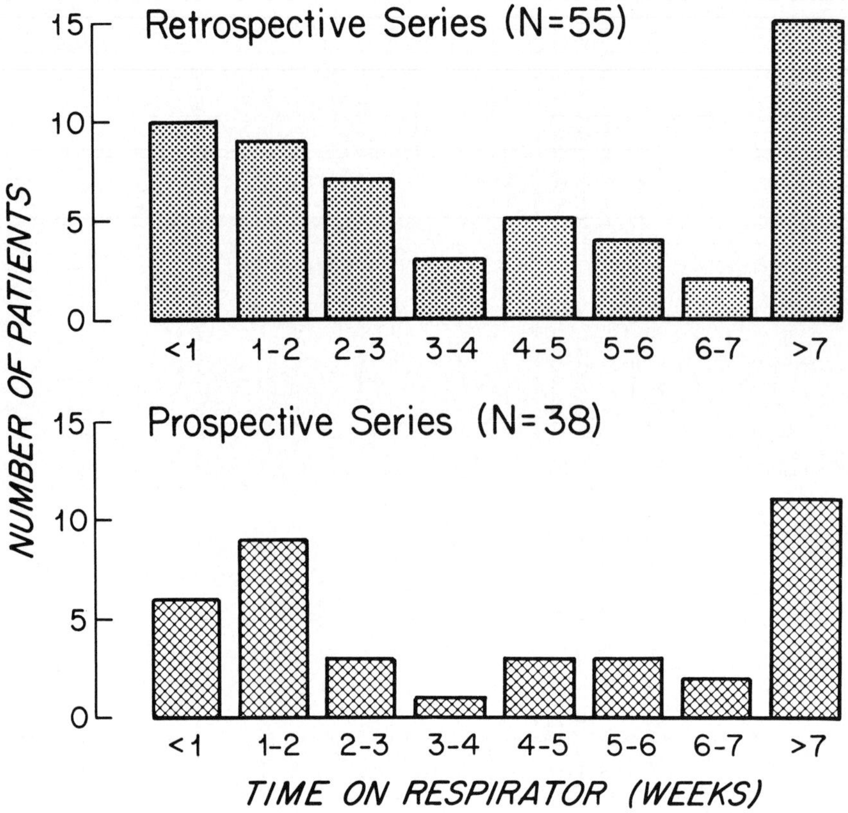

Figure 17–3. Duration of mechanical ventilation in the MGH retrospective and prospective series.

years in a chronic care hospital. The longest time on a ventilator in the MGH experience was 247 days. A reported patient required complete ventilation for 266 days and was then weaned rapidly over 2 weeks.[1276] This relatively rapid period of respiratory improvement has occurred in several patients after months of ventilatory support with spontaneous forced vital capacity (VC) of less than 400 mL (8 mL/kg). Most often, rapid weaning is the result of an ambitious program in a patient who was ready to wean earlier. The durations of mechanical ventilation in the MGH retrospective and prospective series are shown in Figure 17–3.

Pathophysiology and Clinical Features of Mechanical Ventilatory Failure in GBS

Respiratory failure is due primarily to diaphragmatic weakness and is therefore inspiratory in nature. Other features such as intercostal, abdominal, and accessory muscle weakness; airway secretions; atelectasis; and supine posture contribute secondarily. As diaphragmatic weakness progresses and lung volumes diminish, a number of parallel phenomena occur, leading initially to progressive atelectasis and hypoxemia, and later to alveolar hypoventilation and hypercapnia. Figure 17–4 summarizes these events and appropriate therapies at the corresponding VCs.

The patient's overall state, clinical evidence of diaphragmatic fatigue, pulmonary function tests, and arterial blood gases, are combined with the clinician's judgment to determine the timing and need for a ventilator. Respiratory function often deteriorates over several hours, at a time when limb weakness may be stable or deteriorating only slightly. This is apparently the result of diaphragmatic fatigue, a com-

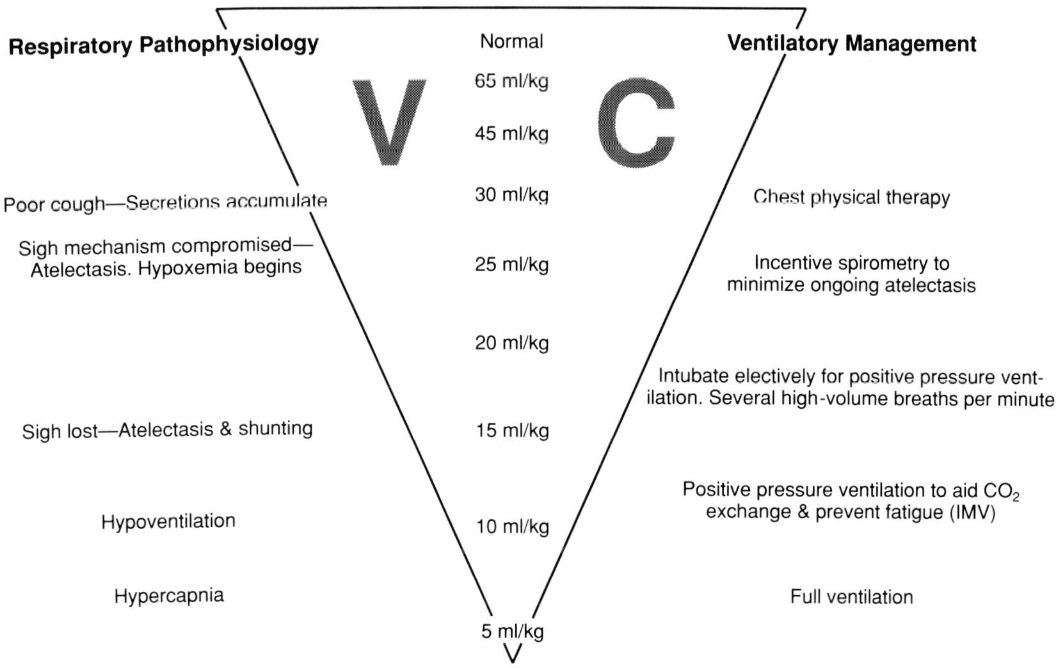

Figure 17–4. Schematic depiction of the pathophysiologic events that occur in mechanical respiratory failure as vital capacity falls, and the therapies appropriate at each stage. (Adapted from Ropper, A, and Kennedy, S, Neurological and Neurosurgical Intensive Care. Aspen Publishers, Rockville, MD, p. 259.

plex phenomenon that results from forcing the respiratory muscles to work excessively outside their normal range of length-tension and energy metabolism.[1031] The early clinical manifestations of respiratory muscle fatigue that are useful in gauging the need for ventilatory assistance include paradoxical breathing (inward movement of the abdomen during inspiration reflecting diaphragmatic fatigue), tachycardia, and brow sweating, probably a result of increased adrenergic activity. Later during deterioration, use of accessory respiratory muscles and respiratory alternans, in which diaphragmatic and intercostal breathing alternate, indicate severe decompensation. Confusion and agitation from hypercapnia are later signs of extreme deterioration. Early during mechanical respiratory failure, when patients may appear to be working harder than usual to breathe, dyspnea is not present and the respiratory rate is only slightly increased. Asthma has preceded GBS in two reported cases.[482a,799a]

PULMONARY FUNCTION TESTS AND ARTERIAL BLOOD GASES

The effect of GBS on lung volumes has not been studied as extensively as in other neurological diseases such as amyotrophic lateral sclerosis (ALS).[344,444,647,836] There is probably little change in functional residual capacity in GBS, while residual volume eventually increases, mainly due to weakness of the expiratory muscles (intercostals and abdominal musculature). Static lung compliance remains normal unless there is extensive atelectasis.[647] Spirometric volumes, however, are prominently reduced in GBS, generally in proportion to respiratory muscle weakness, making bedside testing of these volumes a convenient method of assessing pulmonary function. The main abnormality is inspiratory (diaphragmatic) weakness, reflecting abnormal phrenic nerve function. Inspiratory, and to a greater extent expiratory, pressures are reduced in neuromuscular respiratory failure. A comparison of spirometric volumes (VC) with inspiratory and expiratory pressures in myasthenia gravis, muscular dystrophies, and ALS[445] concluded that pressure measurements were more sensitive than spirometry to early respiratory weakness. It is not known if the same differences apply to GBS.

The most accurate tests of respiratory failure in GBS are, theoretically, mid-inspiratory flow rates (perhaps the best overall measure of diaphragmatic failure), inspiratory VC,[445] and maximal static inspiratory or expiratory pressure. The more consistent and easier to perform measurement of expiratory VC tends to reflect the volume of the prior forced inspiration and is used more often at the bedside, but it measures diaphragmatic weakness only indirectly. Maximum inspiratory force (MIF) is therefore a useful supplement to expiratory VC. Inspiratory VC, a more direct measurement of diaphragmatic function, and an acceptable bedside test,[445] is altered by many factors, including static lung volumes, and is performed less consistently by patients. Tidal volume is not substantially reduced until respiratory failure is severe. Perhaps the most salient limitation to the use of bedside spirometric (VC) measurements is that the more widely available meters do not record portions of the breath at low flow rates, precisely the problem with diaphragmatic weakness. It is not unusual to see the end of a patient's exhalation fail to move the needle on the meter, especially with VC in the 0.5- to 2.0-L range.

Although various guidelines have been suggested for the initiation of a positive pressure ventilator in patients with neurologic disease,[871] the ones most commonly used have been outlined in classic reviews.[109,110,939–941] They suggest that VC less than 15 mL/kg (less than 20% of predicted) and MIF less than 25 centimeters H_2O indicate severe ventilatory failure that justifies assisted ventilation. In the MGH series, mechanical ventilation began with a mean VC of 14 mL/kg (just below 1 liter). Others[431] have used MIF and maximum expiratory force (MEF) of less than 30 centimeters H_2O with additional blood gas criteria to determine the timing of mechanical ventilation. The ease of performance and consistency in application of these criteria based on forced expiratory VC and MIF have led to their widespread adoption.

The trends of VC and MIF are as important as their absolute value in these decisions (See Tables 16–1 and 16–3). Patients who have rapidly advancing limb weakness usually require VC and MIF measurements taken every 2 or 3 hours; otherwise, less frequent testing is reasonable, especially if it allows patients to sleep for longer periods. Measurements should be repeated with the patient in the same position (preferably sitting at about a 60-degree angle), by an experienced individual, with care to assist in sealing the lips around the mouthpiece if there is facial weakness. Holding the patient's nostrils closed may give more authentic measurements if there is severe velopalatine weakness. Whatever technique is used, consistency among measurements is important.

Arterial blood gas sampling can supplement but not replace clinical assessment and spirometric measurements. The earliest blood gas abnormality is usually reduced Pa_{O_2} tension, reflecting miliary microatelectasis and varying degrees of mild shunting in these regions (there is probably as much ventilation-perfusion mismatching as true increase in the shunt fraction). Atelectasis is enhanced by the inability to cough adequately to clear secretions. The Pa_{O_2} in MGH patients with respiratory failure averaged 72 mm Hg, breathing room air, just prior to intubation.[1013] At that time, Pa_{CO_2} was normal (mean 40 mm Hg). Hypercapnia, reflecting alveolar hypoventilation, usually results from a VC below 5 to 8 mL/kg and is therefore a late finding (see Fig. 17–4). Mechanical ventilation is advisable before this point is reached. The threshold both for changes in clinical signs and for arterial blood gas abnormalities is altered by the coexistence of chronic lung disease or aspiration pneumonia.

Guidelines for Instituting Ventilation

A reasonable summary recommendation of the institution of mechanical ventilation in GBS combines clinical features, pulmonary spirometric and force (pressure) measurements, and the trend of each. Sensitivity to capture all patients in need of assistance is preferable to excessive selectivity. Both aims can generally be achieved by instituting artificial ventilation when the expiratory forced VC falls below approximately 12 to 15 mL/kg, modified by signs of fatigue, the rapidity of clinical and respiratory decline, evidence of mild hypoxemia (Pa_{O_2} less than 75 to 80 mm Hg with inspired room air), and the age and preexisting respiratory health of the patient. This allows elective, safe intubation and ventilation, and rarely results in inappropriate institution of treatment.

Parenchymal Pulmonary Failure

Severe aspiration or bacterial pneumonia may produce the adult respiratory distress syndrome (ARDS) in acute GBS. There were 4 such cases in the MGH prospective series, resulting from aspiration in 3 patients (1 from massive epistaxis) and from gram-negative bacterial pneumonia in 1. One additional patient developed a lung abscess from gram-negative bacterial pneumonia with severe hypoxemia, another had a fatal empyema, and two developed ARDS secondary to urosepsis. The care of these patients is similar to that of patients without mechanical ventilatory failure who have ARDS, as complete artificial ventilation is generally required in both circumstances. The use of large amounts of positive end expiratory pressure (PEEP) and high inspired oxygen tensions, however, are not necessary in GBS without ARDS. Other sources may be consulted for more explicit information on the managment of ARDS.[941,1284] Regular surveillance of sputum cultures weekly and biweekly chest x-ray films are appropriate in intubated ICU patients, but prophylactic antibiotics are not believed to be beneficial.

The important complication of pulmonary embolism in the immobilized GBS patient is discussed in Chapter 16. Rare cases of noncardiogenic pulmonary edema have been reported,[137,249] some poorly described or associated with other acute diseases (see Chapter 7). The association is not yet firm.

VENTILATOR MANAGEMENT

Most modern ventilators have similar characteristics, making the initial choice of machine relatively unimportant. In general, a desirable ventilator has an intermittent mandatory ventilation (IMV) circuit that minimizes the work of spontaneous breathing, and adequate ventilation alarms for patient disconnection, low exhaled volume, apnea, and other mishaps. Completely controlled mandatory ventilation (CMV) may be uncomfortable for patients unless they are completely paralyzed. A completely assisted mode of ventilation allows the patient to institute each ventilator breath, thereby risking overventilation if the patient's spontaneous breathing rate is high, or underventilation if the patient does not trigger the machine. Most ICUs therefore use IMV or one of its variants, delivering a preset number of large tidal volume breaths while allowing the patient to breathe spontaneously between ventilator cycles from a reservoir or parallel gas circuit. Most patients find this mode comfortable once an appropriate ventilator frequency is found. The mechanism may be synchronized to avoid superimposing machine breaths on spontaneous breathing (SIMV), although this offers no major advantage. IMV techniques have the theoretical advantage of continuously "training" the diaphragm by allowing it to perform as much work as tolerated, while avoiding fatigue, atelectasis, and hypoventilation. These ventilator modes were devised to continue diaphragmatic work and avoid atrophy so that weaning could commence earlier.[290] No definite advantage in weaning has been shown for IMV, however, and it is widely used in these circumstances mainly because of patient comfort and ease of operation. The IMV mode may be supplemented or, in limited circumstances, replaced by other techniques such as "pressure support," a method that raises the pressure in the ventilator circuit to a preset value to encourage comfortable spontaneous breathing by decreasing respiratory work; this is essentially a form of intermittent positive pressure ventilation (IPPV).

Ventilator tidal volumes of 12 to 14 mL/kg are used with all these machine modes to prevent atelectasis. It is unnecessary to overventilate patients, which in effect removes their respiratory drive and obviates the spontaneous breathing circuit. Patients with VC of 8 to 12 mL/kg usually require 2 to 5 breaths per minute; from 4 to 8 mL/kg, 6 to 10 breaths per minute; and less than 4 mL/kg, full ventilation of 10 to 14 breaths per minute. The patient should be observed while the physician adjusts the ventilator rate to allow comfortable spontaneous breaths for up to 15 minutes without signs of fatigue or anxiety. The arterial Pco_2 tension should be checked when a comfortable rate has been determined. Values between 35 and 42 mm Hg are desirable. Occasionally patients become anxious and air hungry after endotracheal intubation and may require additional ventilation and sedation. Sustained air hunger should not, however, be attributed to anxiety; other causes such as pneumothorax, cuff leakage, or right bronchial main-stem intubation should be sought.

The major complications of mechanical ventilation, in addition to pneumonia, are those resulting from barotrauma. Induced pneumothorax in particular can precipitate hypotension, shock, dyspnea, and worsening lung compliance and oxygenation. Subcutaneous and mediastinal emphysema, and the less-common pneumoperitoneum, are less dramatic and do not require treatment but must be observed carefully for progression. Pressure support-assisted ventilation, described earlier, does have the advantage of reducing mean airway pressure and minimizing barotrauma.

Ventilated patients have a propensity to become hyponatremic (see Table 16–4). Serum sodium concentrations less than 132 mEq/L occurred in 42% of MGH ventilated patients, compared with 20% of nonventilated patients.

Negative pressure, tank, or cuirass ventilators, the original methods of supporting patients with neurologic respiratory failure from polio (see Chapter 1), are potentially employable when ventilatory failure is mild and airway protection is not an issue. These devices can generate −15 to −45 centimeters H_2O negative pressure, but their inconsistent breath-to-breath efficiency, cumbersome nature, inability to assist in airway clearing, and restriction of access to the patient have allowed only limited interim use in patients with GBS.[517,670] They are more appropriate for patients with stable, slowly progressive or incomplete neuromuscular failure, such as nighttime ventilation for ALS or muscular dystrophy patients, but their potential may not yet have been fully explored.

CHEST PHYSICAL THERAPY

As VC drops below approximately 20 mL/kg and MEF rates diminish so that coughing is compromised, pulmonary secretions collect in small airways. Clearing these secretions is aided by frequent changes in body position, chest percussion and vibration, and specifically encouraging coughing. Atelectasis is prevented by these maneuvers and by incentive spirometry, one of numerous techniques that encourage deep breathing. The proper technique for suctioning the airway is discussed in Chapter 16.

Chapter 18

OUTCOME AND REHABILITATION

OUTCOME

"... Monsieur J. A. Barré et moi-même avons toujours insisté sur le caractère favorable du pronostic prognostique; la guérison est en général plus ou moins rapide, mais complète. Seule l'abolition des réflexes peut persister longtemps ..." G. Guillain[460]

This fundamental characteristic of GBS, spontaneous improvement in most cases, remains one of the main features that distinguishes it from other polyneuropathies. Despite Gullain's optimism, many reports and series have documented frequent residual weakness, and in a smaller percentage, severe persistent paresthesias, ataxia, a chair- or bed-bound state, or fatal outcome. Muscle strength may take 1½ to 2 years to reach its best state with an intensive rehabilitation program. A well-planned rehabilitation program requires the cooperative efforts of physiatrists, physical and occupational therapists, social workers, and the primary neurologist. Patients who make incomplete recoveries often are disabled just enough to prevent resuming some portion of their previous lifestyles, a state at times more vexing than more severe fixed disabilities. The desire of incompletely recovered GBS patients to continue improving and to explore various therapeutic options was the basis for their founding the GBS Support Group in 1980.

Table 18–1 DURATION OF HOSPITALIZATION

Series, Year	***No. Patients****	***Hospital Stay (Days)***
McFarland and Heller,[777] 1966	98	75 (mean)
Ravn,[973] 1967	103	78 (mean) (range 7–321)
Osterman et al.,[886] 1984	38	Plasma-exchanged patients: Median 30 Mean 71 Control subjects: Median 78 Mean 105
GBS Study Group,[469] 1985	219	52 (mean) (range 8–245)
French Cooperative Group,[380] 1987	206	Plasma-exchanged patients: Median 28 Control subjects: Median 45
Retrospective MGH Series	167	61 (mean) 30 (median) (range 2–442)
Prospective MGH Series	114	30 (mean) (range 3–259)

*Excludes deaths or unavailable data.

Duration of Hospitalization

Most patients require at least 1 month of hospitalization initially, depending on the severity of illness and on the availability and utilization pattern of rehabilitation hospitals and outpatient services. The average duration of hospitalization at the MGH in the prospective series was 30 days (excluding deaths), and in the GBS Study Group trial,[469] 52 days (Table 18–1). In addition, many Massachusetts General Hospital (MGH) patients spent several days to 2 weeks at referring hospitals prior to transfer. Hospitalization time has probably been reduced by the widespread use of plasma exchange, but resource utilization in GBS has not been studied systematically. The Swedish,[886] French,[380] and North American[469] cooperative studies have shown a decrease in duration of hospital stay of approximately 50% in patients who were given plasma exchanges compared with control subjects.

Patients who require mechanical ventilation are usually hospitalized much longer than those who do not. In the MGH prospective series, ventilated patients had a mean hospital stay of 67 days, with an extreme of 259 days, almost fourfold longer than hospitalization of nonventilated patients. These results are similar to those of series reported before the use of plasma exchange.[431,817] As shown in Table 18–2, the lowest clinical grade during the illness, noted soon after admission, was associated with a longer hospital stay. Patients who remained ambulatory (grade 2) left the hospital within 2 to 3 weeks (see Table 18–2). The duration of mechanical ventilation is discussed in Chapter 17 (see Table 17–1).

Mortality

The causes of death in GBS include pneumonia and adult respiratory distress syndrome (ARDS) from aspiration, sepsis, myocardial infarction, pulmonary embolus, and profound dysautonomia. Mechanical respiratory failure, discussed more extensively in Chapter 17, was commonly fatal prior to the proliferation of respiratory intensive care units (ICUs). For example, most of Haymaker and Kernohan's 50 autopsied patients prior to 1949 died of respiratory failure associated with widespread paralysis and lower cranial nerve involvement, 2 to 46 days after onset of symptoms (mean 4 days).[501] A coexisting bronchopneumonia was found at autopsy in 60%. Focal myocarditis, consisting of lymphocyte and macrophage collections, was reported in 7 of the 50 fatal cases (see Chapter 11).

The overall mortality in GBS has improved considerably since the routine institution of respiratory care and ventilator techniques that were created in response to the polio epidemics of the 1950s. Mortality in large modern series has been 3% to 6%, and in a few series, 10% to 20% (Table 18–3; See also Table 17–1). One retrospective series[968] had a

Table 18–2 DAYS OF HOSPITALIZATION AT MGH IN PROSPECTIVE SERIES, RELATED TO CLINICAL GRADE*

Lowest Clinical Grade (Hughes Disability Scale)	*No. Patients*	Days† *Range*	*Mean*	*Median*
5	35	15–259	67	54
4	50	9–71	15	19
3	18	3–32	14	14
2	11	3–23	9	9
Total	114	3–259	30	—

*Excludes 6 patients who died.
†Excludes acute hospitalization elsewhere before or after MGH admission.

Table 18–3 MORTALITY IN LARGE GBS SERIES

Series, Year	*Period*	*No. Patients*	*Deaths (%)*	*RF/PN*	*PE*	*CA/MI*	*SE*	*Misc*
McFarland and Heller,[777] 1966	1940–1963	100	2 (2)	2	—	—	—	—
Ravn,[973] 1967	1949–1963	127	24 (18)	12	2	6	—	4
Samantray et al.,[1053] 1977	1960–1976	302	12 (4)	12	—	—	—	—
Loffel et al.,[714] 1977	1963–1974	123	3 (2)	1	1	—	1	—
Retrospective MGH Series	1962–1981	169	2 (1)	2	—	—	—	—
GBS Study Group,[469] 1985	1980–1984	245	7 (3)	3	2	1	—	1†
Raphael et al.,[968] 1986	1963–1981	223	23 (10)	5	5	2	2	9‡
French Cooperative Group,[380] 1987	1981–1985	220	14 (6)	NA	NA	NA	1	NA
Winer et al.,[1291] 1988	1983–1984	100	10 (10)§	4	1	4	—	1
Prospective MGH Series‖	1981–1988	120	6 (5)	4	—	1	—	1

†Inflammatory myocarditis.
‡Tracheal hemorrhage[4]; other pulmonary complications, gastric bleed, or sepsis.[5]
§Three unrelated deaths are not included.
‖See Table 18–4.
*RF/PN = Respiratory failure/pneumonia; PE = pulmonary embolus; CA/MI = cardiac arrest/myocardial infarction; SE = sepsis; Misc = miscellaneous; NA = unavailable.

high incidence of cardiac arrest, but the primary event was often aspiration, pulmonary embolus, or myocardial infarction. Dysautonomia, while occasionally life-threatening, is seldom a direct cause of death (exceptions are detailed in Chapter 7). One of the 14 deaths in the French Cooperative Study Group[380] occurred during plasma exchanges that were carried out in the presence of pneumococcal sepsis, but there are few other convincing reports of sudden death during or directly related to plasma exchange in GBS. The majority of deaths in the North American trial[469] were from pulmonary embolus, pneumonia, or sepsis. In the MGH retrospective series 2 patients (1%) died, and in the prospective series 6 (5%) died—all but one, months after the onset of symptoms. The most common proximate cause of death in these series was ARDS, often related to sepsis or aspiration (Table 18–4).

Good Recovery and Mild GBS

At the opposite extreme, approximately 75% of GBS patients recover without important neurologic sequelae, returning to normal life by 6 to 12 months (Table 18–5). The precise time to recover fully depends on the severity of illness. In the MGH experience, less than 15% of patients have had absolutely no residual symptoms. Some patients claim normal strength, but test-

Table 18–4 FATAL GBS IN PROSPECTIVE MGH SERIES

Patient No.	*Age*	*Sex*	*Grade*	*Plasma Exchange*	*ICU Admission*	*Severe Dysautonomia*	*Cause of Death*	*Days after Onset*
1	68	M	5	+	+	No	Myocardial infarction	120
2	69	F	4	−	+	Hypertension	ARDS/sepsis	60
3	74	M	5	−	+	Arrhythmias	ARDS/aspiration	210
4	65	F	4	−	+	Labile blood pressure	ARDS/aspiration	90
5	82	M	4	−	+	No	Brainstem hemorrhage	15
6	84	M	5	+	+	No	ARDS/sepsis	30

Table 18–5 FUNCTIONAL OUTCOME IN LARGE GBS SERIES

Series, Year	***No. of Patients****	***Follow-up***	***Good Recovery† No. Patients (%)***	**Residual Weakness, No. Patients (%)** ***Mild/ Moderate***	***Severe***
Wiederholt et al.,[1278] 1964	89	1–2 yr	61 (69)	28 (31)	0 (0)
McFarland and Heller,[777] 1966	62	mean 7 mo	18 (29)	36 (58)	8 (13)
Ravn,[973] 1967	103	mean 78 days	84 (82)	19 (18)	0 (0)
Samantray et al.,[1053] 1977	290	6 mo	290 (100)	0 (0)	0 (0)
Loffel et al.,[714] 1977	90	0.9–12.3 yr	51 (57)	33 (37)	6 (6)
Raphael et al.,[968] 1986	144	2 yr	104 (72)	31 (22)	9 (6)
Winer et al.,[1291] 1988	83	1 yr	62 (75)	14 (17)	7 (8)

*Excludes deaths or patients lost to follow-up.
†Includes residual symptoms and signs not interfering with normal life.

ing with a hand-held dynamometer reveals mild weakness.[117] Though functioning at everyday chores and work, many patients remain weak proximally or have mild persistent distal paresthesias. Others have a persistent "dead" feeling that impairs their ability to handle small objects (see later). Fatigue is common in the 6 months after discharge but is rarely disabling unless there is associated depression.

In the MGH prospective series, 11 (9%) of 120 patients had very mild but typical GBS, never reaching grade 3 (inability to walk unassisted). These patients experienced their maximum deficit within 2 weeks, and in half cerebrospinal fluid (CSF) protein concentrations were normal. In one, there were various electrophysiologic abnormalities, including severe slowing and sporadic fibrillation potentials. These patients left the hospital within 1 month after onset and recovered completely, usually with the return of some tendon reflexes within 1 to 3 months.

Residual Syndromes

Disabling weakness or sensory symptoms 1 to 2 years after onset of GBS have been reported in up to 15% in some large GBS series, but only 6% to 8% in most others (see Table 18–5). Three residual syndromes have occurred in the MGH experience: severe distal paresthesias or dysesthesias, foot drop and intrinsic hand muscle weakness, or sensory ataxia. These usually occur independently and reflect the major deficits during the peak of illness.

Acral burning dysesthesias precipitated by contact or pressure may occur in patients who have otherwise virtually complete motor recoveries. Paresthesias may be exacerbated slightly by exertion, heat (and less often cold), or acute viral illnesses. The associated sensory loss prevents some patients from using their fingers effectively for fine tasks such as buttoning, sewing, or writing.

A severe bilateral but slightly asymmetric foot drop that impedes walking occurs in only 5% to 10% of patients, but a third of all patients have milder foot weakness requiring a plastic ankle orthosis for several months. There is usually disproportionate weakness of anterior tibial-peroneal compared with gastrocnemius-soleus muscles, but isolated foot drop is uncommon and approximately a third of our patients with foot weakness have had similar degrees of plantarflexion weakness. Unilateral foot drop is rare, suggesting that peroneal pressure palsy is an oversimplified explanation. Forearm muscles seem to recover more rapidly than lower leg muscles, and selective wrist weakness is rare. Approximately 5% of patients have had permanent finger and hand weakness associated with atrophy of intrinsic hand muscle. In the MGH retrospective series, 18% had mild or moderate residual foot drop; in the prospective series, 5% still required ankle splints at 1 year (Table 18–6).

Ataxia seldom persists in GBS, including in patients with Fisher's syndrome, but a few patients with previously severe sensory deficits have residual gait ataxia. Many patients notice some unsteadiness or mild ataxia early in their recovery, but these complaints subside in the majority. The severe persistent ataxia is accompanied by severe large-fiber modality sensory loss.[985,1121,1134] In one report,[1121] muscle weakness resolved, but an ataxic or pseudotabic gait remained 3 to 5 years after onset. Loss of deep sensibility in the distal extremities, pseudoathetotic movements, and moderate limb weakness were present initially. Most of these patients had severe axonal damage and loss of large myelinated fibers on nerve biopsies.

Fatigue is common but rarely disabling, particularly in comparison to a similar fatigue experienced by patients with mutiple sclerosis. Patients with residual disabilities from GBS usually function at the limits of their physical capacities, allowing them to participate enthusiastically in physical therapy. Only when superimposed depression produces mental fatigue and tiredness does the degree of disability exceed weakness. Orthostatic hypotension or other features of severe dysautonomia do not persist much longer than 1 to 3 months, but they may impede physical therapy during that time.

Table 18–6 OUTCOME IN PROSPECTIVE MGH SERIES

Outcome	*No. Patients (%) (N = 111)*	*Follow-up, Range*
Good recovery*	87 (78)	2–17 mo
Walking unsteadily or with splints	5 (5)	≥12 mo
Walking with canes, crutches, braces	7 (6)	6–9 mo
Wheelchair-bound	3 (3)	≥30 mo
Chronic or relapsing course	3 (3)	—
Death	6 (5)	—

*Includes patients with paresthesias, mild facial weakness, and nondisabling weakness of foot elevation.

Severe Disability and Time to Maximal Recovery

We are aware anecdotally of only two patients with acute GBS who have been indefinitely bed-bound, one requiring mechanical ventilation. Even the most severely affected patients recover axial power adequately to sit in a chair and eat with assistive devices. Only 3 of 120 MGH prospective series patients remained wheelchair-bound at 2 to 3 years (Fig. 18–1; see Table 18–6). These patients had become quadriplegic over 2 to 5 days and were attached to a respirator for several months. All had severe residual weakness, distal more than proximal, with atrophy below the knee, but still allowing them to raise their arms for independent eating and washing. Sensory loss was usually mild. As reported in an earlier communication regarding some of these patients,[1007] 3 of 6 who were wheel-chair or bed-bound at 6 months were eventually able to walk with orthotic splints (see Fig. 18–1). Similar to other published experience,[880] wheelchair-bound patients at MGH ceased improving after approximately 18 months. In one report[86] improvement continued until the patient was walking independently 2 years after the onset of severe GBS.

Prognostic Factors

Investigators in at least three large series[780,968,1290] have attempted to identify predictive factors in the first weeks after onset of GBS. These studies generally agree on the following poor prognostic features: the need for ventilatory support, very low distal motor amplitudes (probably reflecting axonal damage), older age, and rapidly progressive

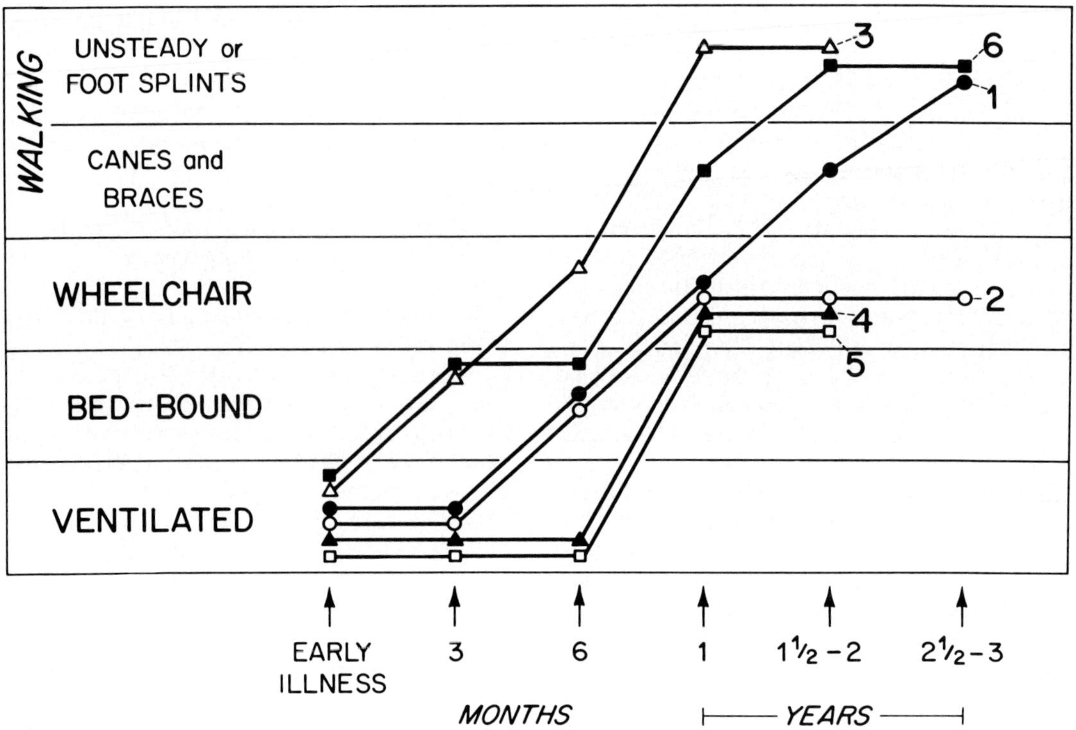

Figure 18–1. Clinical courses of six patients with severe acute GBS who remained bed-bound or chair-bound 6 months after onset. There was negligible improvement after 18 to 24 months. (From Ropper,[1007] p. 430 with permission.)

disease causing quadriparesis within 1 week (Table 18–7). A long plateau phase and the severity of maximal motor deficit have been less convincingly proposed as prognostic factors. Multivariate analysis has demonstrated that plasma exchange improves outcome even when poor prognostic features are present.[780]

Table 18–7 PROGNOSTIC FACTORS FOR RESIDUAL DISABILITY IN GBS IN THREE LARGE SERIES

Raphael et al.,[968] 1986
Plateau duration >1 wk
Severe motor deficit
McKhann et al.,[780] 1988
Age >60 yr
Need for ventilatory support
Time to plateau <7 d
Infection on admission requiring antibiotic treatment
Mean distal motor amplitude ≤20% of lower limit of normal
Winer et al.,[1290] 1985
Age >40 yr
Need for ventilatory support
Grade 4 disability in ≤4 d
Amplitude of median motor nerve ≤1 mV

In the MGH prospective series, most patients who had not required ventilatory support made a complete or good recovery (Table 18–8). Conversely, as in other series, permanent disability, wheelchair-bound state, and death occurred more often in patients who required ventilatory support than in those who did not. Severe disability was associated with ventilatory support only if it was required for more than 1 month ($P < .001$). Following multivariate analysis of prognostic factors in Guillain-Barré Syndrome Study Group trial, a low distal amplitude CMAP (less than 20% of the lower limit of normal) emerged as the most powerful predictor of poor outcome[780] (see Chapter 13). Similar findings have been reported in two other analyses.[800,1291]

Prognosis appeared to worsen with

Table 18–8 VENTILATOR AND OUTCOME IN PROSPECTIVE MGH SERIES (N = 108)*

	Ventilator			
Outcome	**≥1 mo**	**<1 mo**	**No Ventilator**	**Totals**
Good recovery	8	17	62	87
Permanent weakness but ambulatory	5	1	6	12
Wheelchair-bound	3	0	0	3
Death	1	2	3	6
Totals	17	20	71	108

*Excludes 3 patients with chronic inflammatory demyelinating polyneuropathy (CIDP) after acute GBS and 9 patients with incomplete follow-up.

increasing age in two prospective series,[469,1290] but others have not found this association in retrospective reviews.[780,968] In the MGH prospective series, patients older than age 70 generally did worse than younger patients (Table 18–9). No consistent associations with outcome have been reported with gender, CSF protein concentration or cells, dysautonomia, or specific antecedent events.

In the MGH experience, patients with a rapid onset of GBS (plateau within 1 week) had approximately the same distribution of outcomes as those with a longer time to plateau (Table 18–10). This observation counters some other reports but simply reflects the inclusion of many mild cases in both the good and poor outcome groups. When looking for poor prognostic factors the focus should be on patients with severe disease. Patients with milder cases, as a rule, do well no matter what other clinical or electrophysiologic features are found. Although a consistent relationship between outcome and maximal motor deficit has not yet been discovered, an association probably could be demonstrated through more careful scrutiny. Some preliminary serologic evidence has suggested that *Campylobacter jejuni* preceding GBS has been associated with more severe disease[583] but, as discussed in Chapter 6, the MGH experience has not confirmed this.

REHABILITATION

Successful rehabilitation requires an organized program with clear goals and transition points. A rehabilitation team ideally incorporates input from physicians, nurses, and social workers, as well as physical, occupational, speech, and respiratory therapists. Progress in each individual area should be discussed and coordinated regularly. There have been no systematic studies of various rehabilitation programs in GBS, or of the timing of each facet of physical therapy and rehabilitation.

Table 18–9 AGE AND OUTCOME IN PROSPECTIVE MGH SERIES*

	Age (year)			
Outcome	**<60**	**60–70**	**>70**	**Total**
Good recovery	74	12	1	87
Poor outcome	8	1	6	15
Death	0	3	3	6
Totals	82	16	10	108

*Excludes 3 patients with CIDP and 9 with incomplete follow-up.

Table 18–10 RAPIDITY OF ONSET AND OUTCOME IN PROSPECTIVE MGH SERIES*

	Maximal Weakness		
Outcome	**<7 D**	**>7 D**	**Total**
Good recovery	31	56	87
Poor outcome	8	7	15
Death	2	4	6
Totals	41	67	108

*Excludes 3 patients with CIDP after acute GBS and 9 patients with incomplete follow-up.

Most of the interventions that have been used in GBS are derived from practical experience with other similar neurologic and orthopedic diseases. This section therefore presents a practical but general overview of early and later rehabilitation as practiced in most institutions. Respiratory therapy is discussed more extensively in Chapter 17.

Early Physical Therapy

Early physical therapy consultation is required in acute GBS, though not all patients tolerate early limb manipulation. The major features of a physical therapy program are summarized in Table 18–11. The most important early goals of the physiotherapist are to prevent tendon shortening, limb malalignment, and compression neuropathies. Six percent of patients in the MGH retrospective series had one or more (pseudo) contractures that limited rehabilitation.

Table 18–11 PHYSICAL THERAPY MANAGEMENT

Facilitation of pulmonary toilet
Passive range of motion exercises 5 times a week, or more, to maintain mobility
Limb positioning in bed, including splints and wedges
Strengthening exercises after plateau phase
Assisting mobilizing when muscle strength is Medical Research Council grade 3–4
Gait retraining
Instruction in the use of orthotic devices
Pain treatment (TENS, massage, heat)

POSITIONING OF PARALYZED LIMBS

Positioning is determined in part by patient comfort and the severity of weakness. Most patients do not tolerate the prone position despite its advan-

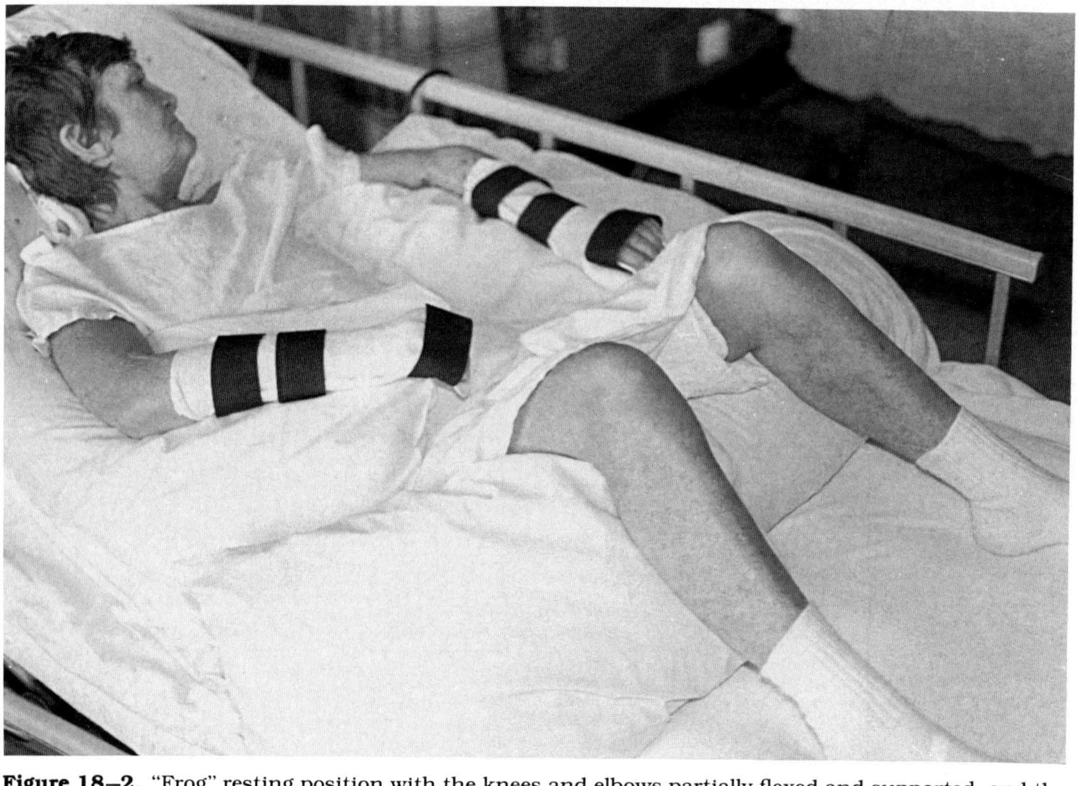

Figure 18–2. "Frog" resting position with the knees and elbows partially flexed and supported, and the shoulders extended. Most patients find this position comfortable for over an hour.

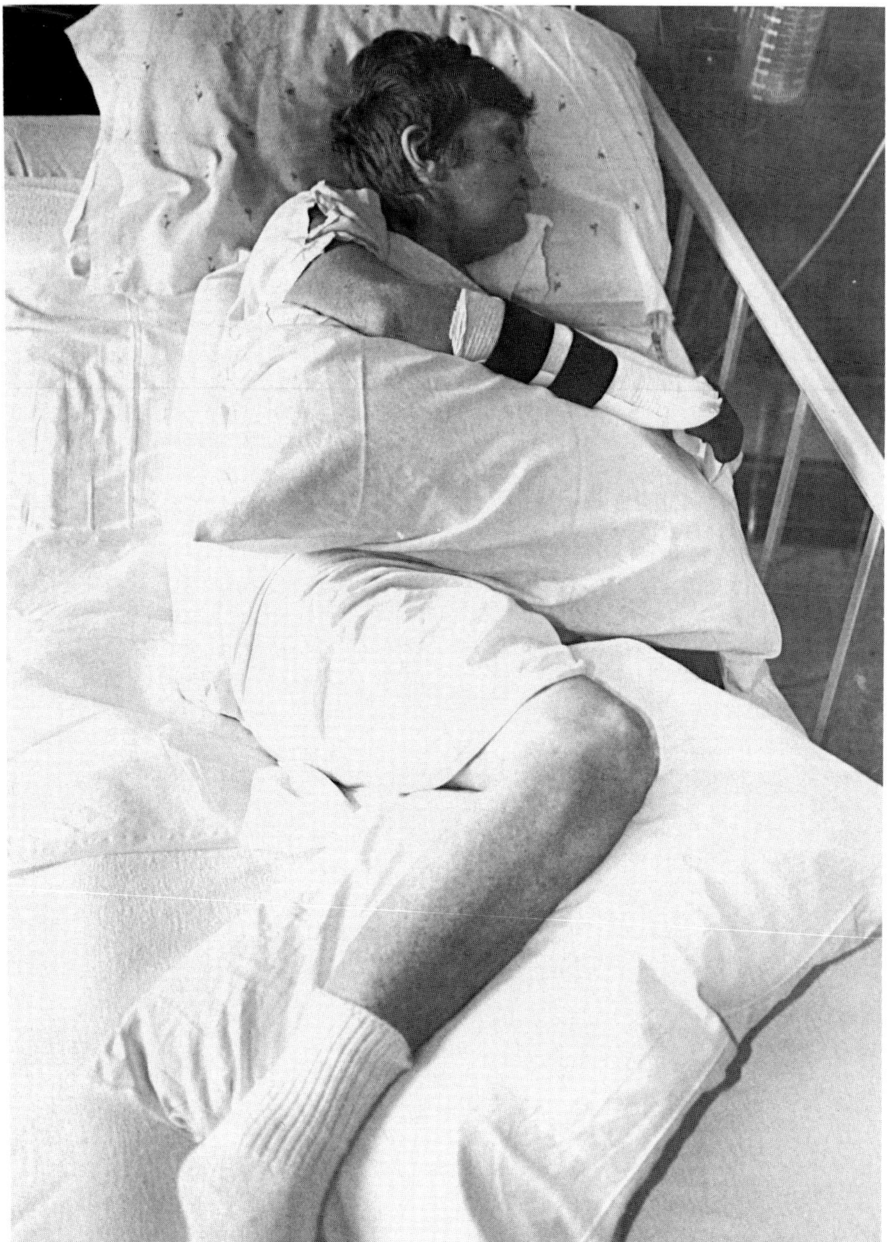

Figure 18–3. Alternative side-lying position to the "frog" position shown in Figure 18–2. This assists pulmonary drainage of one lung but risks atelectasis in the dependent lung. The patient must therefore be shifted to the opposite decubitus position frequently.

tages in maintaining extension of the hips and knees and in reducing skin pressure on posterior bony prominences.

The quadriplegic GBS patient should be turned to a decubitus position frequently, an average of every 1½ hours, for pulmonary toilet and for minimizing pressure on the skin and nerves. Most patients prefer a compromise, tilted position. At night, when pain is usually most severe and sleep should not be interrupted, the frequency of turning may be decreased to every 2 to 3 hours. We have found that a froglike position (legs bent up and apart; arms on two pillows) is comfortable and well tolerated by most quadriplegic patients (Fig. 18–2), but some with severe leg pain prefer to have their legs straightened and separated by a pillow rather than partially flexed.

One comfortable arm position with the patient supine involves 60 degrees of shoulder abduction and slight internal rotation, with 90 degrees of elbow flexion and slight forearm pronation. Alternatively, the shoulder may be externally rotated and slightly abducted, with the elbow extended and the forearm supinated. The arm is usually supported by a soft pillow under the elbow (see Fig. 18–2). An alternative decubitus position is shown in Figure 18–3. The wrists are extended with the fingers slightly flexed and thumb abducted over a hand roll. This position can be alternated with complete extension of the wrist and fingers by means of a palmar splint. Occupational therapists, however, have commented on how often recovered GBS patients have extensor contractures of the metacarpal-phalangeal joints.

Leg positioning prevents hamstring flexion and contractures, which may impede future walking, especially if there is recovery of a strong opposing quadriceps femoris. The knees and hips are therefore extended and the feet placed against a footboard to prevent Achilles tendon contracture (Fig. 18–4).

The risk of pressure sores is minimized by frequent position changes. Soft cloth rolls are usually placed under the trochanters to prevent local pressure and compression of the common peroneal nerve (Fig. 18–5). Partial support with sheepskin over other bony

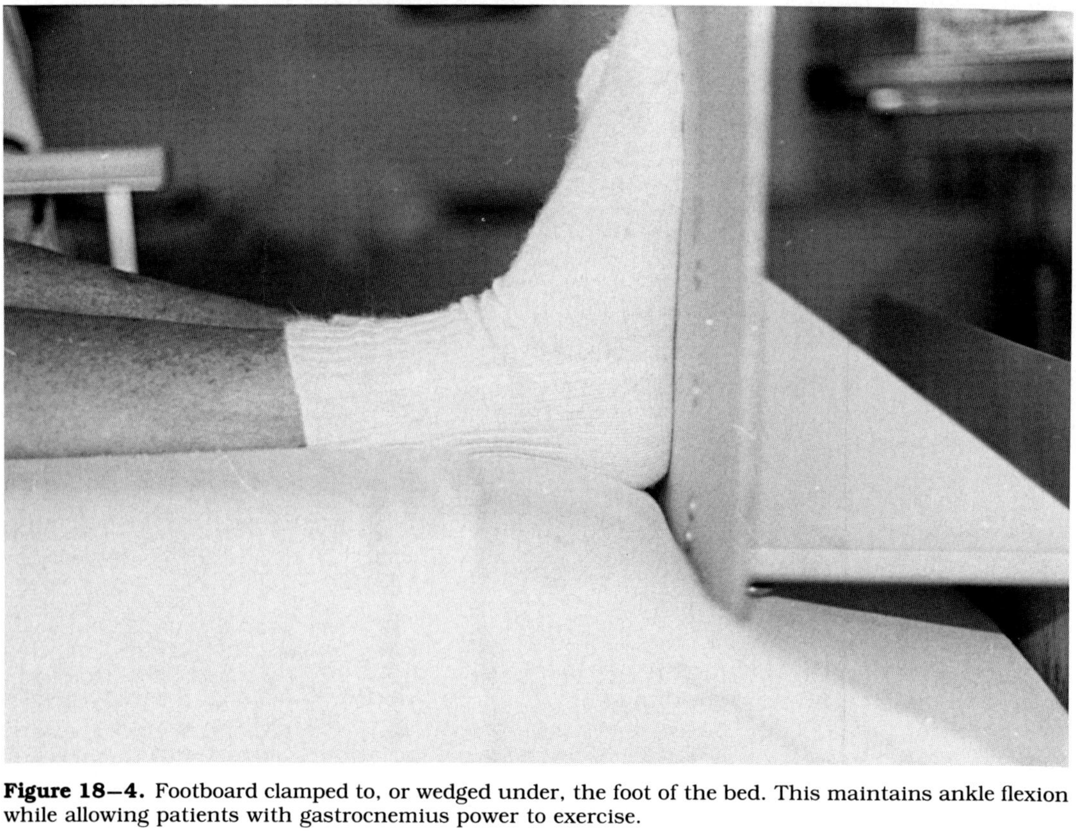

Figure 18–4. Footboard clamped to, or wedged under, the foot of the bed. This maintains ankle flexion while allowing patients with gastrocnemius power to exercise.

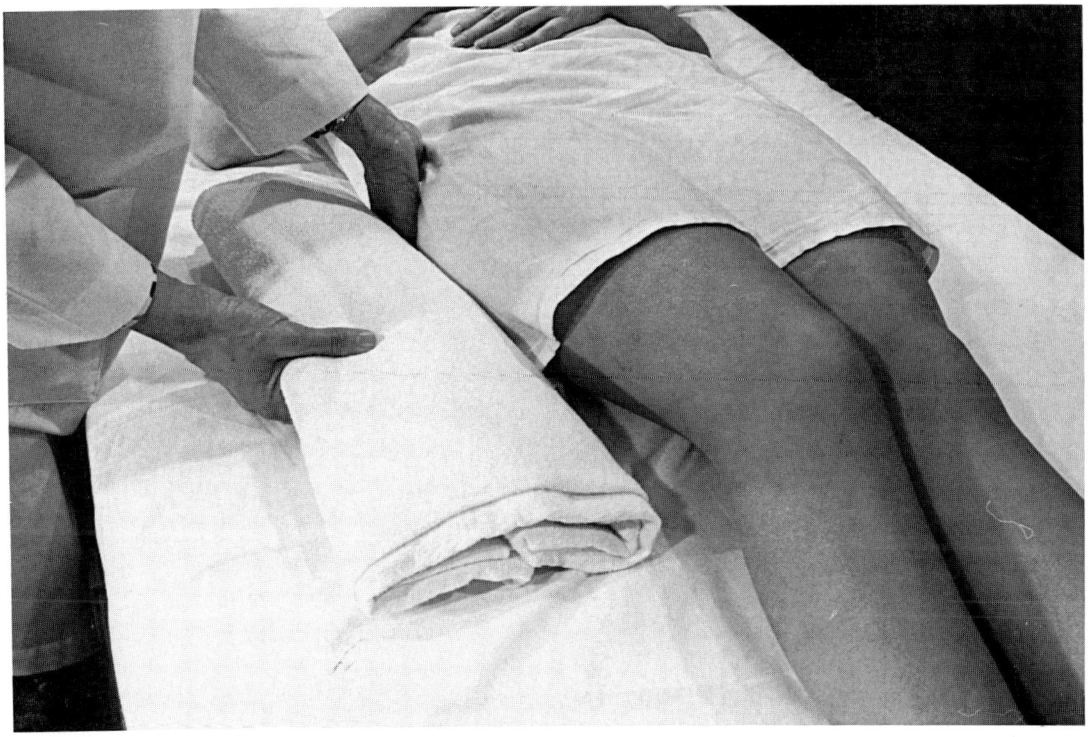

Figure 18–5. A folded bath blanket may be used as a trochanter roll to prevent pressure on the peroneal nerve when the patient is supine. (From Saperstein, AB and Frazier, MA: Introduction to Nursing Practice, F.A. Davis, 1980, p. 506, with permission.)

prominences usually suffices, but the quadriplegic patient may require a flotation of water mattress covered with sheepskin to prevent skin breakdown. Air-fluidized sand beds are seldom used but may be helpful if there have been recurrent multiple pressure sores. Partially immobilized patients have been more comfortable in these types of beds than have completely quadriplegic patients. Mechanized rotating beds for pulmonary toilet are also potentially useful, but only few GBS patients tolerate them for long.

PREVENTION OF COMPRESSION NEUROPATHIES

Foot drop is the most common residual motor deficit in GBS and has been presumed to result from peroneal nerve compression, as noted earlier, the usual symmetric deficit suggests this is an oversimplified explanation. Some electrodiagnostic series have nevertheless reported a high incidence of nerve conduction slowing across the fibular neck and at the elbow. Poor bed positioning and infrequent turning therefore may be sufficient explanations for persistent foot drop in some patients. In one small series,[153] 56% had peroneal nerve slowing, and 60% ulnar nerve slowing across pressure sites. Others[324] have reported much lower incidences of approximately 20%. Pure wrist drop has not been reported, although an uncommon bilateral posterior interosseus nerve compression has been described in GBS, thought to result from edema within an anatomically narrowed supinator space.[1159]

PASSIVE RANGE OF MOTION

Early evaluation of the range of motion of several joints allows an assessment of the likelihood of contractures. A 360-degree goniometer may be used to measure flexion and extension, rota-

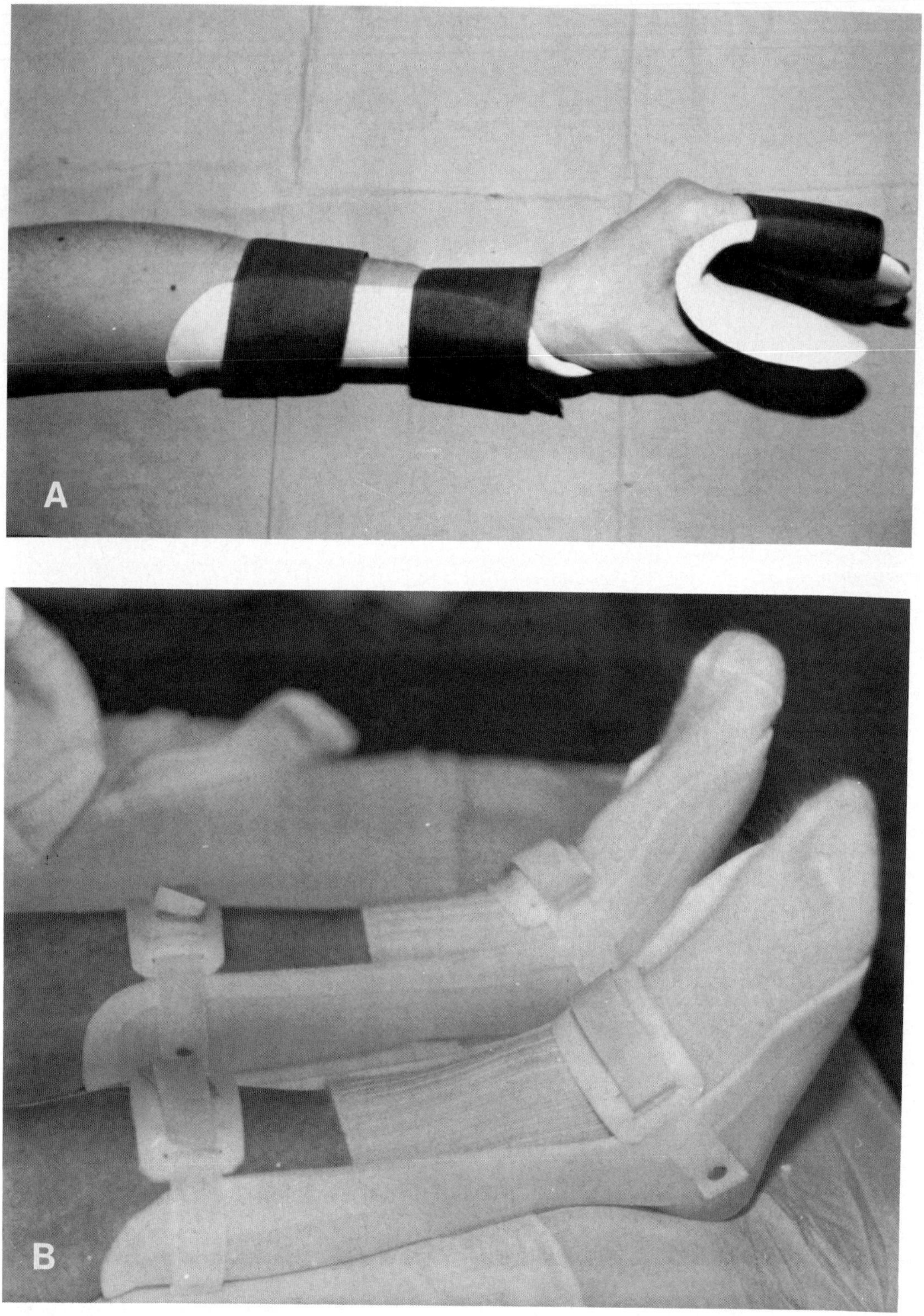

Figure 18–6. (A) Molded wrist and hand splints. (B) Acrylic foot supports with adhesive straps for use in bed (also see Figure 18–10).

tion, pronation, and supination. In the progressive phase of illness, passive range of motion exercises should be instituted to prevent muscle shortening. Persistent proximal weakness can cause significant shoulder range deficits and may produce pain when passive motion exercises are begun later. The use of overstretching, slightly beyond the normal active extension of a joint, is controversial because its value in preventing contractures has not been demonstrated definitely.[1235] Exercises should be done slowly and deliberately and repeated several times. To be effective they must be done for at least 15 minutes, 3 to 5 times a week. Mechanical aids to passive motion are discussed later (see Fig. 18–11). Until the plateau phase of GBS, passive movement exercises are usually used, and active strengthening is avoided because it often induces discomfort at night. As mentioned farther on, overly ambitious exercise anecdotally increases weakness (though there is no systematic confirmation of this).

A program of short, active restricted exercises can be initiated during the plateau or recovery phases of the illness (see Chapter 7 for definitions of these phases), mainly to prevent disuse atrophy. These exercises must be active but can be performed isometrically if motion induces muscle pain. Resistance may be added gradually as strength improves.

SPLINTING

GBS patients with quadriparesis or quadriplegia require splints to prevent flexion contractures in the resting position. A plaster wrist splint that holds the wrist and fingers slightly flexed may be applied to maintain the hands in a functional position, though these have been used infrequently at the MGH. The proper positioning for molded wrist and hand splints, of the type used most often, is shown in Figure 18–6*A*. Molded ankle splints are popular (Fig. 18–6*B*); an alternative is snug-fitting, high-laced shoes or high sneakers for 1 to 2 hour intervals, with the patient supine.

Later Rehabilitation and Physiotherapy

Active resistance strength training and mobilization generally should begin when some muscle power has returned and pain is minimal. Careful timing of exercises prevents an excessive workload, which may cause pain, cramps, or fatigue. There is no clinical evidence that strenuous exercise causes a relapse, but many patients treated ambitiously in the first 2 to 3 weeks after onset seem weaker after physical therapy. Bed-bound patients can strengthen their hand muscles by squeezing a rubber ball, and can exercise proximal muscles by using a restorator (a device with variable resistance that allows the patient to make cycling movements in bed). Such patients can also perform leg-lifting exercises with increasing weights.

Mobilization from bed is managed in defined increments. Increasing mobility begins with rolling in bed, often facilitated by first crossing the patient's ankles. Next, the patient may sit up from lying by grasping the siderails of the bed, dangling, and later continue with assisted transfer to a chair and returning to the lying position. Similar position changes are then performed on a mat.

Gait retraining should start with upright activities on the parallel bars once the patients has progressed through a program of preambulation mat exercises. These may be preceded by standing against an elevated table (Fig. 18–7*A*). Parallel bar activities include stepping forward and backward, turning, and standing pushups (Fig. 18–7*B*). Postural dizziness from orthostatic hypotension may occur when a patient has been confined to bed or a wheelchair for a long time. These complaints usually subside after a few days and a tilt table is therefore seldom needed.

Assistive devices are frequently used

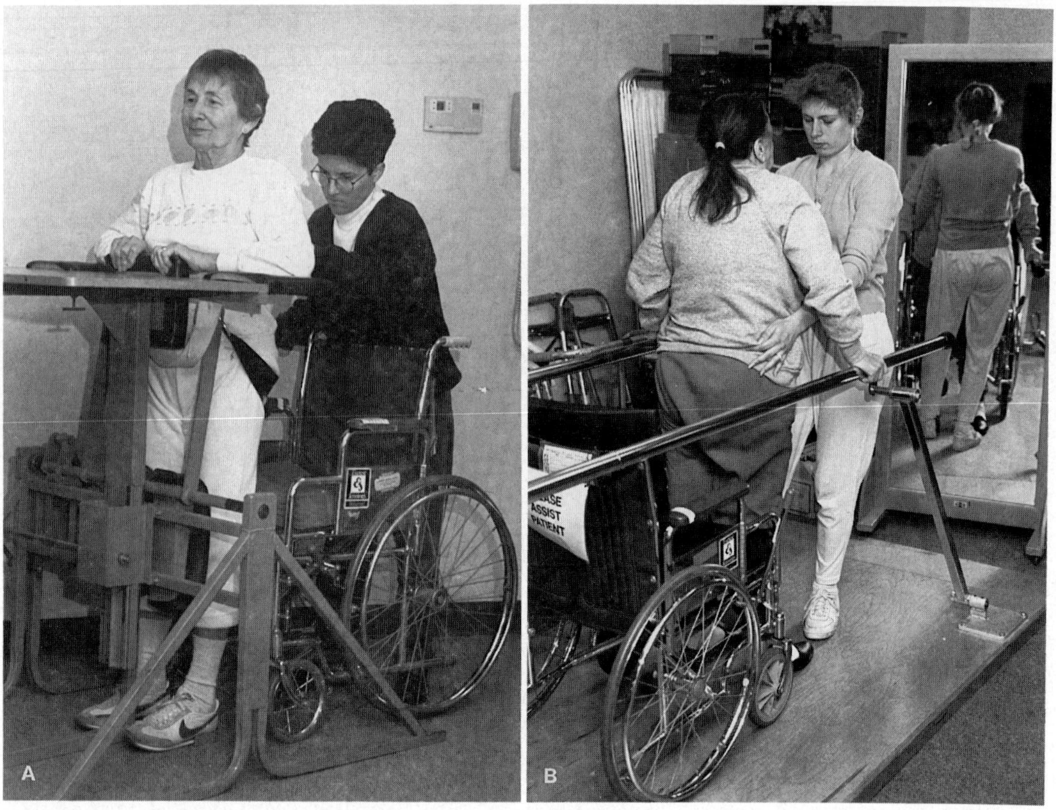

Figure 18–7. (A) Elevated tray table used for standing exercises as a prelude to walking. (B) Parallel bars are used to train walking. Patients must have enough power to elevate each leg off the bed when supine before progressing to this stage. (Courtesy of New England Rehabilitation Hospital, Woburn, MA.)

during the recovery phase. Many patients who have been completely paralyzed will have a sense of well-being during improvement and their residual symptoms may be exacerbated by overexertion. Therefore, gradual progression from a walker to crutches and then to canes is useful. The physical therapist generally gauges the extent of position sense loss and takes appropriate precautions when mobilizing patients. Experienced physiotherapists are excellent judges of the patient's ability to progress to the next phase of rehabilitation. The neurologist should assist by informing therapists of severe large-fiber deficits before therapy begins. The temporary use of a wheelchair for walking support is helpful to patients with ataxia. Finally, patients practice activities such as climbing stairs under observation. Some physiotherapists prefer a pool, when available, to retrain walking (Fig. 18–8). Walking in waist-deep water has been an excellent way to improve stamina and flexibility.

Patients who remain severely disabled, with little improvement in lower-limb strength, require training in wheelchair transfer and transport. Virtually all patients can eventually use a transfer board to move almost independently from a chair to a bed.

Biofeedback Treatment and Acupuncture

In two uncontrolled studies,[206,556] the efficacy of biofeedback was evaluated to improve power in GBS. Surface elec-

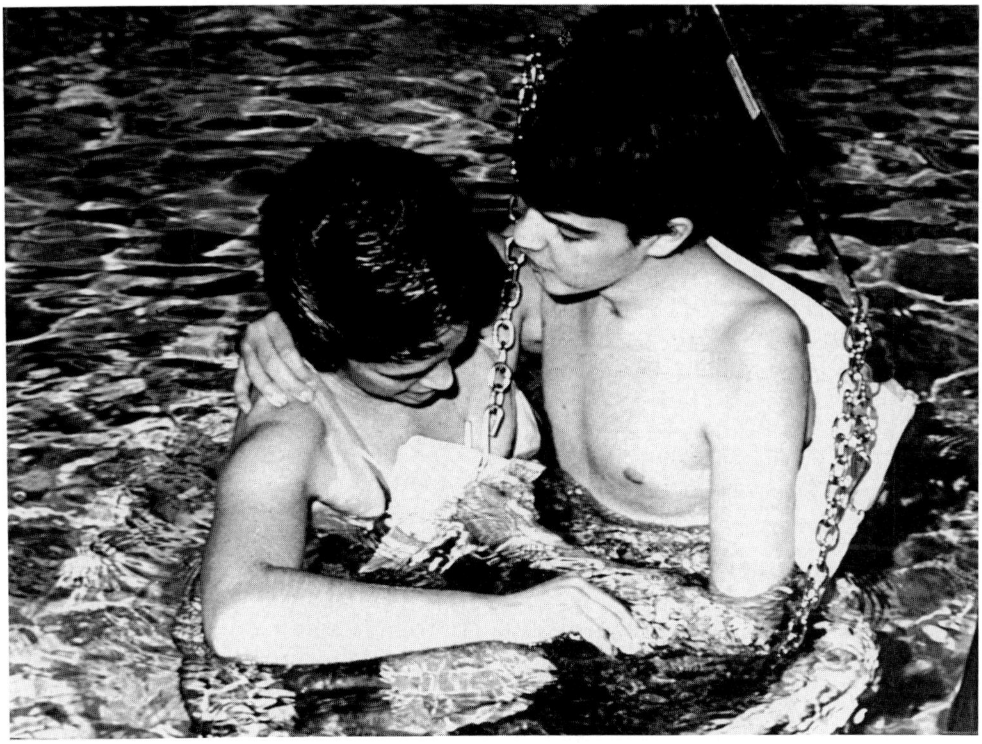

Figure 18–8. Gait and endurance training in a pool. The patient is lowered into the water with a lift and stands with the assistance of a therapist. The water offers graded resistance with increasing effort. (Courtesy of New England Rehabilitation Hospital, Woburn, MA.)

trodes placed over muscles allowed patients to increase muscle activity by observing electromyogram (EMG) interference patterns. Measurable improvement in the power of stimulated muscles was observed in two cases, but functional improvement was minimal.[556] Any advantage over conventional voluntary and assisted exercise remains to be demonstrated.

There are no systematic reports on the beneficial effects of acupuncture on GBS pain, but it may be an alternative to medications in selected patients. One uncontrolled and unconventional study from China[653] claimed improvement in muscle power with multiple acupuncture treatments in 24 patients. There were two deaths, however, and seven showed only "some improvement," which is probably worse than expected. (This paper is interesting reading for the traditional Chinese medical explanations of GBS symptoms.)

Pain Management

Severe muscle pain (see Chapter 16) usually subsides as muscle strength improves; pain is later commonly hyperesthetic or dysesthetic with paroxysmal jabs. Persistent disabling pain is uncommon, but pain remained a problem for a few patients in the prospective series despite virtually complete recovery of power and return of reflexes. Transcutaneous electrical stimulation (TENS) may provide relief in some patients.[769] Several stimulus frequencies (1 to 100 pulses per second) reportedly have been helpful both during the period of stimulation and for approximately 1 hour afterwards. After several treatments, some MGH patients have reported that TENS worsens the pain. The potential for acupuncture treatment is mentioned above.

Phenytoin, carbamazepine, or clonazepam have been inconsistently helpful in treating sharp lancinating pains, and have generally been ineffective for the more common late spontaneous or contact-induced dysesthetic burning sensations. Antidepressant drugs can be tried; one randomized, double-blind cross-over study[766] showed relief of pain in patients with diabetic neuropathy without associated mood improvement, although side effects occurred frequently. Some MGH patients have had modest improvement in nighttime dysesthesias with 50 to 150 milligrams of amitryptiline. Capsaicin has been anecdotally helpful. Hypnotherapy has been tried for pruritis, a residual symptom we have no experience with.[1053a]

Occupational Therapy

The valuable contributions of the occupational therapist are restoration of finger precision and grip power, assessment and instruction in the use of orthotic devices (discussed later), and training in self-care. The occupational therapy (OT) approach is staged to meet the patient's needs at each stage of recuperation. The initial approach is to establish ideal positioning and maintain hand joint mobility. As the patient gains strength, active exercises are used. In later rehabilitation, precision hand use and larger functional activities are taught, such as driving. There is probably a premium on establishing hand and finger positioning as soon as possible, even in the first few days of intensive care.

Many simple daily activities are impeded when thumb opposition is weak. A basic opponens orthosis places the hand in a useful position and prevents web space contracture. Special feeding aids have been developed such as utensil-holding devices for patients with limited grip power or range (Fig. 18–9). Similar cube- or hexagon-shaped wooden blocks with a hole for

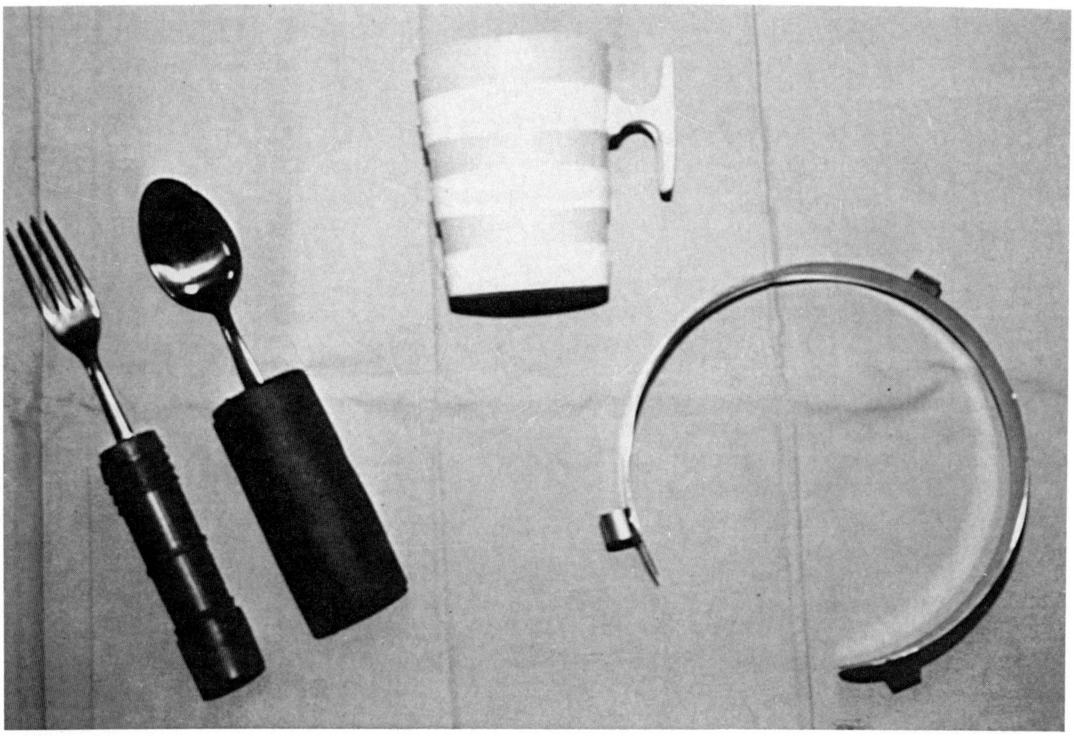

Figure 18–9. Utensils with large handles used by patients with hand weakness, under the supervision of an OT.

pencils can be helpful for writing. Patients with severe quadriplegia may require a full upper limb orthotic system to control a wheelchair motor.

Important aspects in improving independent daily function in severely disabled GBS patients include (1) transfer in and out of bed or from chairs, toilet, car, and wheelchair—sometimes requiring special equipment (eg, toilet seat attachments); (2) dressing and personal hygiene, requiring hand joint movement; and (3) communication, requiring evaluation by a speech therapist in previously intubated patients (see letter board, Fig. 16–6). Fortunately, even the most severely disabled patients usually regain the ability to lift their arms to the level of the mouth to facilitate feeding, and recover enough oropharyngeal function to speak.

Orthosis

Orthotic devices are used to assist patients with persistent regional muscle weakness or to begin ambulation when recovery is still in progress. Ankle-foot orthoses help approximate the normal biomechanical action of walking. Contemporary ankle-foot orthotic splints are molded from polyethylene, polypropylene, or acrylic. These thermoplastics are heated and reshaped to a plaster model of the leg (Fig. 18–10).[779] The flexibility of the ankle orthosis helps dorsiflex the foot during the swing-phase of walking, and assists plantarflexion during heel strike. Patients lacking voluntary knee extension are managed by anterior extension of the brace above the knee.

Upper limb orthoses are used to assist thumb opposition and to preserve the ability to grip with a pincer movement. Several mechanical systems have been developed to improve hand function.[419] For example, rubberbands on hooks cemented to nails and connected to splints allow finger exercises and hold the wrist and fingers in extension. Other mechanized devices may be used

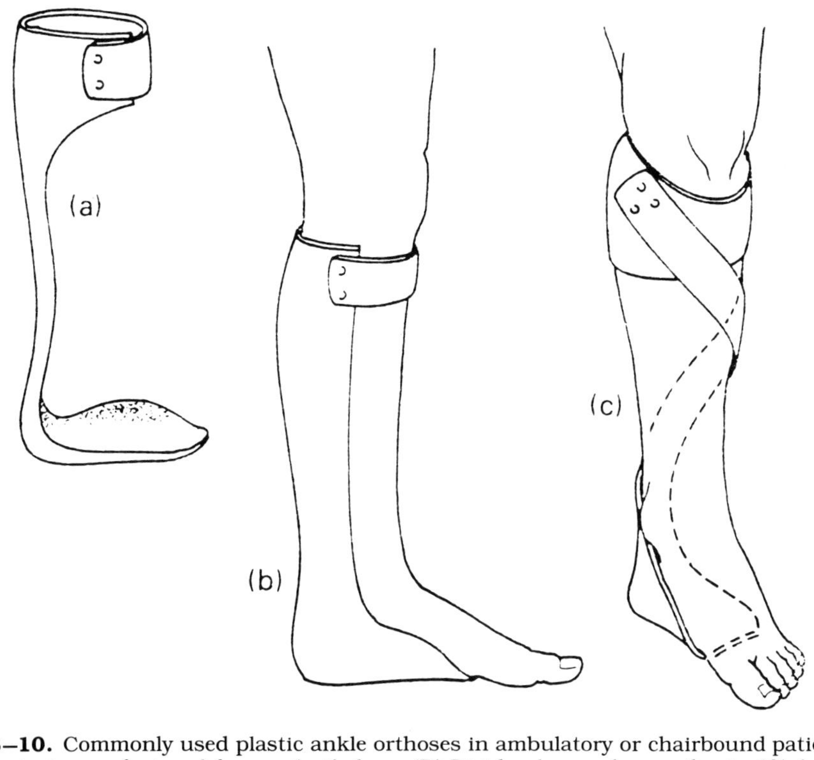

Figure 18–10. Commonly used plastic ankle orthoses in ambulatory or chairbound patients. (A) Posterior leaf spring manufactured from polyethylene. (B) Rigid polypropylene orthosis. (C) Acrylic spiral orthosis. (From McHugh and Campbell,[779] pp. 380–385, with permission.)

to move the fingers passively through an almost natural range of motion (Fig. 18–11).

Social and Psychologic Rehabilitation

After re-entry into the community, most patients take at least a year to resume a normal life. Physical fatigue is common, though, as noted earlier, rarely disabling, and may last 6 to 8 months after discharge from the hospital. Easy physical exhaustion is usually associated with some proximal leg weakness, difficulty arising from chairs, and mild paresthesias.

Mild depression is identifiable by the mental fatigue it causes, in addition to physical complaints. Two severely depressed MGH patients with GBS have required medication in addition to psychologic treatment. A patient committed suicide 40 weeks after onset of GBS in one large series,[1291] and another suicide was reported in a British steroid trial.[547]

Patients with moderate or severe disability may be unable to resume prior work. In a 2-year follow-up series of 38 ventilated GBS patients,[260] approximately one third did not return to prior work and 12% became unemployed. The national social welfare system, age, proximity to retirement, family fi-

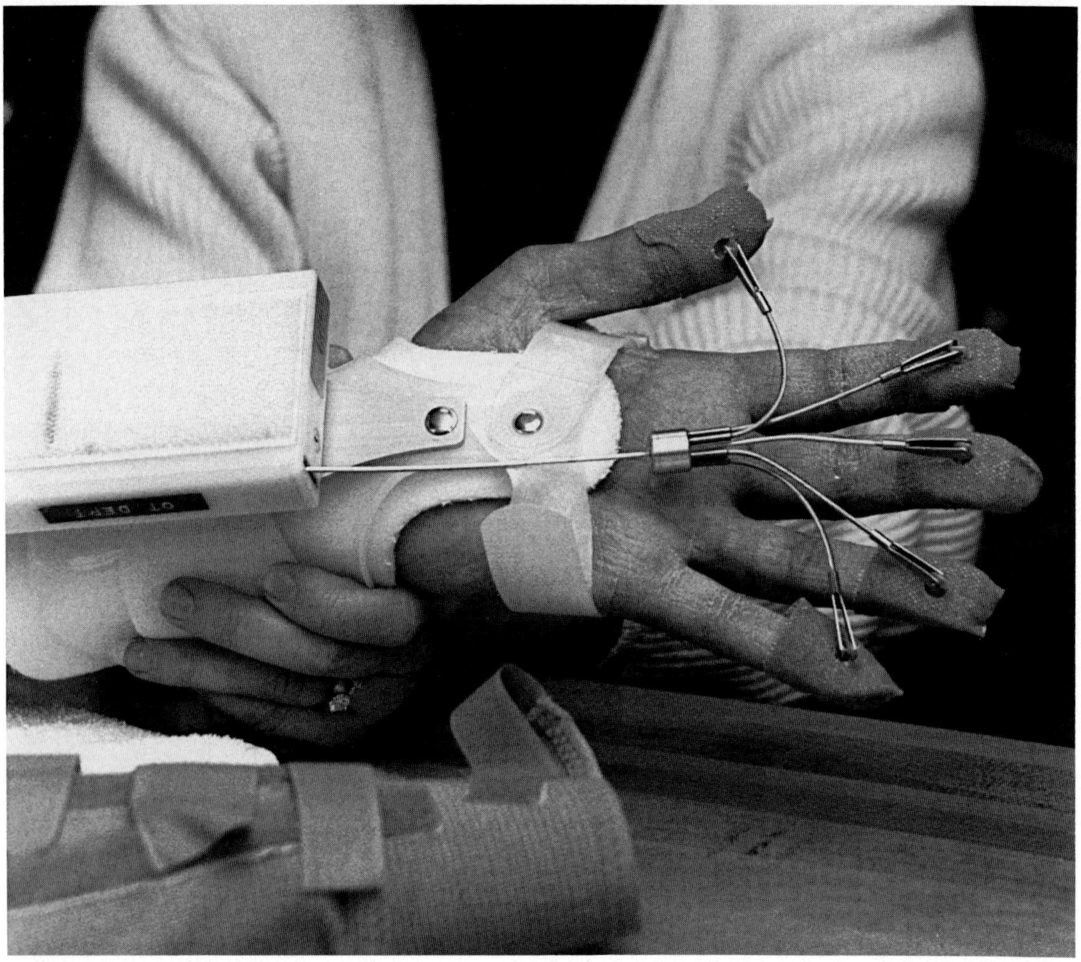

Figure 18–11. Motorized spring mechanism that passively exercises the fingers to maintain range of motion. Flexion contractures and extensor subluxations are major late rehabilitation problems that may be avoided with early attention. (Courtesy of New England Rehabilitation Hospital, Woburn, MA.)

nances, and previous job satisfaction all enter into the timing of returning to work. Patients who are physically able should be encouraged to try part-time work for 6 to 12 weeks before deciding on future plans. All MGH patients who have had professions or who were the owners of small businesses have returned to work, sometimes with additional staff to compensate for physical limitations. Local disability regulations often dictate short-term directions about returning to work. A 6- to 12-month period of total disability is often required for patients to receive compensation. It is often possible to obtain Worker's Compensation (a United States federal insurance) for nurses or physicians whose GBS has followed a cytomegalovirus (CMV) or Epstein-Barr virus (EBV) infection, particularly nurses in ICUs, dialysis units, or blood banks.

Most patients are anxious to drive as soon as possible or are obliged to drive to work. If foot power is good enough to allow independent walking without orthotic splints, driving is usually safe. Otherwise, a driving safety evaluation by a therapist is advisable.

A coordinated approach to rehabilitation, patience on the part of the patient and physician, and some creativity are required for an optimal program in any case of GBS. As with acute medical management, there is a virtue in referring these patients to individuals who embody knowledge of these various disciplines as they pertain to GBS.

REFERENCES

1. Abbas, DH, Schlagenhauff, RE, and Strong, HE: Polyradiculoneuropathy in Addison's disease. Neurology 27:494–495, 1977.
2. Abbott, KH: Tick paralysis: A review. I. Proc Mayo Clin 18:39–45, 1943.
3. Abramsky, O, Korn-Lubetzky, I, and Teitelbaum, D: Association of autoimmune diseases and cellular immune response to the neuritogenic protein in Guillain-Barré syndrome. Trans Am Neurol Assoc 105:350–354, 1980.
4. Adams, D, Festenstein, H, Gibson, JP, Hughes, RAC, Jaraquemada, J, Papasteriadis, C, Sachs, J, and Thomas, PK: HLA antigens in chronic relapsing idiopathic inflammatory polyneuropathy. J Neurol Neurosurg Psychiatry 42:184–186, 1979.
5. Adams, D, Gibson, JD, Thomas, PK, Batchelor, JR, Hughes, RAC, Kennedy, L, Festenstein, H, and Sachs, J: HLA antigens in Guillain-Barré syndrome. Lancet 2:504–505, 1977.
6. Addison, RM, Griswold, K, Huggins, CE, Hunt, JV, Kosinski, KS, and Ropper, AH: Plasma exchange in the treatment of acute Guillain-Barré syndrome (AGBS) (letter). Transfusion 22:435, 1982.
7. Adlakha, A, Phillip, PJ, and Dhar, KL: Guillain-Barré syndrome as a sequela of organophosphorus poisoning. J Assoc Physicians India 35:665–666, 1987.
8. Adler A and Hoff, H: Gehauftes auftreten von polyneuritiden unter dem Bild der Landryschen paralyse. Dtsch Med Wochenschrift 55:1880–1882, 1929.
9. Ahlberg, G and Ahlmark, G: The Landry-Guillain-Barré syndrome and pregnancy. Acta Obstet Gynecol Scand 57:377–380, 1978.
10. Ahmad, J, Kham, AS, and Siddiqui, MA: Estimation of plasma and urinary catecholamines in Guillain-Barré syndrome. Jpn J Med 24:24–29, 1985.
11. Alajouanine, TH: Necrologie, Georges Guillain (1876–1961). Bull Acad Nat Med 146:18–26, 1962.
12. Alajouanine, T, Thurel, R, Hornet, T, and Boudin, G: La polyradiculonevrite aigue generalisée avec diplegie faciale et paralysie terminale des muscles respiratoires et avec dissociation albumino-cytologique. Étude anatomique. Rev Neurol 65:681–697, 1936.
13. Albala, M, McNamara, ME, Sokol, M, and Wyshock, E: Improvement of neurologic function in chronic inflammatory demyelinating polyradiculoneuropathy following intravenous gamma-globulin infusion (letter). Arch Neurol 44:248, 1987.
14. Albers, JW, Donofrio, PD, and McGonagle, TK: Sequential electrodiagnostic abnormalities in acute inflammatory demyelinating polyradiculoneuropathy. Muscle Nerve 8: 528–539, 1985.
15. Albers, JW and Kelly, JJ: Acquired inflammatory demyelinating polyneuropathies: Clinical and electrodiagnostic features. Muscle Nerve 12:435–451, 1989.
16. Albers, JW and Kelly, JJ: Electrodiagnostic findings in acute porphyric neuropathy. Muscle Nerve 1:292–296, 1978.
17. Albert, RK and Condie, F: Handwashing patterns in medical inten-

sive-care units. N Engl J Med 304:1465–1466, 1981.
18. Al Deeb, SM, Yaqub, BA, Sharif, HS, and Phadke, JG: Neurobrucellosis: Clinical characteristics, diagnosis, and outcome. Neurology 39:498–501, 1989.
19. Al-Din, AN: The nosological position of the ophthalmoplegia, ataxia and areflexia syndrome: "The spectrum hypothesis." Acta Neurol Scand 75:287–294, 1987.
20. Al-Din, AN, Anderson, M, Bickerstaff, ER, and Harvey, I: Brainstem encephalitis and the syndrome of Miller Fisher. A clinical study. Brain 105:481–495, 1982.
21. Alfrey, AC, Terman, DS, Brettschneider, L, Simpson, KM, and Odgen, DA: Hypermagnesemia after renal homotransplantation. Ann Intern Med 73:367–371, 1980.
22. Allen, N, Mendell, JR, Billmaier, DJ, Fontaine, RE, and O'Neill, J: Toxic polyneuropathy due to methyl *n*-butyl ketone. Arch Neurol 32:209–218, 1975.
23. Allman, RM, Laprade, CA, Noel, LB, Walker, JM, Moorer, CA, Dear, MR, and Smith, CR: Pressure sores among hospitalized patients. Ann Intern Med 105:337–342, 1986.
24. Al-Qudah, AA, Shahar, E, Logan, WJ, and Murphy, GE: Neonatal Guillain-Barré syndrome. Pediatr Neurol 4:255–256, 1988.
25. Altenkirch, H, Mager, J, Stoltenburg, G, and Helmbrecht, J: Toxic polyneuropathies after sniffing a glue thinner. J Neurol 214:137–152, 1977.
26. Amarenco, P, Sauron, B, Schuller, E, Chain, F, and Castaigne, P: Serum and CSF humoral immunity in Guillain-Barré syndrome: Clinical correlations. J Neurol Sci 80:129–142, 1987.
27. Amundson, DE and Goodman, JC: Hodgkin's disease in association with Guillain-Barré-Strohl syndrome: Case report. Milit Med 148, 512–513, 1983.
28. Andersen, O, Lindberg, J, Modigh, K, and Reske-Nielsen, E: Subacute dysautonomia with incomplete recovery. Acta Neurol Scand 48:510–519, 1972.
29. Anderson, LJ, Nicholson, KG, Tauxe, RV, and Winkler, WG: Human rabies in the United States, 1960–1979: Epidemiology, diagnosis and prevention. Ann Intern Med 100:728–735, 1984.
30. Anderson, NE, Rosenblum, MK, Graus, F, Wiley, RG, and Posner, JB: Autoantibodies in paraneoplastic syndromes associated with small-cell lung cancer. Neurology 38:1391–1398, 1988.
31. Andersson, T and Siden, A: A clinical study of the Guillain-Barré syndrome. Acta Neurol Scand 66:316–327, 1982.
32. Antony, JH, Pollard, JD, and McLeod, JG: Effects of plasmapheresis on the course of experimental allergic neuritis in rabbits. J Neurol Neurosurg Psychiatry 44:1124–1128, 1981.
33. Appenzeller, O: "Pure pan-dysautonomia." A newly discovered syndrome. Calif Med 117:18–23, 1972.
34. Appenzeller, O, Arnason, BG, and Adams, RD: Experimental autonomic neuropathy: An immunologically induced disorder of reflex vasomotor function. J Neurol Neurosurg Psychiatry 28:510–515, 1965.
35. Appenzeller, O and Kornfeld, M: Acute pandysautonomia. Clinical and morphologic study. Arch Neurol 29:334–339, 1973.
36. Appenzeller, O and Marshall, J: Vasomotor disturbance in Landry-Guillain-Barré syndrome. Arch Neurol 9:368–372, 1963.
37. Applebaum, E, Greenberg, M, and Nelson, J: Neurological complications following antirabies vaccination. JAMA 151:188, 1953.
38. Argov, Z and Mastaglia, FL: Disorders of neuromuscular transmission caused by drugs. N Engl J Med 301:409–413, 1979.
39. Aring, CD: Infectious polyneuritis. Clinics 4:263, 1945.
40. Arnason, BGW: Acute inflammatory demyelinating polyradiculoneuropa-

thies. In Dyck, PJ, Thomas, PK, Lambert, EH, and Bunge, R (eds): Peripheral Neuropathy, ed 2. Vol I. WB Saunders, Philadelphia, 1984, pp 2050–2100.

41. Arnason, BG and Asbury, AK: Idiopathic polyneuritis after surgery. Arch Neurol 18:500–507, 1968.
42. Arnason, BG, Winkler, GF, and Hadler, NM: Cell-mediated demyelination of peripheral nerve in tissue culture. Lab Invest 21:1–10, 1969.
43. Arnold, AG, Lawrence, DS, and Corbitt, G: Cytomegalovirus infection and the Guillain-Barré syndrome. Postgrad Med J 54:112–114, 1978.
44. Arnon, SS, Midura, TF, Clay, SA, Wood, RM, and Chin, J: Infant botulism. Epidemiological, clinical, and laboratory aspects. JAMA 237: 1946–1951, 1977.
45. Arnould G, Tridon, P, Schmitt, J, and Guerci, O: Polyradiculonevrite aigue curable a forme ophthalmoplegique. Rev Otoneuroophtalmol 32:425–428, 1960.
46. Aromaa, U and Kalima, RV: Ranitidine and prevention of pulmonary aspiration syndrome. Acta Anaesthesiol Scand 30:10–12, 1986.
47. Arora, NS and Rochester, DF: Respiratory muscle strength and maximal voluntary ventilation in undernourished patients. Am Rev Respir Dis 126:5–8, 1982.
48. Arrowsmith, JB, Milstein, JB, Kuritsky, JN, and Murano, G: Streptokinase and the Guillain-Barré syndrome (letter). Ann Intern Med 103:302, 1985.
49. Arrowsmith, WA, Smithells, RW, and Congdon, PJ: Temporary paralysis after infection by respiratory syncytial virus (letter). Lancet 1:743, 1975.
50. Arstila, AU, Riekkinen, PJ, Rinne, UK, Pelleniemi, TT, and Nevalainen, R: Guillain-Barré syndrome. Neurochemical and ultrastructural study. Eur Neurol 5:257–269, 1971.
51. Asbury, AK: Diagnostic considerations in Guillain-Barré syndrome. Ann Neurol (Suppl) 9:1–5, 1981.
52. Asbury, AK, Arnason, BG, and Adams, RD: The inflammatory lesion in idiopathic polyneuritis. Medicine 48:173–215, 1969.
53. Asbury, AK, Arnason, BG, Karp, HR, and McFarlin, DE: Criteria for diagnosis of Guillain-Barré syndrome. Ann Neurol 3:565–566, 1978.
54. Ashworth, B: Ophthalmoplegia in the Guillain-Barré syndrome. Trans Ophthalmol Soc UK 93:207, 1973.
55. Ashworth, B and Smyth, GE: Relapsing motor polyneuropathy. Acta Neurol Scand 45:342–350, 1969.
56. Astrom, KE, Webster, H deF, and Arnason, BG: The initial lesion in experimental allergic neuritis. A phase and electron microscopic study. J Exp Med 128:469–482, 1968.
57. Atkinson, AB, Brown, JJ, Lever, AF, McAreavey, D, Robertson, JIS, Behan, PO, Melville, ID, and Weir, AI: Neurological dysfunction in two patients receiving captopril and cimetidine. Lancet 2:36–37, 1980.
58. Atwall, AJS, Smith, BH, and Dickenson, ES: Pseudo-internuclear ophthalmoplegia in polyneuritis (letter). Arch Neurol 33:457, 1976.
59. Auld, PAM, Kevy, SV, and Eley, RC: Poliomyelitis in children. Experience with 956 cases in the 1955 Massachusetts epidemic. N Engl J Med 263:1093–1100, 1960.
60. Austin, JH: Recurrent polyneuropathies and their corticosteroid treatment. With five-year observations of a placebo-controlled case treated with corticotrophin, cortisone, and prednisone. Brain 81:157–192, 1958.
61. Avasthi, G and Aggarwal, SP: Plasmodium falciparum malaria associated with Guillain-Barré syndrome. J Indian Med Assoc 83:360, 1985.
62. Aylett, P: Five cases of acute infective polyneuritis (Guillain-Barré syndrome) in children. Arch Dis Child 29:531–536, 1954.
63. Bachman, DS, Paulson, GW, and Mendell, JR: Acute inflammatory polyradiculoneuropathy following hymenoptera stings. JAMA 247:1443–1445, 1982.
64. Baer, GM, Shaddock, JH, Houff, SA, Harrison, AK, and Gardner, JJ: Human rabies transmitted by corneal

transplant. Arch Neurol 39:103–107, 1982.

65. Bahemuka, M: Guillain-Barré syndrome in Kenya: A clinical review of 54 patients. J Neurol 235:418–421, 1988.
66. Baier, S and Zimmeth, Schomaker, M: Woman in Bed Number 10. CRC Press, Boca Raton, 1985.
67. Bailey, P and Ewing, J: A contribution to the study of acute ascending (Landry's) paralysis, with exhibition of specimens stained by Nissl method. J Nerv Ment Dis 23:316–322, 1896.
68. Bak, P: Guillain-Barré syndrome in a Danish county. Neurology 35:207–211, 1985.
69. Bale, JF, Rote, NS, Bloomer, LC, and Bray, PF: Guillain-Barré–like polyneuropathy after renal transplant. Possible association with cytomegalovirus infection (case report). Arch Neurol 37:784, 1980.
70. Banerjee, AK and Chopra, JS: Paralytic rabies. Neurol India 22:83–86, 1974.
71. Banerji, NK and Millar, JHD: Guillain-Barré syndrome in children, with special reference to serial nerve conduction studies. Dev Med Child Neurol 14:56–63, 1972.
72. Bank, WJ, Pleasure, DE, Suzuki, K, Nigro, M, and Katz, R: Thallium poisoning. Arch Neurol 26:456–464, 1972.
73. Bannwarth, A: Chronische lymphocytare meningitis entzundliche polyneuritis und rheumatismus. Arch f Psychiat Nervenkr 113:284–376, 1941.
74. Bannwarth A: Die entzundliche polyneuritis mit dem liquorsyndrom von Guillain und Barré (polyradiculitis) un Rahinen einer biologischen krankheitsz-betrachtung. Arch f Psychiat Nervenkr 115:566–672, 1943.

74a. Bannwarth, A: Neuritis und polyneuritis nach Typhus-Paratyphus-Schutzimpfung. Ein Weiterer Beclrag zum Thema: "Allergie" und Nervensystem." Arch f Psychiat Nervenkr 118–180:531–568, 1948.

75. Bansal, BC, Sood, AK, and Jain, SK: Dysautonomia in Guillain-Barré syndrome. J Assoc Physicians India 35:417–419, 1987.
76. Baoxun, Z, Yang, Y, Huang, H, and Liu, X: Acute polyradiculitis (Guillain-Barré syndrome): An epidemiological study of 156 cases observed in Beijing. Ann Neurol (Suppl) 9:146–148, 1981.
77. Barale, F, Bourgeois, F, Lazar, JP, Daoudal, P, and Becque, O: Entrainement electrosystolique endocavitaire au cours d'une polyradiculonevrite ascendante. Nouv Presse Med 7:1749, 1978.
78. Barbano, AJ and Lifshutz, S: Guillain-Barré syndrome complicating puerperium. Am J Obstet Gynecol 71:893–894, 1956.
79. Barber, HS: Polyradiculoneuritis (Guillain-Barré's syndrome) in East Anglia. Lancet 2:548–550, 1940.
80. Barohn, RJ, Kissel, JT, Warmolts, JR, and Mendell, JR: Chronic inflammatory demyelinating neuropathy. Arch Neurol 46:878–884, 1989.
81. Barontini, F, Sita, D, and Giordano, G: A reappraisal of Fisher's syndrome based on clinical and CT findings in 3 cases. With a relapse in the first case. In Huber, A and Klein, D (eds): Neurogenetics and Neuro-ophthalmology. Elsevier/North-Holland Biomedical Press, Amsterdam, 1981, pp 65–69.
82. Bartlett, JG, O'Keefe, P, Tally, FP, Louie, TJ, and Gorbach, SL: Bacteriology of hospital-acquired pneumonia. Arch Intern Med 146:868–871, 1986.
83. Beale, EO and Miller, MT: The Guillain-Barré Syndrome. A review of admissions to an intensive care unit over 8 years. S Afr Med J 67:10–12, 1985.
84. Beattie, AD, Briggs, JD, Canavan, JSF, Doyle, D, Mullin, PJ, and Watson, AA: Acute lead poisoning. Five cases resulting from self-injection of lead and opium. Q J Med 44:275–284, 1975.
85. Becker, WJ, Walters, GV, and Humphreys, P: Fisher syndrome in childhood. Neurology 31:555–560, 1981.
86. Becker-Casademont, R and Eber, B: Verlauf und prognose der rehabilita-

tion von patienten nach akuter polyneuritis. Rehabilitation 25:160–165, 1986.
87. Beckett, VL and Dinn, JJ: Segmental demyelination in rheumatoid arthritis. Q J Med 4:71–80, 1972.
88. Beghi, E, Kurland, LT, Mulder, DW, and Wiederholt, WC: Guillain-Barré syndrome. Clinicoepidemiologic features and effect of influenza vaccine. Arch Neurol 42:1053–1057, 1985.
89. Behan, PO, Behan, WMH, Feldman, RG, and Kies, MW: Cell-mediated hypersensitivity to neural antigens. Occurrence in human patients and non-human primates with neurological disease. Arch Neurol 27:145–152, 1972.
90. Behan, PO, Lamarche, JB, Feldman, RG, and Sheramata, WA: Lymphocyte transformation in the Guillain-Barré syndrome. Lancet 1:421, 1970.
91. Behan, PO, Lessel, S, and Roche, M: Optic neuritis in the Landry-Guillain-Barré syndrome. Br J Ophthalmol 60:58–59, 1976.
92. Behan, PO, Lowenstein, LM, Stilmant, M, and Sax, DS: Landry-Guillain-Barré-Strohl syndrome and immune-complex nephritis. Lancet 1:850–854, 1973.
93. Bell, W, Van Allan, M, and Blackman, J: Fisher syndrome in childhood. Dev Med Child Neurol 12:758–766, 1970.
94. Berardi, VP, Weeks, KE, and Steere, AC: Serodiagnosis of early Lyme disease: Analysis of IgM and IgG antibody responses to using an antibody-capture enzyme immunoassay. J Infect Dis 158:754–760, 1988.
95. Berger, AR, Logigian, EL, and Shahani, BT: Reversible proximal conduction block underlies rapid recovery in Guillain-Barré syndrome. Muscle Nerve 11:1039–1042, 1988.
96. Berger, JR, Ayyar, DR, and Kaszovitz, B: Guillain-Barré syndrome complicating typhoid fever. Ann Neurol 20:649–650, 1986.
97. Berger, JR, Ayyar, DR, and Sheremata, WR: Guillain-Barré syndrome complicating acute hepatitis B. (A case with detailed electrophysiological and immunological studies.) Arch Neurol 38:366–368, 1981.
98. Bernhardt, M: Beitrag zur Lehre von den acuten allemeinen Paralyse. Berliner Klinische Wochenschrift 8:561–564, 1871.
99. Bernsen, HJJA, Van Loon, AM, Poels, RFJ, Verhagen, WIM, and Frenken, CWGM: Herpes simplex virus specific antibody determined by immunoblotting in cerebrospinal fluid of a patient with the Guillain-Barré syndrome. J Neurol Neurosurg Psychiatry 52:788–791, 1989.
100. Bertrand, A, Janbon, F, Clot, J, Milane, J, and Bosc, E: Guillain-Barré polyradiculoneuritis and influenza virus. Presse Med 79:2328, 1971.
101. Bettinelli, A, Giani, M, Rossi, L, Bardare, M, Longarett, A, Ghio, L, Mazzucchi, E, Paterlini, GL, Edefonti, A, and Mihatsch, MJ: Ex novo episodes of acute glomerulonephritis and Guillain-Barré syndrome: A case report. Clin Nephrol 31:269–273, 1989.
102. Beukelman, D and Garret, K: Augmentive and alternative communication for adults with acquired communication disorders. Augmentive Alternative Communications 4:104–121, 1988.
103. Bienfang, DC, Kantrowitz, FG, Noble, JL, and Raynor, AM: Ocular abnormalities after influenza immunization (letter). Arch Ophthalmol 96:1649, 1977.
104. Bignami, A and Servi, M: Acute internal and external ophthalmoplegia with muscle weakness (letter). Lancet 1:1110, 1963.
105. Birchfield, RI and Shaw C: Postural hypotension in the Guillain-Barré syndrome. Arch Neurol 10:149–157, 1964.
106. Birket-Smith, E and Olivarius BF: Polyradiculo-myopathia in transient thyrotoxicosis. Dan Med Bull 4:217–219, 1957.
107. Bishopric, G, Bruner, J, and Butler, J: Guillain-Barré syndrome with cytomegalovirus infection of peripheral nerves. Arch Pathol Lab Med 109:1106–1108, 1985.
108. Blachley, JD and Knochel, JP: To-

bacco chewer's hypokalemia: Licorice revisited. N Engl J Med 302:784–785, 1980.

109. Black, LF and Hyatt, RE: Maximal respiratory pressures: Normal values and relationship to age and sex. Am Rev Respir Dis 99:696–702, 1969.
110. Black, LF and Hyatt, RE: Maximal static respiratory pressures in generalized neuromuscular disease. Am Rev Respir Dis 103:641–650, 1971.
111. Blackburn, GL, Maini, BS, and Pierce, EC: Nutrition in the critically ill patient. Anesthesiology 47:181–194, 1977.
112. Blanc, PL, Thomas, L, Holzapfal, L, Gerard-Boncompain, M, Robert, D, and Bouillat, J: Entrainement electrosystolique endo-cavitaire temporaire au cours d'un syndrome de Guillain et Barré. Nouv Presse Med 7:123, 1978.
113. Blaser, MJ and Reller, LB: Campylobacter enteritis. N Engl J Med 305:1444–1452, 1981.
114. Blaser, MJ, Wells, JG, Feldman, RA, Pollard, RA, Allen, JR, and the Collaborative Diarrheal Disease Study Group: *Campylobacter* enteritis in the United States. A multicenter study. Ann Intern Med 98:360–365, 1983.
115. Blau, I, Casson, I, Lieberman, A, and Weiss, E: The not-so-benign Miller Fisher syndrome: a variant of the Guillain-Barré syndrome. Arch Neurol 37:384–385, 1980.
116. Blood, A, Locke, W, and Carabasi, R: Corticotropin therapy in Guillain-Barré syndrome. JAMA 152:139–140, 1953.
117. Bohannon, RW and Dubuc, WE: Documentation of the resolution of weakness in a patient with Guillain-Barré syndrome. A clinical report. Phys Ther 64:1388–1389, 1984.
118. Bolton, CF, Gilbert, JJ, Hahn, AF, and Sibbald, WJ: Polyneuropathy in critically ill patients. J Neurol Neurosurg Psychiatry 47:1223–1231, 1984.
119. Bolton, CF, Laverty, DA, Brown, JD, Witt, NJ, Hahn, AF, and Sibbald, WJ: Critically ill polyneuropathy. Electrophysiological studies and differentiation from Guillain-Barré syndrome. J Neurol Neurosurg Psychiatry 49:563–573, 1986.
120. Bronkowsky, HL and Schady, W: Neurologic manifestations of acute porphyria. Seminars in Liver Disease 2:108–124, 1982.
121. Borit, A and Altrocchi, PH: Recurrent polyneuropathy and neurolymphomatosis. Arch Neurol 24:40–48, 1971.
122. Bos, AP, van der Meche, FGA, Witsenburg, M, and van der Voort, E: Experiences with Guillain-Barré syndrome in a pediatric intensive care unit. Intensive Care Med 13:328–331, 1987.
123. Bosch, VV, Dowling, PC, and Cook, SD: Hepatitis A virus immunoglobulin M antibody in acute neurological disease. Ann Neurol 14:685–687, 1983.
124. Boshes, B and Sherman, IC: Variability of the course of the Guillain-Barré syndrome. Neurology 3:789–799, 1953.
125. Boucharlat, J, Groslambert, R, and Chateau, R: Polyradiculoneuritis as a symptom of varicella (a case report). J Med Lyon 49:1443, 1968.
126. Bouche, P, Bousser, M-G, Peytour, MA, and Cathala, HP: Perhexiline maleate and peripheral neuropathy. Neurology 29:739–743, 1979.
127. Boucher, CAB, de Gans, J, van Oers, R, Danner, S, and Goudsmit, J: Transmission of HIV and AIDS by plasmapheresis for Guillain-Barré syndrome. Case report. Clin Neurol Neurosurg 90:235–236, 1988.
128. Bouchez, B, Poirriez, J, Arnott, GE, Fourrier, F, Chopin, C, and Blondel, M: Acute polyradiculoneuritis during toxoplasmosis (letter). J Neurol 231:347, 1985.
129. Bower, BD and Newsholme, EA: Treatment of idiopathic polyneuritis by a polyunsaturated fatty-acid diet. Lancet 1:583–585, 1978.
130. Bowes, D: The doctor as patient: An encounter with Guillain-Barré syndrome. Can Med Assoc J 131:1343–1348, 1984.
131. Bradford, JR, Bashford, EF, and Wilson, JA: Acute infectious polyneuritis. Q J Med 12:88–126, 1918.

132. Bradford, JR, Bashford, EF, and Wilson, JA: Acute infectious polyneuritis by a polyunsaturated fatty-acid diet. Lancet 1:583, 1978.
133. Bradley, SG and Klika, LJ: A fatal poisoning from the Oregon rough-skinned newt *(Taricha granulosa)*. JAMA 246:241, 1981.
134. Brashear, JR, Bonnin, JM, and Login, IS: Encephalomyeloneuritis simulating Guillain-Barré syndrome. Neurology 35:1146–1151, 1985.
135. Bravo, RH, Katz, M, Inturrisi, M, and Cohen, NH: Obstetric management of Landry-Guillain-Barré syndrome: A case report. Am J Obstet Gynecol 142:714–715, 1982.
136. Brechenmacher, C, Vital, C, Deminiere, C, Laurentjoye, L, Castaing, Y, Gbikpi-Benissan, G, Cardinaud, JP, and Favarel-Garrigues, JP: Guillain-Barré syndrome: An ultrastructural study of peripheral nerve in 65 patients. Clin Neuropathol 6:19–24, 1987.
137. Bredin, DP: Guillain-Barré syndrome: The unresolved cardiac problems. Ir J Med Sci 146:273–279, 1977.
138. Breman, JG and Hayner, NS: Guillain-Barré syndrome and its relationship to swine influenza vaccination in Michigan, 1976–1977. Am J Epidemiol 119:880–889, 1984.
139. Bresalier, RS, Grendell, JH, Cello, JP, and Meyer, AA: Sucralfate suspension versus titrated antacid for the prevention of acute stress-related gastrointestinal hemorrhage in critically ill patients. Am J Med 83:110–116, 1987.
140. Bresler, R and Johnson CT: Cushing's syndrome and the Guillain-Barré syndrome. Ann Intern Med 50:1298–1303, 1959.
141. Brettle, RP, Gross, M, Legg, NJ, Lockwood, M, and Pallis, C: Treatment of acute polyneuropathy by plasma exchange. Lancet 2:1100, 1978.
142. Brewis, M, Poskanzer, DC, and Rolland, C: Neurological disease in an English city. Acta Neurol Scand (Suppl)24:12–89, 1966.
143. Briscoe, DM, McMenamin, JB, and O'Donohoe NV: Prognosis in Guillain-Barré syndrome. Arch Dis Child 62:733–735, 1987.
144. Brodie, ED: Toxic salamanders. JAMA 247:1408, 1982.
145. Bronsky, D, Kaganiec, GI, and Waldstein, SS: An association between the Guillain-Barré syndrome and hyperthyroidism. Am J Med Sci 247:196–200, 1964.
146. Brosnan, CF, Lyman, WD, Tansey, FA, and Carter, TH: Quantitation of mast cells in experimental allergic neuritis. J Neuropathol Exp Neurol 44:196–203, 1985.
147. Brosnan, CF and Tansey, FA: Delayed onset of experimental allergic neuritis in rats treated with reserpine. J Neuropathol Exp Neurol 43:84–93, 1984.
148. Brosnan, JV, Craggs, RI, King, RHM, and Thomas, PK: Attempts to suppress experimental allergic neuritis in the rat by pretreatment with antigen. Acta Neuropathol 64:153–160, 1984.
149. Brosnan, JV, Craggs, RI, King, RHM, and Thomas, PK: Reduced susceptibility of T cell-deficient rats to induction of experimental allergic neuritis. J Neuroimmunol 14:267–282, 1987.
150. Brown, JR and Baker, AB: The diagnosis of Guillain-Barré disease. Am J Med 2:45–52, 1947.
151. Brown, MJ, Rosen, JL, and Lisak, RP: Demyelination in vivo by Guillain-Barré syndrome and other human serum. Muscle Nerve 10:263–271, 1987.
152. Brown, MR: The mechanism involved in polyneuritis as exemplified by post-diphtheritic polyneuritis. Ann Intern Med 36:786–791, 1952.
153. Brown, WF and Feasby, TE: Conduction block and denervation in Guillain-Barré polyneuropathy. Brain 107:219–239, 1984.
154. Brown, WF and Feasby, TE: Sensory evoked potentials in Guillain-Barré polyneuropathy. J Neurol Neurosurg Psychiatry 47:288–291, 1984.
155. Brunet, P, Binet, JL, and Saxce, H: Neuropathies au cours de la lympha-

denopathie angio-immunoblastique. Rev Neurol 137:503–515, 1981.

156. Brussilowski, L: Zur lehre von der akuten aufsteigenden Landryschen paralyse. Zentralblatt für die Gesamte Neurologie und Psychiatrie 111:515–528, 1927.
157. Brust, JCM, Hammer, JS, Challenor, Y, Healton, EB, and Lesser, R: Acute generalized polyneuropathy accompanying lithium poisoning. Ann Neurol 6:360–362, 1979.
158. Bryceson, ADM, Greenwood, BM, Warrell, DA, Davidsion, NM, Pope, HM, Lawrie, JH, Barnes, HJ, Bailie, WE, and Wilcox, GE: Demonstration during life of rabies antigen in humans. J Infect Dis 131:71–74, 1975.
159. Buchsbaum, JW and Gallo, AE: Polyneuritis, papilledema and lumboperitoneal shunt. Arch Neurol 21:253–257, 1969.
160. Buge, A, Rancure, G, Brault, JL, and Guillemaud-Schadek, B: Acute polyradiculoneuritis of the ophthalmoplegic type. Recurrence after 12 years (letter). Nouv Presse Med 11:281, 1982.
161. Buruma, OJS and Schipperheyn, JJ: Periodic paralysis. In Vinken, PH and Bruyn, GW (eds): Handbook of Clinical Neurology. North Holland Publishing, Amsterdam, 1979, pp 147–174.
162. Byers, RK and Taft, LT: Chronic multiple peripheral neuropathy in childhood. Pediatrics 20:517–537, 1957.
163. Cabrera, J, Griffin, DE, and Johnson, RT: Unusual features of the Guillain-Barré syndrome after rabies vaccine prepared in suckling mouse brain. J Neurol Sci 81:239–245, 1987.
164. Calderon-Gonzalez, R and Rizzi-Hernandez, H: Buckthorn neuropathy. N Engl J Med 277:69–71, 1967.
165. Calvin, WH, Devor, M, and Howe, JF: Can neuralgias arise from minor demyelination? Spontaneous firing, mechanosensitivity, and after discharge from conducting axons. Exp Neurol 75:755–763, 1982.
166. Cambier, J and Schott, B: Nosologie des polyradiculonevrites inflammatoires. Rev Neurol (Paris) 115:811, 1966.
167. Cameron, DG, Howell, DA, and Hutchison, JL: Acute peripheral neuropathy in Hodgkin's disease. Report of a fatal case with histologic features of allergic neuritis. Neurology 8:575–577, 1958.
168. Campistol, JM, Montoliu, J, Blesa, R, and Revert, L: Crisis hipertensiva como manifestacion inicial en el sindrome de Guillain-Barré-Landry. Med Clin (Barc) 89:558–560, 1987.
169. Canedo J and Sanders, DB: Peripheral electrophysiological studies in ciguatera (abstr). Neurol (Suppl) 383:308, 1988.
170. Cannon, LA, Heiselman, D, Gardner, W, Jones, J: Prophylaxis of upper gastrointestinal tract. Bleeding in mechanically ventilated patients. A randomized study comparing the efficacy of sulcralfate, cimetidine and antacids. Arch Intern Med 147: 2102–2106, 1987.
171. Caplan, ES and Hoyt, NJ: Nosocomial sinusitis. JAMA 247:639–641, 1982.
172. Caputy, AJ, Kim, YI, and Sanders, DB: The neuromuscular blocking effects of therapeutic concentrations of various antibiotics on normal rat skeletal muscle: A quantitative comparison. J Pharmacol Exp Ther 217:369–378, 1981.
173. Carpenter, S: An ultrastructural study of an acute fatal case of the Guillain-Barré syndrome. J Neurol Sci 15:125–140, 1972.
174. Carroll, JE, Jedziniak, M, and Guggenheim, MA: Guillain-Barré syndrome. Another cause of the "floppy infant." Am J Dis Child 131:699–700, 1977.
175. Carroll, WM and Mastaglia, FL: Ocular motor involvement in post-infective polyneuropathy. Proc Aust Assoc Neurol 14:66–74, 1977.
176. Carroll, WM and Mastaglia, FL: "Locked-in coma" in postinfective polyneuropathy. Arch Neurol 36:46–47, 1979.

177. Casey, EB, Jellife, AM, Le Quesne, PM, and Millett, YL: Vincristine neuropathy. Clinical and electrophysiological observations. Brain 96:69–86, 1973.
178. Castaigne, P, Brunet, P, Moulias, R, Goust, J-M, and Delrieu, F: Polyradiculonevrites inflammatoires et immunite cellulaire: Etude de la reponse immunitaire cellulaire envers des antigens de nerf peripherique par le test de migration des leucocytes. Nouv Presse Med 1:2445–2449, 1972.
179. Castaigne, P, Brunet, P, and Nouailhat, F: Enquete clinique sur les polyradiculonevrites inflammatoires en France. Rev Neurol (Paris) 115:849–872, 1966.
180. Castlebaum, AR, Donofrio, PD, Walker, FO and Troost, BT: Laxative abuse causing hypermagnesemia and neuromuscular junction defect. Neurology 39:746–747, 1989.
181. Cavanagh, JB, Fuller, NH, Johnson, HRM, and Rudge, P: The effects of thallium salts, with particular reference to the nervous system changes. Q J Med 43:293–319, 1974.
182. Cendrowski, W: Treatment of polyneuropathy with azathioprine and adrenal steroids. Acta Med Pol 18:147–156, 1977.
183. Chakraborty, TK and Ruddell, WSJ: Guillain-Barré neuropathy during treatment with captopril. Postgrad Med J 63:221–222, 1987.
184. Chanmugam, D and Waniganetti, A: Guillain-Barré syndrome associated with typhoid fever. Br Med J 1:95–96, 1969.
185. Charbonnel A, Feve, J-R, and Blineau, M-F: Les signes oculaires des polyradiculonévrites aiguës inflammatoires. Cahiers de Medecine 11:505–518, 1970.
186. Charous, DI and Saxe, BI: The Landry-Guillain-Barré syndrome in infectious mononucleosis. Report of a case with recovery following administration of cortisone. Arch Intern Med 92:438–441, 1953.
187. Charous, DI and Saxe, BI: The Landry-Guillian-Barré syndrome. Report of an unusual case, with a comment on Bell's palsy. N Engl J Med 267:1334–1338, 1962.
188. Chen, KM, Brody, JA, and Kurland, LT: Patterns of neurologic diseases on Guam. I. Epidemiologic aspects. Arch Neurol 19:573–578, 1968.
189. Cherington, M: Botulism. Ten-year experience. Arch Neurol 30:432–437, 1974.
190. Cherington, M: Locked-in syndrome after "swine flu" inoculation (letter). Arch Neurol 34:258, 1977.
191. Cherington, M and Snyder, RD: Tick paralysis. Neurophysiologic studies. N Engl J Med 278:95–97, 1968.
192. Chia, JK, Clark, JB, Ryan, CA, and Pollack, M: Botulism in an adult associated with food-borne intestinal infection with clostridium botulinum. N Engl J Med 315:239–241, 1986.
193. Chiappa, KH and Young, RR: A case of paracarcinomatous pandysautonomia. Neurology 23:423, 1973.
194. Chomel, AF: J Hebd de Med 1:333, 1828. De l'épidémie actuellement régnante à Paris. Journal Hebdomadaire de Medécine.
195. Chopra, JS, Banerjee, AK, Murthy, JMK, and Pal, SR: Paralytic rabies. A clinico-pathological study. Brain 103:789–802, 1980.
196. Chretien, JH, Fermaglich, J, and Garagusi, VF: Ciguatera poisoning. Presentation as a neurological disorder. Arch Neurol 38:783, 1981.
197. Church, AE and Biggs, PM: Agent of Marek's disease in tissue culture. Nature 215:528–530, 1967.
198. Chutkow, JG: Magnesium ions. In Boulton, AA, Baker, GB, and Walz, W (eds): Neuromethods. Vol 9. Neuronal Microenvironment. Humana Press, Clifton, NJ, 1988, pp 691–715.
199. Chuttani, PN, Chawla, LS, Chugh, KS, and Singh H: Landry-Guillain-Barré-Strohl syndrome in India. J Neurol Sci 7:581–592, 1968.
200. Chuttani, PN, Chawla, LS, and Sharma, TD: Arsenical neuropathy. Neurology 17:269–274, 1967.
201. Cicale, MJ: Guillain-Barré syndrome

after streptokinase therapy (letter). South Med J 80:1068, 1987.

202. Clarke, E, Bayliss, RIS, and Cooper, R: Landry-Guillain-Barré syndrome: Cardiovascular complications. Treatment with ACTH and cortisone. Br Med J 2:1504–1507, 1954.

203. Clavelou, P, Beytout, J, Vernay, D, Aumaitre, O, Dordain, G, and Tournilhac, M: Neurologic manifestations of Lyme disease in the northern part of the Auvergne (abstr). Neurology (Suppl)39:350, 1989.

204. Clavelou, P, Beytout, J, Gourdiat, A, Garandeau, A, Deffond, D, and Tournilhac, M: Atteintes neurologiques au decours d'infections a campylobacter. Clinq cas. Rev Neurol (Paris) 145:208–214, 1989.

205. Coe, CJ: Guillain-Barré syndrome in Korean children. Yonsei Med J 30:81–87, 1989.

206. Cohen, BA, Crough, RH, and Thompson, SN: Electromyographic biofeedback as a physical therapeutic adjunct in Guillain-Barré syndrome. Arch Phys Med Rehabil 58:582–584, 1977.

207. Colan, RV, Snead, OC, III, Oh, SJ, and Benton, JW, Jr: Steroid-responsive polyneuropathy with subacute onset of childhood. J Pediatr 97: 374–377, 1980.

208. Colan, RV, Snead, OC, Oh, SJ, and Kashlan, MB: Acute autonomic and sensory neuropathy. Ann Neurol 8:441–444, 1980.

209. Cole, GF and Matthew, DJ: Prognosis in severe Guillain-Barré syndrome. Arch Dis Child 62:288–291, 1987.

210. Colin-Jones, DG and Heathfield, KWG: 6-Mercaptopurine in polyradiculoneuropathy (letter). Lancet 2: 739, 1965.

211. Collens, WS and Rabinowtiz, MA: Mumps polyneuritis quadriplegia with bilateral facial paralysis. Arch Intern Med 41:61, 1928.

211a. Collier, J: Oculomotor palsies resulting from infective and toxic processes. Trans Ophthalmol Soc UK 50:244–252, 1930.

212. Collins, R, Scrimgeour, A, Yusuf, S, and Peto, R: Reduction of fatal pulmonary embolism and venous thrombosis by perioperative administration of subcutaneous heparin. N Engl J Med 318:1162–1173, 1988.

213. Congy, F, Hauw, JJ, Wang, A, and Moulias, R: Influenzal acute myositis in the elderly. Neurology 30:877–878, 1980.

214. Conn, DL and Dyck, PJ: Angiopathic neuropathy in connective tissue diseases. In Dyck, PJ, Thomas, PK, and Lambert, EH (eds): Peripheral Neuropathy, ed 2. WB Saunders, Philadelphia, 1984, pp 2027–2043.

214a. Conlon, CP: HIV infection presenting as Guillain-Barré syndrome in Luska, Zambia. Trans R Soc Trop Med Hyg 83:109, 1989.

215. Constant, OC, Bentley, CC, Denman, AM, Lehane, JR, and Larson, HE: The Guillain-Barré syndrome following Campylobacter enteritis with recovery after plasmapheresis. J Infect 6:89–91, 1983.

216. Cook, JD, Tindal, RAS, Walker, J, Khan, A, and Rosenberg, R: Plasma exchange as a treatment of acute and chronic idiopathic immune polyneuropathy: Limited success. Neurology 30:361–362, 1980.

217. Cook, SD and Dowling, PC: The role of autoantibody and immune complexes in the pathogenesis of Guillain-Barré syndrome. Ann Neurol (Suppl)9:70–79, 1981.

218. Cook, SD, Dowling, P, Murray, MR, and Whitaker, JN: Circulating demyelinating factors in acute idiopathic polyneuropathy. Arch Neurol 24: 136–144, 1971.

219. Cook, SD, Murray, MR, Whitaker, JN, and Dowling, P: Myelinotoxic antibody in the Guillain-Barré syndrome. Neurology 19:284, 1969.

220. Cornblath, DR, Griffin, JW, and Tennekoon, GI: Immunoreactive myelin basic protein in cerebrospinal fluid of patients with peripheral neuropathies. Ann Neurol 20:370–372, 1986.

221. Cornblath, DR, McArthur, JC, Kennedy, PGE, Witte, AS, and Griffin, JW: Inflammatory demyelinating pe-

ripheral neuropathies associated with human T-cell lymphotropic virus type III infection. Ann Neurol 21:32–40, 1987.

222. Cornblath, DR, Mellits, ED, Griffin, JW, McKhann, GM, Albers, JW, Miller, RG, Feasby, TE, Quaskey, SA, and the Guillain-Barré Syndrome Study Group: Motor conduction studies in Guillain-Barré syndrome: Description and prognostic value. Ann Neurol 23:354–359, 1988.

223. Corston, RN: Temporal arteritis in association with the Guillain-Barré syndrome. Br Med J 280:292–293, 1980.

224. Corston, RN, McGale, EHF, Stonier, C, Aber, GM, and Hutchinson, EC: Abnormalities of cerebrospinal fluid amino acids in patients with the Guillain-Barré syndrome. J Neurol Neurosurg Psychiatry 44:86–89, 1981.

225. Cosnett, JE: Wardrop-Landry-Guillain-Barré-Strohl (letter). Lancet 1:861–862, 1987.

226. Costantino, T and Weintraub, A: The Guillain-Barré syndrome as a complication of the postperfusion syndrome. Am Heart J 84:678–680, 1972.

227. Couchot, J, Pennaforte, F, Leroux, B, Ferrand, O, and Rullier, J: Syndrome de Guillain-Barré au decours d'une varicelle (letter). Nouv Presse Med 7:47, 1978.

228. Craggs, RI, King, RHM, and Thomas, PK: The effect of suppression of macrophage activity on the development of experimental allergic neuritis. Acta Neuropathol 62:316–323, 1984.

229. Cream, JJ, Hern, JEC, Hughes, RAC, and Mackenzie, ICK: Mixed or immune complex cryoglobulinemia and neuropathy. J Neurol Neurosurg Psychiatry 37:82–87, 1974.

230. Crozier, RE and Ainley, AB: The Guillain-Barré syndrome. N Engl J Med 252:83–88, 1955.

231. Culbertson, LR: A case of Landry's disease with involvement of the eye muscles. Am J Ophthalmol 19:113–114, 1902.

232. Culp, WJ and Ochoa, J: Abnormal Nerves and Muscles as Impulse Generators. Oxford University Press, New York, 1982.

233. Cummings, JF and Haas, DC: Coonhound paralysis. An acute idiopathic polyradiculoneuritis in dogs resembling the Landry-Guillain-Barré syndrome. J Neurol Sci 4:51–81, 1967.

234. Cummings, JF, de Lahunta, A, Holmes, DF, and Schultz, RD: Coonhound paralysis. Further clinical studies and electron microscopic observations. Acta Neuropathol 56: 167–178, 1982.

235. Cunningham, JM, Powers, JM, and Brostoff, SW: Prevention of experimental allergic neuritis in the Lewis rat with bovine P2 protein. Brain Res 258:285–289, 1983.

235a. Currie, DM, Nelson, MR, Buck, BC: Guillain-Barré syndrome in children: Evidence of axonal degeneration and long-term follow-up. Arch Phys Med Rehabil 71:244–247, 1990.

236. Currie, S and Henson, RA: Neurological syndromes in the reticuloses. Brain 94:307–320, 1971.

237. Currie, S and Knowles, M: Lymphocyte transformation in the Guillain-Barré syndrome. Brain 94:109–116, 1971.

238. Curtis, BM, Forno, LY, and Smith, ME: Reactivation of neuritogenic activity of P2 protein from rabbit PNS myelin. Brain Res 175:387–391, 1979.

239. Dalakas, MC: Chronic idiopathic ataxic neuropathy. Ann Neurol 19:545–554, 1986.

240. Dalakas, MC and Engel, WK: Chronic relapsing (dysimmune) polyneuropathy: Pathogenesis and treatment. Ann Neurol (Suppl)9:134–145, 1981.

241. Dalakas, MC and Engel, WK: Polyneuropathy with monoclonal gammopathy: Studies of 11 patients. Ann Neurol 10:45–52, 1981.

242. Dalakas, MC, and Hallett, M: The Post-Polio Syndrome. In Plum, F (ed): Advances in Contemporary Neurology. FA Davis, Philadelphia, 1988, pp 51–94.

243. Dalos, NP, Borel, C, and Hanley, DF: Cardiovascular autonomic dysfunc-

tion in Guillain-Barré syndrome. Therapeutic implications of Swan-Ganz monitoring. Arch Neurol 45:115–117, 1988.

244. D'Ambrosio, G and De Angelis, G: Syndrome de Guillain-Barré au cours de la grossesse. Rev Neurol (Paris) 141:33–36, 1985.

245. D'Ambrosio, G, De Angelis, G, and Vizioli, R: Epidemiology of Guillain-Barré syndrome in Campania (South Italy). Preliminary results. Acta Neurol (Napoli) 5:245–252, 1983.

246. Daube, JR, Kelly, JJ, and Martin, RA: Facial myokymia with polyradiculoneuropathy. Neurology 29:662–669, 1979.

247. Davidson, DLW and Jellinek, EH: Hypertension and papilloedema in the Guillain-Barré syndrome. J Neurol Neurosurg Psychiatry 40:144–148, 1977.

248. Davidson, GP and Abbot, K: Guillain-Barré syndrome. Med J Aust 146:401, 1987 (letter).

249. Davies, AG: Inappropriate secretion of antidiuretic hormone in Guillain-Barré syndrome. Postgrad Med J 47:651–655, 1971.

250. Davies, AG and Dingle, HR: Observations on cardiovascular and neuroendocrine disturbances in the Guillain-Barré syndrome. J Neurol Neurosurg Psychiatry 35:176–179, 1972.

251. Davies, J and Rowlatt, RJ: Transient severe hypertension and polyradiculitis after chickenpox. Br Med J 2:1608, 1978.

252. Davis, LE, Standefer, JC, Kornfeld, M, Abercrombie, DM, and Butler, C: Acute thallium poisoning: Toxicological and morphological studies of the nervous system. Ann Neurol 10:38–44, 1981.

253. Dawson, DM, Samuels, MA, and Morris, J: Sensory form of acute polyneuritis. Neurology 38:1728–1731, 1988.

254. Dayan, AD, Ogul, E, and Graveson, GS: Polyneuritis and herpes zoster. J Neurol Neurosurg Psychiatry 35:170–175, 1972.

255. Dean, G: Seven cases of barium carbonate poisoning. Br Med J 2:817–818, 1950.

256. De Bont, B, Matthews, N, Abbot, K, and Davidson, GP: Guillain-Barré syndrome associated with Campylobacter enteritis in a child. J Pediatr 109:660–662, 1986.

257. Debre, RL and Thieffry, S: Remarques sur le syndrome de Guillain-Barré chez L'enfant (a propos de 32 observations personnelles). Arch Fr Pediatr 8:357, 1951.

258. Dehaene, I, Martin, JJ, Geens, K, and Cras, P: Guillain-Barré syndrome with ophthalmoplegia: Clinicopathological study of the central and peripheral nervous systems, including the oculomotor nerves. Neurology 36:851–854, 1986.

259. de Jager, AEJ: Het syndroom van Guillain, Barré en Strohl. Ned Tijdschr Geneeskd 124:1187–1192, 1980.

260. de Jager, AEJ: Residual symptoms in Guillain-Barré syndrome. Thesis, Groningen, Netherlands, 1988.

261. de Jager, AEJ, The, TH, Smit Simbing, CT, and Das, PC: Plasma exchange in Guillain-Barré. Br Med J 283:794–795, 1981.

262. Dejerine, J: Recherches sur les lesions du systeme nerveux dans la paralysie ascendante aigue. These de Paris, No 72, Paris, 1879.

263. Dejerine, J and Goetz, C: Note sur un cas de paralysie ascendante aigue. Archives de Physiologie 8:312, 1876.

264. DeJong, RN: Guillain-Barré syndrome. Polyradiculoneuritis with albuminocytologic dissociation. Arch Neurol Psychiatr 44:1044–1068, 1940.

265. de la Monte, SM, Ropper, AH, Dickersin, GR, Harris, NL, Ferry, JA, and Richardson, EP: Relapsing central and peripheral demyelinating diseases. Unusual pathologic features. Arch Neurol 43:626–629, 1986.

266. de la Monte, SM, Gabuzda, DH, Ho, DD, Brown, RH, Jr, Hedley-Whyte, ET, Schooley, RT, Hirsch, MS, and Bhan, AK: Peripheral neuropathy in the acquired immunodeficiency syndrome. Ann Neurol 23:485–492, 1988.

267. Denny-Brown, DE: The changing pattern of neurologic medicine. N Engl J Med 246:839–846, 1952.

268. Derakhshan, I, Lotfi, J, and Kaufman, B: Ophthalmoplegia, ataxia and hyporeflexia (Fisher's syndrome). With a midbrain lesion demonstrated by CT scanning. Eur Neurol 18:361–366, 1979.
269. DeRosayro, M and Healy, TEJ: Tobramycin and neuromuscular transmission in the rat isolated phrenic nerve–diaphragm preparation. Br J Anaesth 50:251–254, 1978.
270. Descamps, C, VandenBroucke, JM, and van Ypersele de Strihou, C: Rhabdomyolysis and acute tubular necrosis associated with carbenoxolone and diuretic treatment. Br Med J 1:272, 1977.
271. Desgrez, H: André Strohl (1887–1977). Bull Acad Nat Med 161:563–571, 1977.
272. Deutschman, CS, Wilton, P, Sinow, J, Dibbel D, Konstantinides, BS, and Cerra, FB: Paranasal sinusitis associated with nasotracheal intubation: A frequently unrecognized and treatable source of sepsis. Crit Care Med 14:111–114, 1986.
273. Devere, R and Bradley, WG: Polymyositis: Its presentation, morbidity, and mortality. Brain 98:637–666, 1975.
274. DeVivo, DC and Engel, WK: Remarkable recovery of a steroid-responsive recurrent polyneuropathy. J Neurol Neurosurg Psychiatry 33:62–69, 1970.
275. Diamond, S, Schear, HE, and Leeds, MF: Pseudointernuclear oculomotor ophthalmoplegia secondary to Guillain-Barré polyneuritis simulating myasthenia gravis in an air transport pilot. Aviat Space Environ Med 46:204–107, 1975.
276. Dick, DJ and Raman, D: The Guillain-Barré syndrome following gold therapy. Scand J Rheumatol 11: 119–120, 1982.
277. Diller, TH: A study of Landry's paralysis, with a report of three nonfatal cases. J Nerv Ment Dis 29:577, 1902.
278. Diller, Th and Myer, A: A case of Landry's paralysis, with autopsy. Am J Med Sci 111:1–10, 1896.
279. Dolman, CL and Allan, BM: Relapsing hypertrophic neuritis. Arch Neurol 28:351–353, 1973.
280. Donaghy, M and Earl, CJ: Ocular palsy preceding chronic relapsing polyneuropathy by several weeks. Ann Neurol 17:49–50, 1985.
281. Donaghy, M, Hall, P, Gawler, J, Gregson, NA, Leibowitz, S, Jitpimolmard, S, King, RHM, and Thomas, PK: Peripheral neuropathy associated with Castleman's disease. J Neurol Sci 89:253–267, 1989.
282. Donofrio, PD, Tandan, R, and Albers, JW: Plasma exchange in chronic inflammatory demyelinating polyradiculoneuropathy. Muscle Nerve 8: 321–327, 1985.
283. Donofrio, PD, Wilbourn, AJ, Albers, JW, Rogers, L, Salanga, V, Greenberg, HS: Acute arsenic intoxication presenting as Guillain-Barré–like syndrome. Muscle Nerve 10:114–120, 1987.
284. Donoso, R: Guillain-Barré syndrome following typhoid fever (letter). Ann Neurol 23:627, 1988.
285. Dowling, PC, Bosch, VV, and Cook, SD: Possible beneficial effect of high-dose intravenous steroid therapy in acute demyelinating disease and transverse myelitis. Neurology 30: 33–36, 1980.
286. Dowling, PC and Cook, SD: Role of infection in Guillain-Barré syndrome: Laboratory confirmation of herpes viruses in 41 cases. Ann Neurol (Suppl)9:44–55, 1981.
287. Dowling, PC, Cook, SD, and Whitaker, JN: Cold agglutinin positive Guillain-Barré syndrome. Trans Am Neurol Assoc 95:234–235, 1970.
288. Dowling, PC, Menonna, JP, and Cook, SD: Cytomegalovirus complement fixation antibody in Guillain-Barré syndrome. Neurology 27: 1153–1156, 1977.
289. Dowling, PC, Menonna, JP, and Cook, SD: Guillain-Barré syndrome in Greater New York–New Jersey. JAMA 238:317–318, 1977.
290. Downs, JB, Klein, EF, Desautels, D, Modell, JH, and Kirby, RR: Intermittent mandatory ventilation: A new

approach to weaning patients from mechanical ventilators. Chest 64: 331–335, 1973.

291. Drachman, DA, Paterson, PY, Berlin, BS, and Roguska, J: Immunosuppression and the Guillain-Barré syndrome. Arch Neurol 23:385–393, 1970.

292. Draganesco, S and Claudian, J: Sur un cas de radiculo-nevrite curable (syndrome de Guillain et Barré) apparue au cours d'une osteo-myelite du bras. Rev Neurol 2:517–521, 1927.

293. Drew, AL and Magee, KR: Papilledema in the Guillain-Barré syndrome. AMA Arch Neurol Psychiat 66:744–751, 1951.

294. Driks, MR, Craven, DE, Celli, BR, Manning, M, Burke, RA, Garvin, GM, Kunches, LM, Farber HW, Wedel, SA, and McCabe, WR: Nosocomial pneumonia in intubated patients given sucralfate as compared with antacids or histamine type 2 blockers. The role of gastric colonization. N Engl J Med 317:1376–1382, 1987.

295. Drueke, TB, Pujade-Lauraine, E, Poisson, M, Zingraff, J, Ulmann, A, and Crosnier, J: Measles virus and Guillain-Barré syndrome during long-term hemodialysis. Am J Med 60:444–446, 1976.

296. Dubois-Dalcq, M, Buyse, M, Buyse, G, and Gorce F: The action of Guillain-Barré syndrome serum on myelin: A tissue culture and electron miscroscopic analysis. J Neurol Sci 13:67–83, 1971.

297. Duménil, L: Paralysie peripherique du mouvement et du sentiment portant sur les quatres membres. Atrophie des rameaux nerveux des parties paralysees. Gazzette Hebdomadaire de Medécine 1:203–206, 1864.

298. Dummolard, A, Sarrouy, J, Schonshoe, R, and Baredoux, N: Polyradiculonevrite avec hyperalbuminose du liquide cephalorachidien sans reaction cellulaire et nevrite optique—evolution rapide, vers le guerison (Guillain-Barré). Rev Otoneuroophtal (Paris) 15:26–28, 1938.

299. Duncan, R and Kennedy, PGE: Guillain-Barré syndrome following acute head trauma. Postgrad Med J 63:479–480, 1987.

300. Dunn, WJ and McConahey, WM: Cushing's syndrome complicated by Guillain-Barré syndrome and thrombocytopenia with purpura. Proc Staff Meet, Mayo Clin 31:322–324, 1956.

301. Dupont, JR and Earle, KM: Human rabies encephalitis. A study of forty-nine fatal cases with a review of the literature. Neurology 15:1023–1034, 1965.

302. Dureux, JB, Gerard, A, Roche, G, Leheup, B, Canton, P, Schooneman, F, Jannot, C, and Streiff, F: Traitement du syndrome de Guillain et Barré par echange plasmatique. 6 observations. Nouv Presse Med 9: 3696–3697, 1980.

303. Durocher, A, Servais, B, Caridroix, M, Chopin, C, and Wattel, F: Autonomic dysfunction in the Guillain-Barré syndrome. Hemodynamic and neurochemical studies. Intensive Care Med 6:3–6, 1980.

304. Durward, WF, Burnett, AK, Watkins, R, and Reid, JM: Plasma exchange in Guillain-Barré syndrome (letter). Br Med J 283:794, 1981.

305. Dyck, PJ, Benstead, TJ, Conn, DL, Stevens, JC, Windebank, AJ, and Low, PA: Nonsystemic vasculitic neuropathy. Brain 110:843–854, 1987.

306. Dyck, PJ, Conn, D, and Okazaki, H: Necrotizing angiopathic neuropathy: Three-dimensional morphology of fiber degeneration related to sites of occluded blood vessels. Mayo Clin Proc 47:461–475, 1972.

307. Dyck, PJ, Daube, J, O'Brien, P, Pineda, A, Low, PA, Windebank, AJ, and Swanson, C: Plasma exchange in chronic inflammatory demyelinating polyradiculoneuropathy. N Engl J Med 314:461–465, 1986.

308. Dyck, PJ and Kurtzke, JF: Plasmapheresis in Guillain-Barré syndrome. Neurology 35:1105–1107, 1985.

309. Dyck, PJ, Lais AC, Hansen, SM, Sparks, MF, Low, PA, Parthasarathy, S, and Baumann, WJ: Technique assessment of demyelination from en-

doneurial injection. Exp Neurol 77:359–377, 1982.

310. Dyck, PJ, Lais, AC, Ohta, M, Bastron, JA, Okazaki, H, and Groover, RV: Chronic inflammatory polyradiculoneuropathy. Mayo Clin Proc 50: 621–637, 1975.
311. Dyck, PJ, O'Brien, PC, Oviatt, KF, Dinapoli, RP, Daube, JR, Bartleson, JD, Mokri, B, Swift, T, Low, PA, and Windenbank, AJ: Prednisone improves chronic inflammatory demyelinating polyradiculoneuropathy more than no treatment. Ann Neurol 11:136–141, 1982.
312. Dyck, PJ, O'Brien, PC, Swanson, C, Low, P, and Daube, J: Combined azathioprine and prednisone in chronic inflammatory-demyelinating polyneuropathy. Neurology 35:1173–1176, 1985.
313. Dyck, PJ, Oviatt, KF, and Lambert, EH: Intensive evaluation of referred unclassified neuropathies yields improved diagnosis. Ann Neurol 10: 222–226, 1981.
314. Dyck, PJ, Swanson, CJ, Low, PA, Bartleson, JD, and Lambert, EH: Prednisone-responsive hereditary motor and sensory neuropathy. Mayo Clin Proc 57:239–246, 1982.
315. Dynes, JB: Cushing's syndrome associated with Guillain-Barré syndrome. Lahey Clinic Bulletin 9:145–148, 1955.
316. Eaton, OM, Stevens, H, and Silver, HM: Respiratory failure in polyradiculoneuritis associated with infectious mononucleosis. JAMA 194: 609–611, 1965.
317. Eberle, E, Brink, J, Azen, S, and White, D: Early predictors of incomplete recovery in children with Guillain-Barré polyneuritis. J Pediatr 86:356–359, 1975.
318. Edelman, J, Gubbay, SS, and Zilko, PJ: Acute pandysautonomia due to mixed connective tissue disease. Aust NZ J Med 11:68–70, 1981.
319. Eden, KV: Possible association of Guillain-Barré syndrome with thrombolytic therapy (letter). JAMA 249:2020–2021, 1983.
320. Editorial: Guillain-Barré syndrome: Ascending knowledge? Lancet 2: 243–244, 1978.
321. Edmonds, ME and Sturrock, RD: Autonomic neuropathy in the Guillain-Barré syndrome (letter). Br Med J 2:668, 1979.
322. Eiben, RM and Gersony, WM: Recognition, prognosis and treatment of the Guillain-Barré syndrome (acute idiopathic polyneuritis). Med Clin North Am 47:1371–1380, 1963.
323. Eichorst, H: Neuritis acuta progressiva. Virchows Arch [Pathol Anat] 69:265–274, 1877.
324. Eisen, A and Humphreys, P: The Guillain-Barré syndrome. A clinical and electrodiagnostic study of 25 cases. Arch Neurol 30:438–443, 1974.
325. Eisendrath, SJ, Matthay, MA, Dunkel, JA, Zimmerman, JK, and Layzer, RB: Psychosomatics 24:465–475, 1983.
326. Eisenlohr, C: Zur lehre von der acuten spinalen Paralyse. Arch f Psychiatr 5:219–228, 1874.
327. Elizan, TS, Spire, JP, Andiman, RM, Baughman, FA, Jr, and Lloyd-Smith, DL: Syndrome of acute idiopathic ophthalmoplegia with ataxia and areflexia. Neurology 21:281–292, 1971.
328. Emmons, PR, Blume, WT, and DuShane, J: Cardiac monitoring and demand pacemaker in Guillain-Barré syndrome. Arch Neurol 32:59–61, 1975.
329. Emser, W: Hypermagnesemic periodic paralysis. Treatment with digitalis and lithium carbonate. Arch Neurol 39:727–730, 1982.
330. Endtz, LJ and Hers, JFP: Radiculonevrite causee par Mycoplasma pneumoniae avec presentation d'un cas. Rev Neurol (Paris) 114:141–146, 1966.
331. Endtz, LJ and Hers, JFP: Mycoplasma pneumoniae polyradiculitis. Lancet 1:358, 1970.
332. Epstein, L, Blumberg, B, Crowley, J, Samuel, K, Goudsmit, J, Cook, S, and Dowling, P: Serum antibodies to

HTLV-I in human demyelinating disease. Acta Neurol Scand 75:231–233, 1987.

333. Erb, W: Diseases of the peripheral cerebrospinal nerves. In von Ziemmsen, H (ed): Cyclopaidia of the Practice of Medicine. Vol XI. Samson Low, Maston, Seaile and Rivington, London, 1876.
334. Estol, C and Fromm, GH: Treatment of Guillain-Barré syndrome during pregnancy with plasmapheresis: A report of two cases (abstr). Ann Neurol 24:165, 1988.
335. Estrada-Gonzalez, R and Mas, P: Virological studies in acute polyradiculoneuritis-LGBS type. Various findings in relation to Coxsackie A4 virus. Neurologia Neurocirugia Psiquiatria (Suppl 2–3)18:527, 1977.
336. Evans, JH: Neurological complications of glandular fever. II. Review of the literature. Ulster Med J 32:35, 1963.
337. Eylan, EH, Toro-Goyco, E, Kessler, MJ, and Szymanska, I: Induction of allergic neuritis in Rhesus monkeys. J Immunol 3:91–98, 1982.
338. Fadul, CE, Lemann, W, Thaler, HT, and Posner, JB: Perforation of the gastrointestinal tract in patients receiving steroids for neurologic disease. Neurology 38:348–352, 1988.
339. Faed, JM, Day, B, Pollock, M, Taylor, PK, Nukada, H, and Hammond-Tooke, GD: High-dose intravenous human immuno-globulin in chronic inflammatory demyelinating polyneuropathy. Neurology 39:422–425, 1989.
340. Fagius, J, Osterman, PO, Siden, A, and Wiholm, B-E: Guillain-Barré syndrome following zimeldine treatment. J Neurol Neurosurg Psychiatry 48:65–69, 1985.
341. Fagius, J and Wallin, BG: Microneurographic evidence of excessive sympathetic outflow in the Guillain-Barré syndrome. Brain 106:589–600, 1983.
342. Fagius, J, Wallin, BG, Sundlof, G, Nerhed, C, and Englesson, S: Sympathetic outflow in man after anaesthesia of the glossopharyngeal and vagus nerves. Brain 108:423–438, 1985.
343. Fagius, J, Westerber, C-E, and Olsson, Y: Acute pandysautonomia and severe sensory deficit with poor recovery. A clinical neurophysiological and pathological case study. J Neurol Neurosurg Psychiatry 46:725–733, 1983.
344. Fallat, RJ, Jewitt, B, Bass, M, Kamm, B, and Norris, FH, Jr: Spirometry in amyotrophic lateral sclerosis. Arch Neurol 36:74–80, 1979.
345. Faraq, SS and Gelles, BD: Yersinia arthritis and Guillain-Barré syndrome (letter). N Engl J Med 307: 755, 1982.
346. Farrell, K, Hill, A, and Chuang, S: Papilledema in Guillain-Barré syndrome. A case report. Arch Neurol 38:55–57, 1981.
347. Favre, H, Foex, P, and Guggisberg, M: Use of demand pacemaker in a case of Guillain-Barré syndrome. Lancet 1:1062–1063, 1970.
348. Feasby, TE, Gilbert, JJ, Brown, WF, Bolton, CF, Hahn, AF, Koopman, WF, and Zochodne, DW: An acute axonal form of Guillain-Barré polyneuropathy. Brain 109:1115–1126, 1986.
349. Feasby, TE, Gilbert, JJ, Hahn, AF, and Neilson, M: Complement depletion suppresses Lewis rat experimental allergic neuritis. Brain Res 419:97–103, 1987.
350. Feasby, TE, Hahn, AF, and Gilbert, JJ: Passive transfer studies in Guillain-Barré polyneuropathy. Neurology 32:1159–1167, 1982.
351. Feeley, TW, Du Moulin, GC, Hedley-Whyte, J, Bushnell, LS, Gilbert, JP, and Feingold, DS: Aerosol polymyxin and pneumonia in seriously ill patients. N Engl J Med 293:471–475, 1975.
352. Feer: Veranderungen des liquor cerebrospinalis bei diphtheritischen Lahmungen. Dtsch Med Wochenschr 1:967, 1910.
353. Feibel, JH and Campa, JF: Thyrotoxic neuropathy (Basedow's paraple-

gia). J Neurol Neurosurg Psychiatry 39:491–497, 1976.
354. Feiden, W, Gerhard, L, and Borchard, F: Neuritis cordis due to the acute polyneuritis of the Guillain-Barré syndrome. Virchows Arch [A] 413:573–580, 1988.
355. Feinglass, EJ, Arnett, FC, Dorsch, CA, Zizic, TM, and Stevens, MB: Neuropsychiatric manifestations of systemic lupus erythematosus: Diagnosis, clinical spectrum, and relationship to other features of the disease. Medicine 55:323–339, 1976.
356. Feit, H, Tindall, RSA, and Glasberg, M: Sources of error in the diagnosis of Guillain-Barré syndrome. Muscle Nerve 5:111–117, 1982.
357. Feldman, RG, Niles, CA, Kelly-Hayes, M, Sax, DS, Dixon, WJ, Thompson, DJ, and Landau, E: Peripheral neuropathy in arsenic smelter workers. Neurology 29:939–944, 1979.
357a. Feldman, JM: Cardiac arrest after succinylcholine administration in a pregnant patient recovered from Guillain-Barré syndrome. Anesthesiology 72:942–944, 1990.
358. Feldon, SE, Stark, L, Lehman, SL, and Hoyt, WF: Oculomotor effects of intermittent conduction block in myasthenia gravis and Guillain-Barré syndrome. An oculographic study with computer simulations. Arch Neurol 39:497–503, 1982.
359. Fenichel, GM: Neurological complications of immunization. Ann Neurol 12:119–128, 1982.
360. Fergusson, RJ, Wright, DJ, Willey, RF, Crompton, GK, and Grant, IWB: Suxamethonium is dangerous in polyneuropathy. Br Med J 282:298–299, 1981.
361. Ferreiro, JE, Arguelles, DJ, and Rams, H: Thyrotoxic periodic paralysis. Am J Med 80:146–150, 1986.
362. Feutren, G, Gerbal, J, Allinquant, B, and Schuller, E: Association of Guillain-Barré syndrome and B-Virus hepatitis: Simultaneous presence of anti-DS-DNA antibodies and HBS antigen in cerebrospinal fluid. Clin Lab Immunol 11:161–164, 1983.
363. Finkel, MF: Lyme disease and its neurologic complications. Arch Neurol 45:99–104, 1988.
364. Fiorini, G, Bigig, G, Parachini, ML, Marini, GC, and Gibelli, A: Immunological monitoring of a patient with Guillain-Barré syndrome successfully treated with plasma exchange. Vox Sang 42:304–307, 1982.
365. Fisher, CM: An unusual variant of acute idiopathic polyneuritis (syndrome of ophthalmoplegia, ataxia and areflexia). N Engl J Med 255: 57–65, 1956.
366. Fisher, CM: Adams, RD: Diphtheritic polyneuritis—A pathological study. J Neuropathol Exp Neurol 15:243–268, 1956.
367. Fisher, JR: Guillain-Barré syndrome following organophosphate poisoning. JAMA 238:1950–1951, 1977.
368. Fishman, RA: Neurological aspects of magnesium intoxication. Arch Neurol 12:562–569, 1965.
369. Fleischauer, P, Huber, V, Mertens, H, Sethi, KK, and Thurmann, D: Nachweis von mycoplasma pneumoniae in liquor bie akuter polyneuritis. Dtsch Med Wochenschr 97: 678, 1972.
370. Forbes, SJ, Brumlik, J, and Harding, HB: Acute ascending polyradiculomyelitis associated with ECHO 9 virus. Dis Nerve Syst 28:537, 1967.
371. Ford, RE and Walsh, FB: Guillain-Barré syndrome (acute infective polyneuritis) with increased intracranial pressure and papilledema. Report of 2 cases. Bull Johns Hopkins Hosp 73:391–395, 1943.
372. Forrester, C and Lascelles, RG: Association between polyneuritis and multiple sclerosis. J Neurol Neurosurg Psychiatry 42:864–866, 1979.
373. Forster, FM, Brown, M, and Meritt, HH: Polyneuritis with facial diplegia. A clinical study. N Engl J Med 225:51–56, 1941.
374. Foutch, PG, Woods, CA, Talbert, GA, and Sanowski, RA: A critical analysis of the Sacks-Vine gastrostomy tube: A review of 120 consecutive procedures. Am J Gastroenterol 83:812–815, 1988.

375. Fowler, H, Vulpe, M, Marks, G, Egoif, C, and Dau, PC: Recovery from chronic progressive polyneuropathy after treatment with plasma exchange and cyclophosphamide (letter). Lancet 1:1193, 1979.
376. Frampton, G, Winer, JB, Cameron, JS, and Hughes, RAC: Severe Guillain-Barré syndrome: An association with IgA anti-cardiolipin antibody in a series of 92 patients. J Neuroimmunol 19:133–139, 1988.
377. Francois, ZG and Montus, G: Sur un cas de polyradiculo-nevrite curable avec dissociation albumino-cytologique. Syndrome de Guillain et de Barré. Rev Neurol 1:95–99, 1929.
378. Fraser, DM, Campbell, IW, and Miller, HC: Peripheral and autonomic neuropathy after treatment with perhexiline maleate. Br Med J 2:675–676, 1977.
379. Freddo, L, Ariga, T, Saito, M, Macala, LC, Yu, RK, and Latov, N: The neuropathy of plasma cell dyscrasia: Binding of IgM M-proteins to peripheral nerve glycolipids. Neurology 35:1420–1424, 1985.
380. French Cooperative Group on Plasma Exchange in Guillain-Barré Syndrome: Efficiency of plasma exchange in Guillain-Barré syndrome: Role of replacement fluids. Ann Neurol 22:753–761, 1987.
381. Frick, E and Anstwurm, H: Zur kortikosteroid-behandlung der idiopathischen polyneuritis. München Medisiniche Wochenschrift 110:1265, 1968.
382. Fried-Oken, M, Howard, JM, and Stewart, SR: Personal communication, 1989.
383. Frison, JC, Sanchez, L, Garnacho, A, Bofill, J, Olivero, R, and Miguel, C: Heart rate variations in the Guillain-Barré syndrome. Br Med J 281:649, 1980.
384. Froelich, CJ, Searles, RP, Davis, LE, and Goodwin, JS: A case of Guillain-Barré syndrome with immunologic abnormalities. Ann Intern Med 93:563–565, 1980.
385. Fross, RD and Daube, JR: Neuropathy in the Miller Fisher syndrome: Clinical and electrophysiologic findings. Neurology 37:1493–1498, 1987.
386. Furlan, AJ, Hanon, M, Copperman, A, and Farmer, RG: Acute areflexic paralysis. Arch Neurol 32:706–707, 1975.
387. Gabreels-Festen, AAWM, Hageman, ATM, Gabreels, FJM, Joosten, EMG, Renier, W, Weemaes, CMR, and Ter Laak, HJ: Chronic inflammatory demyelinating polyneuropathy in two siblings. J Neurol Neurosurg Psychiatry 49:152–156, 1986.
388. Gamstorp, I, Aronsson, S, and Linquist, B: Mercaptopurine in polyradiculoneuropathy. Lancet 1:99–100, 1966.
389. Ganji, S and Frazier, E: Somatosensory evoked potential studies in acute Guillain-Barré syndrome. Electromyogr Clin Neurophysiol 28:313–317, 1988.
389a. Garcia, T, Sanchez, JC, Maestre, JF, Guisado, F, Vilches, RM, Morales, B. Brucellosis and acute inflammatory polyradiculoneuropathy. Neurologia 4:145–147, 1990.
390. Garcia-Albea, E: Severe aggravation of blepharospasm in Fisher's syndrome (letter). J Neurol Neurosurg Psychiatry 52:130, 1989.
391. Garcia-Bragado, F, Fernandez, JM, Navarro, C, Villar, M, and Bonaventura, I: Peripheral neuropathy in essential mixed cryoglobulinemia. Arch Neurol 45:1210–1214, 1988.
392. Gardner, WJ, Spitler, DK, and Whitten, C: Increased intracranial pressure caused by increased protein content in the cerebrospinal fluid. N Engl J Med 250:932–936, 1954.
393. Garibaldi, RA, Burke, JP, Dickman, ML, and Smith, CB: Factors predisposing to bacteriuria during indwelling urethral catheterization. N Engl J Med 291:215–219, 1974.
394. Garvey, PH, Jones, N, and Warren, SL: Polyradiculoneuritis (Guillain-Barré syndrome) following the use of sulfanilamide and fever therapy. JAMA 115:1955–1959, 1940.
395. Gautier-Smith, PC: Neurological complications of glandular fever (in-

fectious mononucleosis). Brain 88: 323–334, 1965.
396. Gecow, A and Pawela, I: Autonomic disturbances in the Guillain-Barré-Strohl syndrome in children. Pol Med J 10:1230–1235, 1971.
397. Geczy, C, Raper, R, Roberts, IM, Meyer, P, and Bernard, CCA: Macrophage procoagulant activity as a measure of cell-mediated immunity to P2 protein of peripheral nerves in the Guillain-Barré syndrome. J Neuroimmunol 9:179–191, 1985.
398. Genis, D, Busquets, C, Manubens, E, Davalos, A, Baro, J, and Oterino, A: Epidural morphine analgesia in Guillain-Barré syndrome. J Neurol Neurosurg Psychiatry 52:999–1001, 1989.
399. Gens, RD and Beecham, HJ: Meningoencephalitis after influenza inoculation (letter). N Engl J Med 299:721, 1978.
400. George, J and Twomey, JA: The Guillain-Barré syndrome in the elderly: Clinical and electrophysiological features of five cases. Age Ageing 14:216–219, 1985.
401. Gerard, A: Successful plasmapheresis in the Miller-Fisher syndrome. Br Med J 282:1627, 1981.
402. Gerken, G, Trautmann, F, Kohler, H, Falke, D, Bohl, J, Nix, W, and Meyer zum Buschenfelde, K-H: Rare association of herpes simplex virus IgM-specific antibodies and Guillain-Barré syndrome successfully treated with plasma exchange and immunosuppression. Klin Wochenschr 63: 468–474, 1985.
403. Gibbels, E, Toyka, KV, Borberg, H, Haupt, WF, and Hann, P: Plasmaaustauschbehandlung bei chronischen polyneuritiden vom typ Guillain-Barré. Nervenarzt 57:129–139, 1986.
404. Gibberd, FB: Ophthalmoplegia in acute polyneuritis. Arch Neurol 23: 161–164, 1970.
405. Gibberd, FB and Kelly, RE: Acute internal and external ophthalmoplegia with polyradiculitis of probable virus etiology. Brain 87:657–664, 1964.
406. Gilmartin, RC and Ch'ien, LT: Guillain-Barré syndrome with hydrocephalus in early infancy. Arch Neurol 34:567–569, 1977.
407. Gilmartin, RC, Jabbour, J, and Duenas, D: Rubella vaccine myeloradiculitis. J Pediatr 80:406–412, 1972.
408. Gilpin, SF, Moersch, FP, and Kernohan, JW: Polyneuritis: A clinical and pathologic study of a special group of cases frequently referred to as instances of neuronitis. Archives of Neurology and Psychiatry (Chicago) 35:937–963, 1936.
409. Glaser, R, Brennan, R, and Berlin, CM: Guillain-Barré syndrome associated with Epstein-Barr virus in the cytomegalovirus-negative patient. Dev Med Child Neurol 21:787–807, 1979.
410. Gledhill, RF, Verburgh, AP: Exacerbation of Guillain-Barré syndrome following metrizamide myelography (letter). S Afr Med J 69:663–664, 1986.
411. Glikmann, G, Svehag, S-E, Hansen, E, Hansen, O, Husby, S, Nielsen, H, and Farrell, C: Soluble immune complexes in cerebrospinal fluid of patients with multiple sclerosis and other neurological diseases. Acta Neurol Scand 61:333–343, 1980.
412. Gode, GR, Raju, AV, Jayalakshmi, TS, Kaul, HL, and Bhide, NK: Intensive care in rabies therapy. Clinical observations. Lancet 2:6–8, 1976.
412a. Godwin, JE, and Sahn, SA: Sarcoidosis presenting as progressive ascending lower extremity weakness and asymptomatic meningitis with hypoglycorrhea. Chest 97:1263–1265, 1990.
413. Goebel, W: Uber Landrysche Paralyse. München Medesiniche Wochenschrift 45:956–1000, 1031, 1898.
414. Goldberg, A: Acute intermittent porphyria. A study of 50 cases. Q J Med 28:183–209, 1959.
415. Goldberg, M and Chitanondh, H: Polyneuritis with albuminocytologic dissociation in the spinal fluid in systemic lupus erythematosus. Report of a case, with review of pertinent literature. Am J Med 27:342–350, 1959.
416. Goldschmidt, B, Menonna, J, Fortu-

nato, J, Dowling, P, and Cook, S: Mycoplasma antibody in Guillain-Barré syndrome and other neurological disorders. Ann Neurol 7:108–112, 1980.
417. Good, AE, Christopher, RP, Koepke, GH, Bender, LF, and Tarter, ME: Peripheral neuropathy associated with rheumatoid arthritis. A clinical and electrodiagnostic study of 70 consecutive rheumatoid arthritis patients. Ann Intern Med 63:87–99, 1965.
418. Goodall, JAD, Kosmidis, JC, and Geddes, AM: Effect of corticosteroids on course of Guillain-Barré syndrome (letter). Lancet 1:524, 1974.
419. Goodgold, J: Rehabilitation Medicine. CV Mosby, St Louis, 1988.
420. Gordon, G: Pins and needles. Nature 6:742–743, 1948.
421. Gordon, SL, Morris, WT, Stoner, MA, and Greer, RB, III: Residua of Guillain-Barré polyneuritis in children. J Bone Joint Surg 59-A:193–197, 1977.
422. Gorodezky, C, Varela, B, Castro-Escobar, LE, Chavez-Negrete, A, Escobar-Gutierrez, A, and Martinez-Mata, J: HLA-DR antigens in Mexican patients with Guillain-Barré syndrome. J Neuroimmunol 4:1–7, 1983.
423. Goto, I, Matsumura, M, Inoue, N, Murai, Y, Shida, K, Santa, T, and Kuroiwa, Y: Toxic polyneuropathy due to glue sniffing. J Neurol Neurosurg Psychiatry 37:848–853, 1974.
424. Gottschlich, MM, Warden, GD, Michel, M, Havens, P, Kopcha, R, Jenkins, M, and Alexander, JW: Diarrhea in tube-fed burn patients: Incidence, etiology, nutritional impact, and prevention. JPEN 12:338–345, 1988.
425. Gould, DB, Sorrell, MR, and Lupariello, AD: Barium sulfide poisoning. Arch Intern Med 132:891–894, 1973.
426. Goulon, M, Nouaihat, F, Babinet, P, Grosbuis, S, Barois, A, Raphael, JC, and Gajdos, PL: La dysautonomie des polyradiculonévrites aigües primitives. Rev Neurol (Paris) 131:95–119, 1975.
427. Goulon, M, Mouaihat, F, Grosbuis, S, and Gajdos, PL: Hypotension orthostatique a pouls invariable. Rev Neurol (Paris) 125:257–272, 1971.
428. Goulon, M, Raphael, J-C, Gajdos, PH, and Patte, D: Bradycardie et reflexe oculo-cardiaque au cours du syndrome de Landry-Guillain-Barré. Presse Med 7:1866, 1978.
429. Gourie-Devi, M and Ganapathy, GR: Phrenic nerve conduction time in Guillain-Barré syndrome. J Neurol Neurosurg Psychiatry 48:245–249, 1985.
430. Goust, JM, Chenais, F, Carnes, JE, Hames, CG, Fudenberg, HH, and Hogan, EL: Abnormal T cell subpopulations and circulating immune complexes in the Guillain-Barré syndrome and multiple sclerosis. Neurology 28:421–425, 1978.
431. Gracey, DR, McMichan, JC, Divertie, MB, and Howard, FM: Respiratory failure in Guillain-Barré syndrome. A 6-year experience. Mayo Clin Proc 57:742–746, 1982.
432. Graham, WGB and Bradley, DA: Efficacy of chest physiotherapy and intermittent positive-pressure breathing in the resolution of pneumonia. N Engl J Med 299:624–627, 1978.
433. Grant, H and Leopold, HN: Guillain-Barré syndrome occurring during cortisone therapy. JAMA 155:252–253, 1954.
434. Graves, RJ: Clinical Lectures on the Practice of Medicine, ed 2. New Sydenham Society, London, 1884, p 574.
435. Graveson, GS: The use of steroids in the treatment of the Guillain-Barré syndrome. Proc Roy Soc Med 54:575–576, 1961.
436. Green, D: Infectious polyneuritis and Professor André Strohl—A historical note. N Engl J Med 267:821–822, 1962.
437. Green, SH: Polyradiculitis (Landry-Guillain-Barré syndrome) with total ophthalmoplegia: Encephalo-myelo-radiculo-neuropathy. Dev Med Child Neurol 18:369–380, 1976.
438. Greenberg, C, Davies, S, McGowan, T, Schorer, A, Drage, C: Acute respiratory failure following severe arsenic poisoning. Chest 76:596–598, 1979.
439. Greenfield, JG and Carmichael, EA:

The cerebro-spinal fluid in clinical diagnosis. Macmillan, London, 1925, p 160.
440. Greenland, P and Griggs, RC: Arrhythmic complications in the Guillain-Barré syndrome. Arch Intern Med 140:1053–1055, 1980.
441. Greenwood, AG, Barker, J, and McLeish, I: Neuritis of the cauda equina in a horse. Equine Vet J 5:111–115, 1973.
442. Greenwood, RJ, Hughes, RAC, Bowden, AN, Gordon, NS, Millac, P, Newsom-Davis, J, Aslan, S, Chadwick, DW, McLellan, DL, and Stott, RB: Controlled trial of plasma exchange in acute inflammatory polyradiculoneuropathy. Lancet 1:877–879, 1984.
443. Griffin, JW, Thompson, RW, Mitchinson, MJ, de Kiewiet, JC, and Welland, FH: Lymphomatous leptomeningitis. Am J Med 51:200–208, 1971.
444. Griggs, RC and Donohoe, KM: Emergency Management. In Henning, RJ and Jackson, DL (eds): Handbook of Critical Care Neurology and Neurosurgery. Praeger, New York, 1985, pp 201–225.
445. Griggs, RC, Donohoe, KM, Utell, MJ, Goldblatt, D, and Moxley, RT: Evaluation of pulmonary function in neuromuscular disease. Arch Neurol 38:9–12, 1981.
446. Griswold, K, Guanci, MM, and Ropper, AH: An approach to the care of patients with Guillain-Barré syndrome. Heart Lung 13:66–72, 1984.
447. Grose, C, Henle, W, Henle, G, and Feorino, PM: Primary Epstein-Barr virus infections in acute neurologic disease. N Engl J Med 292:392–395, 1975.
448. Grose, C and Spigland, I: Guillain-Barré syndrome following administration of live measles vaccine. Am J Med 60:441–443, 1976.
449. Gross, EG, Dexter, JD, and Roth, RG: Hypokalemic myopathy with myoglobinuria associated with licorice ingestion. N Engl J Med 274:602–606, 1966.
450. Gross, MLP, Graggs, RI, King, RHM, and Thomas, PK: The treatment of experimental allergic neuritis by plasma exchange. J Neurol Sci 61:149–160, 1983.
451. Gross, MLP, Legg, NJ, Lockwood, MC, and Pallis, C: The treatment of inflammatory polyneuropathy by plasma exchange. J Neurol Neurosurg Psychiatry 45:675–679, 1982.
452. Gross, MLP, Sweny, P, and Legg, NJ: Successful plasmapheresis in the Miller-Fisher syndrome. Br Med J 282:1394, 1981.
453. Gross, MLP and Thomas, PK: The treatment of chronic relapsing and chronic progressive idiopathic inflammatory polyneuropathy by plasma exchange. J Neurol Sci 52:69–78, 1981.
454. Grover, B, Dalessandro, L, Sanders, JG, Walter, MH, O'Meara, TF, and Redmond, J: Severe viral hepatitis A infection, Landry-Guillain-Barré syndrome, and hereditary elliptocytosis. South Med J 79:251–252, 1986.
455. Grunnet, ML and Lubow, M: Ascending polyneuritis and ophthalmoplegia. Am J Ophthalmol 74:1155–1160, 1972.
456. Guarda, LA, Luna, MA, Smith, JL, Jr, Mansell, PW, Gyorkey, F, and Roca, AN: Acquired immune deficiency syndrome: Postmortem findings. Am J Clin Pathol 81:549–557, 1984.
457. Gudmundsson, KR: Prevalence and occurrence of some rare neurological diseases in Iceland. Acta Neurol Scand 45:114–118, 1969.
458. Guidon, C, Granthil, C, Djiane, P, and Francois, G: Dysautonomie en deux temps au cours d'un syndrome de Guillain-Barré. Ann Fr Anesth Reanim 5:447–449, 1986.
459. Guillain, G: Radiculoneuritis with acellular hyperalbuminosis of the cerebrospinal fluid. Arch Neurol Psychiat 36:975–990, 1936.
460. Guillain, G: Synthese generale de la discussion. Journal belge de neurologie et de psychiatrie 38:323–329, 1938.
461. Guillain, G: Notice necrologique sur M. Harvey Cushing (1869–1939).

Bull Acad Natl Med (Paris) 122:582–586, 1939.
462. Guillain, G, Alajouanine, Th, and Perisson, J: Sur le syndrome de radiculo-nevrite aigue curable avec dissociation albumino-cytologique du liquide cephalo-rachidien (deux observations). Rev Neurol (Paris) 41:492–496, 1925.
463. Guillain, G and Barré, JA: Paralysie ascendante aigue de Landry consecutive a une vaccination antityphoidique. Rev Neurol (Paris) (Jull 3):595–598, 1919.
464. Guillain, G and Barré, JA: Travaux neurologiques de guerre. Masson et Cie (Paris), 1920.
465. Guillain, G and Barré, JA: Quelques remarques sur notre "syndrome de radiculo-nevrite avec hyperalbuminose du liquide cephalo-rachidien sans reaction cellulaire." Rev Neurol (Paris) 65:573–582, 1936.
466. Guillain, G, Barré, JA, and Strohl, A: Sur un syndrome de radiculo-nevrite avec hyperalbuminose du liquide cephalo-rachidien sans reaction cellulaire. Remarques sur les caracteres clinques et graphiques des reflexes tendineux. Bulletins et memories de la societe medicale des hopitaux de Paris, Masson et Cie 40:1462–1470, 1916.
467. Guillain, G, Barré, JA, and Strohl, A: On a syndrome of radiculoneuritis with hyperalbuminosis of the cerebrospinal fluid without a cellular reaction: Remarks on the clinical characteristics and tracings of the tendon reflexes. In Rottenberg, DA and Hochberg, FH (eds): Neurological Classics in Modern Translation. Hafner Press, New York, 1977, p 309.
468. Guillain-Barré Syndrome: Proceedings of a conference sponsored by the Kroc Foundation. Ann Neurol (Suppl)9:1–148, 1981.
469. Guillain-Barré Syndrome Study Group: Plasmapheresis and acute Guillain-Barré syndrome. Neurology 35:1096–1104, 1985.
470. Guiloff, RJ: Peripheral nerve conduction in Miller Fisher syndrome. J Neurol Neurosurg Psychiatry 40:801–807, 1977.
471. Gunderman, JR: Guillain-Barré syndrome. Occurrence following combined mumps-rubella vaccine. Am J Dis Child 125:834–835, 1973.
472. Haas, A, Trabert, W, Grebnich, N, and Schimrigk, K: High-dose steroid therapy in Guillain-Barré syndrome. J Neuroimmunol 20:305–308, 1988.
473. Haas, DC and Tatum, AH: Plasmapheresis alleviates neuropathy accompanying IgM anti-myelin–associated glycoprotein paraproteinemia. Ann Neurol 23:394–396, 1988.
474. Haberman, S, Benjamin, B, Capildeo, R, and Clifford Rose, F: North West Thames registry of neurological disease. J R Soc Med 75:443–449, 1982.
475. Hafez, M, Nagaty, M, Al-Tonbary, Y, el-Shennawy, FA, el-Mongui, A, el-Sallab, S, and Attia, S: HLA-antigens in Guillain-Barré syndrome. J Neurogenet 2:285–290, 1985.
476. Hafler, DA, Johnson, D, Kelly, JJ, Panitch, H, Kyle, R, and Weiner, HL: Monoclonal gammopathy and neuropathy: Myelin-associated glycoprotein reactivity and clinical characteristics. Neurology 36:75–78, 1986.
477. Hagberg, L, Malmvall, B-E, Svennerholm, L, Alestig, K, and Norkrans, G: Guillain-Barré syndrome as an early manifestation of HIV central nervous system infection. Scand J Infect Dis 18:591–592, 1986.
478. Hahn, AF, Feasby, TE, and Gilbert, JJ: Blood-nerve barrier studies in experimental allergic neuritis. Acta Neuropathol (Berl) 68:101–109, 1985.
479. Hakamada, S, Watanabe, K, Hara, K, Miyazaki, S, Sato, I, Tanaka, E, Yamazaki, T, Kajita, Y, and Maehara, M: Guillain-Barré syndrome presenting with signs of ophthalmoplegia. Brain Dev 2:407–409, 1980.
480. Halls, J, Bredkjaer, C, and Friis, ML: Guillain-Barré syndrome: Diagnostic criteria, epidemiology, clinical course and prognosis. Acta Neurol Scand 78:118–122, 1988.
481. Halperin, JJ and Dattwyler, RJ: Pe-

ripheral nervous system manifestations of Lyme disease (abstr). Neurology (Suppl)39:304, 1989.
482. Halperin, JJ, Little, BW, Coyle, PK, and Dattwyler, RJ: Lyme disease: Cause of a treatable peripheral neuropathy. Neurology 37:1700–1706, 1987.
482a. Hamilton, RJ, Puckett, R, and Bazemore, WC: Ventilator dependence in acute severe asthma due to a variant presentation of Guillain-Barré syndrome. Chest 96:1205–1206, 1989.
483. Hand, M and Rudoy, M: The prognostic significance of the "Guillain-Barré syndrome." Ann Intern Med 29:91–102, 1948.
484. Hankey, GJ: Guillain-Barré syndrome in Western Australia, 1980–1985. Med J Aust 146:130–133, 1987.
485. Hansen, LA, Harrison, BM, Pollard, JD, and McLeod, JG: Peripheral nerve demyelination induced by serum from patients with Guillain-Barré syndrome (abstr). J Neuroimmunol (Suppl 1):525, 1982.
486. Harik, SI, Ghandour, MH, Farah, FS, and Afifi, AK: Postganglionic cholinergic dysautonomia. Ann Neurol 1:393–396, 1977.
487. Harris, EN, Englert, H, Derue, G, Hughes, GRU, and Gharavi, A: Antiphospholyside antibodies in acute Guillain-Barré syndrome. Lancet 2:1361–1362, 1983.
488. Harrison, BM, Hansen, LA, Pollard, JD, and McLeod, JC: Demyelination induced by serum from patients with Guillain-Barré syndrome. Ann Neurol 15:163–170, 1984.
489. Hart, IK and Kennedy, PGE: Guillain-Barré syndrome associated with cytomegalovirus infection. Q J Med 67:425–430, 1988.
490. Hart, MN, Hanks, DT, and MacKay, R: Ultrastructural observations in Guillain-Barré syndrome. Arch Pathol 93:552–555, 1972.
491. Hartung, HP, Schafer, B, Diamantstein, T, Fierz, W, Heininger, K, and Toyka, KV: Suppression of P2-T-cell line mediated experimental autoimmune neuritis by interleukin-2 receptor blockade. Ann NY Acad Sci 540:563–565, 1988.
492. Hartung, HP, Schafer, B, Fierz, W, van der Meide, P, Heininger, K, and Toyka, KV: EAN: Monoclonal antibody to IFN-gamma protects rats from pathogenic effects of autoreactive P2 specific T-helper line cells (abstr). Neurology 39:288, 1989.
493. Hartung, HP, Schafer, B, Heininger, K, Stoll, G, and Toyka, KV: The role of macrophages and eicosanoids in the pathogenesis of experimental allergic neuritis, serial clinical electrophysiological, biochemical and morphological observations. Brain 111:1039–1059, 1988.
494. Hartung, HP, Schafer, B, Heininger, K, and Toyka, KV: Suppression of experimental autoimmune neuritis by the oxygen radical scavengers superoxide dismutase and catalase. Ann Neurol 23:453–460, 1988.
495. Hartung, HP, Schwenke, C, Bitter-Suermann, D, and Toyka, KV: Guillain-Barré syndrome: Activated complement components C3a and C5a in CSF. Neurology 37:1006–1009, 1987.
495a. Hartung, HP and Toyka, KV: T-cell and macrophage activation in experimental autoimmune neuritis and Guillain-Barré syndrome. Ann Neurol 27(Suppl):S57–S63, 1990.
496. Harvey, GK, Schindhelm, K, Anthony, JH, and Pollard, JD: Membrane plasma exchange in experimental allergic neuritis: Effect on antibody levels and clinical course. J Neurol Sci 88:207–218, 1988.
497. Hassin, GB: Landry's paralysis: Its clinical and pathologic features. J Neuropathol Exp Neurol 2:293–300, 1943.
498. Hauser, SL, Ropper, AH, Perlo, VP, Reinherz, EL, Scholossman, SF, and Weiner, HL: T-cell subsets in human autoimmune diseases. Neurology 22:1320–1321, 1982.
499. Hausmanowa-Petrusewicz, I, Emeryk, B, Rowinska-Marcinska, K, and Jedrzejowska, H: Nerve conduction in the Guillain-Barré-Strohl syn-

drome. J Neurol 220:169–184, 1979.
500. Haymaker, W: Jean Baptiste Octave Landry De Thezillat (1826–1865). In Haymaker, W and Schiller, F (eds): The Founders of Neurology, ed 2. Charles C Thomas, Springfield, IL, 1970, p 466.
501. Haymaker, W, and Kernohan, JW: The Landry-Guillain-Barré syndrome: Clinicopathologic report of fifty fatal cases and a critique of the literature. Medicine 28:59–141, 1949.
502. Heath, JW, Ueda, S, Bornstein, MB, Daves, GD, and Raine, CS: Buckthorn neuropathy in vitro: Evidence of a primary neuronal effect. J Neuropathol Exp Neurol 41:204–220, 1982.
503. Hedley-Whyte, J, Burgess, G, Feely, T, and Miller, M: Applied Physiology of Respiratory Care. Little, Brown, Boston, 1976.
504. Heffner, JE, Miller, KS, and Sahn, SA: Tracheostomy in the intensive care unit. Part 1: Indications, technique, management. Chest 90:269–274, 1986.
505. Heffner, JE, Miller, KS, and Sahn, SA: Tracheostomy in the intensive care unit. Part 2: Complications. Chest 90:430–436, 1986.
506. Heinonen, E, Molnar, G, Lang, H, and Valimaki, I: Computer-assisted monitoring of heart rate variation as a method of following the autonomic symptoms of the Guillain-Barré syndrome. Acta Neurol Scand (Suppl 90)65:232–233, 1982.
507. Heller, GL and DeJong, RN: Treatment of the Guillain-Barré syndrome. Use of corticotropin and glucocorticoids. Arch Neurol 8:179–193, 1963.
508. Heller, J and Vogel, S: No Laughing Matter. GP Putnam, New York, 1986.
509. Hemachudha, T, Griffin, DE, Chen, WW, and Johnson, RT: Immunologic studies of rabies vaccination-induced Guillain-Barré syndrome. Neurology 38:375–378, 1988.
510. Hemachudha, T, Phanuphak, P, Johnson, RT, Griffin, DE, Ratanavongsiri, J, and Siriprasomsup, W: Neurologic complications of Semple-type rabies vaccine: Clinical and immunologic studies. Neurology 37:550–556, 1987.
511. Henriet, M and Jacquy, J: Facial myokymia in Guillain-Barré (letter). Neurology 33:1534, 1983.
512. Henson, RA and Urich, H: Cancer and the nervous system. The neurological manifestations of systemic malignant disease. Blackwell Scientific, Oxford, 1982, p 387.
513. Henze, T, Prange, HW, and Ritter, G: Vegetative funktionsstorungen bei schwer verlaufender polyradikulitis Guillain-Barré-Strohl. Dtsch Med Wochenschr 111:1050–1054, 1986.
514. Heptinstall, RH and Sowry, GSC: Peripheral neuritis in systemic lupus erythematosus. Br Med J 1:525–527, 1952.
515. Hewer, RL, Hilton, PJ, Crampton-Smith, A, and Spalding, JMK: Acute polyneuritis requiring artificial respiration. Q J Med 37:479–491, 1968.
516. Heyman, A, Pfeiffer, JB, Willett, RW, and Taylor, HM: Peripheral neuropathy caused by arsenical intoxication. A study of 41 cases with observations on the effects of BAL (2,3 Dimercapto-Propanol). N Engl J Med 254:401–409, 1956.
517. Hill, NS: Clinical applications of body ventilators. Chest 90:897–905, 1986.
518. Hinman, RC and Magee, KR: Guillain-Barré syndrome with slow progressive onset and persistent elevation of spinal fluid protein. Ann Intern Med 67:1007–1012, 1967.
519. Hirano, A, Cooks, SD, Whitaker, JN, Dowling, PC, and Murray, MR: Fine structual aspects of demyelination in vitro: The effects of Guillain-Barré serum. J Neuropathol Exp Neurol 30:249–265, 1971.
520. Ho, DD, Rota, TR, Schooley, RT, Kaplan, JC, Allan, JD, Groopman, JE, Resnick, L, Felsenstein, D, Andrews, CA, and Hirsch, MS: Isolation of HTLV-III from cerebrospinal fluid and neural tissues of patients with neurologic syndromes related to the

acquired immunodeficiency syndrome. N Engl J Med 313:1493–1497, 1985.
521. Hobday, JD and Baker, AJ: Guillain-Barré syndrome complicated by hypertension and ileitis. Med J Aust 2:536–538, 1968.
522. Hochman, MS, Kobetz, SA, and Handwerker, JV: Inappropriate secretion of antidiuretic hormone associated with Guillain-Barré syndrome (letter). Ann Neurol 11:322–323, 1982.
523. Hodges, GR and Perkins, RL: Landry-Guillain-Barré syndrome associated with Mycoplasma pneumoniae infection. JAMA 210:2088–2090, 1969.
524. Hodson, AK, Hurwitz, BJ, and Albrecht, R: Dysautonomia in Guillain-Barré syndrome with dorsal root ganglioneuropathy, Wallerian degeneration, and fatal myocarditis. Ann Neurol 15:88–95, 1984.
525. Hoerlein, BF: Canine Neurology. WB Saunders, Philadelphia, 1971, p 174.
526. Hoff, SD and Rowlands, BJ: Guillain-Barré syndrome due to hypophosphatemia following intravenous hyperalimentation. JPEN 12:414–416, 1988.
527. Hogg, JE, Korbin, DE, and Schoenberg, BS: The Guillain-Barré syndrome epidemiologic and clinical features. J Chron Dis 32:227–231, 1979.
528. Holmdahl, R, Olsson, T, Moron, T, and Klareskog, L: In vivo treatment of rats with monoclonal anti T cell antibodies immunohistochemical and functional analysis in normal rats and in experimental allergic neuritis (EAN). Scand J Immunol 22:157–169, 1985.
529. Holmes, DF and deLahunta, A: Experimental allergic neuritis in the dog and its comparison with the naturally occurring disease; coonhound paralysis. Acta Neuropathol 30:329–337, 1974.
530. Holmes, DF, Schultz, RD, Cummings, JF, and deLahunta, A: Experimental coonhound paralysis: Animal model of Guillain-Barré syndrome. Neurology 29:1186–1187, 1979.
531. Holmes, G: Acute febrile polyneuritis. Br Med J 2:37–39, 1917.
532. Hopkins, A, Neville, B, and Bannister, R: Autonomic neuropathy of acute onset. Lancet 1:769–771, 1974.
533. Hopkins, IJ, Shield, LK, and Harris, M: Subacute cholinergic dysautonomia in childhood. Clin Exp Neurol 17:147–151, 1980.
534. Horwich, MS, Cho, L, Porro, RS, and Posner, JB: Subacute sensory neuropathy: A remote effect of carcinoma. Ann Neurol 2:7–19, 1977.
535. Hory, B, Blanc, D, Boillot, A, and Panouse-Perrin, J: Guillain-Barré syndrome following danazol and corticosteroid therapy for hereditary angioedema. Am J Med 79:111–114, 1985.
536. Houff, SA, Burton, RC, Wilson, RW, Henson, TE, London, WT, Baer, GM, Anderson, LJ, Winkler, WG, Madden, DL, and Sever, JL: Human-to-human transmission of rabies virus by corneal transplant. N Engl J Med 300:603–604, 1979.
537. Howard, BD and Gundersen, CB: Effects and mechanisms of polypeptide neurotoxins that act presynaptically. Ann Rev Pharmacol Toxicol 20:307–336, 1980.
538. Hudgson, P: Polymyositis and dermatomyositis in adults. Clin Rheum Dis 10:85–93, 1984.
539. Huestis, DW: Mortality in therapeutic haemapheresis (letter). Lancet 1:1043, 1983.
540. Huet, P-M, Layrargues, GP, Lebrun, LH, and Richer, G: Hepatitis B surface antigen in the cerebrospinal fluid in a case of Guillain-Barré syndrome. Can Med Assoc J 122:1157–1159, 1980.
541. Hugh-Jones, T, Kanis, JA, and Yates, AJP: Hypercalcaemia complicating polyneuropathy (letter). J Neurol Neurosurg Psychiatry 48:390, 1985.
542. Hughes, JM, Blumenthal, JR, Merson, MH, Lombard, GL, Dowell, VR,

and Gangarosa, ED: Clinical features of Types A and B food-borne botulism. Ann Intern Med 95:442–445, 1981.

543. Hughes, JM and Merson, MH: Fish and shellfish poisoning. N Engl J Med 295:1117–1120, 1976.

544. Hughes, RAC, Gray, IA, Gregson, NA, Kadlubowski, M, Kennedy, M, Leibowitz, S, and Thompson, H: Immune responses to myelin antigens in Guillain-Barré syndrome. J Neuroimmunol 6:303–312, 1984.

545. Hughes, RAC, Kadlubowksi, M, Gray, IA, and Leibowitz, S: Immune responses in experimental allergic neuritis. J Neurol Neurosurg Psychiatry 44:565–569, 1981.

546. Hughes, RAC, Kadlubowksi, M, and Hufschmidt, A: Treatment of acute inflammatory polyneuropathy. Ann Neurol (Suppl)9:125–133, 1981.

547. Hughes, RAC, Newsom-Davis, JM, Perkin, GD, and Pierce, JM: Controlled trial of prednisolone in acute polyneuropathy. Lancet 2:750–753, 1978.

548. Hughes, RAC and Winer, JB: Guillain-Barré syndrome. In Mathews, WB and Glaser, GD (eds): Recent Advances in Clinical Neurology 4. Churchill Livingstone, Edinburgh, 1984, pp 19–48.

549. Humphrey, GL and Constantine, DG: Rabies. In Hoeprich, PD (ed): Infectious Diseases, ed 3. Harper and Row, Philadelphia, 1983, pp 1089–1100.

550. Humphrey, JG: Toronto study: The utility of therapeutic plasmapheresis for neurological disorders. NIH Consensus Development Conference, 1986.

551. Hurst, EW and Pawan, JL: An outbreak of rabies in Trinidad. Without history of bites, and with the symptoms of acute myelitis. Lancet 2: 622–628, 1931.

552. Hurwitz, ES, Holman, RC, Nelson, DB, and Schonberger, LB: National surveillance for Guillain-Barré syndrome. January 1978–March 1979. Neurology 33:150–157, 1983.

553. Hutchinson, EC, Leonard, BJ, Maudsley, C, and Yates, PO: Neurological complications of the reticuloses. Brain 81:75–93, 1958.

554. Igbal, A, Oger, JJ-F, and Arnason, BGW: Cell-mediated immunity in idiopathic polyneuritis. Ann Neurol (Suppl)9:65–69, 1981.

555. Ilyas, AA, Willison, HJ, Quarles, RH, Jungalwala, FB, Cornblath, DR, Trapp, BD, Griffin, DE, Griffin, JW, and McKhann, GM: Serum antibodies to gangliosides in Guillain-Barré syndrome. Ann Neurol 23:440–447, 1988.

556. Ince, LP and Leon, MS: Biofeedback treatment of upper extremity dysfunction in Guillain-Barré syndrome. Arch Phys Med Rehabil 67:30–33, 1986.

557. Irvine, AT and Tibbles, J: Treatment of Fisher's variant of Guillain-Barré syndrome by exchange transfusion. Can J Neurol Sci 8:49–50, 1981.

557a. Iwatsubu, T, Sakanaka, C, Obi, T, Takeda, K, and Sakuta, M: Chronic inflammatory demyelinating polyradiculoneuropathy of acute onset: Relapse after temporary improvement by plasma exchange.

558. Jackman, RL and Jones, RE: Hyperthyroidism and periodic paralysis. Arch Intern Med 113:657–664, 1964.

559. Jackson, AL: A clinical study of the Landry-Guillain-Barré syndrome with reference to aetiology, including the role of coxsackie virus infections. S Afr Med J 7:121–137, 1961.

560. Jackson, RN, Miller, H, and Schapira, K: Polyradiculitis (Landry-Guillain-Barré syndrome). Treatment with cortisone and corticotropin. Br Med J 1:480–484, 1957.

561. Jamal, GA and Ballantyne, JP: The localization of the lesion in patients with acute ophthalmoplegia, ataxia and areflexia (Miller Fisher syndrome). A serial multimodal neurophysiological study. Brain 111:95–114, 1988.

562. Jamal, GA and McLeod, WN: Electrophysiologic studies in Miller Fisher syndrome. Neurology 34:685–688, 1984.

563. Jampel, RS and Haidt, SJ: Bell's phenomenon and acute idiopathic polyneuritis. Am J Ophthalmol 74: 145–153, 1972.

564. Janeway, R and Kelly, DL, Jr: Papilledema and hydrocephalus associated with recurrent polyneuritis. Arch Neurol 15:507–514, 1966.

565. Janny, P, Chazal, J, Colent, G, Irthum, B, and Georget, AM: Benign intracranial hypertension and disorders of CSF absorption. Surg Neurol 15:168–174, 1981.

566. Jenkins, RB and Toole, JF: Polyneuropathy following exposure to insecticides. Arch Intern Med 13:69–695, 1964.

567. Johanson, WG, Pierce, AK, and Sanford, JP: Changing pharyngeal bacterial flora of hospitalized patients. Emergence of gram-negative bacili. N Engl J Med 281:1137–1140, 1969.

568. Johnson, DE: Guillain-Barré syndrome in the US Army. Arch Neurol 39:21–24, 1982.

569. Johnson, D, Seeldrayers, PA, and Weiner, HL: The role of mast cells in demyelination. 1. Myelin proteins are degraded by mast cell proteases and myelin basic protein and P2 can stimulate mast cell degranulation. Brain Res 444:195–198, 1988.

570. Johnson, EW, Guyton, JD, and Olsen, KJ: Motor nerve conduction velocity studies in poliomyelitis. Arch Phys Med Rehabil 41:185–190, 1960.

571. Johnson, RH and Spalding, JMK: Disorders of the Autonomic Nervous System. FA Davis, Philadelphia, 1974, p 98.

572. Johnson, RT and Richardson, EP: The neurological manifestations of systemic lupus erythematosus: A clinical-pathological study of 24 cases and review of the literature. Medicine 47:337–369, 1968.

573. Johnston, CLW, Schwartz, M, and Wansbrough-Jones, MH: Acute inflammatory polyradiculoneuropathy following type A viral hepatitis. Postgrad Med J 57:647–648, 1981.

574. Jones, HR: Acute ataxia associated with ciguatera-type (grouper) tropical fish poisoning. Ann Neurol 7:491, 1980.

575. Joynt, RJ: The mechanism of production of papilledema in the Guillain-Barré syndrome. Neurology 8:8–12, 1958.

576. Julien, J, Vital, C, Aupy, G, Lagueny, A, Darriet, D, and Brechenmacher, C: Guillain-Barré syndrome and Hodgkin's disease. Ultrastructural study of a peripheral nerve. J Neurol Sci 45:23–27, 1980.

577. Kabins, S, Keller, R, Peitchel, R, and Ali, MA: Acute idiopathic polyneuritis caused by cytomegalovirus. Arch Intern Med 136:100–101, 1976.

578. Kadlubowski, M and Hughes, RAC: Identification of the neuritogen for experimental allergic neuritis. Nature 277:140–141, 1979.

579. Kadlubowski, M and Ingram, PL: Circulating antibodies to the neuritogenic myelin protein P2, in neuritis of the cauda equina of the horse. Nature 293:299–300, 1981.

580. Kaeser, HE, Richter, HR, and Wuthrich, R: Les dyscinesies faciales. Rev Neurol 108:538–541, 1963.

581. Kahler, O and Pick, A: Weitere Beitrage zur Pathologie und pathologischen Anatomie des Centralnervensystems. Arch f Psychiat 10:297, 1880.

582. Kaiser-Smith, and Barrone: Relapsing polyneuritis following classic Miller Fisher syndrome. J Neurol Neurosurg Psychiatry 52:802–803, 1989.

583. Kaldor, J and Speed, BR: Guillain-Barré syndrome and Campylobacter jejuni: A serological study. Br Med J 288:1867–1870, 1984.

584. Kalimo, H, Molnar, GK, Saksa, M, and Riekkinen, PJ: Involvement of autonomic nervous system in experimental allergic neuritis. J Neuroimmunol 2:9–19, 1982.

585. Kammer, GM and Hamilton, CR: Acute bulbar muscle dysfunction and hyperthyroidism. Am J Med 56:464–470, 1974.

586. Kanda, T, Hayashi, H, Tanabe, H, Tsubaki, T, and Oda, M: A fulminant case of Guillain-Barré syndrome: To-

pographic and fibre size related analysis of demyelinating changes. J Neurol Neurosurg Psychiatry 52: 857–864, 1989.

587. Kaplan, JE, Greenspan, JR, Bomgaars, M, Wiebenga, N, Bart, RD, Robbins, K, Wiebe, R, Tabrah, F, Stewart, J, and Schonberger, LB: Simultaneous outbreaks of Guillain-Barré syndrome and Bell's palsy in Hawaii in 1981. JAMA 250:2635–2640, 1983.
588. Kaplan, JE, Poduska, PJ, McIntosh, GC, Hopkins, RS, Ferguson, SW, and Schonberger, LB: Guillain-Barré syndrome in Larimer County, Colorado: A high-incidence area. Neurology 35:581–584, 1985.
589. Kaplan, JE, Schonberger, LB, Hurwitz, ES, and Katona, P: Guillain-Barré syndrome in the United States, 1978–1981: Additional observations from the national surveillance system. Neurology 33:633–637, 1983.
590. Kaplan, JG, Schaumburg, HH, and Sumner, A: Relapsing ophthalmoparesis-sensory neuropathy syndrome. Neurology 35:595–596, 1985.
591. Kashihara, K and Yabuki, S: Cold-induced dysaesthesia in acute idiopathic polyneuritis. J Neurol 235: 53–55, 1987.
592. Kashihara, K, Yabuki, S, Mimori, Y, Yamazaki, My, and Yamashita, M: An outbreak of Guillain-Barré syndrome with ophthalmoplegia in Kochi. Rinsho Shinkeigaku 27:305–309, 1987.
593. Kaslow, RA, Sullivan-Bolyai, JZ, Hafkin, B, Schonberger, LB, Kraus, L, Moore, MJ, Yunis, E, and Williams, RM: HLA antigens in Guillain-Barré syndrome. Neurology 34:240–242, 1984.
594. Kaslow, RA, Sullivan-Bolyai, JZ, Holman, RC, Hafkin, B, Dicker, RC, and Schonberger, LB: Risk factors for Guillain-Barré syndrome. Neurology 37:685–688, 1987.
595. Katrak, SM, Pollock, M, O'Brien, CP, Nukada, H, Allpress, S, Calder, C, Palmer, DG, Grennan, DM, McCormack, PL, and Laurent, MR: Clinical and morphological features of gold neuropathy. Brain 103:671–693, 1980.
596. Katznelson, D, Gross, S, and Sack, J: Polyneuritis following BCG revaccination. Postgrad Med J 58: 496–497, 1982.
597. Kaufman, MD, Hopkins, LC, and Hurwitz, BJ: Progressive sensory neuropathy in patients without carcinoma: A disorder with distinctive clinical and electrophysiological findings. Ann Neurol 9:237–242, 1981.
598. Keane, JR: Lid-lag in the Guillain-Barré syndrome. Arch Neurol 32:478–479, 1975.
599. Keane, JR and Finstead, BA: Upward gaze paralysis as the initial sign of Fisher's syndrome. Arch Neurol 39:781–782, 1982.
600. Keenlyside, RA, Schonberger, LB, Bregman, DJ, and Bolyai, JZS: Fatal Guillain-Barré syndrome after the National Influenza Immunization Program. Neurology 30:929–933, 1980.
601. Keller, AJ, Chirnside, A, and Urbaniak, SJ: Coagulation abnormalities produced by plasma exchange on the cell separator with special reference to fibrinogen and platelet levels. Br J Haematol 42:593–602, 1979.
602. Kelly, JJ, Adelman, LS, Berkman, E, and Bhan, I: Polyneuropathies associated with IgM monoclonal gammopathies. Arch Neurol 45:1355–1359, 1988.
603. Kelly, JJ, Kyle, RA, Miles, JM, and Dyck, PJ: Osteosclerotic myeloma and peripheral neuropathy. Neurology 33:202–210, 1983.
604. Kennard, C, Newland, AC, and Ridley, A: Treatment of the Guillain-Barré syndrome by plasma exchange. J Neurol Neurosurg Psychiatry 45:847–850, 1982.
605. Kennedy, P and Cavanagh, JB: Spinal changes in the neuropathy of thallium poisoning. A case with neuropathological studies. J Neurol Sci 29:295–301, 1976.
606. Kennedy, RH, Danielson, MA,

Mulder, DW, and Kurland, LT: Guillain-Barré syndrome. A 42-year epidemiologic and clinical study. Mayo Clin Proc 53:93–99, 1978.

606a. Khaldi, F, Larnaout, A, Miladi, N, and Bennaceur, B: Guillain-Barré syndrome and idiopathic thrombocytopenic purpura. Can J Neurol Sci 17:95, 1990 (letter).

607. Khatri, BO, Flamini, R, Baruah, JK, Dobyson, WB, and Konkol, RJ: Plasmapheresis in children with acute polyneuropathy (abstr). Neurology (Suppl)38:238, 1988.

608. Khosla, SN, Srivasta, SC, and Gupta, S: Neuropsychiatric manifestations of thyphoid. J Trop Med Hyg 80:95–98, 1977.

609. Khouri, SA: Guillain-Barré syndrome: Epidemiology of an outbreak. Am J Epidemiol 107:433–438, 1978.

610. Kurana, RK, Koski, CL, and Mayer, RF: Dysautonomia in Eaton-Lambert syndrome. Ann Neurol 14:123, 1983.

611. Kibel, MA: Guillain-Barré syndrome in childhood (letter). S Afr Med J 63:715, 1983.

612. Kilroy, AW, Schaffner, W, Fleet, WF, Lefkowitz, LB, Karzon, DT, and Fenichel, GM: Two syndromes following rubella immunization. JAMA 214: 2287–2292, 1970.

613. Kimura, J: An evaluation of the facial and trigeminal nerves in polyneuropathy: Electrodiagnostic study in Charcot-Marie-Tooth disease, Guillain-Barré syndrome and diabetic neuropathy. Neurology 21:747–753, 1971.

614. Kimura, J: Proximal versus distal slowing of motor nerve conduction velocity in the Guillain-Barré syndrome. Ann Neurol 3:344–350, 1978.

615. Kimura, J and Butzer, JF: F-wave conduction velocity in Guillain-Barré syndrome. Assessment of nerve segment between axilla and spinal cord. Arch Neurol 32:524–529, 1975.

616. King, RHM, Craggs, RI, Gross, MLP, and Thomas, PK: Effects of glucocorticoids on experimental allergic neuritis. Exp Neurol 87:9–19, 1985.

617. King, RHM, Craggs, RI, Gross, MLP, Tompkins, C, and Thomas, PK: Suppression of experimental allergic neuritis by cyclosporin-A. Acta Neuropathol 59:262–268, 1983.

618. Kingma, FJ and Catcott, EJ: A paralytic syndrome in coonhounds. North American Veterinarian 35: 115–117, 1954.

619. Kinnunen, E, Farkkila, M, Hovi, T, Juntunen, J, and Weckstrom, P: Incidence of Guillain-Barré syndrome during a nationwide oral poliovirus vaccine campaign. Neurology 39: 1034–1036, 1989.

620. Kirby, RS, Fowler, CJ, Gosling, JA, and Bannister, R: Bladder dysfunction in distal autonomic neuropathy of acute onset. J Neurol Neurosurg Psychiatry 48:762–767, 1985.

621. Kissel, JT, Slivka, AP, and Mendell, JR: The spectrum of peripheral neuropathies with necrotizing angiopathy. Ann Neurol 14:122–123, 1983.

622. Klastersky, J, Hensgens, C, Noterman, J, Monawad, E, and Mennier-Carpentier, F: Endotracheal antibiotics for the prevention of tracheobronchial infections in tracheotomized unconscious patients. Chest 68:302–306, 1975.

623. Klemola, E, Weckman, N, Haltia, K, and Kaariainen, L: The Guillain-Barré syndrome associated with acquired cytomegalovirus infection. Acta Scand 181:603–607, 1967.

624. Kleyweg, RP, van der Meche, FGA, and Meulstee, J: Treatment of Guillain-Barré syndrome with high-dose gammaglobulin. Neurology 38:1639–1641, 1988.

625. Klick, JM, du Moulin, GC, Hedley-Whyte, J, Teres, P, Bushnell, LS, and Feingold, DS: Prevention of gram-negative bacillary pneumonia using polymyxin aerosol as prophylaxis. II. Effect on the incidence of pneumonia in seriously ill patients. J Clin Invest 55:514–519, 1975.

626. Klingon, GH: The Guillain-Barré syndrome associated with cancer. Cancer 18:157–163, 1965.

627. Knezevic, W, Quintner, J, Mastaglia, FL, and Zilko, PJ: Guillain-Barré syndrome and pemphigus foliaceus associated with D-penicillamine ther-

apy. Aust NZ J Med 14:50–52, 1984.
628. Knochel, JP: The pathophysiology and clinical characteristics of severe hypophosphatemia. Arch Intern Med 137:203–220, 1977.
629. Knochel, JP: Neuromuscular manifestations of electrolyte disorders. Am J Med 72:521–535, 1982.
630. Knox, DL, Clark, DB, and Schuster, FF: Benign VI nerve palsies in children. Pediatrics 40:560–564, 1967.
631. Knox, JDE, Levy, R, and Simpson, JA: Herpes zoster and the Landry-Guillain-Barré syndrome. J Neurol Neurosurg Psychiatry 24:167–172, 1961.
632. Knutti, RE: Acute ascending paralysis and myelitis due to the virus of rabies. JAMA 93:754–758, 1929.
633. Kocen, RS: Diabetes mellitus with acute polyneuritis. Br Med J 2:100–101, 1957.
634. Koch, J, Sagartz, JW, Davidson, DE, and Lawhaswasdi, K: Diagnosis of human rabies by the cornea test. Am J Clin Pathol 63:509–515, 1975.
635. Koenig, MG, Drutz, DJ, Mushlin, AI, Schaffner, W, and Rogers, DE: Type B botulism in man. Am J Med 42:208–219, 1967.
636. Koenig, MG, Spickard, A, Cardella, MA, and Rogers, DE: Clinical and laboratory observations on Type E botulism in man. Medicine 43:517–545, 1964.
637. Kogan, BA, Solomon, MH, and Diokno, AC: Urinary retention secondary to Landry-Guillain-Barré syndrome. J Urol 126:643–644, 1981.
638. Kohler, A, de Torrente, A, and Inderwildi, B: Fisher's syndrome associated with Campylobacter jejuni infection. Eur Neurol 28:150–151, 1988.
639. Kohler, PC and Goldblatt, D: Guillain-Barré syndrome following Campylobacter jejuni enteritis (letter). Arch Neurol 44:1219, 1987.
640. Koizumi, K, Cannan, H, and Yamashite, H: The Role of Baroreceptors in Control of Hypothalamic Neurosecretory Cells. In Sleight, P (ed): Arterial Baroreceptors and Hypertension. Oxford University Press, Oxford, 1988, pp 193–201.
641. Korn-Lubetzki, I and Abramsky, O: Acute and chronic demyelinating inflammatory polyradiculoneuropathy. Association with autoimmune diseases and lymphocyte response to human neuritogenic protein. Arch Neurol 43:604–608, 1986.
642. Koski, CL: Complement-fixing antiperipheral myelin antibodies and C9 neoantigen in serum of patients with Guillain-Barré syndrome: Quantitation, kinetics, and clinical correlation. Ann NY Acad Sci 540:319–325, 1988.
643. Koski, CL, Gratz, E, Sutherland, J, and Mayer, RF: Clinical correlation with anti-peripheral-nerve myelin antibodies in Guillain-Barré syndrome. Ann Neurol 19:573–577, 1986.
644. Koski, CL, Jungalwala, FB, and Chou, D: Anti-peripheral nerve myelin antibodies in Guillain-Barré syndrome bind a neutral glycolipid of peripheral nerve myelin and cross-react with Forssman antigen (abstr). Ann Neurol 24:122, 1988.
645. Koski, CL, Sanders, ME, Swoveland, PT, Lawley, TJ, Shin, ML, Frank, MM, and Joiner, KA: Activation of terminal components of complement in patients with Guillain-Barré syndrome and other demyelinating neuropathies. J Clin Invest 80:1492–1497, 1987.
646. Kotsoris, H, Schleifer, L, Menken, M, and Plum, F: Total locked-in state resembling brain death in polyneuropathy (abstr). Ann Neurol 16:150, 1984.
647. Kreitzer, SM, Saunders, NA, Tyler, HR, and Ingram, RH: Respiratory muscle function in amyotrophic lateral sclerosis. Am Rev Respir Dis 117:437–447, 1978.
648. Krendel, DA, Parks, HP, Anthony, DC, St Clair, MB, and Graham, DG: Sural nerve biopsy in chronic inflammatory demyelinating polyradiculoneuropathy. Muscle Nerve 12: 257–264, 1989.
649. Krone, A, Reuther, P, and Fuhrmeister, U: Autonomic dysfunction in polyneuropathies: A report of 106 cases. J Neurol 230:111–121, 1983.

650. Krucke, W: Die primar-entzundliche polyneuritis unbekannter Ursache. In Lubarsch, O, Henke, F, and Rossle, G (eds): Handbuch des speziellen pathologischen Anatomie und Histologie. Band 13, Teil 5, Springer Verlag, Berlin, 1955, p 164.
651. Kruger, H, Engler, D, and Pflughaupt, KW: Demonstration of oligoclonal immunoglobulin G in Guillain-Barré syndrome and lymphocyte meningoradiculitis by isoelectric focusing. J Neurol 226:15–24, 1981.
652. Krull, F, Schuchardt, V, Haupt, WF, and Mewes, J: Prognosis of acute polyneuritis requiring artificial ventilation. Intensive Care Med 14:388–392, 1988.
653. Kuishan, Z, Junjiang, Z, Zhaomin, M, and Junpeng, A: Acupuncture treatment in 24 cases of infectious neuritis. J Tradit Chin Med 6:29–30, 1986.
654. Kunin, CM: Can we build a better urinary catheter? (Editorial) N Engl J Med 319:365–366, 1988.
655. Kunst, H and Grosser, KD: Das elektrokardiogramm bei idiopathischen polyneuritiden. Dtsch Med Wochenschr 99:1350–1354, 1974.
656. Kurdi, A and Abdul-Kader, M: Clinical and electrophysiological studies of diphtheritic neuritis in Jordan. J Neurol Sci 42:243–250, 1979.
657. Kurland, LT: Descriptive epidemiology of selected neurologic and myopathic disorders with particular reference to a survey in Rochester, Minnesota. J Chron Dis 8:378–418, 1958.
658. Kurland, LT, Wiederholt, WC, Kirkpatrick, JW, Potter, HG, and Armstrong, P: Swine influenza vaccine and Guillain-Barré syndrome. Epidemic or artifact? Arch Neurol 42:1089–1090, 1985.
659. Kyrieleis, W: Augenveranderungen bei entzundlichen Erkrankungen des Zentral-Systems. D. Die Landrysche Paralyse (akut aufsteigende Spinalparalyse). In Schieck, F and Bruckner, A (eds): Kurzes Handbuch der Ophthalmologie. Vol 6. Julius Springer, Berlin, 1931, pp 742–743.
660. Lachman, T, Shahani, BT, and Young, RR: Late responses as aids to diagnosis in peripheral neuropathy. J Neurol Neurosurg Psychiatry 43:156–162, 1980.
661. Lam, AM, Grace, DM, Penny, FJ, and Venzina, WC: Prophylactic intravenous cimetidine reduces the risk of acid aspiration in morbidly obese patients. Anesthesiology 65:684–687, 1986.
662. Lambert, EH and Mulder, DW: Nerve conduction in the Guillain-Barré syndrome (abstr). Electroencephalogr Clin Neurophysiol 17:86, 1964.
663. Lambregts, PCLA and Op de Coul, AAW: Hartritmestoornissen bij het syndroom van Guillain-Barré-Strohl. Ned Tijdschr Geneeskd 129:260–264, 1985.
664. Lampert, PW: Mechanism of demyelination in experimental allergic neuritis. Electron-microscopic studies. Lab Invest 20:127–138, 1969.
665. Lamy, M, Aussannaire, M, Nick, J, and Jammet, ML: Polyradiculonevrite varicelleuse a forme pseudo-myopathique. Arch Fr Pediatr 9:976–978, 1952.
666. Landau, WM, Glenn, C, and Dust, G: MRI in Miller-Fisher variant of Guillain-Barré syndrome (letter). Neurology 37:1431, 1987.
667. Landry, O: Comments of Dr. Landry immediately following Dr. Foville's paper. In Wolf, JK (ed): The Classical Brain Stem Syndromes. Translations of the Original Papers with Notes on the Evolution of Clinical Neuroanatomy. Charles C Thomas, Springfield, IL, 1971, p 46.
668. Landry, O: Note sur la paralysie ascendante aigue. Gazette Hebdomadaire 6:472–474, 1859.
669. Landry, O: A note on acute ascending paralysis. In Rottenberg, DA and Hochberg, FH (eds): Neurological Classics in Modern Translation. Hafner Press, New York, 1977, p 298.
670. Lands, L and Zinman, R: Maximal static pressures and lung volumes in a child with Guillain-Barré syndrome ventilated by a cuirass ventilator. Chest 89:757–760, 1986.
671. Langer, T and Levy RI: Acute muscular syndrome associated with admin-

istration of clofibrate. N Engl J Med 279:856–858, 1968.
672. Langmuir, AD, Bregman, DJ, Kurland, LT, Nathanson, N, and Victor, M: An epidemiologic and clinical evaluation of Guillain-Barré syndrome reported in association with the administration of swine influenza vaccines. Am J Epidemiol 119:842–879, 1984.
673. Larsen, JP, Kvale, G, and Nyland, H: Epidemiology of the Guillain-Barré syndrome in the county of Hordaland, Western Norway. Acta Neurol Scand 71:43–47, 1985.
674. Larson, DE, Burton, DD, Schroeder, KW, and DiMagno, E: Percutaneous endoscopic gastrostomy. Gastroenterology 93:48–52, 1987.
675. Lassmann, H, Budka, H, and Schnaberth, G: Inflammatory demyelinating polyradiculitis in a patient with multiple sclerosis. Arch Neurol 38:99–102, 1981.
675a. Latov, N: Neuropathy and anti-GM1 antibodies. Ann Neurol 27(Suppl): 541–543, 1990.
676. Latov, N, Gross, RB, Kastelman, J, Flanagan, T, Lamme, S, Alkaitis, DA, Olarte, MR, Sherman, WH, Chess, L, and Penn, AS: Complement-fixing antiperipheral nerve myelin antibodies in patients with inflammatory polyneuritis and with polyneuropathy and paraproteinemia. Neurology 31:1530–1534, 1981.
677. Latov, N, Sherman, WH, Nemni, R, Galassi, G, Shyong, JS, Penn, AS, Chess, L, Olarte, MR, Rowland, LP, and Osserman, EF: Plasma-cell dyscrasia and peripheral neuropathy with a monoclonal antibody to peripheral-nerve myelin. N Engl J Med 303:618–621, 1980.
678. Latovitzki, N, Suciu-Foca, N, Penn, AS, Olarte, MR, and Chutorian, AM: HLA typing and Guillain-Barré syndrome. Neurology 29:743–745, 1979.
679. Laufenburg, HF and Sirus, SR: Guillain-Barré syndrome in pregnancy. Am Fam Physician 39:147–150, 1989.
680. Laufer, J, Passwell, J, Keren, G, Brandt, N, and Cohen, BE: Raised plasma renin activity in the hypertension of the Guillain-Barré syndrome. Br Med J 282:1272, 1981.
681. Laville, M, Blanc, PL, Robert, D, and Lemelin, J-P: Complexes immuns circulants au cours des polyradiculonevrites. Frequence et signification. Nouv Presse Med 10:3825–3829, 1981.
682. Leaf, DA, MacDonald, I, Kliks, B, Wilson, R, and Jones, SR: Streptokinase and the Guillain-Barré syndrome (letter). Ann Intern Med 100:617, 1984.
683. Lecour, H, Ramos, H, Almeida, B, and Barbosa, R: Food-borne botulism. A review of 13 outbreaks. Arch Intern Med 148:578–580, 1988.
684. Lehrich, JR and Arnason, BG: Suppression of experimental allergic neuritis in rats by prior immunization with nerve in saline. Acta Neuropathol 18:144–149, 1971.
685. Le Luyer, B, Devaux, AM, Dailly, R, and Ensel, P: Polyradiculonevrite revelatrice d'une sarcoidose de l'enfant. Arch Fr Pediatr 40:175–178, 1983.
686. Leneman, F: The Guillain-Barré syndrome: Definition, etiology, and review of 1100 cases. Arch Intern Med 118:139–114, 1966.
687. Lesser, RP, Hauser, WA, Kurland, LT, and Mulder, DW: Epidemiologic features of the Guillain-Barré syndrome. Experience in Olmsted County, Minnesota, 1935 through 1968. Neurology 23:1269–1272, 1973.
688. Levy, RL: Panautonomic dysfunction and Guillain-Barré syndrome. JAMA 243:1895, 1980.
689. Levy, RL, Newkirk, R, and Ochoa, J: Treating chronic relapsing Guillain-Barré syndrome by plasma exchange. Lancet 2:259–260, 1979.
690. Lewi, Z and Bar-Khayim, Y: Food poisoning from barium carbonate. Lancet 2:342–343, 1964.
691. Lewis, DC: Systemic lupus and polyneuropathy. Arch Intern Med 116:518–522, 1965.
692. Lewis, RA, Sumner, AJ, Brown, MJ, and Asbury, AK: Multifocal demyelinating neuropathy with persistent

conduction block. Neurology 32: 958–964, 1982.

693. Lewis, T, Pickering, GW, and Rothschild, P: Centripetal paralysis arising out of arresting blood flow to the limb, including notes on the form of tingling. Heart 16:1–32, 1931.
694. LeWitt, PA: The neurotoxicity of the rat poison vacor. A clinical study of 12 cases. N Engl J Med 302:73–77, 1980.
695. Leyden, E: Ueber poliomyelitis und neuritis. Zeitschrift für Klinische Medizin (Berlin) 1:387–434, 1880.
696. Leys, D, Pasquier, F, Lamblin, MD, Dubois, F, and Petit, H: Acute polyradiculoneuropathy after amitriptyline overdose. Br Med J 294:608, 1987.
697. Lichtenfeld, P: Autonomic dysfunction in the Guillain-Barré syndrome. Am J Med 50:772–780, 1971.
698. Lidin-Janson, G and Strannegard, O: Two cases of Guillain-Barré syndrome and encephalitis after measles (case reports). Br Med J 2:572, 1972.
699. Light, WC, Reisman, RE, Shimizu, M, and Arbesman, CE: Unusual reactions following insect stings. Clinical features and immunological analysis. J Allergy Clin Immunol 59:391–397, 1977.
700. Lim, TC and Hoh, TK: The Landry-Guillain-Barré-Strohl syndrome or polyradiculoneuropathy with extraocular muscle involvement in two children. Singapore Med J 7:34–37, 1966.
701. Linden, MA, Manton, WI, Stewart, RM, Thal, ER, and Feit, H: Lead poisoning from retained bullets. Pathogenesis, diagnosis, and management. Ann Surg 195:305–313, 1982.
702. Lindesmith, LA, Baines, RD, Bigelow, DB, and Petty, TL: Reversible respiratory paralysis associated with polymyxin therapy. Ann Intern Med 68:318–327, 1968.
703. Lindqvist, T and Stenstrom, N-M: A case of Guillain-Barré's syndrome following vaccination against smallpox. Acta psychiatrica et neurologica 23:279–283, 1948.
704. Link, H: Immunoglobulin abnormalities in the Guillain-Barré syndrome. J Neurol Sci 18:11–23, 1973.
705. Link, H: Demonstration of oligoclonal immunoglobulin G in Guillain-Barré syndrome. Acta Neurol Scand 52:111–120, 1975.
706. Links, TP, Zwarts, MJ, and Oosterhuis, HJGH: Improvement in muscle strength in familial hypokalemic periodic paralysis with acetazolamide. J Neurol Neurosurg Psychiatry 51:1142–1145, 1988.
707. Lisak, RP, Mitchel, M, Zweiman, B, Orrechio, E, and Asbury, AK: Guillain-Barré syndrome and Hodgkin's disease: Three cases with immunological studies. Ann Neurol 1:72–78, 1977.
708. Lisak, RP, Zweiman, B, Guerrero, F, and Moskovitz, AR: Circulating T-cell subsets in Guillain-Barré syndrome. J Neuroimmunol 8:93–101, 1985.
709. Little, JR, Dale, AJD, and Okazaki, H: Meningeal carcinomatosis. Clinical manifestations. Arch Neurol 30:138–143, 1974.
710. Littlewood, R and Bajada, S: Successful plasmapheresis in the Miller-Fisher syndrome (letter). Br Med J 282:778, 1981.
711. Liu, HM: Ultrastructure of remyelination of peripheral nerves in Landry-Guillain-Barré syndrome. Acta Neuropathol 16:262–265, 1970.
712. Livingstone, IR and Cumming, WJK: Hyperkalemic paralysis resembling Guillain-Barré syndrome. Lancet 2:963–964, 1979.
713. Lobue, G, Senda, Y, and Matsuoka, Y: Sensory ataxia: A residual disability of Guillain-Barré syndrome. Arch Neurol 40:86–89, 1983.
714. Loffel, NB, Rossi, LN, Mumenthaler, M, Lutschg, J, and Ludin, H-P: The Landry-Guillain-Barré syndrome: Complications prognosis and natural history in 123 cases. J Neurol Sci 33:71–79, 1977.
715. Logothetis, J, Kennedy, WR, Ellington, A, and Williams, RC: Cryoglobulinemic neuropathy. Incidence and clinical characteristics. Arch Neurol 19:389–397, 1968.
716. Loizou, LA and Boddie, HG: Polyradiculoneuropathy associated with

heroin abuse. J Neurol Neurosurg Psychiatry 41:855–857, 1978.

717. Long, SS: Epidemiologic study of infant botulism in Pennsylvania: Report of the Infant Botulism Study Group. Pediatrics 75:928–934, 1985a.

718. Long, SS, Gajewski, JL, Brown, LW, and Gilligan, PH: Clinical, laboratory, and environmental features of infant botulism in Southeastern Pennsylvania. Pediatrics 75:935–941, 1985b.

719. Longe, RL: Current concepts in clinical therapeutics: Pressure sores. Clin Pharm 5:669–681, 1986.

720. Lopez, F, Lopez, JH, Holguin, J, and Flewett, TH: An outbreak of acute polyradiculoneuropathy in Colombia in 1968. Am J Epidemiol 98:226–230, 1973.

721. Lopez-Lozano, JJ, Merino, AG, and Liano, H: Bilateral facial paralysis secondary to trichinosis. Acta Neurol Scand 78:194–197, 1988.

722. Love, SV: Paralytic rabies. Review of the literature and report of a case. J Pediatr 24:312–325, 1944.

723. Low, NL, Schneider, J, and Carter, S: Polyneuritis in children. Pediatrics 22:972–990, 1958.

724. Low, PA, Casey, PE, Tuck, RR, Fealey, RD, and Dyck, PJ: Quantitative sudomotor axon reflex test in normal and neuropathic subjects. Ann Neurol 14:573–580, 1983.

725. Low, PA, Schmelzer, J, and Dyck, PJ: Results of endoneural injection of Guillain-Barré serum in Lewis rats. Mayo Clin Proc 57:360–364, 1982.

726. Low, PA, Schmelzer, J, Dyck, PJ, and Kelly, JJ: Endoneurial effects of sera from patients with acute inflammatory polyradiculoneuropathy: Electrophysiologic studies on normal and demyelinated rat nerves. Neurology 32:720–724, 1982.

727. Low, PA, Zimmerman, BR, and Dyck, PJ: Comparison of distal sympathetic with vagal function in diabetic neuropathy. Muscle Nerve 9: 592–596, 1986.

728. Lucchesi, PF: Poliomyelitis. A study of 410 patients at the Philadelphia Hospital for Contagious Diseases. Am J Med Sci 188:515–522, 1934.

729. Luijten, JAFM and Baart De La Faille-Kuyper, EH: The occurrence of IgM and complement factors along myelin sheaths of peripheral nerves. An immunohistochemical study of the Guillain-Barré syndrome (preliminary communication). J Neurol Sci 15:219–224, 1972.

730. Luijten, JAFM, De Jong, WAC, Demel, RA, Heijnen, CJ, and Ballieux, RE: Peripheral nerve P2 basic protein and the Guillain-Barré syndrome. J Neurol Sci 66:209–216, 1984.

731. Luijten, JAFM, Reijneveld-De Jong, SD, Teerlink, T, Camps, VTM, Osterhaus, ADME, and UytdeHaag, AGCM: Monoclonal antibodies to P2 basic protein and their use in the investigation of some aspects of the Guillain-Barré syndrome. J Neurol Sci 86:265–276, 1988.

732. Lundkvist, I, van Doorn, PA, Vermeulen, M, van Lint, M, van Rood, JJ, and Brand, A: Regulation of autoantibodies in inflammatory demyelinating polyneuropathy: Spontaneous and therapeutic. Immunol Rev 110:105–117, 1989.

733. Lycklama, A, Nijeholt, J, and Troost, J: Critical Illness Polyneuropathy. In Matthews, WB (ed): Handbook of Clinical Neurology. Elsevier Science Publishers, Amsterdam, BV, 1987, p 575.

734. Maas, AIR, Busch, HEM, and van der Heul, C: Plasma infusion and plasma exchange in chronic idiopathic polyneuropathy (letter). N Engl J Med 305:344, 1981.

735. Macay, A, Roig, M, Fernandex, JM, and Boronat, M: Pseudotumor cerebri, spinal and radicular pain, and hyporeflexia: A clinical variant of the Guillain-Barré syndrome? Pediatr Neurol 4:120–121, 1988.

736. MacDonald, KL, Rutherford, GW, Friedman, SM, Dietz, JR, Kaye, BR, McKinley, GF, Tenney, JH, Cohen, ML: Botulism and botulism-like illness in chronic drug abusers. Ann Intern Med 102:616–618, 1985.

737. MacGregor, GA: Familial Guillain-

Barré syndrome. Lancet 2:1296, 1965.
738. MacLeod, WN: Sporadic Non-A, Non-B hepatitis and Epstein-Barr hepatitis associated with the Guillain-Barré syndrome. Arch Neurol 44: 438–442, 1987.
739. MacLeod, W and Cherryman, GR: MRI and electrophysiologic evidence suggesting a secondary functional disturbance of the central nervous system in Fisher's syndrome (abstr). Neurology (Suppl)37:366, 1987.
740. Maki, DG, Weise, CE, and Sarafin, HM: A semiquantitative culture method for identifying intravenous-catheter-related infection. N Engl J Med 296:1305–1309, 1977.
741. Mamdan, MB, Walsh, RL, Rubino, FA, Brannegan, RT, and Hwang, MH: Autonomic dysfunction and Eaton-Lambert syndrome. J Auton Nerv Syst 12:315–320, 1985.
742. Mancardi, GL, Del Sette, M, Primavera, A, Farinelli, M, and Fumarola, D: A prospective study of acute idiopathic neuropathy II antecedent events (letter). J Neurol Neurosurg Psychiatry 52:424–425, 1989.
743. Marek, J: Multiple nerven entzundung (polyneuritis) bein Huhnern Deutsch. Tierartzl Wschr 15:417–421, 1907.
744. Mares-Segura, R, Sola-Lamoglia, R, Soler-Singla, L, and Pou-Serradell, A: Guillain-Barré syndrome associated with hepatitis A (letter). Ann Neurol 19:100, 1986.
745. Marie, P and Chatelin, Ch: Note sur un syndrome de paralysie flasque plus ou moins generalisee avec abolition des reflexes, hyperalbuminose massive et xanthochromie du liquide cephalo-rachidien, evoluant spontanement vers la guerison et de nature indeterminee. Rev Neurol (Paris) 2:564–565, 1916.
746. Markland, LD and Riley, HD, Jr: The Guillain-Barré syndrome in childhood. A comprehensive review, including observations on 19 additional cases. Clin Pediatr 6:162–170, 1967.
747. Markovitz, M: Acute intermittent porphyria: A report of five cases and a review of the literature. Ann Intern Med 41:1170–1188, 1954.
748. Marks, HG, Augustyn, P, and Allen, RJ: Fisher's syndrome in children. Pediatrics 60:726–729, 1977.
749. Marks, JS and Halpin, TJ: Guillain-Barré syndrome in recipients of A–New Jersey influenza vaccine. JAMA 243:2490–2494, 1980.
750. Marshall, AJ and Rogerson, FE: Severe Guillain-Barré syndrome following urethritis with cardiovascular and ophthalmic involvement. Postgrad Med J 51:643–645, 1975.
751. Marshall, J: The Landry-Guillain-Barré syndrome. Brain 86:55–66, 1963.
752. Martens, R, Stewart, J, and Eichholtz, D: Clinico-pathologic conference. J Am Vet Med Assoc 156:478–487, 1970.
753. Marthedal, AFNJ and Fisch-Thomson, J: Legionairsygdon med Guillain-Barré syndrome. Ugeskr Laeger 10:625, 1981.
754. Martin, JJ: Polyradiculonevrite aigues et subaigues. I Formes ataxiques des polyradiculonevrites aigues et subaigues (surtout de type Guillain-Barré: etude anatomoclinique. Acta Neurologica et Psychiatricia Belgica 60:1087–1101, 1960.
755. Martin, JJ: Polyradiculonevrite avec dissociation albuminocytologique (du type Guillain-Barré) et atteinte optique. (Contribution anatomo-clinique.) Psychiatria et Neurologia (Basel) 142:265–292, 1961.
756. Martinez, AC, Anciones, B, Ferrer, MT, Tejedor, ED, Conde, MCP, and Bescansa E: Electrophysiologic study in benign human botulism Type B. Muscle Nerve 8:580–585, 1985.
757. Martinez-Figueroa, A, Hansen, S, and Ballantyne, JP: A quantitative electrophysiological study of acute idiopathic polyneuritis. J Neurol Neurosurg Psychiatry 40:156–161, 1977.
758. Maselli, R, Jacobsen, JH, and Spire, J-P: Edrophonium: An aid in the diagnosis of acute organophosphate poisoning. Ann Neurol 19:508–510, 1986.
759. Massion-Verniory, L: Formes pseudo-

myastheniques, a debut ophtalmoplegique, du syndrome radiculonevritique dc Guillain et Barré. J Belge de neurol et de Psychiat 6:294–309, 1940.

760. Mastaglia, FL and Ojeda, VJ: Inflammatory myopathics: Part 1. Ann Neurol 17:215–227, 1985.

761. Masucci, EF and Kurtzke, JF: Diagnostic criteria for the Guillain-Barré syndrome. An analysis of 50 cases. J Neurol Sci 13:483–501, 1971.

762. Masucci, EF and Kurtzke, JF: Dissociated quadriceps-hamstring weakness: A clue to the clinical diagnosis of Guillain-Barré syndrome. Ann Neurol 9:96–97, 1981.

763. Matsuyama, H and Haymaker, W: Distribution of lesions in the Landry-Guillain-Barré syndrome, with emphasis on involvement of the sympathetic system. Acta Neuropathol 8:230–241, 1967.

764. Matthews, WB, Howell, DA, and Hughes, RC: Relapsing corticosteroid-dependent polyneuritis. J Neurol Neurosurg Psychiatry 33: 330–337, 1970.

765. Mattucci, KF and Chodosh, PL: Vocal cord paralysis in Guillain-Barré syndrome. Eye, Ear, Nose and Throat Monthly 49:318–321, 1970.

765a. Mauro, G: A case of Guillain-Barré syndrome treated with intravenous high doses of immunoglobulins. Rev Neurol 145:731–732, 1989.

766. Max, MB, Culnane, M, Schafer, SC, Gracely, RH, Walther, DJ, Smoller, B, and Dubner, R: Amitriptyline relieves diabetic neuropathy pain in patients with normal or depressed mood. Neurology 37:589–596, 1987.

766a. Mayatal, J, Eviatar L, Brunson, SC, and Gootman, N: Use of demand pacemaker in children with Guillain-Barré syndrome. Pediatr Neurol 5:303–305, 1989.

767. Mayer, RF and Feldman, RG: Observations on the nature of the F-wave in man. Neurology 17:147–156, 1967.

768. McCain, MA: Guillain-Barré–associated diarrhea. Dig Dis Sci 30:1112–1113, 1985.

769. McCarthy, JA and Zigenfus, RW: Transcutaneous electrical nerve stimulation: An adjunct in the pain management of Guillain-Barré syndrome. Phys Ther 58:23–24, 1978.

770. McCleave, DJ, Fletcher, J, and Cruden, LC: The Guillain-Barré syndrome in intensive care. Anaesth Intensive Care 4:46–52, 1976.

771. McCombe, PA, Clark, P, Frith, JA, Hammond, SR, Stewart, GJ, Pollard, JD, and McLeod, JG: Alpha-1 antitrypsin phenotypes in demyelinating disease: An association between demyelinating disease and the allele PiM3. Ann Neurol 18:514–516, 1985.

772. McCombe, PA, McManis, PG, Frith, JA, Pollard, JD, and McLeod, JG: Chronic inflammatory demyelinating polyradiculoneuropathy associated with pregnancy. Ann Neurol 21:102–104, 1987.

773. McCombe, PA, Pollard, JD, and McLeod, JG: Chronic inflammatory demyelinating polyradiculoneuropathy. A clinical and electrophysiological study of 92 cases. Brain 110:1617–1630, 1987.

774. McDonald, WI: The effects of experimental demyelination on conduction in peripheral nerves: A histological and electrophysiological study. I. Clinical and histological observations. Brain 86:501–524, 1963.

775. McDonald, WI and Kocen, RS: Diphtheritic neuropathy. In Dyck, PJ, Thomas, PK, and Lambert, EH (eds): Peripheral Neuropathy, ed 2. WB Saunders, Philadelphia 1984, pp 2010–2017.

776. McFadzean, AJS and Yeung, R: Periodic paralysis complicating thyrotoxicosis in Chinese. Br Med J 1:451–455, 1967.

777. McFarland, HR and Heller, GL: Guillain-Barré disease complex; a statement of diagnostic criteria and analysis of 100 cases. Arch Neurol 14:196–201, 1966.

778. McGuire, EJ: Editorial. J Urol 126:644, 1981.

779. McHugh, B and Campbell, J: Below-knee orthoses. Physiotherapy 73: 380–385, 1987.

780. McKhann, GM, Griffin, JW, Corn-

blath, DR, Mellits, ED, Fisher, RS, Quaskey, SA, and the Guillain-Barré Syndrome Study Group: Plasmapheresis and Guillain-Barré syndrome: Analysis of prognostic factors and the effect of plasmapheresis. Ann Neurol 23:347–353, 1988.

781. McLeod, JG: Electrophysiological studies in the Guillain-Barré syndrome. Ann Neurol (Suppl)9:20–27, 1981.

782. McLeod, JC and Walsh, JC: Peripheral neuropathy associated with lymphomas and other reticulosis. In Dyck, PJ, Thomas, PK, Lambert, EH, and Bunge, R (eds): Peripheral Neuropathy. Vol 2. WB Saunders, Philadelphia, 1984, p 2192.

783. McLeod, JC, Walsh, JC, Prineas, JW, and Pollard, JD: Acute idiopathic polyneuritis. A clinical and electrophysiological follow-up study. J Neurol Sci 27:145–162, 1976.

784. McQuillan, JJ and Bullock, RF: Extreme labile blood pressure in Guillain-Barré syndrome. Lancet 2:172–173, 1988.

785. McQuillen, MP: Idiopathic polyneuritis: Serial studies of nerve and immune functions. J Neurol Neurosurg Psychiatry 34:607–615, 1971.

786. McQuillen, MP, Cantor, HE, and O'Rourke, JR: Myasthenic syndrome associated with antibiotics. Arch Neurol 18:402–415, 1968.

787. McWey, RE, Curry, NS, Schabel, SI, and Reines, HD: Complications of nasoenteric feeding tubes. Am J Surg 155:253–257, 1988.

788. Means, ED, Barron, KD, and Van Dyne, BJ: Nervous system lesions after sting by yellow jacket. A case report. Neurology 23:881–890, 1973.

789. Meienberg, O: Lesion site in Fisher's syndrome. Arch Neurol 41:250–251, 1984.

790. Meienberg, O and Ryffel, E: Supranuclear eye movements disorders in Fisher's syndrome of ophthalmoplegia ataxia and areflexia. Report of a case and literature review. Arch Neurol 40:402–405, 1983.

791. Melnick, SC: Thirty-eight cases of the Guillain-Barré syndrome: An immunological study. Br Med J 1:368–373, 1963.

792. Mclnick, SC and Flewett, TH: Role of infection in the Guillain-Barré syndrome. J Neurol Neurosurg Psychiatry 27:395–407, 1964.

793. Mendell, JR, Kissel, JT, Kennedy, MS, Sahenk, KZ, Grinvalsky, HT, Pittman, GL, Kyler, RS, Roelofs, RI, Whitaker, JN, and Bertorini, TE: Plasma exchange and prednisone in Guillain-Barré syndrome: A controlled randomized trial. Neurology 35:1551–1555, 1985.

794. Mendell, JR, Kolkin, S, Kissel, JT, Weiss, KL, Chakeres, DW, and Rammohan, KW: Evidence for central nervous system demyelination in chronic inflammatory demyelinating polyradiculoneuropathy. Neurology 37:1291–1294, 1987.

795. Menonna, J, Goldschmidt, B, Haidri, N, Dowling, P, and Cook, S: Herpes simplex virus-IgM specific antibodies in Guillain-Barré syndrome and encephalitis. Acta Neurol Scand 56:223–231, 1977.

796. Merrington, WR and Nathan, PW: A study of post-ischaemic paraesthesias. J Neurol Neurosurg Psychiatry 12:1–18, 1959.

797. Merson, MH and Dowell, VR: Epidemiologic, clinical and laboratory aspects of wound botulism. N Engl J Med 289:1005–1010, 1973.

798. Meythaler, JM, Korkor, AB, Nanda, T, Kumar, NA, and Fallon, M: Immobilization hypercalcemia associated with Landry-Guillain-Barré syndrome. Successful therapy with combined calcitonin and etidronate. Arch Intern Med 146:1567–1571, 1986.

799. Mikati, MA and DeLong, GR: Childhood Guillain-Barré syndrome masquerading as a protracted pain syndrome. (Letter to the Editor.) Arch Neurol 42:839, 1985.

799a. Millar, AB, Clarke, SW, Davis, SN, and Gross, ML: Prolonged ventilation in acute severe asthma caused by the Guillain-Barré-Strohl syndrome. J Roy Soc Med 77:965–966, 1984.

800. Miller, GM, Peterson, GW, Daube,

JR, and Albers, JW: Prognostic value of electrodiagnosis in Guillain-Barré syndrome. Muscle Nerve 11:769–774, 1988.

801. Miller NR: Walsh and Hoyt's Clinical Neurophthalmology, ed 4. Williams & Wilkins, Baltimore, 1982, p 241.

802. Miller, RG, Parry, G, Lang, W, Lippert, R, and Kiprov, D: AIDS-related inflammatory polyradiculoneuropathy: Successful treatment with plasma exchange. Neurology (Suppl) 36:206, 1986.

803. Miller, RG, Peterson, C, and Rosenberg, NL: Electrophysiologic evidence of severe distal nerve segment pathology in the Guillain-Barré syndrome. Muscle Nerve 10:524–529, 1987.

803a. Miller, R, Sheron, N, and Semple, S: Sarcoidosis presenting with an acute Guillain-Barré syndrome. Postgrad Med J 65:756–757, 1989.

804. Millette, TJ, Subramony, SH, Wee, AS, and Harisdangkul, V: Systemic lupus erythematosus presenting with recurrent acute demyelinating polyneuropathy. Eur Neurol 25:397–402, 1986.

805. Mills, AR, and Passmore, R: Pelagic paralysis. Lancet 1:161–164, 1988.

806. Mills, CK and Spiller, WG: On Landry's paralysis, with the report of a case. J Nerv Ment Dis 25:365–391, 1898.

807. Mills, KR and Murray, NMF: Proximal conduction block in early Guillain-Barré syndrome (letter). Lancet 2:659, 1985.

808. Mirus, E: Beitrag zur frage der stellung des Guillain-Barreschen syndroms im rahmen der polyneuritis. Deutsche Zeitschrift für Nervenheilkunde. 150:39–69, 1939–1940.

809. Mishra, BB, Sommers, W, Koski, CL, and Greenstein, JI: Acute inflammatory demyelinating polyneuropathy in the acquired immune deficiency syndrome (abstr). Ann Neurol 18:131–132, 1985.

810. Mitchel, GW, Bosch, EP, and Hart, MN: Response to immunosuppressive therapy in patients with hereditary motor and sensory neuropathy and associated dysimmune neuromuscular disorders. Eur Neurol 27:188–196, 1987.

811. Mitchel, GW, Bosch, P, Williams, GS, and Hart, MN: Class II antigen expression in peripheral neuropathies (abstr). Neurology 39:392, 1989.

812. Mitchell, PL and Meilman, E: The mechanism of hypertension in the Guillain-Barré syndrome. Am J Med 42:986–995, 1967.

813. Mittal, MM, Bhargava, SP, and Sharma, ML: The Landry-Guillain-Barré syndrome survey and clinical report of 45 cases. J Assoc Physicians India 17:57–67, 1969.

814. Miyakawa, T, Murayama, E, Sumiyoski, S, Deshimaru, M, Kamano, A, Miyakawa, K, and Tatetsu, S: A biopsy of Landry-Guillain-Barré syndrome. Acta Neuropathol 17:181–187, 1971.

815. Mohamed, SD, Chapman, RS, and Crooks, J: Hypokalemia, flaccid quadriparesis, and myoglobinuria with carbenoxolone (biogastrone). Br Med J 1:1581–1582, 1966.

816. Molnar, GK, Mertsola, J, and Erkko, M: Guillain-Barré syndrome associated with Campylobacter infection (letter). Br Med J 285–652, 1982.

817. Moore, P and James, O: Guillain-Barré syndrome: Incidence, management and outcome of major complications. Crit Care Med 9:549–555, 1981.

818. Moore, PM and Fauci, AS: Neurologic manifestations of systemic vasculitis. A retrospective and prospective study of the clinicopathologic features and responses to therapy in 25 patients. Am J Med 71:517–524, 1981.

819. Moreau, BA, Schuller, E, and Georges, B: Case report: Association of Guillain-Barré syndrome and Henoch-Schönlein purpura: Is immunoglobulin A responsible for the neurologic syndrome? Am J Med Sci 296:198–201, 1988.

820. Morgan, AG and Cawich, F: Ascending polyneuropathy in leptospirosis—a case study. Ann Trop Med Parasitol 74:567–568, 1980.

821. Mori, E, Yoshida, T, Ohsumi, Y, Tabuchi, M, and Yamadori, A: Beneficial effects of plasma exchange in acute Guillain-Barré syndrome: Comparison with methylprednisolone pulse therapy. Clin Neurol 28:196–203, 1988.
822. Morley, JB and Reynolds, EH: Papilloedema and the Landry-Guillain-Barré syndrome. Brain 80:205–222, 1966.
823. Moses, H: Thallium poisoning. Johns Hopkins Med J 142:27–31, 1978.
824. Moskowitz, LB, Gregorios, JB, Hensley, GT, and Berger, JR: Cytomegalovirus-induced demyelination association with acquired immune deficiency syndrome. Arch Pathol Lab Med 108:873–877, 1984.
825. Mouren, P, Vital-Berard, P, Poinso, Y, Giudicelli, S, Fresco, R, De Bisschop, G, and Scarone, JJ: Nevrite optique retro-bulbaire au cours d'un syndrome de Guillain-Barré. Rev otoneuroophthalmol 43:216–221, 1971.
826. Mozes, B, Pines, A, Sayar, Y, Kaplinsky N, and Frankl, O: Guillain-Barré syndrome associated with acute cytomegalovirus mononucleosis syndrome. Eur Neurol 23:237–239, 1984.
827. Mueller, JM and Flaherty, MJ: Vincristine-induced quadriparesis. South Med J 71:1310–1311, 1978.
828. Munch, JC, Ginsburg, HM, and Nixon, CE: The 1932 thallatoxicosis outbreak in California. JAMA 100:1315–1319, 1933.
829. Munsat, TL and Barnes, JE: Relation of multiple cranial nerve dysfunction to the Guillain-Barré syndrome. J Neurol Neurosurg Psychiatry 28:115–120, 1965.
830. Murphy, BF, Gonzales, MF, Ebeling, P, Fairley, KF, and Kincaid-Smith, P: Membranous glomerulonephritis and Landry-Guillain-Barré syndrome. Am J Kidney Dis 8:267–270, 1986.
831. Murray, A, Ewing, JD, Campbell, IW, Neilson, JMM, and Clarke, BF: RR interval in young male diabetics. Br Med J 37:882–885, 1977.
832. Murray, NMF, Miles, CM, Karni, Y, and Newsom-Davis, J: Intensive plasma exchange in acute inflammatory polyneuropathy (letter). Ann Med Interne (Paris) 135:144, 1984.
833. Murray, NMF and Wade, DT: The sural sensory action potential in Guillain-Barré syndrome (letter). Muscle Nerve 3:444, 1980.
834. Mushinski, JF, Taniguchi, RM, and Stiefel, JW: Guillain-Barré syndrome associated with ulceroglandular tularemia. Neurology 14:877–879, 1964.
835. Naiditch, MJ and Bower, AG: Diphtheria. A study of 1,433 cases observed during a ten-year period at the Los Angeles County Hospital. Am J Med 17:229–245, 1954.
836. Nakano, KK, Bass, H, Tyler, HR, and Carmel, RJ: Amyotrophic lateral sclerosis: A study of pulmonary function. Dis Nerv Sys 37:32–35, 1976.
837. Namba, T, Nolte, CT, Jackrel, J, and Grob, D: Poisoning due to organophosphate insecticides. Acute and chronic manifestations. Am J Med 50:475–492, 1971.
838. Nass, R and Chutorian, A: Dysaesthesias and dysautonomia: A self-limited syndrome of painful dysaesthesias and autonomic dysfunction in childhood. J Neurol Neurosurg Psychiatry 45:162–165, 1982.
839. Necrologie (Anonymous): Georges Guillain. Presse Med 69:1695–1696, 1961.
840. Neetens, A and Smet, H: Lid lag in Guillain-Barré-Strohl syndrome. Arch Neurol 45:1046–1047, 1988.
841. Negishi, T, Yamashita, T, Nomura, K, Hosokawa, T, Ohno, R, Hamaguchi, K, and Uyemura, K: Serum Antibodies to peripheral nerve antigens in Guillain-Barré syndrome. Ann NY Acad Sci 540:376–377, 1988.
842. Nelson, KR, Gilmore, RL, and Massey, A: Acoustic nerve conduction abnormalities in Guillain-Barré syndrome. Neurology 38:1263–1266, 1988.
843. Neubert, FR: Complete ophthalmoplegia in acute toxic polyneuritis. Br J Ophthalmol 42:632–633, 1958.

844. Newey, JA and Lubin, RI: Corticotropin therapy in Guillain-Barré syndrome. JAMA 152:137–139, 1953.
845. Newland, AC, Treleaven, JG, Minchinton, RM, and Waters, AH: High-dose intravenous IgG in adults with autoimmune thrombocytopenia. Lancet 1:84–87, 1983.
846. Newman, GC, Newman, EJ, Hospod, FE, and Bogoch, S: Simple language system for speechless, handicapped patients. Ann Neurol 26:156, 1989.
847. Newman, JH, Neff, TA, and Ziporin, P: Acute respiratory failure associated with hypophosphatemia. N Engl J Med 296:1101–1103, 1977.
848. Newsom-Davis, J: Phrenic nerve conduction in man. J Neurol Neurosurg Psychiatry 30:420–426, 1967.
849. Newsom-Davis, J: Lambert-Eaton myasthenic syndrome. Springer Semin Immunopathol 8:129–140, 1985.
850. Newsum, JK, Smith, RM, and Crocker, D: Intubation for acute respiratory failure in Guillain-Barré syndrome. JAMA 242:1650–1651, 1979.
851. Newton, N and Janati, A: Guillain-Barré syndrome after vaccination with purified tetanus toxoid. South Med J 80:1053–1054, 1987.
852. Newton-John, H: Prevention of pulmonary complications in severe Guillain-Barré syndrome by early assisted ventilation. Med J Aust 142:444–445, 1985.
853. Ng, PL, Powell, LW, and Campbell, CB: Guillain-Barré syndrome during the pre-icteric phase of acute type B viral hepatitis. Aust NZ J Med 5:367–369, 1975.
854. Niermeijer, P and Gips, CH: Guillain-Barré syndrome in acute HBsAg-positive hepatitis. Br Med J 4:732–733, 1975.
855. Nikoskelainen, E and Riekkinen, P: Retrobulbar neuritis as an early symptom of Guillain-Barré syndrome. Report of a case. Acta Ophthalmol 50:111–115, 1972.
856. Nixon, RA: Quinine sulfate for pain in the Guillain-Barré syndrome. Ann Neurol 4:386–387, 1978.
857. Krowane, BM, Wassilak, SGF, Orenstein, WA, Bart, KJ, Schonberger, LB, Hinman, AR, and Kew, OM: Vaccine-associated paralytic poliomyelitis. United States: 1973 through 1984. JAMA 257:1335–1340, 1987.
858. Nobile-Orazio, E, Baldini, L, Barbieri, S, Marmiroli, P, Spagnol, G, Francomano, E, and Scarlato, G: Treatment of patients with neuropathy and anti-MAG IgM M-proteins. Ann Neurol 24:93–97, 1988.
859. Nobile-Orazio, E, Latov, N, Hays, AP, Takatsu, M, Abrams, GM, Sherman, WH, Miller, JR, Messito, M-J, Saito, T, Tahmoush, A, Lovelace, RE, and Rowland, LP: Neuropathy and anti-MAG antibodies without detectable serum M protein. Neurology 34:218–221, 1984.
860. Nolte, J, Thoden, U, Herkel, L, Mobius, W, and Gerok, W: Akute polyneuroradikulitis. Verlauf und Komplikationen bein 30 patienten mit schwerem krankheitsbild. Innere Medizin 8:320–327, 1979.
861. Norman, M, Elinder, G, and Finkel, Y: Vincristine neuropathy and a Guillain-Barré syndrome: A case with acute lympathic leukemia and quadriparesis. Eur J Haematol 39:75–76, 1987.
862. Northington, JW, Brown, MJ, Farnbach, GC, and Steinberg, SA: Acute idiopathic polyneuropathy in the dog. J Am Vet Med Assoc 179:375–379, 1981.
863. Novak, DJ and Johnson, KP: Relapsing idiopathic polyneuritis during pregnancy. Immunological aspects and literature review. Arch neurol 28:219–223, 1973.
864. Nowack, WJ, French, MW, and Gilmor, R: Central nervous system lesions in Fisher syndrome: Report of a case with CT findings. J Indiana State Med Assoc 75:623–624, 1982.
865. Nukada, H, Pollock, M, and Haas, LF: Is ischemia implicated in chronic multifocal demyelinating neuropathy? Neurology 39:106–110, 1989.
866. Nyland, H and Aarli, JA: Guillain-Barré syndrome: Demonstration of antibodies to peripheral nerve tissue. Acta Neurol Scand 58:35–43, 1978.

867. Nyland, H, Matre, R, and Mork, S: Immunological characterization of sural nerve biopsies from patients with Guillain-Barré syndrome. Ann Neurol (Suppl)9:80–86, 1981.
868. Nystrom, B, Frederici, H, and von Euler, C: Bacterial colonization and infection in an intensive care unit. Intensive Care Med 14:34–38, 1988.
869. Oakley, CM: The heart in Guillain-Barré syndrome (letter). Br Med J 288:94, 1984.
870. Ochoa, JL and Torebjork, HE: Paresthesias from ectopic impulse generation in human sensory nerves. Brain 103:835–853, 1980.
871. O'Donohue, WJ, Baker, JP, Bell, GM, Muren, Parker, CL, and Patterson, JL: Respiratory failure in neuromuscular disease. JAMA 235:733–735 1976.
872. Oh, ST: Subacute demyelinating polyneuropathy responding to corticosteroid treatment. Arch neurol 35:509–516, 1978.
873. Ohno, R, Hamaguchi, K, Nomura, K, Negishi, T, Suzuki, M, and Uyemura, K: Cellular hypersensitivity to nervous antigens in Guillain-Barré syndrome. Neurochem Pathol 4:119–126, 1986.
873a. Okada, F: Acute pandysautonomia and acute autonomic and sensory neuropathy. Hokkaido-Igaku-Zasshi 64:4–9, 1989.
874. Okada, F, Yamashita, I, and Suwa, N: Two cases of acute pandysautonomia. Arch Neurol 32:146–151, 1975.
875. Olivarius Bent de Fine, O and Buhl, M: Herpes simplex virus and Guillain-Barré polyradiculitis. Br Med J 1:192–193, 1975.
876. Ollivier, CP: Traite des maladies de la moelle epiniere. Mequignon-Marvis Pere et fils. Vol 2. Paris, 1837, pp 51, 73.
877. Olson, ME, Chernik, NL, and Posner, JB: Infiltration of the leptomeninges by systemic cancer. A clinical and pathologic study. Arch Neurol 30:122–137, 1974.
878. Op de Coul, AAW, Lambregts, PCLA, Koeman, J, Van Puyenbroek, MJE, Ter Laak, HJ, and Gabreels-Festen, AAWM: Neuromuscular complications in patients given Pavulon (pancuronium bromide), during artificial respiration. Clin Neurol Neurosurg 87:17–22, 1985.
879. Openshaw, H and Lieberman, JS: Vaccine-related poliomyelitis. Arch Intern Med 142:1617, 1982.
880. Oppenheimer, DR and Spalding, JMK: Late residua of acute idiopathic polyneuritis. J Neurol Neurosurg Psychiatry 36:978–988, 1973.
881. O'Reilly, MJ, Reddick, EJ, Black, W, Carter, PL, Erhardt, J, Fill, W, Maughn, D, Sado, A, and Klatt, GR: Sepsis from sinusitis in nasotracheally intubated patients. Am J Surg 147:601–604, 1984.
882. Osler, LD and Sidell, AD: The Guillain-Barré syndrome. The need for exact diagnostic criteria. N Engl J Med 262:964–969, 1960.
883. Osterman, PO, Fagius, J, Safwenberg, J, Danersund, A, Wallin, BG, and Nordesjo, L-O: Treatment of the Guillain-Barré syndrome by plasmapheresis. Arch Neurol 39:148–154, 1982.
884. Osterman, PO, Fagius, J, Safwenberg, J, Danielson, BG, and Wikstrom, B: Early relapses after plasma exchange in acute inflammatory polyradiculoneuropathy (letter). Lancet 2:1161, 1986.
885. Osterman, PO, Fagius, J, Safwenberg, J, and Wikstrom, B: Early relapse of acute inflammatory polyradiculoneuropathy after successful treatment with plasma exchange. Acta Neurol Scand 77:273–277, 1988.
886. Osterman, PO, Lundemo, G, Pirskanen, R, Fagius, J, Pihlstedt, P, Siden, A, and Safwenberg, J: Beneficial effects of plasma exchange in acute inflammatory polyradiculoneuropathy. Lancet 2:1296–1312, 1984.
887. Osterman, PO, Vedeler, CA, Ryberg, B, Fagius, J, and Nyland, H: Serum antibodies to peripheral nerve tissue in acute Guillain-Barré syndrome in relation to outcome of plasma exchange. J Neurol 235:285–289, 1988.
888. Osuntokun, BO and Agbebi, K: Prog-

nosis of Guillain-Barré syndrome in the African: The Nigerian experience. J Neurol Neurosurg Psychiatry 36:478–483, 1973.

889. Osuntokun, BO, Bademosi, O, Ogunremi, K, and Wright, SG: Neuropsychiatric manifestations of typhoid fever in 959 patients. Arch neurol 27:7–13, 1972.

890. Ott, T: Un cas de polyradiculonevrite ascendante subacute avec dissociation albumino-cytologique. Etude anatomoclinique. Schweiz Arch Neurol Psychiatr 48:83–105, 1941.

891. Pace, NL: Cardiac monitoring and demand pacemaker in Guillain-Barré syndrome. Arch Neurol 22:374, 1976.

892. Pachner, AR and Steere, AC: The triad of neurologic manifestations of Lyme disease: Meningitis, cranial neuritis, and radiculoneuritis. Neurology 35:47–53, 1985.

893. Padmini, R and Maheshwari, MC: P. vivax malaria complicated by peripheral neuropathy with electrophysiological studies. J Assoc Physicians India 28:153–156, 1980.

894. Paley, RG and Truelove, SC: Diphtheria in the Army in the United Kingdom. A study of its complications. J R Army Med Corps 90:109–116, 1948.

895. Pall, PS and William, AC: Subacute polyradiculopathy with optic and auditory nerve involvement. Arch Neurol 44:885–887, 1987.

896. Palmer, KN: Polyradiculoneuropathy (Guillain-Barré syndrome) treated with 6-mercaptopurine. Lancet 1: 733–734, 1965.

897. Palosuo, T, Vaarala, O, and Kinnunen, E: Anticardiolipin antibodies in Guillain-Barré syndrome (letter). Lancet 2:839, 1985.

898. Pandolfi, C and Filipi, C: Guillain-Barré syndrome associated with hypothyroidism. Reports of a case. Minerva Med 80:1129–1131, 1989.

898a. Panegyres, PK, Mastaglia, FL: Guillain-Barré syndrome with involvement of the central nervous system. Med J Aust 150:655–659, 1989.

899. Parry, GJ and Heiman-Patterson, TD: Pregnancy and autoimmune neuromuscular disease. Semin Neurol 8:197–204, 1988.

900. Paterson, PY: Cyclophosphamide treatment of experimental allergic encephalomyelitis in Lewis rats. J Immunol 106:1473–1479, 1971.

901. Pathy, MS: Varicella with neurological complications in an adult (letter). Br Med J 1:1324, 1955.

902. Paulson, GW: The Landry-Guillain-Barré-Strohl syndrome in childhood. Dev Med Child Neurol 12:604–607, 1970.

903. Payne, LN, Frazier, JA, and Powell, PC: Pathogenesis of Marek's disease. Int Rev Exp Pathol 16:59–154, 1976.

904. Pearn, J: Neuromuscular paralysis caused by tick envenomation. J Neurol Sci 34:37–42, 1977.

905. Pearson, CM: The periodic paralyses: Differential features and pathological observations in permanent myopathic weakness. Brain 87:341–354, 1964.

906. Peiris, JB, Wickremasinghe, HR, and Chandrasekara, MA: Tuberculous polyradiculitis. Br Med J 4:107, 1974.

907. Pellegrino-Levi: Contribution a l'etude de la paralysie ascendante aiguë ou extenso-progressive aigue. Arch gen de med 6e serie, vol 1:129–147, 1865.

908. Penner, E, Maida, E, Mamoli, B, and Gangl, A: Serum and cerebrospinal fluid immune complexes containing hepatitis B surface antigen in Guillain-Barré syndrome. Gastroenterology 82:576–580, 1982.

909. Penney, MD, Murphy, D, and Walters, G: Resetting of osmoreceptor response as a cause of hyponaetremia in acute idiopathic polyneuritis. Br Med J 2:1474–1476, 1979.

910. Perez-Perez, GI, Dworkin, BM, Chodos, JE, and Blaser, MJ: Campylobacter pylori antibodies in humans. Ann Intern Med 109:11–17, 1988.

911. Persson, A and Solders, G: R-R variations in Guillain-Barré syndrome: A test of autonomic dysfunction. Acta Neurol Scand 67:294–300, 1983.

912. Pessin, MS: Transient diabetes insipidus in thc Landry-Guillain-Barré syndrome. Arch Neurol 27:85–86, 1972.
913. Pestronk, A, Cornblath, DR, Ilyas, AA, Baba, H, Quarles, RH, Griffin, JW, Alderson, K, and Adams, RN: A treatable multifocal motor neuropathy with antibodies to GMl ganglioside. Ann Neurol 24:73–78, 1988.
914. Petch, CP: Guillain-Barré . . . and Strohl (letter). Lancet 2:380, 1978.
915. Peterman, AF, Daly, DD, Dion, FR, and Keith, HM: Infectious neuronitis (Guillain-Barré syndrome) in children. Neurology 9:533–539, 1959.
916. Peters, DK, Sevitt, LH, Direkze, M, and Bayliss, SG: Landry-Guillain-Barré-Strohl polyneuritis and the nephrotic syndrome. Lancet 1:1183–1184, 1973.
917. Pette, H and Kornyey, S: Zur histologie und pathogenese der akutentzundlichen formen der Landryschen paralyse (letter). Z Ges Neurol Psychiat 128:390–412, 1930.
918. Petty, TL, Lakshminarayan, S, Salon, SA, Zwillich, CW, Nett, LM: Intensive respiratory care unit—A review of ten years experience. JAMA 233:34–37, 1975.
919. Phanthumchinda, K, Intragumtornchai, T, and Kasantikul, V: Guillain-Barré syndrome and optic neuropathy in acute leukemia. Neurology 38:1324–1326, 1988.
920. Phelan, DM and Hagley, SR and Guerin, MD: Is hypokalemia the cause of paralysis in barium poisoning? Br Med J 289:882, 1984.
921. Phillips, MS, Steward, S, and Anderson, JR: Neuropathological findings in Miller Fisher syndrome. J Neurol Neurosurg Psychiatry 47:492–495, 1984.
922. Phillips, OC, Ebner, H, Nelson, AT, and Black, MH: Neurologic complications following spinal anesthesia with lidocaine: A prospective review of 10,440 cases. Anaesthesiology 30:289, 1969.
923. Phillips, PE: Guillain-Barré syndrome and Epstein-Barr virus. Lancet 1:720, 1973.
924. Phillips, RE, Theakston, RDG, Warrell, DA, Galigedera, Y, Abeyshekera, DTDJ, Dissanayaka, P, Hutton, PA, and Aloysius, DJ: Paralysis, rhabdomyolysis and haemolysis causcd by bites of Russell's viper (Vipera russelli pulchella) in Sri Lanka: Failure of Indian (Haffkine) antivenom. Q J Med 68:691–716, 1988.
925. Pickney, C: Acute infective polyneuritis with a report of 5 cases. Br Med J 2:333–335, 1936.
926. Pierides, AM, Alvarez, Ude, F, Kerr, DNS, and Skillen, AW: Clofibrate-induced muscle damage in patients with chronic renal failure. Lancet 2:1279–1282, 1975.
927. Piette, AM, Tusseau, F, Vignon, D, Chapman, A, Parrot, G, Leibowitch, J, and Montagnier, L: Acute neuropathy coincident with seroconversion for anti-LAV/HTLV-III (letter). Lancet 1:852, 1986.
928. Pillay, N and Oliver, S: Evoked potentials in Fisher's syndrome (abstr). Can J Neurol Sci 11:341, 1984.
929. Pittinger, CB, Eryasa, Y, and Adamson, R: Antibiotic-induced paralysis. Anesth Analg 49:487–501, 1970.
930. Platt, R, Polk, BF, Murdock, B, and Rosner, B: Mortality associated with nosocomial urinary-tract infection. N Engl J Med 307:637–642, 1982.
931. Platt, R, Polk, BF, Murdock, B, and Rosner, B: Reduction of mortality associated with nosocomial urinary tract infection. Lancet 1:893–897, 1983.
932. Pleasure, DE, Lovelace, RE, and Dovoisin, RC: The prognosis of acute polyradiculoneuritis. Neurology 18: 1143–1148, 1968.
933. Plum, F: Technics for minimizing trauma to the tracheobronchial tree after tracheotomy. N Engl J Med 254:193–200, 1956.
934. Plum, F: Multiple symmetrical polyneuropathy treated with cortisone. Neurology 3:661–667, 1961.
935. Pollard, JD, Baverstock, J, and McLeod, JG: Class II antigen expression and inflammatory cells in the Guillain-Barré syndrome. Ann Neurol 21:337–341, 1987.
936. Pollard, JD, McLeod, JG, Gatenby, P, and Kronenberg, H: Prediction of

response to plasma exchange in chronic relapsing polyneuropathy. (A clinico-pathological correlation.) J Neurol Sci 58:269–287, 1983.

937. Pollard, JD and Selby, G: Relapsing neuropathy due to tetanus toxoid. J Neurol Sci 37:113–125, 1978.
938. Pollock, M, Calder, C, and Allpress, S: Peripheral nerve abnormality in multiple sclerosis. Ann Neurol 2:41–48, 1977.
939. Pontoppidan, H, Geffin, B, and Lowenstein, E: Acute respiratory failure in the adult (second of three parts). N Engl J Med 287:743–752, 1972.
940. Pontoppidan, H, Geffin, B, and Lowenstein, E: Acute respiratory failure in the adult (third of three parts) N Engl J Med 287:799–806, 1972.
941. Pontoppidan, H, Wilson, RS, Rie, MA, and Schneider, RC: Respiratory intensive care. Anaesthesiology 47:96–116, 1977.
942. Porst, H, Hentschel, R, Sauerman, W, Lehmann, H, Lohmann, J, and Schentke, K: Polyradikulitis Guillain-Barré bei akuter virus hepatitis B. Dtsch Z Verdau Stoffwechselkr 43:146–149, 1983.
943. Poser, CM and Fowler, CW: The nosologic situation of the Landry-Guillain-Barré syndrome. Acta Neurol Scand 39:187–201, 1963.
944. Poser, CM: Criteria for the diagnosis of the Guillain-Barré syndrome. A critique of the NINCDS Guidelines. J Neurol Sci 52:191–199, 1981.
945. Poser, CM: Swine influenza vaccination. Truth and consequences. 42:1090–1092, 1985.
946. Poskanzer, DC and Kerr, DNS: A third type of periodic paralysis, with normokalemia and favorable response to sodium chloride. Am J Med 31:328–342, 1961.
947. Posner, JB, Ertel, NH, Kossmann, RJ, and Scheinberg, LC: Hyponatremia in acute polyneuropathy. Arch Neurol 17:530–541, 1967.
948. Potz, G and Neundorfer, B: Polyradicular neuritis and Hashimoto's thyroiditis. J Neurol 210:283–289, 1975.
949. Pouget, J, Weiller, PJ, Harle, JR, Pellissier, P, Valentin, P, and Serratrice, G: Acute pandysautonomia with subclinical involvement of somatic fibers (abstr). Neurology (Suppl)39:137, 1989.
950. Powell, HC, Braheny, SL, Myers, RR, Rodriguez, M, and Lambert, PW: Early changes in experimental allergic neuritis. Lab Invest 48:332–338, 1983.
951. Powles, RL and Malpas, JS: Guillain-Barré syndrome associated with chronic lymphatic leukaemia. Br Med J 3:286–287, 1967.
952. Poyart, C and Pocidalo, JJ: Hyponatremie avec natriurie conservee par trouble de l'elimination de l'eau libre au cours d'un syndrome de Guillain-Barré. Revue Francaise d'etudes Cliniques et Biologiques (Paris) 9:1068–1071, 1964.
953. Price, RL, O'Connor, PS, and Rothner, AD: Acute ophthalmoplegia, ataxia and areflexia (Fisher syndrome) in childhood. Cleve Clin Q 45:247–252, 1978.
954. Priebe, HJ, Skillman, JJ, Bushnell, LS, Long, PC, and Silen, W: Antacid versus cimetidine in preventing acute gastrointestinal bleeding. A randomized trial in 75 critically ill patients. N Engl J Med 302:426–430, 1980.
955. Prineas, JW: Acute idiopathic polyneuritis. An electron microscope study. Lab Invest 26:133–147, 1972.
956. Prineas, JW: Pathology of the Guillain-Barré syndrome. Ann Neurol (Suppl)9:6–19, 1981.
957. Prineas, JW and McLeod, JG: Chronic relapsing polyneuritis. J Neurol Sci 27:427–458, 1976.
958. Prineas, JW and Wright, RG: The fine structure of peripheral nerve lesions in a virus-induced demyelinating disease in fowl (Marek's disease). Lab Invest 26:548–557, 1972.
959. Pryor, WM, Freiman, JS, Gillies, MA, and Tuck, RR: Guillain-Barré syndrome associated with Campylobacter infection. Aust NZ J Med 14:687–688, 1984.
960. Przedborski, S, Liesnard, C, Voordecker, P, Gerard, JM, Taelman, H, Sprecher, S, Goldman, M, and Hilde-

brand, J: Inflammatory demyelinating polyradiculoneuropathy associated with human immunodeficiency virus infection. J Neurol 235:359–361, 1988.
961. Queckenstedt, HG, Uber veranderungen der spinalflussigkeit bei erkrankunger peripherer nerven, insbesondere bei polyneuritis und bei ischias. Deutsche Ztschr f Nervenh 57:316–329, 1917.
962. Radman, HM: Guillain-Barré disease complicating pregnancy. Md State Med J 26:54–56, 1967.
963. Raman, PT and Taori, GM: Prognostic significance of electrodiagnostic studies in the Guillain-Barré syndrome. J Neurol Neurosurg Psychiatry 39:163–170, 1976.
964. Raman, RK, Blake, JA, and Harris, TM: Pulmonary embolism in Landry-Guillain-Barré-Strohl syndrome. Chest 60:555–556, 1971.
965. Ramanathan, J, Sibai, BM, Pillai, R, and Angel, JJ: Neuromuscular transmission studies in preeclamptic women receiving magnesium sulfate. Am J Obstet Gynecol 158:40–46, 1988.
966. Ramos-Alvarez, M, Bessudo, L, and Sabin, AB: Paralytic syndromes associated with non-inflammatory cytoplasmic or nuclear neuronopathy. Acute paralytic disease in Mexican children neuropathologically distinguishable from Landry-Guillain-Barré syndrome. JAMA 207:1481–1492, 1969.
967. Randall, RE, Cohen, MD, Spray, CC, and Rossmeisl, EC: Hypermagnesemia in renal failure. Etiology and toxic manifestations. Ann Intern Med 61:73–88, 1964.
968. Raphael, JC, Masson, C, Morice, V, Brunel, D, Gajdos, Ph, Barois, A, and Goulon, M: Le syndrome de Landry-Guillain-Barré. Etude des facteurs prognostiques dans 223 cas. Rev Neurol (Paris) 142:613–624, 1986.
969. Rapoport, S and Watkins, PB: Descending paralysis resulting from occult wound botulism. Ann Neurol 16:359–361, 1984.
970. Rasminsky, M: Ephaptic transmission between single nerve fibers in spinal nerve roots of dystrophic mice. J Physiol 305:151–169, 1980.
971. Rasminsky, M and Sears, TA: Internodal conduction in undissected demyelinated nerve fibers. J Physiol (Lond) 227:323–350, 1972.
972. Rasminsky, M and Sumner, AJ: Development of conduction block in single rate spinal root fibers locally exposed to antigalactocerebroside serum (abstr). Neurology 30:371, 1980.
973. Ravn, H: The Landry-Guillain-Barré syndrome: A survey and a clinical report of 127 cases. Acta Neurol Scand (Suppl)43:1–64, 1967.
974. Razavi-Encha, F, Fleury-Feith, J, Gherardi, R, and Bernaudin, J-F: Cytologic features of cerebrospinal fluid in Lyme disease. Acta Cytol 31:439–440, 1987.
975. Rechthand, E, Cornblath, DR, Stern, BJ, and Meyerhoff, JO: Chronic demyelinating polyneuropathy in systemic lupus erythematosus. Neurology 34:1375–1377, 1984.
976. Reed, D, Crawley, J, Faro, SN, Pieper, SJ, and Kurland, LT: Thallotoxicosis. Acute manifestations and sequelae. JAMA 183:516–522, 1963.
976a. Regev, I, Bornstein, N, Carasso, R, and Vardi, Y: Acute polyneuropathy combined with myasthenia gravis. Acta Neurol Scand 65:681–682, 1982.
977. Reich, SG: Harvey Cushing's Guillain-Barré syndrome: An historical diagnosis. Neurosurgery 21:135–141, 1987.
978. Reid, HA: Cobra-bites. Br Med J 2:540–545, 1964.
979. Remlinger, P: J-B Octave Landry (1826–1865). Presse Med 11:227–229, 1933.
980. Renlund, DG, Hanley, DF, and Traill, TA: Guillain-Barré syndrome following coronary artery bypass surgery. Am Heart J 113:844–845, 1987.
981. Rhodes, KM and Tattersfield, AE: Guillain-Barré syndrome associated with Campylobacter infection. Br Med J 285:173–174, 1982.
982. Ribera, EF and Dutka, AJ: Polyneu-

ropathy associated with administration of hepatitis B vaccine (letter). N Engl J Med 309:614, 1983.

983. Rice, D: Landry-Guillain-Barré syndrome: Personal experience of acute ascending paralysis. Br Med J 1: 1330–1332, 1977.
984. Richards, AM, Nicholls, MG, Beard, MEJ, Parkin, PJ, and Espiner, EA: Severe hypertension and raised haematocrit: Unusual presentation of Guillain-Barré syndrome. Postgrad Med J 61:53–55, 1985.
985. Richter, RB: The ataxic form of polyradiculoneuritis (Landry-Guillain-Barré syndrome). J Neuropathol Exp Neurol 21:171–184, 1962.
986. Richter, RW, Pearson, J, Bruun, B, Challenor, YB, Brust, JCM, and Baden, MM: Neurological complications of addition to heroin. Bull NY Acad Med 49:3–21, 1973.
987. Ricker, K and Hertel, G: Electrophysiological findings in the syndrome of acute ocular muscle palsy with ataxia (Fisher syndrome). J Neurol 214:35–44, 1976.
988. Ricker, W, Blumberg, A, Peters, CH, and Widerman, A: The association of the Guillain-Barré syndrome with infectious mononucleosis with a report of two fatal cases. Blood 2:217–226, 1947.
989. Ridley, A: The neuropathy of acute intermittent porphyria. Q J Med 38:307–333, 1969.
990. Ridley, A: Porphyric Neuropathy. In Dyck, PJ, Thomas, PK, and Lambert, EH (eds): Peripheral Neuropathy, ed 2. WB Saudners, Philadelphia, 1984, pp 1704–1716.
991. Ridley, A, Hierons, R, and Cavanaugh, JB: Tachycardia and the neuropathy of porphyria. Lancet 2:708–710, 1968.
992. Riggs, JE, Whited, JD, and Gutmann, L: Guillain-Barré syndrome (GBS): Another immune-mediated neurologic disease with a predilection for young women (abstr). Neurology (Suppl)38:312, 1988.
993. Riser et Planques: Les polyradiculonevrites aiques. J belge de neurol et de psychiat 38:264–275, 1938.
994. Ritch, PS, Hansen, RM, and McQuillen, MP: Transient polyradiculoneuropathy following a febrile transfusion reaction. Arch Neurol 39: 597–598, 1982.
995. Robertson, GL, Bhoopalam, N, and Zelkowitz, LJ: Vincristine neurotoxicity and abnormal secretion of antidiuretic hormone. Arch Intern Med 132:717–720, 1973.
996. Roche, J: Notice necrologique, André Strohl (1887–1977). Comptes rendus des seances de societe de biologie et de ses fiales. CR Soc Biol (Paris) 171:1161–1162, 1977.
997. Rocklin, RF, Sheremata, WA, Feldman, RG, Kies, MW, and David, JR: The Guillain-Barré syndrome and multiple sclerosis. In vitro cellular responses to nervous-tissue antigens. N Engl J Med 284:803–808, 1971.
998. Rodriguez-Iturbe, B, Garcia, R, Rubio, L, Zabala, J, Moros, G, and Torres, R: Acute glomerulonephritis in the Guillain-Barré syndrome. Ann Intern Med 78:391–395, 1973.
999. Roemheld, L: Zur Klinik postdiphtherischer pseudotabes; liquorbefunde bei postdiphtherischer Lahmung. Dtsch Med Wochenschr 35:669–671, 1908.
1000. Rolleston, JD: Clinical observations on diphtheritic paralysis. Practitioner 2:597–623, 1904.
1001. Roman, G, Phillips, A, and Poser, CM: Parainfluenza virus type 3. Isolation from CSF of a patient with Guillain-Barré syndrome. JAMA 240:1613–1615, 1978.
1002. Rombeau, JL and Barot, LR: Enteral nutritional therapy. Surg Clin North Am 61:605–620, 1981.
1003. Ropper, AH: The CNS in Guillain-Barré syndrome. Arch Neurol 40: 397–398, 1983.
1004. Ropper, AH: Preservation of jaw power in Guillain-Barré syndrome (letter). Lancet 1:961, 1984.
1005. Ropper, AH: Guillain-Barré syndrome: Management of respiratory failure. Neurology 35:1662–1665, 1985.
1006. Ropper, AH: Controversely about Fisher's syndrome (letter). Arch Neurol 43:543–544, 1986.
1007. Ropper, AH: Severe acute Guillain-

Barré syndrome. Neurology 36:429–432, 1986.
1008. Ropper, AH: Unusual clinical variants and signs in Guillain-Barré syndrome. Arch Neurol 43:1150–1152, 1986.
1009. Ropper, AH: Campylobacter diarrhea and Guillain-Barré syndrome. Arch Neurol 45:655–656, 1988.
1010. Ropper, AH: Three patients with Fisher's syndrome and normal MRI. Neurology 38:1630–1631, 1988.
1011. Ropper, AH, Albers, JW, and Addison, R: Limited relapse in Guillain-Barré syndrome after plasma exchange. Arch Neurol 45:314–315, 1988.
1012. Ropper, AH and Chiappa, KH: Evoked potentials in Guillain-Barré syndrome. Neurology 36:587–590, 1986.
1013. Ropper, AH and Kehne, SM: Guillain-Barré syndrome: Management of respiratory failure. Neurology 35:1662–1665, 1985.
1014. Ropper, AH and Marmarou, A: Mechanism of pseudotumor in Guillain-Barré syndrome. Arch Neurol 41:259–261, 1984.
1015. Ropper, AH and Poskanzer, DC: The prognosis of acute and subacute transverse myelopathy based on early signs and symptoms. Ann Neurol 4:51–59, 1978.
1016. Ropper, AH and Shahani, BT: Proposed mechanism of ataxia in Fisher's syndrome. Arch Neurol 40:537–538, 1983.
1017. Ropper, AH and Shahani, BT: Pain in Guillain-Barré syndrome. Arch Neurol 41:511–514, 1984.
1018. Ropper, AH, Shahani, BT, and Huggins, CE: Improvement in 4 patients with acute Guillain-Barré syndrome after plasma exchange (abstr). Neurology 30:361, 1980.
1019. Ropper, AH, Wechsler, LR, and Wilson, LS: Carotid bruit and the risk of stroke in elective surgery. N Engl J Med 307:1388–1390, 1982.
1020. Ropper, AH and Wijdicks, EFM: Blood pressure fluctuations in the dysautonomia of Guillain-Barré syndrome. Arch Neurol 27:337–338, 1990.
1021. Ropper, AH, Wijdicks, EFM, and Shahani, BT: Electrodiagnostic changes in early Guillain-Barré. A prospective study in 113 patients. Arch Neurol 47:881–887, 1990.
1022. Roquer, J, Herraiz, J, Maymo, J, Olive, A, and Carbonell, J: Miller-Fisher syndrome (Guillain-Barré syndrome with ophthalmoplegia) during treatment with gold salts in a patient with rheumatoid arthritis. Arthritis Rheum 28:838–839, 1985.
1023. Roseman, E and Aring, CD: Infectious polyneuritis, acute polyneuritis with facial diplegia, Guillain-Barré syndrome, Landry's paralysis, etc. Medicine 20:463–494, 1941.
1024. Rosen, AD and Vastola, EF: Clinical effects of cyclophosphamide in Guillain-Barré polyneuritis. J Neurol Sci 30:179–187, 1976.
1025. Rosenfeld, B, Borel, C, and Hanley, D: Epidural morphine treatment of pain in Guillain-Barré syndrome. Arch Neurol 43:1194–1196, 1986.
1026. Ross, J and Bury, JS: On Peripheral Neuritis; A Treatise. Griffin, London, 1893.
1027. Rossi, LN, Mumenthaler, M, Lutschg, J, and Ludin, HP: Guillain-Barré syndrome in children with special reference to the natural history of 38 personal cases. Neuropadiatrie 7:42–51, 1976.
1028. Rostami, AM, Ventura, E, Kimura, H, Brown, MJ, and Pleasure, DE: Induction of severe experimental allergic neuritis (EAN) with a synthetic peptide corresponding to the 53-78 amino acid sequence of the myelin P2 protein (abstr). Neurology (Suppl) 38:375, 1988.
1029. Rothrock, JF, Johnson, PC, Rothrock, SM, and Merkley, R: Fulminant polyneuritis after overdose of disulfiram and ethanol. Neurology 34:357–359, 1984.
1030. Rotteveel, JJ, Mullaart, RA, Weemaes, CMR, and Van Empelen, R: Plasmaferese bij twee kinderen met het Guillain-Barré syndroom. Tijd Kindergeneeskd 51:57–62, 1983.
1031. Roussos, CS and Macklem, PT: The respiratory muscles. N Engl J Med 307:786–797, 1982.

1032. Rubenstein, AE, Horowitz, SH, and Bender, AN: Cholinergic dysautonomia and Easton-Lambert syndrome. Neurology 29:720–723, 1979.

1033. Rudolph, JH, Norris, FH, Jr, Gravey, PH, and Friederich, M: The Landry-Guillain-Barré syndrome in pregnancy: A review. Obstet Gynecol 26:265–217, 1965.

1034. Rudolph, SH, Montesinos, C, and Shanzer, S: Abnormal brain stem auditory evoked potentials in Fisher syndrome (abstr). Neurology (Suppl) 35:70, 1985.

1035. Rumpl, E, Mayr, U, Gertstenbrand, F, Hackl, JM, Rosmanith, P, and Aichner, F: Treatment of Guillain-Barré syndrome by plasma exchange. J Neurol 225:207–217, 1981.

1036. Russell, WO and Moore, WL: Permanent damage to the nervous system following an attack of polyradiculoneuritis (Guillain-Barré syndrome). Report of a case with necropsy. Arch Neurol and Psychiat 49:895–903, 1943.

1037. Ryberg, B: Clonal restriction of complement-fixing antineural antibodies in the Guillain-Barré syndrome. Ann NY Acad Sci 540:384–386, 1988.

1038. Sabin, AB and Aring, CD: Visceral lesions in infectious polyneuritis. (Infectious neuronitis, acute polyneuritis with facial diplegia, Guillain-Barré syndrome, Landry's paralysis.) Am J Pathol 17:469–481, 1941.

1039. Sabin, TD, Geschwind, N, and Waxman, SA: Patterns of Clinical Deficit in Peripheral Nerve Disease. In Waxman, SG (ed): Physiology and Pathobiology of Axons. Raven Press, New York, 1978, p 431.

1040. Saeed, AA and Lange, LS: Guillain-Barré syndrome after rubella. Postgrad Med J 54:333–334, 1978.

1041. Sahashi, K, Takahashi, A, Ibi, T, Gotoh, S, and Matsui, T: Acute predominantly sensory neuropathy. Klin Wochenschr 63:319–324, 1985.

1042. Said, G: Perhexiline neuropathy: A clinicopathological study. Ann Neurol 3:259–266, 1978.

1043. Saida, K, Mendell, JR, and Sahenk, Z: Peripheral nerve changes induced by local application of bee venom. J Neuropathol Exp Neurol 36:783–796, 1977.

1044. Saida, K, Saida, T, Brown, MJ, and Silberberg, DH: In vivo demyelination induced by intraneural injection of anti-galactocerebroside serum. Am J Pathol 95:99–116, 1979.

1045. Saida, K, Saida, T, Goban, Y, Ozawa, K, Kawanishi, T, and Nishitani, H: The role of macrophages in serum-induced demyelination. Ann Neurol 16:139–140, 1984.

1046. Saida, T, Saida, K, Dorfman, SH, Silberberg, DH, Sumner, AJ, Manning, MC, Lisak, RP, and Brown, MJ: Experimental allergic neuritis induced by sensitization with galactocerebroside. Science 204:1103–1106, 1979.

1047. Saida, T, Saida, K, Lisak, RP, Brown, MJ, Silberberg, DH, and Asbury, AK: In vivo demyelinating activity of sera from patients with Guillain-Barré syndrome. Ann Neurol 11:69–75, 1982.

1048. Saida, T, Saida, K, Silberberg, DH, and Brown, MJ: Experimental allergic neuritis induced by galactocerebroside. Ann Neurol (Suppl)9:87–191, 1981.

1049. Sakamoto, Y, Lockey, RF, and Krzanowski, JJ: Shellfish and fish poisoning related to the toxic dinoflagellates. South Med J 80:866–872, 1987.

1050. Saksa, M, Molnar, GK, and Riekkinen, PJ: Bradycardic response to respiratory strain as a measure of autonomic dysfunction in experimental allergic neuritis. Acta Neurol Scand (Suppl 90) 65:234–235, 1982.

1051. Salata, RA, Lederman, MM, Shlaes, DM, Jacogs, MR, Eckstein, E, Tweardy, D, Toossi, Z, Chmielewski, R, Marino, J, King, CH, Graham, RC, and Ellner, JJ: Diagnosis of nosocomial pneumonia in intubated, intensive care unit patients. Am Rev Respir Dis 135:426–432, 1987.

1052. Salisachs, P and Lapresle, J: Upper lid jerks in the Fisher syndrome. Eur Neurol 15:237–240, 1977.

1053. Samantray, SK, Johnson, SC, Mathai, KV, and Pulimood, BM: Landry-Guillain-Barré-Strohl syndrome. A study of 302 cases. Med J Aust 2:84–91, 1977.

1053a. Sampson, RN: Hypnotherapy in a case of pruritis and Guillain-Barré syndrome. Am J Clin Hypn 32:168–173, 1990.

1054. Sanders, EACM, Yewdall, VMA, Hughes, RAC, and Cameron, JS: Absence of complement activation in demyelinating polyradiculoneuropathies (letter). Ann Neurol 23:102–103, 1988.

1055. Sandu L: Corticosteroids in Landry-Guillain-Barré-Strohl syndrome (letter). Lancet 2:662, 1974.

1056. Saunders, M and Rake, M: Familial Guillain-Barré syndrome. Lancet 2:1106–1107, 1965.

1057. Sauron, B, Bouche, P, Cathala, H-P, Chain, F, and Castaigne, P: Miller Fisher syndrome: Clinical and electrophysiologic evidence of peripheral origin in 10 cases. Neurology 34:953–956, 1984.

1058. Saxenhofer, H, Weidman, P, Shaw, S, Sulzer, M, Sregrist, P, and Staubli, M: Atrial natriuretic factor in the Landry-Guillain-Barré syndrome (letter). N Engl J Med 319:448, 1988.

1059. Schaeffer, AJ: Catheter-associated bacteriuria. Urol Clin North Am 13:735–747, 1986.

1060. Schaltenbrand, G and Bammer, H: La clinique et le traitement des polynevrites inflammatoiries ou sereuses aiguës. Rev Neurol 115:783–810, 1966.

1061. Schapira, AHV and Thomas, PK: A case of recurrent idiopathic ophthalmoplegic neuropathy (Miller Fisher syndrome). J Neurol Neurosurg Psychiatry 49:463–464, 1986.

1062. Schaumburg, HH, Spencer, PS, and Thomas, PK: Disorders of Peripheral Nerve. FA Davis, Philadelphia, 1983, p 31.

1063. Schaumburg, HH and Spencer, PS: Human Toxic Neuropathy Due to Industrial Agents. In Dyck, PJ, Thomas, PK, and Lambert, EH (eds): Peripheral Neuropathy, ed 2. WB Saunders, Philadelphia, 1984, p 2115.

1064. Scheid, W: Diphtherial paralysis. An analysis of 2,292 cases of diphtheria in adults, which included 174 cases of polyneuritis. J Nerv Ment Dis 116:1095–1101, 1952.

1065. Scheinberg, L: Polyneuritis in systemic lupus erythematosus: Review of the literature and report of a case. N Engl J Med 255:416–421, 1956.

1066. Schiff, JA, Cracco, RQ, and Cracco, JB: Brainstem auditory evoked potentials in Guillain-Barré syndrome. Neurology 35:771–773, 1985.

1067. Schlumpf, U, Meyer, M, Ulrich, J, and Friede, RL: Neurological complications induced by gold treatment. Arthritis Rheum 26:825–831, 1983.

1068. Schmaus, H: Die Landry'schen paralyse. Ergebn d allg Path u path Anat 9:396–422, 1904.

1069. Schmitz, H and Enders, G: Cytomegalovirus as a frequent cause of Guillain-Barré syndrome. J Med Virol 1:21–27, 1977.

1070. Schneck, SA and Claman, HN: CSF immunoglobulins in multiple sclerosis and other neurological diseases: Measurement by electroimmuno diffusion. Arch Neurol 20:132–139, 1969.

1071. Scholz, DG, Olson, JM, Thurber, DL, and Larson, DE: Tetanus: An uncommon cause of dysphagia. Mayo Clin Proc 64:335–338, 1989.

1072. Schonberger, LB, Bregman, DJ, Sullivan-Bolyai, JZ, Keenlyside, RA, Ziegler, DW, Retailliau, HF, Eddins, DL, and Bryan, JA: Guillain-Barré syndrome following vaccination in the national influenza immunization program, United States, 1976–1977. Am J Epidemiol 110:105–123, 1979.

1073. Schoolmeester, WL and White, DR: Arsenic poisoning. South Med J 73:198–208, 1980.

1074. Schooneman, F, Janot, C, Streiff, F, Gerard, A, Dureux, JB, Canton, P, Roche, G, and Aubrun, P: Plasma exchange in Guillain-Barré syndrome: Ten cases. Plasma Therapy 2:117–122, 1981.

1075. Schorder, P: Contribution a l'etude des formes ataxiques du syndrome de

Guillain et Barré. These Université Nancy, 1949–1950.

1076. Schott, B: Histoire du syndrome de Guillain et Barre. Rev Neurol 138:931–938, 1982.

1077. Schott, B, Michel, D, Lejeune, E, Bouvier, M, Vauzelle, J-L, Girard, R, Roumagoux, J, Ramel, P, and Bouvier, S: Polyradiculonévrites au cours de la maladie de Besnier-Boeck-Schaumann. Le Journal de Medicien de Lyon 49:931–937, 1968.

1078. Schrade, H: Ein fall von Guillain-Barré syndrom nach Cholera-Schutzimpfung. A Case of Guillain-Barré syndrome following Cholera vaccination. J Neurol 209:69–74, 1975.

1079. Schweiger, L: Uber veranderungen der spinalganglien in einem fall von Landryschen paralyse (mit status hypoplasticus). Deutsch Ztschr f Nervenh 37:35, 1909.

1080. Seeldrayers, P, Johnson, D, and Weiner, HL: Treatment of experimental allergic neuritis with a mast cell stablizing drug (abstr). Neurology (Suppl 1)38:238, 1988.

1081. Segurado, OG, Kruger, H, and Mertens, HG: Clinical significance of serum and CSF findings in the Guillain-Barré syndrome and related disorders. J Neurol 233:202–208, 1986.

1081a. Seibert, DG and Seals, JE: Polyneuropathy after herpes simplex type 2 meningitis. South Med J 77:1476–1477, 1984.

1082. Selmaj, K and Raine, CS: Tumor necrosis factor mediates myelin and oligodendrocyte damage in vitro. Ann Neurol 23:339–346, 1988.

1083. Senanayake, N and Karalliedde, L: Neurotoxic effects of organophosphorus insecticides. An intermediate syndrome. N Engl J Med 316:761–763, 1987.

1084. Server, AC, Lefkowith, J, Brian, H, and McKhann, GM: Treatment of chronic relapsing inflammatory polyradiculoneuropathy by plasma exchange. Ann Neurol 6:258–261, 1979.

1085. Seyal, M, Ziegler, DW, and Couch, JR: Recurrent Guillain-Barré syndrome following influenza vaccine. Neurology 28:725–726, 1978.

1085a. Shahani, BT, Day, TJ, Cros, D, Khalil, N, and Kneebone, CS: RR interval variation and the sympathetic skin response in the assessment of autonomic function in peripheral neuropathy. Arch Neurol 47:659–664, 1990.

1086. Shahani, BT, Halperin, JJ, Boulu, P, and Cohen, J: Sympathetic skin response—A method of assessing unmyelinated axon dysfunction in peripheral neuropathies. J Neurol Neurosurg Psychiatry 47:536–542, 1984.

1087. Shahani, BT, Potts, F, and Dominque, J: F-response studies in peripheral neuropathies (abstr). Neurology 30:409, 1980.

1088. Shahani, BT and Sumner, AJ: Electrophysiological studies in peripheral neuropathy: Early detection and monitoring. In Stalberg, E and Young, RR (eds): Clinical Neurophysiology. Butterworths, London, 1981, p 117.

1089. Shahani, BT and Young, RR: Human orbicularis oculi reflexes. Neurology 22:149–154, 1972.

1090. Shahani, BT, Young, RR, and Adams, RD: The tremor in Roussy-Levy syndrome. Neurology 23:425–426, 1973.

1090a. Sahar, E, Murphy, EG, and Roifman, CM: Benefit of intravenously administered immune serum globulin in patients with Guillain-Barré syndrome. J Pediatr 116:141–144, 1990.

1091. Shankle, R and Keane, JR: Acute paralysis from inhaled barium carbonate. Arch Neurol 45:579–580, 1988.

1092. Shaw, FE, Graham, DJ, Guess, HA, Milstien, JB, Johnson, JM, Schatz, GC, Hadler, SC, Kuritsky, JN, Hiner, EE, Bregman, DJ, and Maynard, JE: Postmarketing surveillance for neurologic adverse events reported after hepatitis B vaccination: Experience of the first three years. Am J Epidemiol 127:337–352, 1988.

1093. Shearn, MA and Shearn, L: A personal experience with Guillain-Barré syndrome: Are the psychologic needs of patients and family being met? South Med J 79:800–803, 1986.

1094. Sheremata, W, Colby, S, Lusky, G, and Cosgrove, JBR: Cellular hypersensitization to peripheral nervous antigens in the Guillain-Barré syndrome. Neurology 25:833–839, 1975.

1095. Shim, C, Fine, N, Fernandez, R, and Williams, MH: Cardiac arrhythmias resulting from tracheal suctioning. Ann Intern Med 71:1149–1153, 1969.

1096. Shlim, DR and Cohen, MT: Guillain-Barré syndrome presenting as high-altitude cerebral edema. N Engl J Med 321:545, 1989.

1097. Shumak, KH, Humphrey, JG, Chin, JY, Routledge, ML, Elphick, M, and Humphrey, HE: The effect of the replacement solution (plasma or albumin) on the response of acute Guillain-Barré syndrome to plasma exchange. Plasma Therapy 6:427–431, 1985.

1098. Shumak, KH, Humphrey, JG, Chin, JY, Routledge, ML, and Humphrey, HE: Toronto General Hospital controlled trial on plasma exchange in Guillain-Barré syndrome (letter). Ann Med Interne 135:33, 1984.

1099. Shumak, KH and Rock, GA: Therapeutic plasma exchange. N Engl J Med 310:762–771, 1984.

1100. Shy, GM and McEachern, D: Further studies on the effect of cortisone and ACTH in neurological disorders. Brain 74:354–362, 1951.

1101. Sigwald, J: Notice necrologique; J. A. Barré (1880–1967). Rev Neurol (Paris) 17:412–415, 1967.

1102. Silberberg, DH, Manning, MC, and Schreiber, AD: Tissue culture demyelination by normal human serum. Ann Neurol 15:575–580, 1984.

1103. Silvis, SE and Paragas, PD: Paresthesias, weakness, seizures, and hypophosphatemia in patients receiving hyperalimentation. Gastroenterology 62:513–520, 1972.

1104. Simmons, BP: CDC guidelines for the prevention and control of nosocomial infections. Guidelines for hospital environmental control. Am J Infect Control 11:97–120, 1983.

1105. Simpson, LL: The origin, structure, and pharmacological activity of botulinum toxin. Pharmacol Rev 33:155–188, 1981.

1106. Singer, JI and Back, K: Postural guarding and hypertension as initial manifestations of Guillain-Barré syndrome. Am J Emerg Med 7:177–179, 1989.

1107. Singh, A, Jolly, SS: Landry-Guillain-Barré syndrome. Report of 25 cases. Ind J M Sc 12:347–350, 1958.

1108. Singh, NK, Jaiswal, AK, Misra, S, and Srivastava, PK: Assessment of autonomic dysfunction in Guillain-Barré syndrome and its prognostic implications. Acta Neurol Scand 75:101–105, 1987.

1108a. Singh, S, and Sinhi, S: Recovery from respiratory paralysis caused by Guillain-Barré syndrome in an infant after repeated exchange transfusions. Clin Pediatr 28:480–481, 1989.

1109. Sitzmann, JA, Townsend, TR, Siler, MC, and Bartlett, JG: Septic and technical complications of central venous catheterization. Ann Surg 202:766–770, 1985.

1110. Sklar, FH: Non-steady state measurements of CSF dynamics. In Wood, J (ed): Neurobiology of Cerebrospinal Fluid. Plenum Press, New York, 1980, p 365.

1111. Sladky, JT: Neuropathy in childhood. Semin Neurol 7:67–75, 1987.

1112. Sladky, JT, Brown, MJ, and Berman, PH: Chronic inflammatory demyelinating polyneuropathy of infancy: A corticosteroid-responsive disorder. Ann Neurol 20:76–81, 1986.

1113. Slavik, HE and Shapiro, RA: Fisher's syndrome associated with Epstein-Barr virus. Arch Neurol 38:134–135, 1981.

1114. Slavin, ML: Gaze palsy associated with viral syndrome. Am J Ophthalmol 100:468–473, 1985.

1115. Sliman, NF: Outbreak of Guillain-Barré syndrome associated with water pollution. Br Med J 1:751–752, 1978.

1116. Smith, IS, Kahn, SN, Lacey, BW, King, RHM, Eames, RA, Whybrew,

DJ, and Thomas, PK: Chronic demyelinating neuropathy associated with benign IgM paraproteinaemia. Brain 106:169–195, 1983.

1117. Smith, JL and Walsh, FB: Syndrome of external ophthalmoplegia, ataxia and areflexia (Fisher). AMA Arch Ophthalmol 58:109–114, 1957.

1118. Smith, SA and Smith, SE: Heart rate variations in Guillain-Barré syndrome. Br Med J 281:1099, 1980.

1119. Smith, WR and Wilson, AF: Guillain-Barré syndrome in heroin addiction. JAMA 231:1367–1368, 1975.

1120. Sneck, SA and Claman, HN: CSF immunoglobulins in multiple sclerosis and other neurological diseases; measurements by electroimmuno diffusion. Arch Neurol 20:132–139, 1969.

1121. Sobue, G, Senda, Y, Matsuoka, Y, and Sobue, I: Sensory ataxia: A residual disability of Guillain-Barré syndrome. Arch Neurol 40:86–89, 1983.

1122. Soffer, D, Feldman, S, and Alter, M: Clinical features of the Guillain-Barré syndrome. J Neurol Sci 37:135–143, 1978.

1123. Soffer, D, Feldman, S, and Alter, M: Epidemiology of Guillain-Barré syndrome. Neurology 28:686–690, 1978.

1124. Solders, G, Persson, A, Kristensson, K, and Hansson, S: Autonomic dysfunction in experimental allergic neuritis. Acta Neurol Scand 72:18–25, 1985.

1125. Soliven, B, Maselli, R, Jaspan, J, Green, A, Graziano, H, Petersen, M, and Spire, J-P: Sympathetic skin response in diabetic neuropathy. Muscle Nerve 10:711–716, 1987.

1126. Somjen, G, Hilmy, M, and Stephen, CR: Failure to anesthetize human subjects by intravenous administration of magnesium sulfate. J Pharmacol Exp Ther 154:652–659, 1966.

1127. Sonnabend, WF, Sonnabend, OA, Grundler, P, and Ketz, E: Intestinal toxicoinfection by Clostridium botulinum Type F in an adult. Case associated with Guillain-Barré syndrome. Lancet 1:357–360, 1987.

1128. Sorensen, AWS and With, TK: Persistent pareses after porphyric attacks. Acta Med Scand 190:219–222, 1971.

1129. Soria, ED, Candaras, MM, and Truax, BT: Impairment of taste in the Guillain-Barré syndrome. Clin Neurol Neurosurg 92:75–79, 1990.

1130. Southcott, RV: Intoxications of the Nervous System. In Vinken, PJ and Bruyn, GW (eds): Handbook of Clinical Neurology, Part II. Vol 37. Elsevier/North-Holland Biomedical Press, Amsterdam, 1979, pp 27–106.

1131. Sovilla, J-Y, Regli, F, and Francioli, PB: Guillain-Barré syndrome following Campylobacter jejuni enteritis. Report of three cases and review of the literature. Arch Intern Med 148:739–741, 1988.

1132. Spaans, F: Guillain-Barré syndrome with exclusively motor involvement. Electroencephalogr Clin Neurophysiol 61:15–16p, 1985.

1133. Spaar, FW and Orthner, H: Adrenalitis inclusio-necroticans in Landry-Guillain-Barré syndrome. Deutsch Z Nervenheilk 193:195–218, 1968.

1134. Spector, S: Guillain-Barré syndrome; a case with ataxia as initial and most prominent symptom. New York State J Med 42:1959–1961, 1942.

1135. Speed, BR, Kaldor, J, Watson, J, Newton-John, H, Tee W, Noonan, D, and Dwyer, BW: Campylobacter jejuni/Campylobacter coli–associated Guillain-Barré syndrome. Med J Aust 147:13–16, 1987.

1136. Spencer, PS, Schaumburg, HH, Raleigh, RL, and Terhaar, CJ: Nervous system degeneration produced by the industrial solvent methyl *n*-butyl ketone. Arch Neurol 32:219–222, 1975.

1137. Spillane, JD: The Evolution of the Concepts of Peripheral Paralysis and of Sensory Ataxia in the 19th Century. In Clifford Rose, F and Bynum, WF (eds): Historical Aspects of the Neurosciences. Raven Press, New York, 1981.

1138. Stahnke, HL, Heffron, WA, and Lewis, DL: Bite of the Gila monster. Rocky Mountain Medical Journal 67:25–30, 1970.

1138a. Stambough, JL, Quinlan, JG, and

Swanson, JD: Guillain-Barré syndrome following spinal fusion for adult scoliosis. Spine 15:45–46, 1990.

1139. Stamm, WE: Guidelines for prevention of catheter-associated urinary tract infections. Ann Intern Med 82:386–390, 1975.

1140. Stanbury, JB and Huyck, JH: Tick paralysis: A critical review. Medicine 24:219–242, 1945.

1141. Stapleton, FB, Skoglund, RR, and Daggett, RB: Hypertension associated with the Guillain-Barré syndrome. Pediatrics 62:588–590, 1978.

1142. Stauffer, JL, Olson, DE, and Petty, TL: Complications and consequences of endotracheal intubation and tracheotomy. A prospective study of 150 critically ill adult patients. Am J Med 70:65–76, 1981.

1143. Steck, AJ and Schleup, M: Neuromuscular Manifestations of Plasma Cell Dyscrasias. In Appel, SH (ed): Current Neurology. Vol 9. Year Book Medical Publishers, Chicago, 1989, pp 219–244.

1144. Steck, AJ, Murray, N, Dellagi, K, Brouet, J-C, and Seligmann, M: Peripheral neuropathy associated with monoclonal IgM autoantibody. Ann Neurol 22:764–767, 1987.

1145. Stein, JA and Tschudy, DP: Acute intermittent porphyria. A clinical and biochemical study of 46 patients. Medicine 49:1–16, 1970.

1146. Steiner, I, Argov, Z, Cahan, C, and Abramsky, O: Guillain-Barré syndrome after epidural anesthesia: Direct nerve root damage may trigger disease. Neurology 35:1473–1475, 1985.

1147. Steiner, I, Wirguin, I, and Abramsky, O: Appearance of Guillain-Barré syndrome in patients during corticosteroid treatment. J Neurol 233: 221–223, 1986.

1148. Sterman, AB, Nelson, S, and Barclay, P: Demyelinating neuropathy accompanying Lyme disease. Neurology 32:1302–1305, 1982.

1149. Sterman, AB, Schaumberg, HH, and Asbury, AK: The acute sensory neuronopathy syndrome: A distinct clinical entity. Ann Neurol 7:354–358, 1980.

1150. Stevens, JG, Prepose, JS, and Cook, ML: Marek's disease: A natural model for the Landry-Guillain-Barré syndrome. Ann Neurol (Suppl)9: 102–106, 1981.

1151. Stevens, AR and Wolff, HG: Magnesium intoxication. Absorption from the intact gastrointestinal tract. Archives of Neurology and Psychiatry 63:749–759, 1950.

1152. Stewart, AF, Adler, M, Byers, CM, Segre, GB, and Broadus, AE: Calcium homeostasis in immobilization: An example of resorptive hypercalcinuria. N Engl J Med 306:1136–1140, 1982.

1153. Stewart, GJ, Pollard, JD, McLeod, JG, and Wolnizer, CM: HLA antigens in the Landry-Guillain-Barré syndrome and chronic relapsing polyneuritis. Ann Neurol 4:285–289, 1978.

1154. Stillman, JS, and Ganong, WF: The Guillain-Barré syndrome: Report of a case treated with ACTH and cortisone. N Engl J Med 246:293–298, 1952.

1155. Stoll, G, Schwendemann, G, Heininger, K, Kohne, W, Hartung, H-P, Seitz, R, and Toyka, KV: Relation of clinical serological, morphological, and electrophysiological findings in galactocerebroside-induced experimental allergic neuritis. J Neurol Neurosurg Psychiatry 49:258–264, 1986.

1155a. Storgion, SA, Igarashi, M, May WN, and Stidman, GL: Plasmapheresis for Guillain-Barré syndrome. Pediatr Neurol 5:389–390, 1989.

1156. Strickland, GT and Moser, KM: Sarcoidosis with a Landry-Guillain-Barré syndrome and clinical response to corticosteroids. Am J Med 43:131–135, 1967.

1157. Strigard, K, Brismar, T, Olsson, T, Kristensson, K, and Klareskog, L: T-lymphocyte subsets, functional deficits and morphology in sciatic nerves during experimental allergic neuritis. Muscle Nerve 10:329–337, 1987.

1158. Strigard, K, Olsson, T, Larsson, P, Holmdahl R, and Klareskog, L: Modulation of experimental allergic neuritis in rats by in vivo treatment with monoclonal anti T cell antibodies. J Neurol Sci 83:283–291, 1988.

1159. Sucher, BM and Cavanaugh, JA: Guillain-Barré syndrome with secondary bilateral posterior interosseous nerve syndrome. Arch Phys Med Rehabil 63:184–187, 1982.

1160. Sudo, N and Weingold, AB: Obstetric aspects of the Guillain-Barré syndrome. Obstet Gynecol 45:39–43, 1975.

1161. Sullivan, R and Reeves, A: Normal cerebrospinal fluid protein, increased intracranial pressure and the Guillain-Barré syndrome. Ann Neurol 1:108–109, 1977.

1162. Summers, Q and Harris, A: Autonomic neuropathy after rubella infection. Med Aust 147:353–355, 1987.

1163. Sumner, AJ: The physiological basis for symptoms in Guillain-Barré syndrome. Ann Neurol (Suppl)9:28–30, 1981.

1164. Sumner, AJ: Chronic Demyelinating Neuropathies. In Asbury, AK and Gilliatt, RW (eds): Peripheral Nerve Disorders: A Practical Approach. Butterworths, London, 1984, p 46.

1165. Sunderrajan, EV and Davenport, J: The Guillain-Barré syndrome: Pulmonary-neurologic correlations. Medicine 64:333–341, 1985.

1166. Susac, JO and Hoyt, WF: Inferior branch palsy of the oculomotor nerve. Ann Neurol 2:336–339, 1977.

1167. Susman, E and Maddox, K: The Guillain-Barré syndrome. Med J Aust 1:158–162, 1940.

1168. Suzuki, M, Kitamura, K, Uyemura, K, Ogawa, Y, Ishihara, Y, and Matsuyamu, H: Neuritogenic activity of peripheral nerve myelin proteins in Lewis rats. Neurosci Lett 19:353–358, 1980.

1169. Swedberg, J, Wendel, TH, and Deiss, F: Wound botulism. West J Med 147:335–338, 1987.

1170. Swick, HM: Pseudo-internuclear ophthalmoplegia in acute idiopathic polyneuritis (Fisher's syndrome). Am J Ophthalmol 77:725–728, 1974.

1171. Swick, HM and McQuillen, MP: The use of steroids in the treatment of idiopathic polyneuritis. Neurology 26:205–212, 1976.

1172. Swift, TR: Weakness from magnesium-containing cathartics: Electrophysiologic studies. Muscle Nerve 2:295–298, 1979.

1173. Swift, TR: Disorders of neuromuscular transmission other than myasthenia gravis. Muscle Nerve 4:334–353, 1981.

1174. Swift, TR and Ignacio, OJ: Tick paralysis: Electrophysiologic studies. Neurology 25:1130–1133, 1975.

1175. Syrjala, H, Koskela, P, Kujala, P, and Myllyla, V: Guillain-Barré syndrome and tularemia pleuritis with high adenosine deaminase activity in pleural fluid. Infection 17:152–153, 1989.

1176. Tachovsky, TG, Lisak, RP, Koprowsky, H, Theophilopoulos, AN, and Dixon, FJ: Circulating immune complexes in multiple sclerosis and other neurological diseases. Lancet 2:997–999, 1976.

1177. Takeuchi, H, Takahashi, M, Kang, J, Ueno, S, Yamada, A, Miki, H, and Tarui, S: The Guillain-Barré syndrome: Clinical and electroneuromyographic studies. J Neurol 231:6–10, 1984.

1178. Talamo, TS and Borochovitz, D: Membranous glomerulonephritis associated with the Guillain-Barré syndrome. Am J Clin Pathol 78:563–566, 1982.

1179. Tandon, DS, Griffin, JW, Drachman, DE, Price, DL, and Coyle, PL: Studies on the humoral mechanisms of inflammatory demyelinating neuropathies. Neurology 30:362, 1980.

1180. Taverner, D, Zardawi, IM, and Walls, J: Acute ventilatory failure and myoglobinuria. Neurology 34:369–371, 1984.

1181. Taylor, TT: A comparison of two methods of nasogastric feedings. J Neurosurg 14:49–55, 1982.

1182. Ten Eyck, FW, Martin, WJ, and Kernohan, JW: Acute porphyria: Nec-

ropsy studies in nine cases. Mayo Clin Proc 36:409–422, 1961.
1183. Terranova, W, Palumbo, JN, and Breman, JG: Ocular findings in botulism Type B. JAMA 241:475–477, 1979.
1184. Thames, MD and Schmid, PG: Interaction of Arterial Baroreceptors and Cardiopulmonary Receptors with Vagal Afferents in the Control of Vasopressin Secretion. In Sleigth, P (ed): Arterial Baroreceptors and Hypertension. Oxford University Press, Oxford, 1988, pp 186–192.
1185. Thieffry, S, Arthuis, M, Monsallier, F, and Sorrel-Dejerine, J: La Maladie de Guillain-Barré chez l'enfant (95 observations). Journée de Reanimation Neurorespiratoire de L'Hôspital Claude Bernard 95:61–73, 1961.
1186. Thomas, PK, Lascelles, RG, Hallpike, JF, and Hewer, RL: Recurrent and chronic relapsing Guillain-Barré polyneuritis. Brain 92:589–606, 1969.
1187. Thomas, PK and Shield, S: Associated autonomic dysfunction and carcinoma of the pancreas (letter). Br Med J 4:32, 1970.
1188. Thomas, PK, Walker, RWH, Rudge, P, Morgan-Hughes, JA, King, RHM, Jacobs, JM, Mills, KR, Ormerod, IEC, Murray, NMF, and McDonald WI: Chronic demyelinating peripheral neuropathy associated with multifocal central nervous system demyelination. Brain 110:53–76, 1987.
1189. Thomashefsky, AJ, Horwitz, SJ, and Feingold, MH: Acute autonomic neuropathy. Neurology 22:251–255, 1972.
1190. Thorner, MW, Alpers, BJ, and Yaskin, JC: Acute ascending paralysis (Landry's paralysis); clinicopathologic study. Archives of Neurology and Psychiatry 44:17–42, 1940.
1191. Timmis, HH: Tracheostomy: An overview of implications, management and morbidity. Adv Surg 7:199–233, 1973.
1192. Tindall, RSA, Zinn, P, and Rosenberg, RN: Humoral immunity in the Guillain-Barré syndrome: Evidence for circulating IgG and IgM (abstr). Neurology 30:362–363, 1980.
1193. Tong, HI, Devathasan, G, and Wong, PK: Guillain-Barré syndrome in Singapore. The pattern of Guillain-Barré syndrome (acute polyradiculopathy) in Singapore—A critical analysis of 46 cases. Ann Acad Med 8:27–32, 1979.
1194. Tonnessen, TI, Nyland, H, and Aarli, JA: Complement factors and acute phase reactants in the Guillain-Barré syndrome. Eur Neurol 21: 124–128, 1982.
1195. Toro, G, Vergara, I, and Roman, G: Neuroparalytic accidents of antirabies vaccination with suckling mouse brain vaccine. Clinical and pathologic study of 21 cases. Arch Neurol 34:694–700, 1977.
1196. Toshniwal, P: Demyelinating optic neuropathy with Miller-Fisher syndrome. The case for overlap syndromes with central and peripheral demyelination. J Neurol 234:353–358, 1987.
1197. Toyka, KV, Augspach, R, Wietholter, H, Besinger, UA, Haneveld, F, Liebert, UG, Heininger, K, Schwendemann, G, Reiners, K, and Grabensee, B: Plasma exchange in chronic inflammatory polyneuropathy: Evidence suggestive of a pathogenic humoral factor. Muscle Nerve 5:479–484, 1982.
1198. Trapp, BD, Mcintyre, LJ, Quarles, RH, Sternberger, NH, and Webster, H: Immunocytochemical localization of rat peripheral nervous system protein: P2 protein is not a component of all peripheral nervous system myelin sheaths. Proc Natl Acad Sci 76:3552–3556, 1979.
1199. Troni, W, Doriguzzi, C, and Mongini, T: Interictal conduction slowing in muscle fibers in hypokalemic periodic paralysis. Neurology 33:1522–1525, 1983.
1200. Traux, BT: Autonomic disturbances in the Guillain-Barré syndrome. Semin Neurol 4:462–468, 1984.
1201. Traux, BT: Sinus tachycardia in the Guillain-Barré syndrome. Acta Neurol Scand 77:270–271, 1988.
1202. Tryba, M: Risk of acute stress bleeding and nosocomial pneumonia in ventilated intensive care unit pa-

tients. Sucralfate versus antacids. Am J Med 83:117–124, 1987.
1203. Tsairis, P: Infectious Polyneuritis. In Rottenberg, DA and Hochberg, FH (eds): Neurological Classics in Modern Translation. Hafner Press, New York, 1977, p 295.
1204. Tse, KS, Arbesman, CE, Tomasi, TB, and Tourville, D: Demonstration of antimyelin antibodies by immunofluorescence in Guillain-Barré syndrome. Clin Exp Immunol 8:881–887, 1971.
1205. Tsukagoshi, H, Mori, H, Enomoto, A, Nakao, K, and Fukushima, N: Sensory polyradiculoneuropathy following spinal anesthesia. A clinicopathologic study. Neurology 20:266–274, 1970.
1206. Tuck, RR and McLeod, JG: Autonomic dysfunction in the Landry-Guillain-Barré syndrome. Clin Exp Neurol 15:197–203, 1978.
1207. Tyler, HR: Physiologic observations in human botulism. Arch Neurol 9:663–670, 1963.
1208. Uncini, A, Treviso, M, Basciani, M, Onofrj, M, and Gambi, D: Associated central and peripheral demyelination: An electrophysiological study. J Neurol 235:238–240, 1988.
1209. Uprichard, E, Martin, A, and Evans, S: Guillain-Barré syndrome—patients' and nurses perspectives. Intensive Care Nursing 2:123–134, 1987.
1210. Urano, T, Kawase, T, Kodaira, K, Takeuchi, Y, Kikuchi, T, and Kimura, M: Guillain-Barré syndrome associated with Echo virus Type 7 infections. Pediatrics 45:294–295, 1970.
1211. Usui, T, Hamada, Y, and Arita, M: A case of Guillain-Barré syndrome associated with Coxsackie B-5 virus. Tukushima Journal of Experimental Medicine 7:17–19, 1974.
1212. Uyemura, K, Suzuki, M, Kitamura, K, Horie, K, Ogawa, Y, Matsuyama, H, Nozaki, S, and Muramatsu, I: Neuritogenic determinant of bovine P2 protein in peripheral nerve myelin. J Neurochem 39:895–898, 1982.
1213. Vaillant, GI, Sobowall, NL, and McArthur, C: Some psychologic vulnerabilities of physicians. N Engl J Med 287:372–375, 1972.
1214. Valbonesi, M, Garelli, S, Mosconi, L, Zerbi, D, and Celano, I: Plasma exchange as a therapy for Guillain-Barré syndrome with immune complexes. Vox Sang 41:74–78, 1981.
1215. Valbonesi, M, Mosconi, L, Garelli, S, Zerbi, D, and Celano, I: Successful treatment by plasma exchange in Guillain-Barré syndrome with immune complexes. Vox Sang 38:181–184, 1980.
1216. Valenciano, L, Najera, E, Perez Gallardo, F, Gonzalez, A, and Enrech, J: Outbreak of paralytic illness of unknown etiology in Albacete, Spain. Am J Epidemiol 94:450–456, 1971.
1217. Vallat, JM: Sensory Guillain-Barré syndrome (letter). Neurology 39:879, 1989.
1218. Valli, G, Barbieri, S, and Scarlato, G: Neurophysiological tests in human botulism. Electromyogr Clin Neurophysiol 23:3–11, 1983.
1219. Van Allen, MW and MacQueen, JC: Ophthalmoplegia, ataxia and the syndrome of Landry-Guillain-Barré. A report of four cases with comments on the ophthalmoplegia. Trans Am Neurol Assoc 89:99–103, 1964.
1220. Van Bogaert, L, Philips, F, Radermecker, MA, and Versch-Raegen, T: Essai sur un group épidémique de cas de polyradiculonévrite avec dissociation albumino-cytologique de liquid céphalo-rachidrien (type de Guillain et Barré). Chez l'enfant et chez l'adulte. J belge de neurol et de psychiat 38:151–211, 1938.
1221. van der Meche, FGA and Meulstee, J: Guillain-Barré syndrome: A model of random conduction block. J Neurol Neurosurg Psychiatry 51:1158–1163, 1988.
1222. van der Meche, FGA, Meulstee, J, Vermeulen, M, and Kievit, A: Patterns of conduction failure in the Guillain-Barré syndrome. Brain 111: 405–416, 1988.
1223. van Doorn, PA, Brand, A, and Vermeulen, M: Clinical significance of antibodies against peripheral nerve tissue in inflammatory polyneuropa-

thy (letter). Neurology 37:1798–1802, 1987.
1224. van Doorn, PA, Brand, A, and Vermeulen, M: Anti-neuroblastoma cell line antibodies in inflammatory demyelinating polyneuropathy: Inhibition in vitro and in vivo by IV immunoglobulin. Neurology 38:1592–1595, 1988.
1225. Vanguri, P, Koski, CL, Silverman, B, and Shin, ML: Complement activation by isolated myelin: Activation of the classical pathway in the absence of myelin-specific antibodies (Cl activation). Proc Natl Acad Sci 79:3290–3294, 1982.
1226. Van Horn, G, Drori, JB, and Schwartz, FD: Hypokalemic myopathy and elevation of serum enzymes. Arch Neurol 22:335–341, 1970.
1227. Van Zandycke, M, Martin, J-J, Vande Gaer, L, and Van den Heyning, P: Facial myokymia in the Guillain-Barré syndrome: A clinicopathologic study. Neurology 32:744–748, 1982.
1228. Veltri, C and Mamoli, A: Si du un caso di sindrome di Guillain-Barré complicata da diabetes insipido. Riv Neurobiol 14:590–605, 1968.
1229. Venables, GS, Bates, D, Carllidge, NEF, and Hudgson, P: Acute polymyositis with subcutaneous oedema. J Neurol Sci 55:161–164, 1982.
1230. Vendrell, J, Heredia, C, Pujol, M, Vidal, J, Blesa, R, and Graus, F: Guillain-Barré syndrome associated with seroconversion for anti-HTLV-III. Neurology 37:544, 1987.
1231. Ventura, HO, Messerli, FH, and Barron, RE: Norepinephrine-induced hypertension in Guillain-Barré syndrome. J Hypertens 4:265–267, 1986.
1232. Verma, AK, Maheshwari, MC, Chawdhary, C, and Tickoo, S: Acute ascending motor paralysis due to rabies: A clinicopathological report. Eur Neurol 24:160–162, 1985.
1233. Vermeulen, M, van der Meche, FGA, Speelman, JD, Weber, A, and Busch, HFM: Plasma and gamma-globulin infusion in chronic inflammatory polyneuropathy. J Neurol Sci 70:317–326, 1985.
1234. Vernay, D, Dubost, JJ, Thevent, JP, Sauvezie, B, and Rampon, S: "Choree fibrillaire de Morvan" followed by Guillain-Barré syndrome in a patient receiving gold therapy. Arthritis Rheum 29:1413–1414, 1986.
1235. Vignos, PJ: Physical models of rehabilitation in neuromuscular disease. Muscle Nerve 6:323–338, 1983.
1236. Vital, C, Aparicio, M, Brechenmacher, C, and Laurentjoye, L: Improvement of Guillain-Barré syndrome by hemodialysis (letter). Ann Neurol 7:496, 1980.
1237. Vital, C, Brechenmacher, C, Cardinaud, J-P, Manier, G, Vital, A, and Mora, B: Acute inflammatory demyelinating polyneuropathy in a diabetic patient: Predominance of vesicular disruption in myelin sheaths. Acta Neuropathol 67:337–340, 1985.
1238. Vriesendorp, FJ, Rudnicki, S, Mayer, RF, and Koski, CL: Plasma exchange and antibody rebound in the Guillain-Barré syndrome (GBS) (abstr). Neurology (Suppl)39:291, 1989.
1239. Vulpian, A: Maladies du systeme nerveux. Lecons professees a la faculte de medicine. O Doin, Paris, 1879, pp 189–195.
1240. Vyravanathan, S and Senanayake, N: Guillain-Barré syndrome associated with tuberculosis. Postgrad Med J 59:516–517, 1983.
1241. Wadia, RS, Sadagopan, C, Amin, RB, and Sardesai, HV: Neurological manifestations of organophosphorous insecticide poisoning. J Neurol Neurosurg Psychiatry 37:841–847, 1974.
1242. Wadsack: Ein fall von Landry'scher paralyse. Med Klin 6:1933–1979, 1910.
1243. Wahren, B and Link, H: Antibodies to Epstein-Barr virus and cytomegalovirus in Guillain-Barré syndrome. J Neurol Sci 28:129–138, 1976.
1244. Waksman, BH and Adams, RD: Allergic neuritis: An experimental disease of rabbits induced by the injection of peripheral nervous tissue and adjuvants. J Exp Med 102:213–235, 1955.
1245. Wallace, JF: Disorders Caused by Venoms, Bites, and Stings. In Braunwald, E, Isselbacher, KJ, Petersdorf,

RG, Wilson, JD, Martin, JB, and Fauci, AS: Harrison's Principles of Internal Medicine, ed 11. McGraw-Hill, New York, 1978, pp 831–838.

1246. Walle, A and Lehmann, H: Guillain-Barré syndrome and HBS-Ag positive acute viral hepatitis (case report) Hepatogastroenterology 28:305–307, 1981.

1247. Walsh, JC: Gold neuropathy. Neurology 20:455–458, 1970.

1248. Walsh, JC, Yiannikas, C, and McLeod, JG: Abnormalities of proximal conduction in acute idiopathic polyneuritis: Comparison of short latency evoked potentials and F-waves. J Neurol Neurosurg Psychiatry 47:197–200, 1984.

1249. Walshe, FMR: On the pathogenesis of diphtheritic paralysis. Q J Med 11:191–204, 1918.

1250. Walter, FK: Zur frage der lokalisation der polyneuritis. Zeitschrift für die gesamte Neurologie und Psychiatrie 44:150–178, 1918.

1251. Wardrop, J: Clinical observations on various diseases. Lancet 1:390, 1834.

1252. Warembourg, H, Voisin, C, and Furon, D: Neuropathies peripheriques aiqües associees a la brucellose. Lille Med 14:536–539, 1969.

1253. Warner, WA and Sanders, E: Neuromuscular blockade associated with gentamycin therapy. JAMA 215: 1153–1154, 1971.

1254. Warrell, DA: The clinical picture of rabies in man. Trans R Soc Trop Med Hyg 70:188–195, 1976.

1255. Warrell, DA, Davidson, NM, Pope, HM, Bailie, WE, Laurie, JH, Ormerod, LD, Kertesz, A, and Lewis, P: Pathophysiologic studies in human rabies. Am J Med 60:180–190, 1976.

1256. Warrell, DA, Looareesuwan, S, White, NJ, Theakston, RDG, Warrell, MJ, Kosackaran, W, and Reid, HA: Severe neurotoxic envenoming by the Malayan krait bungarus candidus (Linnaeus): Response to antivenom and anticholinesterase. Br Med J 286:678–680, 1983.

1257. Warren, JW, Platt, R, Thomas, RJ, Rosner, B, and Kass, EH: Antibiotic irrigation and catheter-associated urinary-tract infections. N Engl J Med 299:570–573, 1978.

1258. Wasserstrom, WR and Starr, A: Facial myokymia in the Guillain-Barré syndrome. Arch Neurol 34:576–577, 1977.

1259. Watson, WR: Some circulatory responses of Valsalva's manoeuvre in patients with polyneuritis and spinal cord disease. J Neurol Neurosurg Psychiatry 25:19–23, 1962.

1260. Watt, G, Theakston, RDG, Hayes, CG, Yambao, ML, Sangalang, R, Ranoa, CP, Alquizalas, E, and Warrell, DA: Positive response to edrophonium in patients with neurotoxic envenoming by cobras (Naja Naja Philippinensis). A placebo-controlled study. N Engl J Med 315:1444–1448, 1986.

1261. Waxman, SG, Brill, MH, Geschrind, N, Sabin, TB, and Lettvin, JY: Probability of conduction deficit as related to fiber length in random-distribution models of peripheral neuropathies. J Neurol Sci 29:39–53, 1976.

1262. Webster, ADB and Lever, AML: Non-A, non-B hepatitis after intravenous gammaglobulin (letter). Lancet 1:322, 1986.

1263. Wedgwood, J: Diabetes mellitus with acute polyneuritis. Br Med J 1:1346, 1957.

1264. Weinstein, M: Guillain-Barré syndrome and Epstein-Barr virus. Lancet 1:555, 1973.

1265. Weintraub, MI: Hypophosphatemia mimicking acute Guillain-Barré-Strohl syndrome. A complication of parenteral hyperalimentation. JAMA 235:1040–1041, 1976.

1266. Weintraub, MI: External ophthalmoplegia, ataxia, and areflexia complicating acute infectious polyneuritis. Am J Ophthalmol 83:355–357, 1977.

1267. Weintraub, MI: Autonomic failure in Guillain-Barré syndrome—Value of Swan-Ganz catheterization. JAMA 242:513–514, 1979.

1268. Weintraub, MI: Panautonomic dysfunction and Guillain-Barré syndrome. JAMA 243:1895–1896, 1980.

1269. Weise, MJ, Hsieh, D, Hoffman, PM, Powers, JM, and Brostoff, SW: Bovine peripheral nervous system myelin P2 protein: Chemical and immunological characterization of the cyanogen bromide peptides. J Neurochem 35:393–399, 1980.

1270. Welch, RG: Chicken-pox and the Guillain-Barré syndrome. Arch Dis Child 37:557–559, 1962.

1271. Wells, CEC: A neurological note on vaccination against influenza. Br Med J 3:755–756, 1971.

1272. Wells, CEC, James, WRL, and Evans, AD: Guillain-Barré syndrome and virus of influenza A (Asian strain). Report of two fatal cases during the 1957 epidemic in Wales. Arch Neurol Psych 81:699–705, 1959.

1273. Westall, FC and Root-Bernstein, R: Cause and prevention of postinfectious and postvaccinal neuropathies in light of a new theory of autoimmunity. Lancet 2:251–252, 1986.

1274. Westphal, C: Ueber einige Falle von acuter todtlicher Spinallahmung (sogenannter acuter aufsteigender Paralyse) (letter). Arch f Psychiat 6:765, 1876.

1275. White, WA and Berglend, RM: Experimental inappropriate ADH secretion caused by positive pressure respirators. J Neurosurg 63:608–613, 1972.

1276. Whitehouse, AC and Petty, TL: Recovery of Landry-Guillain-Barré syndrome after prolonged respiratory support. Lancet 1:1029–1030, 1969.

1277. Wiederholt, WC and Mulder, DW: Cerebrospinal fluid findings in the Landry-Guillain-Barré-Strohl syndrome. Neurology 15:184–187, 1965.

1278. Wiederholt, WC, Mulder, DW, and Lambert, EH: The Landry-Guillain-Barré-Strohl syndrome or polyradiculoneuropathy. Historical review, report on 97 patients and present concepts. Mayo Clin Proc 39:427–451, 1964.

1279. Wijdicks, EFM and Ropper, AH: Acute relapsing Guillain-Barré syndrome after long asymptomatic intervals. Arch Neurol 47:82–84, 1990.

1280. Wijdicks, EFM and Ropper, AH: Atrial natriuretic factor and blood pressure fluctuations in Guillain-Barré syndrome. Ann Neurol 27:337–338, 1990.

1281. Williams, B, Ghosh, TN, and Stockley, RA: Ophthalmoplegia, amblyopia and diffuse encephalomyelitis associated with pelvic abscess (letter). Br Med J 1:453, 1979.

1282. Williams, D, Brust, JC, Abrams, G, Challenor, Y, and Devereaux, M: Landry-Guillain-Barré syndrome with abnormal pupils and normal eye movements: A case report. Neurology 29:1033–1036, 1979.

1283. Wilson, DJ: Airway Appliances and Management. In Current Respiratory Care. BC Decker, Inc., Toronto, 1988, pp 80–89.

1284. Wilson, RS, Pontoppidan, H, and Rie, MA: Acute Respiratory Failure. In Ropper, AH and Kennedy, SF (eds): Neurological and Neurosurgical Intensive Care. Aspen Publishers, Rockville, MD, 1988, pp 85–97.

1285. Wilson, SAK: Acute Anterior Poliomyelitis. In Wilson, SAK: Neurology, ed 2. Vol 1. Williams & Wilkins, Baltimore, 1955, pp 245–287.

1286. Windebank, AJ, McCall, JT, and Dyck, PJ: Metal Neuropathy. In Dyck PJ, Thomas, PK, and Lambert, RH (eds): Peripheral Neuropathy, ed 2. WB Saunders, Philadelphia, 1984, pp 2133–2161.

1287. Winer, JB, Briggs, D, Welsh, K, and Hughes, RAC: HLA antigens in the Guillain-Barré syndrome. J Neuroimmunol 18:13–16, 1988.

1288. Winer, JB, Gray, IA, Gregson, NA, Hughes, RAC, Leibowitz, S, Shepherd, P, Taylor, WA, and Yewdall, V: A prospective study of acute idiopathic neuropathy. III. Immunological studies. J Neurol Neurosurg Psychiatry 51:619–625, 1988.

1288a. Winer, JB and Hughes, RAC: Identification of patients at risk of arrhythmia in the Guillain-Barré syndrome. Q J Med 68:735–739, 1988.

1289. Winer, JB, Hughes, RAC, Anderson, MJ, Jones, DM, Kangro, H, and Watkins, RPF: A prospective study of acute idiopathic neuropathy. II. Antecedent events. J Neurol Neurosurg Psychiatry 51:613–618, 1988.

1290. Winer, JB, Hughes, RAC, Greenwood, RJ, Perkin, GD, and Healy, MJR: Prognosis in Guillain-Barré syndrome. Lancet 1:1202–1203, 1985.

1291. Winer, JB, Hughes, RAC, and Osmond, C: A prospective study of acute idiopathic neuropathy. I. Clinical features and their prognostic value. J Neurol Neurosurg Psychiatry 51:605–612, 1988.

1292. Wischer, J, Vijayan, N, and Dreyfus, PM: Dysautonomia—Its significance in neurological disease. California Medicine (San Francisco) 17:28–37, 1972.

1293. Wisniewski, H, Terry, RD, Whitaker, JN, Cook, SD, and Dowling, PC: Landry-Guillain-Barré syndrome. Primary demyelinating disease. Arch Neurol 21:269–276, 1969.

1294. Wlodarczyk, S: Un cas de syndrome de Guillain-Barré avec nevrite optique retrobulbaire. En polonais. Neurologia Polska 23:110–115, 1949.

1295. Wochnik-Dyjas, D, Niewiadomska, M, and Kostrzewska, E: Porphyric polyneuropathy and its pathogenesis in the light of electrophysiological investigations. J Neurol Sci 35:243–256, 1978.

1296. Wokke, JHJ, de Koning, J, Stanek, J, and Jennekens, FGI: Chronic muscle weakness caused by Borrelia burgdorferi meningoradiculitis. Ann Neurol 22:389–392, 1987.

1297. Wong, PS, Fothergill, NJ, and Touquet, R: Abdominal pain as a presenting symptom of the Guillain-Barré syndrome. Arch Emerg Med 4:242–245, 1988.

1298. World Health Organization: Weekly Epidem Rec No. 11:82–83, 1979.

1299. Worster-Drought, C and Sargent, F: Muscular fasciculation and reactive myotonia in polyneuritis. Brain 75: 595–560, 1952.

1300. Wroe, SJ and Blumhardt, LD: Acute polyneuritis with cranial nerve involvement following Campylobacter jejuni infection (letter). J Neurol Neurosurg Psychiatry 48:593, 1985.

1301. Wulff, CH and Hansen, K: Miller Fisher syndrom: Oftalmoplegi, ataksi og arefleksi. Ugeskr Laeger 147:515–517, 1985.

1302. Wulff, CH, Hansen, K, Strange, P, and Trojaborg, W: Multiple mononeuritis and radiculitis with erythema, pain, elevated CSF protein and pleocytosis (Bannwarth's syndrome). J Neurol Neurosurg Psychiatry 46:485–490, 1983.

1303. Xie, J, Cai, Y, and Davis, LE: Guillain-Barré syndrome and hepatitis A: Lack of association during a major epidemic (letter). Ann Neurol 24:697–698, 1988.

1304. Yagnik, P, Singh, N, and Burns, R: Peripheral neuropathy with hypophosphatemia in patients receiving intravenous hyperalimentation (abstr). Muscle Nerve 5:562A, 1982.

1305. Yahr, MD and Frontera, AT: Acute autonomic neuropathy. Its occurrence in infectious mononucleosis. Arch Neurol 32:132–133, 1975.

1306. Yao, H, Fukiyama, K, Takada, Y, Fujishima, M, and Omae, T: Neurogenic hypertension in the Guillain-Barré syndrome. Jpn Heart J 26:593–596, 1985.

1307. Yee, RD, Trese, M, Zee, DS, Kollanits, CR, and Cogan, DG: Ocular manifestations of acute pandysautonomia. Am J Ophthalmol 81:740–744, 1976.

1308. Yoshioka, M, Kuroki, S, and Mizue, H: Plasmapheresis in the treatment of the Guillain-Barré syndrome in childhood. Pediatr Neurol 1:329–334, 1985.

1309. Young, RR, Asbury, AK, Adams, RD, and Corbett, JL: Pure pan-dysautonomia with recovery. Trans Am Neurol Assoc 94:355–357, 1969.

1310. Young, RR, Asbury, AK, Corbett, JL, and Adams, RD: Pure pan-dysautonomia with recovery. Description and discussion of diagnostic criteria. Brain 98:613–636, 1975.

1311. Yuill, GM, Swinburn, LA, and Liversedge, LA: Treatment of polyneuropathy with azathioprine. Lancet 2: 854–856, 1970.

1312. Zasorin, NI, Yee, RD, and Baloh, RW: Eye-movement abnormalities in ophthalmoplegia, ataxia and areflexia (Fisher's syndrome). Arch Ophthalmol 103:55–58, 1985.

1313. Zhao, B, Yang, Y, Huang, H, and Liu, X: Acute polyradiculitis (Guillain-Barré syndrome): An epidemiological study of 156 cases observed in Beijing. Ann Neurol (Suppl)9: 146–148, 1981.

1314. Zimmerman, J, Steiner, I, Gavish, D, and Argov, Z: Guillain-Barré syndrome: A possible extraintestinal manifestation of ulcerative colitis. J Clin Gastroenterol 7:301–303, 1985.

1315. Zochodne, DW, Bolton, CF, Wells, GA, Gilbert, JJ, Hahn, AF, Brown, JD, and Sibbald, WA: Critical illness polyneuropathy. A complication of sepsis and multiple organ failure. Brain 110:819–842, 1987.

1316. Zweiman, B, Rostami, A, Lisak, RP, Moskovitz, AR, and Pleasure, DE: Immune reactions to P2 protein in human inflammatory demyelinative neuropathies. Neurology 33:234–237, 1983.

INDEX

A page # followed by an "F" indicates a figure; A "T" following a page # indicates a table.